W9-DFR-182

The Self in Neuroscience and Psychiatry

In recent years the clinical and cognitive sciences and neuroscience have contributed important insights to understanding the self. The neuroscientific study of the self and self-consciousness is in its infancy in terms of established models, available data and even vocabulary. However, there are neuropsychiatric conditions, such as schizophrenia, in which the self becomes disordered and this aspect can be studied against healthy controls through experiments, building cognitive models of how the mind works, and imaging brain states. In this, the first book to address the scientific contribution to an understanding of the self, an eminent, international team focuses on current models of self-consciousness from the neurosciences and psychiatry. These are set against introductory essays describing the philosophical, historical and psychological approaches, making this a uniquely inclusive overview. It will appeal to a wide audience of scientists, clinicians and scholars concerned with the phenomenology and psychopathology of the self.

Tilo Kircher is Senior Lecturer and Consultant Psychiatrist at the Department of Psychiatry at the University of Tübingen.

Anthony David is Professor of Cognitive Neuropsychiatry at the Institute of Psychiatry and Consultant Psychiatrist at the Maudsley Hospital, London.

The Self in Neuroscience and Psychiatry

Edited by

Tilo Kircher
Department of Psychiatry, University of Tübingen, Germany

and

Anthony David
Institute of Psychiatry and Maudsley Hospital, London, UK

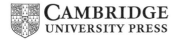
CAMBRIDGE
UNIVERSITY PRESS

PUBLISHED BY THE PRESS SYNDICATE OF THE UNIVERSITY OF CAMBRIDGE
The Pitt Building, Trumpington Street, Cambridge, United Kingdom

CAMBRIDGE UNIVERSITY PRESS
The Edinburgh Building, Cambridge CB2 2RU, UK
40 West 20th Street, New York, NY 10011–4211, USA
477 Williamstown Road, Port Melbourne, VIC 3207, Australia
Ruiz de Alarcón 13, 28014 Madrid, Spain
Dock House, The Waterfront, Cape Town 8001, South Africa

http://www.cambridge.org

First published 2003

Printed in the United Kingdom at the University Press, Cambridge

Typefaces Minion 10.5/14 pt. and Formata   *System* LaTeX 2$_\varepsilon$ [TB]

A catalogue record for this book is available from the British Library

Library of Congress Cataloguing-in-Publication Data
The self in neuroscience and psychiatry / edited by Tilo Kircher and Anthony David.
       p.   cm.
Includes bibliographical references and index.
ISBN 0 521 80387 X – ISBN 0 521 53350 3 (paperback)
1. Self. 2. Psychiatry. 3. Neurosciences.   I. Kircher, Tilo, 1965–   II. David, Anthony S.
RC489.S43 S445 2003
616.89–dc21   2002031550

ISBN 0 521 80387 X hardback
ISBN 0 521 53350 3 paperback

Every effort has been made in preparing this book to provide accurate and up-to-date
information that is in accord with accepted standards and practice at the time of publication. Nevertheless, the authors, editors and publisher can make no warranties that
the information contained herein is totally free from error, not least because clinical
standards are constantly changing through research and regulation. The authors, editors and publisher therefore disclaim all liability for direct or consequential damages
resulting from the use of material contained in this book. Readers are strongly advised
to pay careful attention to information provided by the manufacturer of any drugs or
equipment that they plan to use.

Contents

v

Contents

Contributors

James R Anderson, PhD
University of Stirling
Stirling FK9 4LA
Scotland
UK

Philip J Barnard, BSc, PhD
MRC Cognition and Brain Sciences Unit
15 Chaucer Road
Cambridge CB2 2EF
UK

Richard Bentall, MD
Department of Psychology
University of Manchester
Coupland-1 Building
Oxford Road
Manchester M13 9PL
UK

German E Berrios, BA (Oxford), MD, Dr. Med. *honoris causa* **(Heidelberg; San Marcos), FRCPsych, FBPsS, FMedSci**
Department of Psychiatry
University of Cambridge
Addenbrooke's Hospital
Box 189
Hills Road
Cambridge BC2 2QQ
UK

Sarah Blakemore, BA Hons (Oxon), PhD
Wellcome Department of Cognitive
  Neurology
Institute of Neurology
12 Queen Square
London WC1N 3BG
UK

Elena Daprati, PhD
Institut des Sciences Cognitives – UMR
  5015
67 Boulevard Pinel
69675 Bron Cedex
France

Anthony S David, FRCP, FRCPsych, MD, MSc, FMedSci
Neuropsychiatry and Psychological
  Medicine
Institute of Psychiatry and GKT School of
Medicine
Denmark Hill
London SE5 8AF
UK

Michael Ewers, BA
Department of Psychology
Temple University
Weiss Hall
Philadelphia PA 19122
USA

Chloe Farrer, PhD
Institut des Sciences Cognitives – UMR
  5015
67 Boulevard Pinel
69675 Bron Cedex
France

Pierre Fourneret, MD, PhD
Institut des Sciences Cognitives – UMR
  5015
67 Boulevard Pinel
69675 Bron Cedex
France

Nicolas Franck, MD, PhD
Institut des Sciences Cognitives – UMR
  5015
67 Boulevard Pinel
69675 Bron Cedex
France

Chris Frith, MA, DipPsych, PhD
Wellcome Department of Cognitive
  Neurology
Institute of Neurology
12 Queen Square
London WC1N 3BG
UK

Cynthia HY Fu, MD, MSc, FRCPC
Division of Psychological Medicine
Institute of Psychiatry
Denmark Hill
London SE5 8AF
UK

Shaun Gallagher, PhD
Department of Philosophy and Cognitive
  Science
Canisius College
Buffalo NY 14208
USA

Gordon G Gallup, Jr, PhD
Department of Psychology
State University of New York at Albany
1400 Washington Avenue
Albany NY 12222
USA

Nicolas Georgieff, MD, PhD
Institut des Sciences Cognitives – UMR
  5015
67 Boulevard Pinel
69675 Bron Cedex
France

Alexander Heinzel, MD, PhD
Harvard University
Beth Israel Hospital
Kirstein Building, KS 454
330 Brookline Avenue
Boston MA 00215
USA

Marc Jeannerod, MD
Institut des Sciences Cognitives – UMR
  5015
67 Boulevard Pinel
69675 Bron Cedex
France

Julian Paul Keenan, PhD
Department of Psychology
Montclair State University
219 Dickson Hall
Upper Montclair NJ 07304
USA

Tilo Kircher, MD, PhD
Department of Psychiatry
University of Tübingen
Osiander Str. 24
D-72076 Tübingen
Germany

Ivana S Marková, MPhil (Cantab), MD, MRCPsych
Department of Psychiatry
Coniston House
East Riding Campus
University of Hull
Willerby HU10 6N
UK

Hans J Markowitsch, PhD
Physiological Psychology
Universität Bielefeld
Postfach 10 01 31
Universitätsstr. 25
33501 Bielefeld
Germany

Philip K McGuire, BSc, MB, ChB, PhD, MD, MRCPsych
Division of Psychological Medicine
Institute of Psychiatry
De Crespigny Park
Denmark Hill
London SE5 8AF
UK

Georg Northoff, MD, PhD, PhD
Harvard University
Beth Israel Hospital
Kirstein Building, KS 454
330 Brookline Avenue
Boston MA 00215
USA

Gerard O'Brien, DPhil
Department of Philosophy
University of Adelaide
South Australia 5005
Australia

Jonathan Opie, PhD
Department of Philosophy
University of Adelaide

South Australia 5005
Australia

Jaak Panksepp, PhD
JP Scott Center for Neuroscience, Mind and Behavior
Department of Psychology
Bowling Green State University
Bowling Green OH 43403
USA

Josef Parnas, MD, DrMedSci
Department of Psychiatry
Copenhagen University
Hvidovre Hospital
2650 Hvidovre
Denmark

James Phillips, MD
88 Noble Avenue
Milford CT 06460
USA

Steven M Platek, PhD
Department of Psychology
Drexel University
Philadelphia PA 19102
USA

Andres Posada, PhD
Institut des Sciences Cognitives – UMR 5015
67 Boulevard Pinel
69675 Bron Cedex
France

Louis A Sass, PhD
Rutgers University
GSAPP
152 Frelinghuysen Road
Piscataway NJ 08854-8085
USA

Christian Scharfetter, MD, PhD, Prof. em.
Psychiatric University Hospital
Research Department
Lenggstrasse 31
PB 68
CH-8029 Zurich
Switzerland

Manfred Spitzer, MD
Universitätsklinik für Psychiatrie
Leimgrubenweg 12–14
89075 Ulm
Germany

Maxim I Stamenov, PhD
Seminar für Slavische Philologie
Der Georg-August-Universität Göttingen
Humboldtallee 19
37073 Göttingen
Germany

Kai Vogeley, MD
Department of Psychiatry
Friedrich-Wilhelms-University Bonn

Sigmund Freud Str. 25
53105 Bonn
Germany

Henrik Walter, MD
Universitätsklinik für Psychiatrie
Leimgrubenweg 12–14
89075 Ulm
Germany

Mark A Wheeler, PhD
Department of Psychology
Temple University
Weiss Hall
Philadelphia PA 19122
USA

Dan Zahavi, DrPhil, PhD
Danish National Research Foundation:
Center for Subjectivity Research
University of Copenhagen
Købmagergade 46
DK-1150 Copenhagen K
Denmark

Introduction: the self and neuroscience

Tilo Kircher[1] and Anthony S. David[2]

[1] Department of Psychiatry, University of Tübingen, Germany
[2] Institute of Psychiatry and Maudsley Hospital, London, UK

Who are we and what makes us who we are? Like our world, our self is a construction of our minds. But we do not live in isolation. The self is also a construction of our relations with other selves. And most intriguingly, the self is a construction of its relation with itself. One question is, how does the mind construct this world and ourselves in it? Constantly we think, feel, decide, perceive. Understanding how these things happen is central to our grasp of what kind of being we are. The way our mental life is constituted is also important to our understanding of who we are individually, because the variation of our mental lives constitutes our feeling of differentiation between our fellow humans. Mental states, unlike most other things of our everyday experience, have no spatial characteristics and they do not seem to belong to a world constituted by physical things. How to place our mental experience in the physical universe is therefore perplexing. Mental phenomena also interest us because we infer from ourselves that others have similar mental experiences. Social interactions require us to understand each other's thoughts and feelings. And language would not exist as a medium of expressing our inner world without our elaborate cognitive abilities. We seem to understand the content of our mind readily from our own experience. The problem arises when we try to know objectively, independently from ourselves, what we experience. From this arises the general problem of how the study of mind should proceed.

Much of our knowledge about our mind is immediate, and seems to have some sort of privileged status. That is, only we ourselves really know what is going on in our mind, and nobody else can know exactly what we feel or experience. Nothing seems to mediate between our mental states and knowledge we have of those states; such knowledge seems both direct and automatic. The privilege may not be absolute, it may not mean we are usually correct about our own mental states, nor that what we know about them is all there is to know. But our automatic and immediate access to our own mental states leads to a natural presumption that our beliefs about ourselves are correct. It is tempting to regard this special access as superior to any other sort of knowledge we could have about mind. This tantalizing problem has so far been widely neglected by scientific studies.

What we have said so far brings about two main topics of interest: firstly, the relation between *mind and body*, and secondly the nature of the *self* or *self-consciousness*. The latter is what we are concerned with in this book. What we mean by *self* here is as a first approximation the commonly shared experience, that we know we are the same person across time, that we are the author of our thoughts/actions, and that we are distinct from the environment. It is the immediate, pervasive, automatic feeling of being a whole person, different from others, constant over time, with a physical boundary, the centre of all our experience. These feelings are so fundamental to our human experience that we hardly ever think about them.

These are exciting times for the closer examination of self-consciousness. For many years, the topic has been studied primarily at a philosophical level (Rosenthal, 1991; Metzinger, 1995; Block et al., 1997; Gallagher & Shear, 1999; Zahavi, 2000). More recently, however, progress has been made by linking theories and experimental procedures from psychology to the results of neuroscience. This has allowed us to begin to understand how processing of self-relevant material is taking place on a cognitive and neural level, and how models of self-processing can explain some pathological states of mind.

For every author who has written about the *self* there are as many concepts, so the literature is full of diverse definitions and overcrowded by misunderstandings. The most basic thing to keep in mind is the level of description and study:

1. On a philosophical level, we can distinguish basically between two different schools, phenomenology and philosophy of mind. Phenomenology, in its broadest sense, describes the *essence*, the content and *feel* of a mental state. Philosophy of mind, based on concepts of analytical philosophy, is, for our purposes, mainly concerned with the logical connection and systematization of our knowledge of the mind.

2. Social science, social and personality psychology are concerned with how people regard themselves ('What kind of person am I? How do others see me?'), the different roles one person can have in society (researcher, mother, amateur musician . . .), and how these things interact and change over time.

3. Cognitive science tries to build models of how the mind works, derived from computer simulations as well as experimental data on healthy subjects and patients with brain lesions or mental disorders.

4. The neurosciences try to correlate mental phenomena with brain states and structures, using brain imaging or electrophysiological techniques.

5. The clinical sciences: descriptive psychopathology describes and classifies pathological mental states. Neurology and classical neuropsychology try to relate mental faculties to distinct brain areas by examining patients with cerebral lesions.

When we talk about mental or brain states we always have to be aware which level of investigation we are talking about. Confusion often arises when concepts of different fields are mixed, particularly points 1, 3 and 4, described above. However, often the goal of an enquiry is an explanation of a phenomenon in one field with concepts or results from another. Here it is particularly important to remember that a model from one field (e.g. in cognitive sciences *attention*) does not necessarily have a clearcut correlation with findings from other areas (e.g. a particular brain area). It becomes even more difficult when we cross borders between philosophy and sciences. However, this is what we have tried in this volume for a particular purpose. The neuroscientific study of the self and self-consciousness is in its infancy. There are no established models, very little data and not even the vocabulary to describe neuroscientific notions on these topics. For a start it is therefore necessary to draw from as many sources as possible to form a basis of enquiry. This volume brings together contributions from different fields, but focuses on the cognitive and neurosciences, and particularly pathological states of the self in schizophrenia.

We know that we are the same person across time, that we are the author of our thoughts/actions, and that we are distinct from the environment. This means there is a fundamental, affective tone of mental, emotional and bodily unity, which is so basic to our experience that it is very difficult to grasp. However, there are neuropsychiatric conditions such as schizophrenia where this basic tone of selfhood loses its natural givenness, with subsequent changes in the perception of oneself and the environment. This makes it possible to interview and test patients with impairments in self-experience. We can describe their experiences and compare results from experiments with those of healthy controls and thus generate tentative models of the underlying neurocognitive structure, correlating with the experience.

In this volume, we focus on schizophrenia, because the core pathology of the disorder is a disentanglement of the normal unity of body, thoughts and emotions. Schizophrenia is one of the most interesting and tantalizing of all human diseases, because what is most central to our existence, the mind, is lost or distorted (at least in the severe and acute phases). While it is commonplace in the cognitive neurosciences to draw inferences from the loss or disturbances of functions seen in patients, this is less common in psychiatric patients. However, it is only in disorders such as schizophrenia that the mental architecture underlying the self is so cruelly exposed.

The clinical presentation of schizophrenia varies both between individuals and within the same individual at different stages of the illness. But there are some prevalent features which most frequently comprise acoustic hallucinations (hearing voices) and delusions (false, uncorrectable beliefs, e.g. the ability to control the weather). Other common symptoms are thought withdrawal and insertion (patients have the feeling that their own thoughts and emotions are introduced from out-side), formal thought disorder (language disorder), incongruous affect and negative symptoms (Crow, 1985), such as apathy, social withdrawal and flattened affect (McKenna, 1994; Crow, 1985; Cutting, 1985; American Psychiatric Association, 2000; Gelder et al., 2000). Schizophrenia is a disorder with a worldwide incidence of 2–4 cases per 10 000/year. The lifetime risk is about 1% in the general population; the disease usually starts before the age of 30. It is therefore a common disorder which leads to chronic disability in about one-third of affected patients.

In this volume, we have brought together scholars from different fields of study to present their views on consciousness and self-consciousness, which are probably the most complex phenomena we know of. We focus on the cognitive and neuro-sciences and give special weight to the pathological self-states in schizophrenia. The book is divided into three parts. In the first part (chapters 1–4), some important theoretical and conceptual foundations are laid out. In the second part the cognitive and neurosciences present empirical data and models about the self from its differ-ent aspects (chapters 5–10). In the third part (chapters 11–21), concepts, models and data are presented to explain normal and disturbed self-states, focusing on schizophrenia. In the final chapter, our own integrative view, encompassing most of the aspects dealt with in the previous contributions, is attempted. Most authors agree that there is a feeling of *self* (thoughts, emotions, body, across time), that this is a mental state, that mental states are represented in the brain and that these states can be investigated scientifically.

Berrios and Marková, in their challenging contribution (chapter 1), regard the *self* as a mere construct of western thought that can be traced back to Greek phi-losophy. Consequently, they argue that it is not a natural entity, that it cannot be investigated scientifically, and *self-pathology*, such as passivity phenomena, are pure metaphors. In contrast, Northoff and Heinzel (chapter 2) elaborate the idea put forward above, that it depends on the level of description (or perspective, as they put it) what kind of model is to be applied to describe the self. These different perspectives lead to particular implications regarding notions of the self in the different scientific disciplines, that are not mutually interchangeable. This idea is developed further by Zahavi (chapter 3), who focuses on one particular perspec-tive, the *first-person perspective*, from a phenomenological point of view. He goes on to criticize the higher-order representation theory put forward by the philo-sophy of mind school, which is the basis for the investigations described mainly in chapters 17–21. Stamenov (chapter 4) dissects the relationship between self-awareness, self-consciousness, auditory hallucinations and linguistics. The sym-bolic representation of the self in language is the personal pronoun 'I'. Based on Chomsky's generative grammar, the smallest enactment of the self in the world is a simple sentence.

In chapter 5, O'Brian and Opie, as a linking contribution between philosophy of mind and cognitive science, develop their multitrack model of consciousness. They argue that although we have the feeling of being a mental unity, in fact the underlying mechanism is an aggregate of phenomenal elements (units of experience), each of which is the product of a distinct consciousness-making mechanism in the brain. Barnard (chapter 6) offers a cognitive multilevel theory and argues that the mind has a modular architecture with specialized subsystems to process information. Meaning, such as the representation of self-related material, is created by an emotionally charged interaction of different system levels. Gallup, Anderson and Platek (chapter 7) open up the view to incorporate ontogenetic and phylogenetic aspects of self-awareness. They demonstrate that mirror self-recognition in infants and primates must go hand in hand with a sense of self and with theory of mind abilities. Keenan, Wheeler and Ewers (chapter 8) extend this view to human adults and present experiments on facial self-recognition using different techniques. The memory aspect of our own past, as a constituent of a coherent feeling of self in time, is discussed by Markowitsch (chapter 9). He presents a neuropsychologically based theory of autobiographical memory and integrates levels of psychology, cognitive science, clinical neurology and functional imaging. Yet another important aspect of self-representation is discussed by Panksepp (chapter 10): the emotional aspect, and how this might be implemented on a neural level.

Chapters 11–21 mainly focus on psychopathological states of self-disturbances with an emphasis on schizophrenia. From a phenomenologically oriented position, Parnas (chapter 11) presents detailed clinical descriptions of the disorders of self-experience in patients with schizophrenia spectrum disorders. Further, data on prepsychotic stages demonstrate anomalies of self-aspects already present in the early stages of the disorder. From a similar conceptual background, Sass (chapter 12) argues that some schizophrenic symptoms can be understood as phenomena that would normally be taking place naturally and unnoticed which are instead taken as objects of one's awareness. Similar to Parnas and Sass, Scharfetter (chapter 13) regards a self-disturbance as the core symptomatology of schizophrenia. He presents data on a newly developed rating scale, based on Karl Jaspers' ego-pathology, for the description and classification of severe psychotic experiences. Chapters 14–16 are based on models derived from social and personality psychology to explain some of the symptoms and life courses of patients with schizophrenia. Bentall (chapter 14) introduces a model of self-attribution ('How am I, compared to other people, compared to how I would like to be?') and applies it to paranoid ideation. The way we see ourselves over time and make a coherent story out of it for ourselves is called self-narrative. Phillips (chapter 15) discusses this notion in a broader context of philosophy and the social sciences and introduces histories of patients to show how the disorder might have influenced their course of life. From a more cognitive point of view, Gallagher (chapter 16) defines four capacities that are necessary to construct a coherent self-narrative and tries to link them to cerebral structures. In another overarching attempt, Vogeley (chapter 17) introduces his definition of self-consciousness and applies it in more detail to the symptom of auditory hallucinations. These are thought to arise from a disturbance in a self-produced action-monitoring system, something dealt with in detail in chapters 18–21. Jeannerod and colleagues (chapter 18) and subsequently Blakemore and Frith (chapter 19) unfold their notion of action (and thought) recognition in others and oneself. They present empirical data and conclude that some symptoms in schizophrenia are a result of an alteration in the 'Who is the source of the action?' system. Fu and McGuire (chapter 20) apply these ideas particularly to the auditory and speech system and describe a functional imaging aproach to investigate them. These models cannot explain schizophrenic ego-disturbances (*Ichstörungen*) claim Walter and Spitzer (chapter 21), who present a modified theory based on right hemispheric and dopamine-system dysfunction.

In chapter 22, the final chapter, Kircher and David attempt to integrate most of what has been proposed in this volume by presenting a model of consciousness and self-consciousness. Psychopathological and empirical findings are related to this model.

REFERENCES

American Psychiatric Association (2000). *Diagnostic and Statistical Manual of Mental Disorders* (DSM IV), 4th edn. Washington, DC: American Psychiatric Association.

Block, N., Flanagan, O. & Güzeldere, G. (eds.) (1997). *The Nature of Consciousness.* Cambridge, MA: Bradford Book/MIT Press.

Crow, T.J. (1985). The two syndrome concept: origins and current status. *Schizophrenia Bulletin,* **11**, 471–86.

Cutting, J. (1985). *The Psychology of Schizophrenia.* Edinburgh: Churchill Livingstone.

Gallagher, S. & Shear, J. (eds.) (1999). *Models of the Self.* Thorverton, UK: Imprint Academic.

Gelder, M., Lopez-Ibor, J.J. & Andreasen, N. (2000). *Oxford Textbook of Psychiatry.* Oxford: Oxford University Press.

McKenna, P. (ed.) (1994). *Schizophrenia and Related Disorders.* Oxford: Oxford University Press.

Metzinger, T. (ed.) (1995). *Conscious Experience.* Paderborn: Schöningh-Verlag.

Rosenthal, D. (ed.) (1991). *The Nature of Mind.* Oxford: Oxford University Press.

Zahavi, D. (ed.) (2000). *Exploring the Self.* Amsterdam: John Benjamin.

Part I

Conceptual background

1

The self and psychiatry: a conceptual history

German E. Berrios[1] and Ivana S. Marková[2]

[1] Department of Psychiatry, University of Cambridge, UK
[2] Department of Psychiatry, University of Hull, UK

Abstract

The concept of self is a construct. It is not a 'natural kind' sited somewhere in the human brain. The western concept of self emphasizes individualism and autonomy but this view is cultural and no more scientific or truthful or advanced than the syncytial or collective view of self developed in other cultures and which revolves around family or clan rather than individual. Originally meant by St Augustine to be just a metaphorical or virtual space within which theological models of responsibility, guilt and sin could be played out, the self regained importance in the hands of Luther who started its reification as a private cave where god and man would regularly meet to sort out their differences. During the seventeenth century, the metaphors of the Reformation become secularized and built into liberalism and capitalism. The self survived by becoming a conceptual prop for bourgeois notions such as individual ownership, natural rights and democracy.

Wanting to reinforce the political status quo, nineteenth-century science transformed the political self into a psychological entity and proceeded to 'naturalize it' (i.e. render it into a natural kind). This additional reification engendered curious inferences. One was the belief that a 'self' really existed inside the European mind and brain. This self was characterized as driving, organized, executive and with a capacity for leadership and domination. Another curious inference was that, since the self was an ontological blob, it could be affected by pathological lesions and disease; and that this could be 'visualized' if only the right technique was available.

For a time, alienists took to the self with great gusto. For example, based on the tautological view that the self is truly impaired only in schizophrenia (*Ichstörungen*), much effort was invested in trying to find out whether this disease had to do with a disintegration of the 'boundaries' of the self; a reduction in its power and energy; its incapacity to discriminate between itself and the environment. This debate was harmless enough when played out in the territory of phenomenology or popular existentialist literature. However, during the last 30 years new techniques have encouraged researchers to reify the self further. Unfortunately, no new conceptualization has arisen and hence no interesting questions are being asked.

This is a pity for there is enough historical information available to see that the self is a linguistic trope, a yarn, a mode of talking about people and their reasons for doing things.

The self was never meant to be a solid object like a stone, a horse or a weed, nor even a concept to be considered as semantically tantamount to changes in blood flow or test scores. Of course, patients with disordered minds do sport hurting, afflicted and cursing selves but not as they may do carcinomas or broken legs. Their selves live in the same realm as do their virtues, vices, beliefs and aspirations, and that is where they should remain.

The self and psychiatry: a conceptual history

The term *self*[1] is currently used to refer to a putative *core*,[2] assumedly a defining feature of humanity and responsible; inter alia, for the experience of the so-called *sens intime*.[3] The appearance of the 'self' is part of the wider process whereby 'person-related' concepts (Laurent, 1993)[4] were constructed in western culture.[5] To this day, philosophical, psychological, theological and moral versions of the self vie for supremacy[6] and the debate continues on whether they have a divine, evolutionary or cultural origin[7] (Lévy-Bruhl, 1928; Marsella et al., 1985; Renaut, 1997; Gergen, 1998). Because of its unclear boundaries (Gallagher & Shear, 1999) and voluminous literature, writing on the history of the self is a hard task (Danziger, 1997b). After offering a summary of its history, this chapter will focus on the period during which the self was incorporated into psychiatry.

The beginnings

Plato (McCabe, 1994) and Aristotle[8] (Hartman, 1977) were amongst the first to discuss the need for a theory of *individuation* of objects and entities; indeed, it has been claimed that an inchoate 'form' of self was already present in Aristotle's notion of memory (Annas, 1992). However, the sense in which the self will be discussed in this chapter was only achieved during the post-Aristotelian period (Snell, 1953; Onians, 1954) and it is marked by the moment in which the philosophers of the first Stoa[9] redefined the Platonic term imagination (*phantasia*) as a collection of *individual* imaginations, *phantasiai*. The problem of how, then, did individuals 'recognize' multiple experience as theirs (Sandbach, 1994) was resolved by stating that the *hêgemonikon* (the highest component of the soul)[10] actually tagged up or personalized individual *phantasiai*: 'The *hêgemonikon* provided the Stoics with the concept of unitary self, actively engaged as whole in all moments of an animal's experience' (p. 107, Long, 1991). In Plotinus (1966), the *hêgemonikon* acquired a sense or feeling of 'privacy' and 'interiority'.[11] Concepts such as introspection (Reesor, 1989; Rappe, 2000), consciousness and awareness of function and content of function (O'Meara, 1995) started life during this same period. In his effort to consolidate the idea that man and God needed a private venue to meet,[12] St Augustine (1991) developed the idea of the self as a 'private inner space'.[13] It has been suggested that such a concept was based on Greek notions of 'subjectivity' and 'sin' and on Plotinus' mechanism of self-reflection (Mondolfo, 1955).

The seventeenth century

Descartes (1596–1650) (1967)[14] identified the self with the *res cogitans* (thinking substance) and believed it to be the basis for the belief in the existence of the external world. The legitimacy of this foundationalist claim, the nature of his dualism and the force of 'I think, therefore I am' (*cogito ergo sum*) as a logical entailment have since been subject to scrutiny (Frondizi, 1952).[15] Whether out of conviction or convenience, eighteenth-century neuroscientists followed a naive 'dualist' interpretation of Cartesianism so that they could claim that knowledge gained on the *res extensa* (the brain) had no theological implications (in regards to the soul or *res cogitans*) (Bynum, 1976).[16] The same interpretation of the Cartesian self (as an absolute knower) was built by nineteenth-century alienists into their own concepts of mental symptom and disease.

Descartes restarted the seventeenth century debate on 'interiority', 'self' and 'self-identity' (Garber & Ayers, 1998; Schoenfeldt, 1999). John Locke (1632–1704) (1959), one of the participants in the debate, set the scene in his analysis of the *principium individuationis*:[17]

to find wherein personal identity consists, we must consider what person stands for;- which, I think, is a thinking intelligent being, that has reason and reflection, and can consider itself as itself, the same thinking thing, in different times and places; which it does only by that consciousness which is inseparable from thinking, and, as it seems to me, essential to it: it being impossible for any one to perceive without perceiving that he does perceive. When we see, hear, smell, taste, feel, meditate, or will anything, we know that we do so. Thus it is always as to our present sensations and perceptions: and by this every one is to himself that which he calls self (Locke, 1959, II, xxvii).

John Locke also proposed that the feeling of continuity of the self was based on a concatenation of memories[18]:

Make these intervals of memory and forgetfulness to take their turns regularly by day and night, and you have two persons with the same immaterial spirit, as much as in the former instance two persons with the same body. So that self is not determined by identity or diversity of substance, which it cannot be sure of, but only by identity of consciousness (Locke, 1959, II, xxvii, 23).

However, by suggesting that it was mappable on to a region of the *body*, Locke encouraged the development of a 'psychological' self; indeed, like all other images resulting from perception, the self also revealed itself as a projection on to the camera obscura of the mind – which was the way John Locke was to allegorize its functioning.[19] Via the French version of the *Essay*,[20] Locke's ideas became fundamental to the development of the idea of 'self-awareness' (*sens intime* or *sentiment intérieur*)[21] in the France of the Enlightenment.

The eighteenth century

Locke (1959) equivocated on the *origin* of our knowledge of the *nature* of the self. Since it could not come from either the *senses* or *reflection*,[22] Locke reluctantly agreed with Descartes that knowledge of the self was 'a form' of intuitive, noninferential knowledge. He denied, however, that we can know the nature of the 'thing that thinks'[23]: 'the substance of spirits is unknown to us; and so is the substance of body equally unknown to us' (Locke, 1959, II, xiii, 30).

The two outstanding issues for the eighteenth century were firstly, the origin of our knowledge about the *nature* of self and secondly, the validity of *memory* as an explanation for the feeling of 'continuity' of the self (Perkins, 1969). Both questions were repeatedly analysed by the great thinkers of the Enlightenment[24]: Condillac,[25] Bonnet,[26] Hartley,[27] Helvétius[28] and Rousseau.[29] Hume (1711–76) went further:

> there are some philosophers, who imagine we are every moment intimately conscious of what we call our self; that we feel its existence and its continuance in existence; and are certain, beyond the evidence of a demonstration, both of its perfect identity and simplicity ... unluckily, all these positive assertions are contrary to that very experience, which is pleaded for them, nor have we any idea of self, after the manner it is here exp. For from what impression cou'd this idea be deriv'd? ... it must be some one impression, that gives rise to very real idea. But self or person is not any one impression, but that to which our several impressions and ideas are suppos'd to have reference (p. 251, Hume, 1967).

Then, Hume (1967) attacked the view of the self as substance:

> in order to justify to ourselves this absurdity, we often feign some new and unintelligible principle, that connects the objects together, and prevents their interruption or variation. Thus we feign the continu'd existence of the perceptions of our senses, to remove the interruption; and run into the notion of a *soul*, and *self*, and *substance*, to disguise the variation (p. 254).

After challenging the role of memory,[30] Hume (1967) went on to expound on his own:

> for my part, when I enter most intimately into what I call myself, I always stumble on some particular perception or other ... I never can catch myself at any time without a perception, and never can observe anything but a perception ... [human beings] are nothing but a bundle or collection of different perceptions,[31] which succeed each other with an inconceivable rapidity, and are in a perpetual flux and movement (p. 252).

German philosophy was less welcoming to Cartesianism (Beck, 1996). Kant (1724–1804) claimed that in the expression 'being conscious of myself' there were two components (Mendus, 1984; Kitcher, 1990; Ameriks, 1997, 2000): the empirical, psychological or anthropological self, 'I as object', or 'the object of intuition', and the transcendental or logical subject, the 'I as subject', captured by means of 'apperception'.[32]

However shadowy and abstract, the transcendental self is at the root of all cognitions and mental acts (Brook, 1994). Hence, it can be fallaciously reified into a 'substance'. But doing this is affirming the antecedent (i.e. concluding that it was a 'substance') on the basis of a consequent (the shadowy transcendental self) and this fallacy Kant called 'paralogism'. Kant's diremption of the self[33] provides a frame to understand nineteenth-century developments,[34] for his concept of 'empirical self consciousness' 'characterized [as it was] by a unity of the contents of consciousness that depends for its character on the spatio-temporal context of a particular individual' (p. 82, Keller, 1998) provided the justification for a 'science' of the self.[35]

The nineteenth century

The versions of the 'self' sponsored by the grand philosophical doctrines of the early nineteenth century were not influential on psychiatry. For example, subjectivity and the self played a central role in the work of Hegel (Russon, 1997) and Fichte,[36] but they left only a tenuous mark on early nineteenth-century German psychiatry. In general, European alienists (and those trained in Europe and working in their own country, like Benjamin Rush) repeatedly went back to the simpler ideas of Descartes and Locke.

Parallel versions of the 'self' were entertained in Europe at the time. In France, for example, the established view by the 1850s was a compromise between the Condillacean ideas (originated in John Locke) that had dominated French thinking until the very early nineteenth century (via the Ideologues), Scottish Philosophy of Common Sense (via Royer Collard) and their own brand of Roman Catholic thinking (via Jouffroy and Garnier). Thus, *moi* is defined by Franck (1875) as 'the name given by modern philosophers to the soul insofar as it has consciousness of itself, is familiar with its own operations, or is simultaneously the subject and object of its thought'.[37] This entry also included the claim that the self was not fully 'functional' in early infancy, lethargy, deep sleep and profound idiocy; no mention was made of mental illness.

In Britain, Fleming (1857) did not include an entry on the self and that on the ego consists in few quotations from Reid and Hamilton. The latter philosopher, however, had dedicated one of his *Lectures* to 'mind, soul, ego, I and self' (Hamilton, 1859). Because it cannot be differentiated phonetically from 'the eye', Hamilton claimed, 'I' should not be used: 'the self is more allowable; yet still the expressions ego and non-ego are felt to be less awkward than those of self and non-self' (p. 167). Be that as it may, the word 'self' took long before it entered technical English.[38]

The self in psychiatry

The incorporation of the self into nineteenth-century psychiatry was facilitated by the eventual acceptance of subjectivity and of patients' utterances as a valid source of information; and the development of a working notion of 'coenaesthesis'.

The incorporation of subjectivity

At the beginning of the nineteenth century the view predominated that signs were the direct expression of an anatomical lesion and diseases defined themselves in terms of signs.[39] In the field of alienism this led to a neglect of the study of subjective complaints (i.e. of symptoms). By the middle of the century, however, the acceptance of the self and coenaesthesis as legitimate sources of information and of introspection as a reliable instrument of analysis[40] led to an increasing interest in mental symptoms, i.e. in the utterances of patients, as markers of mental disorder (Berrios, 1996).

This transition was facilitated by the acceptance of a substantialist view of mind which led to a search for anatomical lesions. But postmortem studies rarely showed brain lesions consistently associated with mental symptoms. The day was saved by the growth of neurophysiology, particularly after the acceptance of Müller's view on the functional specificity of the nerves.[41] Subjective complaints were recategorized as resulting from aberrant 'functions' and as not requiring permanent structural foundations. During the second half of the nineteenth century, most of the manifestations of mental disorder were explained in terms of this mechanism. The concept of a physiological lesion itself became even more abstract and by the end of the nineteenth century psychodynamic psychology accounts began to predominate. This is the time when the disorders of the self started to be explained in terms of dissociation and germane mechanisms.

Coenaesthesis

During the eighteenth century, renewed interest had been shown in the classification of sensations. Although the Aristotelian 'five senses' still held firm, attention focused on experiences such as pain, nausea and position of the body and on the *sens intime*, none of which were classifiable or intelligible in terms of the traditional physiology of sensations. In 1794, C.F. Hübner used the term *coenaesthesis*[42] to refer to the bundle of sensations that originated from the body. It has been (wrongly) assumed that this concept is related to the κοινὰ αἰσθητὰ (koina aisteta) of Aristotle. In fact, the latter used 'common sensible' to refer to the perception of movement, rest, number, figure and size, i.e. of stimuli whose understanding required a simultaneous presence to the senses (Lloyd, 1968).

Although there were disagreements as to its referent, coenaesthesis became a popular term during the nineteenth century (Starobinski, 1977; Schiller, 1984).

According to Henle (1841), it referred to the 'tonus of the nerves of sensation and the perception of the state of activity in which the nerves constantly exist'; and Weber (1996) defined it as 'inner sensibility or inner touch' into which fed information from 'mechanical and chemico-organic state of the skin, mucous and serous membranes, viscera, etc.'.

The epistemology of coenaesthesis was discussed by Jouffroy (1826), who considered it to be a direct source of information, as valid as the external senses, but fundamentally different in nature.[43] Reinforced by Müller's theory of 'specific energy' (informational specificity), coenaesthesis was to become a foundational concept for the notions of muscular and joint sense (Bastian, 1887; Jones, 1972). Later in the century, it also provided Schiff (Starobinski, 1977) and Bonnier (1905) with the mould for their concepts of bodily schema. Since the eighteenth century, the self and coenaesthesis had been closely linked and this continued in the following century, giving rise to a 'physiological' definition of the self, particularly amongst those who did not want to be involved in its metaphysical or epistemological aspects which they considered as pertaining to the 'old psychology'.[44]

To create the language of psychiatry and of mental symptoms and diseases, alienists borrowed concepts from psychology, philosophy, medicine, biology and often the *belles lettres*.[45] In this way, various versions of the self came into psychiatry and it is a contention of this chapter that they have not yet been blended into a unitary view of the self.[46] Then and now, dissimilar conceptions of the self were associated with different disorders of the self. For example, the philosophical version that was at the basis of Reil's proposal (1803) that insanity resulted from a disturbance of the self had little to do with the models of the self that emerged from clinical narratives based on expressions of dissatisfaction and unhappiness, unlocated pains, coenaesthesic worries, feelings of depersonalization or disintegration of the unity of the mind and feelings of change of personality. Unattributable to specific mental functions (such as perception or memory), these complaints all became linked to a 'new' model of the the 'self' (or of its physiological equivalent, coenaesthesis) (Starobinski, 1990), whose understandability made it popular, and in due course, provided a platform upon which the versions of 'multiple personality' were to rest (Taylor & Martin, 1944; Carroy, 1993; Goettman et al., 1994; Spanos, 1996).

The disorders of the self

By the end of the nineteenth century, the list of 'disorders of the self' was as long as it was heterogeneous.[47] The old explanations, based on the hypothesis of a duality of the mind (Wigan, 1844) had given way to more 'functional' explanations (often Freudian-like, *avant la lettre*). In spite of its avowed emphasis on nonconscious behaviour and conflict, psychoanalysis allowed the 'conscious' self and associated structures the central stage. 'Disintegration', 'blurring of boundaries' and germane descriptions were made into explanations and reappeared as 'discordance', 'intrapsychical ataxia', 'schizophrenia', and 'dementia sejunctiva' (Lanteri-Laura & Gros, 1984). After the Great War, a group of 'disorders of the self' appeared which for some reason was claimed to be specific of schizophrenia (Spitzer, 1988).

The self and insanity

Reil believed that certain forms of madness resulted from a disorder of the self.[48] The latter, in turn, was the expression of bundled sensations whose integration was mediated by the sympathetic nervous system. Although setting an important frame for an empirical analysis of the self, Reil's view is jejune in regards to linking up specific manifestations of madness to specific disorders of his sympathetic nervous network.[49] von Feuchtersleben (1847) also proposed that coenaesthesic signals became pathological when they were felt 'too strongly, too weakly, erroneously and differently in different parts'. Each of these functional distortions led to a different psychiatric disorder; for example, an 'exalted coenaesthesis' will render the patient oversensitive to his body and this might linger on even if the original case disappeared; a 'depressed coenaesthesis' may deny the individual all information from his own body; an 'altered coenaesthesis' may lead to delusional and hallucinatory interpretations of the state of the body (pp. 215–218). This was the first clinically meaningful treatment of these disorders.

In France, the question concerning the nature of the self and its relationship to insanity was addressed by A. A. Royer-Collard (1843).[50] Applying the doctrine of Maine de Biran[51] to his patients, he objected to the latter's views,[52] believing that it was only in the most extreme cases of mental disorder, i.e. idiocy, that the self was completely lost.[53] In lesser degrees of madness, such as monomanias, the self was affected to various degrees; for example, a disturbance of free will would only affect some ideas and objects, or there could be fluctuations in the disturbance of the self. Importantly, however, Royer-Collard emphasized that the will, though ceasing to be free, could continue to be active. The patient's will would no longer be directed by deliberation or reflection but would be exercised by the deregulated passive faculties, e.g. imagination. The evidence, however, that it was still present, albeit in a disturbed way, came from the observation that at the time the patient was aware of his self, though at the same time aware of his subjugation to his uncontrolled will. Similarly, he argued that, whilst the behaviours of insane patients might be governed by the passive faculties, nevertheless, they would show signs that some intellectual faculties were being exercised because they were able to recognize people and objects seen previously and recall various incidents in which they took part.[54]

Multiple personalities

The concept of multiple personality was born from the interaction of what was called above clinical narratives of the self and the forceful application of theories of dissociation. Ever since, historical accounts have looked at this clinical phenomenon through the lens of hysteria and dissociation.[55] Whilst this provides a reassuring tale of continuity, it suggests that before Eugène Azam (Bourgeois & Geraud, 1990) or Morton Prince,[56] there were no contexts of knowledge and culture worth analysing and that earlier cases can be dismissed as simple 'curiosities'.[57] Dissociation theory and hypnosis have not done that well either, and the genuine nature of some 'classical' cases of multiple personality (e.g. 'Sybil') have since been called into question (Rieber, 1999).

Depersonalization

Reports of behaviours redolent of what later on was to be called depersonalization can be found since early in the nineteenth century. Esquirol, Zeller, Billod and others reported patients with stereotyped complaints that they had lost their capacity to feel, that it was as if they were dead, although they still could think clearly. The first systematic account was Krishaber's (1873), who reported 38 patients with *la névropathie cérebrocardiaque* (cerebrocardiac neuropathy). Over one-third of these patients complained of feelings of unreality. But it was Dugas who coined the term *depersonnalisation* as a derivation of an expression that appeared in the diary of H.F. Amiel. 'Depersonalization' was intended by Dugas to describe 'a state in which there is the feeling or sensation that thoughts and acts elude the self (*le moi sent ses pensées et ses acts lui échapper*) and become strange (*lui devenir étranger*), there is an alienation of personality'. To start off, depersonalization was explained as a disorder of coenaesthesis or of disorders in the sensory apparatus where 'multiple sensory distortions led to strange experiences'. Later on it was believed to be a disorder of recognition memory and/or consciousness or affectivity (for a full history of depersonalization and references quoted in this chapter, see Sierra & Berrios 1996, 1997). With Störring (1900) it became a disorder of 'self-awareness' (*Ichbewußtsein*) and of 'body image'.

Ichstörungen

At the beginning of the twentieth century, Pick (1904) published a paper on the disturbances of the consciousness of the self,[58] reporting a symptom cluster which in due course was to give rise to the German concept of *Ichstörungen* and which included what nowadays would be called passivity feelings (as first-rank symptoms of schizophrenia), disorders of body schema, and even depersonalization. According to Störring (1900), on whose views Pick based his analysis, 'consciousness of the self' (*Ichbewußtsein*) resulted from the combination of the consciousness of one's body, 'feelings of activity', consciousness of the capacity for the actualization of psychic functions (such as the capacity to remember past mental states), and the concatenation of mental processes.[59] This mongrel notion is based on a strange mixture of irreconcilable theories of the self,[60] but based on it clinical phenomena were grouped that to this day remain unrelated neurobiologically and semantically[61] and which had been kept separate in other countries.[62] No wonder current researchers still notice that the *Ichstörungen* are in need of a 'unificatory' theory (e.g. Spitzer, 1988)!

For complex reasons (which are beyond the purview of this chapter), quoting Jaspers has become a canonical act. However, for anyone having more than a superficial acquaintance with his work, the question becomes which version of Jaspers' analysis of the disorders of the perception of the self should be given credence? Should one go for that contained in the first or second edition (which are known to have been written by him alone) or in later editions (which are known to have been edited by Kurt Schneider)? The usual way amongst clinicians is to quote from the English translation of one of the last editions (indeed, it is not yet altogether clear which was used for this purpose) as *if all editions said the same* (on the history of general psychopathology, see Berrios, 1992). However, a comparison of the section on disorders of the self as appeared in the first edition (1913, all written by Jaspers) and in the fifth edition (1946, edited by Schneider) (Jaspers, 1948) shows important differences. For example, there is only one reference to schizophrenia in the first edition and various in the fifth; the model of the self described in the first edition was taken from Störring (1900) and Oesterreich (1910),[63] whilst that used in the fifth edition is redolent of Max Scheler's hierarchical model (Scheler was Schneider's supervisor). Thus, the question remains, which of these two versions of the 'disorders of the self' does best represent Jaspers' thinking?

The issue of whether the disorders of the self are pathognomonic of schizophrenia is in a way easier to handle, for the question only has meaning if the foundational claim is accepted that schizophrenia is a 'natural kind'. But in view of the fact that the official view of the history of schizophrenia is in need of revision, no historian may want to do that[64] (Berrios, 2000). If the view that schizophrenia is a construct turns out to be coherent, then the claim that the disorders of the self are pathognomonic becomes arbitrary and its acceptance will depend upon the social power of whoever is making the claim. Further historical research is needed to develop an alternative narrative and this chapter is not the appropriate place to do so. In the meantime, conventional readers may want to know what Kraepelin, Bleuler and Berze (inter alia) say about the disorders of the self.

Kraepelin published two parallel series of textbooks. The *Manual* started in 1883 and the *Lectures* in 1901.[65] The first time Kraepelin makes the claim that dementia praecox causes a breaking-down of the self can be located against the map of his publications. Kraepelin (1896) introduced the concept of dementia praecox in the fifth edition of the *Manual*. This same edition includes a short section of 'disorders of the awareness of the self' (pp. 163–164) but in it he never mentions dementia praecox; all he does is list epilepsy and degenerative processes (*Verblödungsprocesse*). In the sixth edition of the *Manual* (Kraepelin, 1899) the term 'degenerative process' in this section is replaced by dementia praecox. In the eighth edition, this section is much enlarged and Kraepelin (1909) quotes Pick and Oesterreich and (predictably) includes depersonalization and the fashionable phenomenon of multiple personalities (pp. 333–338). However, in the chapter carrying the long description of dementia praecox, rather intriguingly, Kraepelin does not say anything on the disorders of the self and in the very short section on the 'disorders of consciousness' he only mentions stupor and hypnotic and similar states (p. 684, Kraepelin, 1913).

In his book on schizophrenia, Eugen Bleuler only discussed the disorders of the self in the section on *Die Person* (pp. 117–120, Bleuler 1911), as his view on consciousness was narrow and hence only admitted of clouding, twilight states and the like (pp. 50–51, Bleuler, 1911).[66] His examples of disorders of the person and the self centre on cases suffering from delusions of being someone else or having 'made' emotions, actions and feelings, for example a subject with hebephrenia believed that whatever he did (e.g. scratching his face) was done by someone else (p. 119, Bleuler 1911). Similar points are made in the general psychopathology section of his *Textbook of Psychiatry* (pp. 137–142, Bleuler, 1924).

Based on Brentano's view of the mind as a set of intentional acts,[67] Joseph Berze (1866–1958) avoided the repetitiousness of views on the disorders of the self expressed by Jaspers, Kraepelin and Bleuler (Berze, 1914; Berze & Gruhle, 1929). Emphasis on the structure of the psychological act led Berze to develop the idea of 'insufficient mental activity' which in turn led to a gradual disintegration of consciousness. This ranged from mild to severe, as was the case in schizophrenia. Based on this mechanism, Berze (1987) attempted to explain mild changes in personality, tiredness, irritability, depersonalization and split personality, all of which he considered as disorders of the self.

The self becomes aware of its own disorders: the concept of insight

Debates concerning the question of whether insane patients could have consciousness of their insanity mainly took place towards the end of the nineteenth century (Berrios & Marková, 1998). Whilst some alienists observed that certain insane patients did appear to show some understanding of their madness (Guislain, 1852; Delasiauve, 1870; Prichard, 1835),[68] most alienists by the middle of the century considered loss of awareness to be a necessary feature of madness. Baillarger (1853), for example, emphasized specifically that loss of consciousness was an essential criterion of insanity and that patients who showed awareness of their disorder were not truly insane.[69] Towards the latter part of the century, however, more explicit debates were taking place concerning this issue. Degrees of awareness in patients were being increasingly recognized and Falret (1866) argued specifically against loss of awareness being used as a criterion to separate insanity from reason.

In 'Conscience et aliénation mentale', Dagonet (1881) addressed the concept of consciousness or awareness ('conscience') in relation to mental illness. Based on the ideas of Littré and Despine,[70] Dagonet (1881) defined consciousness as the 'intimate knowledge of ourselves, or the moral and intellectual processes going on within us (p. 370). Thus, like Littré and Despine, he viewed consciousness as an intrinsic aspect of the self which, at the same time, was able to observe its own constituents. However, where the earlier writers had conceptualized the self as comprising no more than the sum of the activities of its operations, Dagonet went further. His elaboration of consciousness as a deeper self-understanding, including 'all the phenomena of our internal life and committing them to memory', that is, it amounted 'to the feeling of totality of the person' (*le sentiment de la personnalité*: p. 370), implied a concept of self that was more than the sum of mental activities, a concept that was of a higher order in the sense that it included judgements of such activities.

Victor Parant (1888) was even more explicit in his analysis of awareness of self in mental illness (*conscience de soi*). He defined this as a 'state [in mental illness] in which the patient can take account of his impressions, his actions, his internal experiences and their resultant effects'. In other words, awareness 'implies not just knowledge of the mental state, but also the capacity, in varying degrees, to judge this' (p. 174). Both Dagonet and Parant argued that patients could show a wide range of awareness or consciousness in relation to their madness. Thus, aspects of the self could be sufficiently intact to be able to judge to varying degrees the disorder affecting the other aspects of self.

Reflecting perhaps the narrower concept of self, Maudsley (1895) expressed scepticism towards the importance and role placed on consciousness in relation to mental function.[71] Like some of the earlier French alienists, Maudsley believed that madness had effects on all mental faculties even if some were more affected than others. Thus, he drew a line between the sane and insane aspects of the mind, with no communication between them. In the same way that the sane man was incapable of judging precisely the behaviours and experiences of an insane man, then, similarly, patients with partial insanity could not judge with their sane mental functions the phenomena produced by their insane mental functions.[72]

Whether the 'self' or aspects of the self, in terms of awareness of self as a thinking and acting individual, could be preserved in the face of madness was an important question in the nineteenth century. This was not only because answers might help inform knowledge about the nature and classification of insanity but also because of the *medical legal issues* at the time and the question of responsibility for criminal acts. In other words, if patients had intact selves, or preserved awareness of their disorder, then they could be held responsible for criminal acts occurring in the context of their madness. This issue was evident at the time of Royer-Collard (Swain, 1978) and continued throughout the century. By the late nineteenth century, it was generally accepted that patients could have degrees of awareness in relation to their conditions but were nevertheless unable to control their insane acts and hence could not be held responsible for such behaviours (Falret, 1866; Morel, 1870; Dagonet, 1881; Parant, 1888).

Conclusions

Although fundamentally a western construct, versions of 'selves' can be found in other cultures. This commonality can be variously explained by means other than neurobiology, i.e. the view that the self perforce reflects a feature of the human brain or some atavistic behaviour with brain representation. This point is important to those who may want to locate the self on the brain *simpliciter*.

The inception of the self can be traced to Hellenistic philosophy. Ever since, it has been saddled with all manner of allegories and roles. St Augustine's view that it provided an inner private space for religious transactions has proved enduring. Taken up by the rhetoric of the Reformation, this view became central to the definitions of identity, responsibility, autonomy and individuality required by political liberalism and capitalism.

To earlier religious, moral and metaphysical versions of the self, the eighteenth century added a psychological one and versions thereof became available to the next century. The anatomoclinical model of disease encouraged a reification of these selves and soon claims started to be made as to their putative brain localization and pathology. This is one of the sources of the so-called clinical disorders of the self.

However, during the nineteenth century there was never a unified view of the self and the disorders in question were but a medley of behaviours and complaints. By the end of the century, a sort of coherence was achieved by claiming that all the disorders of the self resulted from the same abstract mechanism (e.g. dissociation). This delayed much-needed work on the conceptual structure of the self. Current neurobiological approaches alone are unlikely to be more successful.

Following the arrival of the psychological concept of self into psychiatry during the latter part of the nineteenth century, alienists took it up with gusto and soon the concept of 'disorder of the self' made its appearance. What had originally been a religious metaphor (the space where man meets God) was reified into an object with boundaries, content, tension, energy, sufficiency and a developmental history to boot. The old Lockean view that memory was the glue keeping the ingredients of the object together was taken at the foot of the letter and efforts were made, via Semon's concept of 'engram' (Schacter, 1982) to anchor the 'self' on to the brain.

For some reason, schizophrenia has borne the brunt of this speculative enthusiasm. The official justification has been that, whilst the self might be a trifle impaired in all mental disorders, it is truly so only in schizophrenia. Some went on to claim that schizophrenia resulted from a disintegration of the 'boundaries' of the self; others that it had to do with a reduction in its power and energy; others believed that underdeveloped selves were incapable of discriminating between themselves and the environment and got confused, and that this incapacity predictably was a pathognomonic feature of schizophrenia. Once this was fully established, then the rest of the symptoms of schizophrenia were explained on the basis of a basic fault of the self.

By the 1930s all combinations had been completed and the metaphor of the 'disorders of the self' overflowed into fictional literature.[73] Reduced ad absurdum, the metaphor gradually disappeared from science and could only be found in the language of late-hour existentialism, for example, *The Divided Self* (Laing, 1961). Although since the nineteenth century there had been a decent version of neuropsychiatry in Europe (Berrios & Marková, 2002a), a new one (originated in another continent) was to predominate after the 1970s. This was based on a strange version of the views of Kraepelin and Schneider retranslated from a short reprocessing in the English language. Hughlings Jackson was also rediscovered and his views were (wrongly) applied to the symptoms of schizophrenia. In all this, the disorders of the self were nowhere to be seen. European psychiatry accepted all these without much protest, although talk about the self and the subjectivity of the patient with schizophrenia continued behind closed doors, and not in English (see, for example, reviews by Wyrsch, 1949, 1956; Cabaleiro, 1966).

Once again, as happened in the first half of the twentieth century,[74] basic sciences have drawn a blank during the second half and little that is really new has been said about the conventional symptoms of schizophrenia. And once again, as happened in the 1900s, neuropsychology (this time called 'cognitive') has come to the rescue. New psychiatric 'symptoms' were badly needed to expand research and secure funds, and cognitive deficits, depersonalization and insightlessness have of late received much attention. Now it is the turn of the disorders of the self and no doubt neuroimaging, neuropsychology and naive enthusiasm will show that there is a correlation between the noble metaphor of the self and some proxy variable purportedly representing the frontal lobes.

If there was one lesson to be learned from the history of the 'disorders of the self' before the Second World War, it was that such notions can only function properly in the medium of language: they are linguistic tropes, narrative yarns, modes of talking about people and their reasons for doing things, devices to capture meaning, even bridges over fences erected by humans beings. They are *not* like stones, horses or weeds; even less should they be considered as semantically tantamount to anatomical structures or functions, not even to changes in blood flow or test scores. That they may show 'correlations' with proxy variables should not be the motive of excitement, for we do not really know about the epistemic mechanisms responsible for 'significant' correlations (Berrios & Marková, 2002b). At any rate, such correlations will not help clinicians to reconfigure the meaning that guides the life and behaviour of their patients. The lesson has not yet been learned.

REFERENCES

Allen, R.C. (1999). *David Hartley on Human Nature*. New York: State University of New York Press.

Ameriks, K. (1997). Kant and the self: a retrospective. In *Figuring the Self. Subject, Absolute, and Others in Classical German Philosophy*, ed. D.E. Klemm & G. Zöller, pp. 55–72. New York: State University of New York Press.

Ameriks, K. (2000). *Kant's Theory of Mind*, 2nd edn. Oxford: Oxford University Press.

Ameriks, K. & Sturma, D. (1995). *The Modern Subject. Conceptions of the Self in Classical German Philosophy*. New York: State University of New York Press.

Annas, J. (1992). Aristotle on memory and the self. In *Essays on Aristotle's De Anima*, ed. M. Nussbaum & A.O. Rorty, pp. 299–311. Oxford: Clarendon Press.

Arénilla, L. (2000). *Luther et notre Société Liberale*. Paris: L'Harmattan.

Baillarger, J. (1853). Essai sur une classification des différents genres de folie. *Annales Médico-Psychologiques*, **5**, 545–66.

Baker, G. & Morris, K.J. (1996). *Descartes' Dualism*. London: Routledge.

Bakhurst, D. & Sypnowich, C. (eds) (1995). *The Social Self*. London: Sage.

Baldwin, J.M. (1903). *Mental Development in the Child and the Race*. New York: Macmillan.

Bastian, H.C. (1887). The muscular sense: its nature and cortical localization. *Brain*, **10**, 1–137.

Beck, L.W. (1996). *Early German Philosophy*. Bristol: Thoemmes Press.

Bellak, L. (1958). *Schizophrenia*. New York: Logos Press.

Berrios, G.E. (1992). Phenomenology, psychopathology and Jaspers: a conceptual history. *History of Psychiatry*, **3**, 303–27.

Berrios, G.E. (1996). *The History of Mental Symptoms*. Cambridge: Cambridge University Press.

Berrios, G.E. (2000). Schizophrenia: a conceptual history. In *New Oxford Textbook of Psychiatry*, vol. 1, ed. M. Gelder, J.J. López-Ibor & N.C. Andreasen, pp. 567–71. Oxford: Oxford University Press.

Berrios, G.E. (2002). The face in medicine and psychology: a conceptual history. In *The Human Face: Measurement and Meaning*, ed. M. Katsikitis, pp. 49–62. Boston: Kluwer Academic Publishers.

Berrios, G.E. & Marková, I.S. (1998). Insight in the psychosis: a conceptual history. In *Insight in the Psychosis*, ed. A. David & D. Amador, pp. 33–56. New York: Oxford University Press.

Berrios, G.E. & Marková, I.S. (2002a). The concept of neuropsychiatry. A historical overview. *Journal of Psychosomatic Research*, **53**, 629–38.

Berrios, G.E. & Marková, I.S. (2002b). Biological psychiatry: conceptual issues. In *Biological Psychiatry*, ed. H. D'haenen, J.A. den Boer, H. Westenberg & P. Willner, pp. 3–24. New York: Wiley.

Berze, J. (1914). *Die Primäre Insuffizienz der Psychischen Aktivität. Ihr Wesen, ihre Erscheinungen und ihre Bedeutung als Gründstorung der dementia praecox und der Hypophrenien überhaupt.* Leipzig: Franz Deuticke.

Berze, J. (1987). Primary insufficiency of mental activity. In *The Clinical Roots of the Schizophrenia Concept*, ed. J. Cutting & M. Shepherd, pp. 51–8. Cambridge: Cambridge University Press.

Berze, J. & Gruhle, H.W. (1929). *Psychologie der Schizophrenie*. Berlin: Springer Verlag von Julius Springer.

Biro, J. (1993). Hume's new science of the mind. In *The Cambridge Companion to Hume*, ed. D.F. Norton, pp. 33–63. Cambridge: Cambridge University Press.

Bleuler, E. (1911). *Dementia Praecox oder Gruppe der Schizophrenien*. Leipzig: Franz Deuticke.

Bleuler, E. (1924). *Textbook of Psychiatry*. Translated by A.A. Brill. New York: Macmillan.

Blondel, C. (1924). La personnalité. In *Traité de Psychologie*, vol. 2, ed. C. Dumas, pp. 522–74. Paris: Alcan.

Bonnier, P. (1905). L'aschématie. *Revue Neurologique*, **13**, 605–9.

Boring, E.G. (1953). A history of introspection. *Psychological Bulletin*, **50**, 169–89.

Bourgeois, M. & Geraud, M. (1990). Eugène Azam (1822–1899). *Annales Médico-Psychologiques*, **148**, 709–17.

Breazeale, D. (1995). Check or checkmate? The infinitude of the Fichtean self. In *The Modern Subject. Conceptions of the Self in Classical German Philosophy*, ed. K. Ameriks & D. Sturma, pp. 87–114. New York: State University of New York Press.

Brentano, F. (1973). *Psychology from an Empirical Standpoint*. London: Routledge & Kegan Paul.

Bricke, J. (1980). *Hume's Philosophy of Mind*. Princeton: Princeton University Press.

Brook, A. (1994). *Kant and the Mind*. Cambridge: Cambridge University Press.

Burke, P. (1997). Representations of the self from Petrarch to Descartes. In *Rewriting the Self. Histories from the Renaissance to the Present*, ed. R. Porter, pp. 17–28. London: Routledge.

Burns, R.B. (1979). *The Self Concept. Theory, Measurement, Development and Behaviour*. London: Longman.

Bynum, W.F. (1976). Varieties of Cartesian experience in early nineteenth century neurophysiology. In *Philosophical Dimensions of the Neuro-Sciences*, ed. S.F. Spicker & H.T. Engelhardt, pp. 15–33. Dordrecht: Reidel.

Cabaleiro, M. (1966). *Temas Psiquiátricos. Algunas Cuestiones Psicopatológicas Generales*, pp. 321–420. Madrid: Paz Montalvo.

Carlson, E. (1989). Multiple personality and hypnosis. The first one hundred years. *Journal of the History of the Behavioral Sciences*, **25**, 315–22.

Carroy, J. (1993). *Les Personnalités Doubles et Multiples. Entre Science et Fiction*. Paris: Presses Universitaires de France.

Cicchetti, D. & Toth, S.L. (eds) (1994). *Disorders and Dysfunctions of the Self*. New York: University of Rochester Press.

Condillac (1984). *Traité des Sensations*. Paris: Fayard.

Coons, P.M. (1993). L'epidemiologie des personnalités multiples et la dissociation. *Nervure: Journal de Psychiatrie*, **6**, 38–47.

Cutler, B. & Reed, J. (1975). Multiple personalities. *Psychological Medicine*, **5**, 18–26.

Dagonet, M.H. (1881). Conscience et aliénation mentale. *Annales Médico-Psychologiques*, **5**, 368–97; **6**, 19–32.

Danziger, K. (1997a). *Naming the Mind*. London: Sage.

Danziger, K. (1997b). The historical formation of selves. In *Self and Identity*, ed. R.D. Ashmore & L. Jussim, pp. 137–59. Oxford: Oxford University Press.

Davies, C.G. (1990). *Conscience as Consciousness: The Idea of Self-awareness in French Philosophical Writing from Descartes to Diderot*. Oxford: the Voltaire Foundation at the Taylor Institution.

Delasiauve, L.J.F. (1870). Discussion sur les aliénes avec consciences Annales médico-Psycho-logiques, **3**, 103–9, 126–30, 290–1, 307–9.

Des Chene, D. (2000). *Life's Form. Late Aristotelian Conceptions of the Soul*. Ithaca: Cornell University Press.

Descartes (1967). *The Philosophical Works*. Translated by E.S. Haldane and G.R.T. Ross. Cambridge: Cambridge University Press.

Despine, P. (1875). *De la Folie au Point de Vue Philosophique ou plus Spécialement Psychologique*. Paris: Savy.

De Vita, D.J. (1965). *The Concept of Identity*. The Hague: Mouton.

Drever, J. (1965). The historical background for national trends in psychology: on the non-existence of English associationism. *Journal of the History of Behavioral Sciences*, **1**, 123–30.

Falret, J.P. (1866). Discussion sur la folie raisonnante. *Annales Médico-Psychologiques*, **7**, 382–426.

Fleming, W. (1857). *The Vocabulary of Philosophy*. London: Griffin.

Foster, J. (1991). *The Immaterial Self. A Defence of the Cartesian Dualist Conception of the Mind*. London: Routledge.

Foucault, M. (1984). *The Souci de Soi*. Paris: Gallimard.

Franck, A. (1875). *Dictionnaire des Sciences Philosophiques*, 2nd edn., Paris: Hachette.

Frondizi, R. (1952). *Substancia y Función en el Problema del Yo*. Buenos Aires: Editorial Lozada.

Gallagher, S. & Shear, J. (eds) (1999). *Models of the Self*. Thorverton: Imprint Academic.

Garber, D. & Ayers, M. (eds) (1998). *The Cambridge History of Seventeenth Century Philosophy*. Cambridge: Cambridge University Press.

Gergen, K.J. (1998). The ordinary, the original, and the believable in psychology's construction of the person. In *Reconstructing the Psychological Subject. Bodies, Practices and Technologies*, ed. B.M. Bayer & J. Shotter, pp. 111–25. London: Sage.

Gibson, J. (1968). *Locke's Theory of Knowledge and its Historical Relations*. Cambridge: Cambridge University Press.

Ginzo, A. (2000). *Protestantismo y Filosofía. La Recepción de la Reforma en la Filosofía Alemana.* Madrid: Publicaciones de la Universidad de Alcalá.

Goettman, C., Greaves, G.B. & Coones, P.M. (1994). *Multiple Personalities and Dissociation 1791–1992. A Complete Bibliography.* Lutherville: Sidran Press.

Gold, J. (1985). Cartesian dualism and the current crisis in medicine – a plea for a philosophical approach: discussion paper. *Journal of the Royal Society of Medicine*, **78**, 663–6.

Goldstein, J. (2000). Mutations of the self in old regime and post-revolutionary France. In *Biographies of Scientific Objects*, ed. L. Daston, pp. 86–116. Chicago: Chicago University Press.

Gouhier, H. (1978). *Cartésianisme et augustinisme au XVIIᵉ siècle.* Paris: Vrin.

Gueroult, M. (1987). *Étendue et Psychologie chez Malebranche.* Paris: Vrin.

Guislain, J. (1852). *Leçons Orales sur les Phrénopathies, ou Traité Théorique et Pratique des Maladies Mentales.* Gand: Hebbelynck.

Hacking, I. (1992). Multiple personality disorder and its hosts. *History of the Human Sciences*, **5**, 3–31.

Hacking, I. (1995). *Rewriting the Soul. Multiple Personalities and the Sciences of Memory.* Princeton: Princeton University Press.

Hamilton, W. (1859). *Lectures on Metaphysics and Logic*, vol. 1. Edinburgh: William Blackwood.

Hanafi, Z. (2000). *The Monster in the Machine.* Durham: Duke University Press.

Hartle, A. (1983). *The Modern Self in Rousseau's 'Confessions': A Reply to St Augustine.* Indiana: University of Notre Dame Press.

Hartman, E. (1977). *Substance, Body and Soul. Aristotelian Investigations.* Princeton, New Jersey: Princeton University Press.

Helvétius, C.A. (1771). *De l'Esprit.* Amsterdam: Arkstée & Merkus.

Henle, J. (1841). *Allgemeine Anatomie.* Leipzig: Voss.

Hoeldtke, R. (1967). The history of associationism and British medical psychology. *Medical History*, **11**, 46–64.

Hume, D. (1967). *A Treatise of Human Nature.* Selby-Bigge edition. Oxford: Clarendon Press.

Hundert, E.J. (1997). The European enlightenment and the history of the self. In *Rewriting the Self. Histories from the Renaissance to the Present*, ed. R. Porter, pp. 72–83. London: Routledge.

Jaspers, K. (1913). *Allgemeine Psychopathologie*, 1st edn. Berlin: Springer.

Jaspers, K. (1948). *Allgemeine Psychopathologie*, 5th edn. Berlin: Springer.

Jones, E.G. (1972). The development of the 'muscular sense' concept during the nineteenth century and the work of H. Charlton Bastian. *Journal of the History of Medicine*, **27**, 298–311.

Jouffroy, T. (1826). Préface de traducteur. In *Esquisse de Philosophie Morale*, ed. D. Stewart, pp. i–clii. Paris: Johanneau.

Keller, P. (1998). *Kant and the Demands of Self-consciousness.* Cambridge: Cambridge University Press.

Kitcher, P. (1990). *Kant's Transcendental Psychology.* Oxford: Oxford University Press.

Kneller, J.E. (1997). Conceptions of the self in Hölderlin and Novalis. In *Figuring the Self. Subject, Absolute, and Others in Classical German Philosophy*, ed. D.E. Klemm & G. Zöller, pp. 134–48. New York: State University of New York Press.

Kofman, S. (1973). *Camera Obscura.* Paris: Galilée.

Kogan, A.A. (1969). *El Yo y el Sí mismo.* Buenos Aires: Centro Editor de America Latina.

Kraepelin, E. (1883). *Compendium der Psychiatrie*. Leipzig: Abel.

Kraepelin, E. (1887). *Psychiatrie. Ein kurzes Lehrbuch für Studirende und Aertze*, 2nd edn. Leipzig: Abel.

Kraepelin, E. (1896). *Psychiatrie. Ein kurzes Lehrbuch für Studirende und Aertze*, 5th edn. Leipzig: J.A. Barth.

Kraepelin, E. (1899). *Psychiatrie. Ein kurzes Lehrbuch für Studirende und Aertze*, 6th edn. Leipzig: J.A. Barth.

Kraepelin, E. (1901). *Einführung in die psychiatrische Klinik. Dreissig Vorlesungen*. Leipzig: J.A. Barth.

Kraepelin, E. (1909). *Psychiatrie. Ein Lehrbuch für Studirende und Aertze*, vol. 1. Leipzig: J.A. Barth.

Kraepelin, E. (1909–15). *Psychiatrie. Ein Lehrbuch für Studirende und Aertze*. Leipzig: J.A. Barth.

Kraepelin, E. (1913). *Psychiatrie. Ein Lehrbuch für Studirende und Aertze*, vol. 3. Leipzig: J.A. Barth.

Krishaber, M. (1873). *De la Névropathie Cérébro-cardiaque*. Paris: Masson.

Laing, R.D. (1961). *The Divided Self*. London: Tavistock.

Lanteri-Laura, G. & Gros, M. (1984). *La Discordance*. Paris: Unicet.

Laurent, A. (1993). *Histoire de L'Individualisme*. Paris: Presses Universitaires de France.

Levin, J.D. (1992). *Theories of the Self*. Washington: Hemisphere.

Lévy-Bruhl, L. (1928). *The 'soul' of the primitive*. Translated by L.A. Clare. London: George Allen & Unwin.

Lewis, N.D.C. (1936). *Research in Dementia Praecox*. New York: Supreme Council of the North Masonic Jurisdiction of the United States of America.

Littré, E. (1878). *Dictionnaire de la Langue Française*, Paris: Hachette.

Lloyd, G.E.R. (1968). *Aristotle*. Cambridge: Cambridge University Press.

Locke, J. (1959). *An Essay Concerning Human Understanding*. Collated and annotated by A.C. Fraser. New York: Dover Publications.

Long, A.A. (1991). Representation and the self in stoicism. In *Psychology. Companion to Ancient Thought 2*, ed. S. Everson, pp. 102–20. Cambridge: Cambridge University Press.

Lowe, E.J. (1996). *Subjects of Experience*. Cambridge: Cambridge University Press.

Marsella, A.J., DeVos, G. & Hsu, F.L.K. (eds) (1985). *Culture and the Self. Asian and Western Perspectives*. London: Tavistock Publications.

Martin, R. & Barresi, J. (1999). *Naturalization of the Soul: Self and Personal Identity in the Eighteenth Century*. London: Routledge.

Maudsley, H. (1895). *The Pathology of Mind*. London: Macmillan.

McCabe, M.M. (1994). *Plato's Individuals*. Princeton: Princeton University Press.

McCracken, C.J. (1983). *Malebranche and British Philosophy*. Oxford: Oxford University Press.

McGrath, A.E. (1999). *Reformation Thought*. Oxford: Blackwells.

Mendus, S. (1984). Kant's doctrine of the self. *Kant Studien*, **75**, 55–64.

Mischel, T. (ed.) (1977). *The Self. Psychological and Philosophical Issues*. Oxford: Blackwell.

Modell, A.H. (1993). *The Private Self*. Cambridge: Harvard University Press.

Mondolfo, R. (1955). *La Comprensión del Sujeto Humano en la Cultura Antigua*. Buenos Aires: Imán.

Moore, F.C.T. (1970). *The Psychology of Maine de Biran*. Oxford: Clarendon Press.

Morel, B.A. (1870). Discussion sur les aliénés avec conscience. *Annales Médico-Psychologiques*, **3**, 110–19.

Morris, C. (1972). *The Discovery of the Individual 1050–1200*. London: SPCK.

Müller, J.P. (1946). *Los Fenómenos Fantásticos de la Visión*. Translated by J.M. Sacristán. Madrid: Espasa Calpe.

Müller-Sievers, H. (1997). *Self-generation: Biology, Philosophy and Literature Around 1800*. Stanford: Stanford University Press.

Neisser, U. (ed.) (1993). *The Perceived Self*. Cambridge: Cambridge University Press.

Neisser, U. & Fivush, R. (eds) (1994). *The Remembering Self*. Cambridge: Cambridge University Press.

Neuhouser, F. (1990). *Fichte's Theory of Subjectivity*. Cambridge: Cambridge University Press.

O'Meara, D.J. (1995). *Plotinus. An Introduction to the Enneads*. Oxford: Clarendon Press.

Oesterreich, K. (1910). *Die Phänomenologie des Ich in ihren Grundproblemen. First part: Das Ich und das Selbstbewußtsein. Die scheinbare Spaltung des Ich*. Leipzig: J.A. Barth.

Oesterreich, M. (1954). *Traugott Konstantin Oesterreich*. Stuttgart: Fromanns.

Onians, R.B. (1954). *The Origins of European Thought: About the Body, the Mind, the Soul, the World Time, and Fate*. Cambridge: Cambridge University Press.

Parant, V. (1888). *La Raison dans la Folie*. Paris: Doin.

Perkins, J.A. (1969). *The Concept of the Self in the French Enlightenment*. Geneva: Droz.

Perry, J. (1993). *The Problem of the Essential Indexical*. Oxford: Oxford University Press.

Pick, A. (1904). Zur Pathologie des Ich-Bewusstseins. Studie aus der allgemeinen Psychopathologie. *Archiv für Psychiatrie und Nervenkrankheiten*, **38**, 22–33. [See: Pick, A. (1996). On the pathology of the consciousness of the self. Translated by R. Viviani & G.E. Berrios. *History of Psychiatry*, **7**, 324–32.]

Pigeaud, J. (2001). *Aux Portes de la Psychiatrie. Pinel, l'Ancient et le Moderne*. Paris: Aubier.

Plotinus (1966). *Ennead 1*. Translated by A.H. Armstrong. Cambridge: Harvard University Press.

Prichard, J.C. (1835). *A Treatise on Insanity and other Disorders Affecting the Mind*. London: Sherwood, Gilbert and Piper.

Prince, M. (1929). *The Unconscious*, 2nd edn. New York: Macmillan.

Rappe, S. (2000). *Reading Neoplatonism*. Cambridge: Cambridge University Press.

Reesor, M.E. (1989). *The Nature of Man in Early Stoic Philosophy*. London: Duckworth.

Reil, J.C. (1803). *Rhapsodien*. Halle: Unveraenderter Nachdruck der Ausgabe.

Renaut, A. (1997). *The Era of the Individual. A Contribution to the History of Subjectivity*. Translated by M.B. De Bevoise & F. Philip. Princeton: Princeton University Press.

Ribot, T. (1887). *The Diseases of the Personality*. Translated by J. Fitzgerald. New York: Humboldt Library.

Rieber, R.W. (1999). Hypnosis, false memory and multiple personality: a trinity of affinity. *History of Psychiatry*, **10**, 3–11.

Riobó, M. (1988). *Fichte, Filósofo de la Intersubjetividad*. Barcelona: Herder.

Rose, N. (1996). *Inventing our Selves. Psychology, Power and Personhood*. Cambridge: Cambridge University Press.

Rousseau, N. (1986). *Connaissance et Langage chez Condillac*. Geneva: Droz.

Royer-Collard, A.-A. (1843). Examen de la doctrine de Maine de Biran sur les rapports du physique et du moral de l'homme. *Annales Medico-psychologiques*, **2**, 1–45.

Russon, J. (1997). *The Self and its Body in Hegel's Phenomenology of Spirit*. Toronto: Toronto University Press.

Sandbach, F.H. (1994). *The Stoics*, 2nd edn. London: Duckworth.

Sauri, J.J. (1989). *Persona y Personalización*. Buenos Aires: Carlos Lohlé.

Sawday, J. (1997). Self and selfhood in the seventeenth century. In *Rewriting the Self. Histories from the Renaissance to the Present*, ed. R. Porter, pp. 29–48. London: Routledge.

Schacter, D.L. (1982). *Stranger behind the Engram. Theories of Memory and the Psychology of Science*. Hillsdale: Lawrence Erlbaum.

Schiller, F. (1984). Coenesthesis. *Bulletin of the History of Medicine*, **58**, 496–515.

Schmaltz, T.M. (1996). *Malebranche's Theory of the Soul*. Oxford: Oxford University Press.

Schoenfeldt, M.C. (1999). *Bodies and Selves in Early Modern England*. Cambridge: Cambridge University Press.

Sepper, D.L. (1996). *Descartes's Imagination. Proportion, Images, and the Activity of Thinking*. Berkeley: University of California Press.

Sierra, M. & Berrios, G.E. (1996). L. Dugas et un cas de dépersonalisation. *History of Psychiatry*, **7**, 451–62.

Sierra, M. & Berrios, G.E. (1997). Depersonalization: a conceptual history. *History of Psychiatry*, **8**, 213–29.

Snell, B. (1953). *The Discovery of the Mind*. Cambridge, MA: Harvard University Press.

Spanos, N.P. (1996). *Multiple Identities and False Memories*. Washington: American Psychological Association.

Spiegelberg, H. (1972). *Phenomenology in Psychology and Psychiatry*. Evanston: Northwestern University Press.

Spitzer, M. (1988). Ichstörungen: in search of a theory. In *Psychopathology and Philosophy*, ed. M. Spitzer, F.A. Uehlein & G. Oepen, pp. 167–83. Heidelberg: Springer.

Starobinski, J. (1977). Le concept de cénesthésie et les idées neuropsychologiques de Moritz Schiff. *Gesnerus*, **37**, 2–19.

Starobinski, J. (1990). A short history of bodily sensation. *Psychological Medicine*, **20**, 23–33.

St Augustine (1991). *Confessions. A New Translation by Henry Chadwick*. Oxford: Oxford University Press.

Störring, G. (1900). *Vorlesungen über Psychopathologie in irher Bedeutung für die normale Psychologie*. Leipzig: Engelmann.

Strauss, J. & Goethals, G.R. (1991). *The Self: Interdisciplinary Approaches*. Berlin: Springer.

Suber, P. (1990). A case study in *ad hominem* arguments: Fichte's science of knowledge. *Philosophy and Rhetoric*, **23**, 12–42.

Swain, G. (1978). L'aliéné entre le médecin et le philosophe. *Perspectives Psychiatriques*, **1**, 90–9.

Tallon, H.J. (1939). *The Concept of Self in British and American Idealism*. Washington: Catholic University of America Press.

Tauber, A.I. (1997). *The Immune Self*. Cambridge: Cambridge University Press.

Taylor, C. (1989). *Sources of the Self*. Cambridge: Cambridge University Press.

Taylor, W.S. & Martin, M.F. (1944). Multiple personalities. *Journal of Abnormal and Social Psychology*, **39**, 281–300.

Thandeka (1995) *Embodied Self, the Friedrich Schleiermacher's Solution to Kant's Problem of the Emperical self*. New York: State University of New York Press.

Viviani, R. (1998). *The Notion of Self and Mental Automatism in 19th Century French and German Psychopathology*. PhD Dissertation. Cambridge: University of Cambridge.

von Feuchtersleben, E. (1847). *The Principles of Medical Psychology*. Translated by H.E. Evans and B.G. Babington. London: Sydenham Society.

von Krafft-Ebing, R. (1904). *Textbook of Insanity*. Philadelphia: A. Davis.

Weber, M. (1958). *The Protestant Ethic and the Spirit of Capitalism*. Translated by Talcott Parsons. New York: Scribner's.

Weber, E.H. (1996). *On the Tactile senses*, 2nd edn. Translated by H.E. Ross & David J. Murray. Hove: Erlbaum.

Wigan, A.L. (1844). *The Duality of the Mind*. London: Longman, Brown, Green, and Longmans.

Wilson, F. (1991). Mill and Comte on the method of introspection. *Journal of the History of the Behavioral Sciences*, **27**, 107–29.

Wyrsch, J. (1949). *Die Person des Schizophrenen*. Bern: Haupt.

Wyrsch, J. (1956). *Zur Geschichte und Deutung der endogenen Psychosen*. Stuttgart: Thieme.

Yolton, J.W. (1991). *Locke and French Materialism*. Oxford: Clarendon Press.

NOTES

1. The self is also considered as an 'indexical' expression. The latter is defined as expressions whose meaning is determined (to a varied extent) by their context of utterance and include personal pronouns and demonstratives. Expressions such as 'my self', 'your self' fall into this category because sentences containing them mean different things in different contexts (Perry, 1993).

2. This core would: (1) integrate, harmonize and tag all cognitive, emotional and volitional acts performed by each individual; and (2) cause in him/her a feeling of continuity with the past and future and also a sense of autonomy and privacy, i.e. the belief that the said core is only accessible to his/her possessor (and to God, according to the Christian claim).

3. The expression *sens intime* developed in France during the seventeenth century, and refers both to the actual *sensation* of feelings of awareness and of consciousness in general, and beliefs thereof (see Davies, 1990).

4. This family includes concepts such as soul, mind, individual, persona, subject, subjective, subjectivity, self-knowledge, consciousness, awareness, self-awareness, insight, agency, identity, will and interiority (Saurí, 1989; De Vita, 1965).

5. Broad as it is, the meaning of self used in this chapter is narrower than the one used by Foucault (1984) or Rose (1998).

6. Assumptions made in regard to the 'nature' of the self affect the behaviour of users. For example, the view that the self is a substance or object invites questions as to its neurological 'localization' and its 'disorders' (Cicchetti & Toth, 1994) or its 'development' (Baldwin, 1903; De Vita, 1965). This ontological view of the self is ideally served by a historiographical approach that is linear, progressist and justificatory and which endeavours to show how scientists are

getting 'ever closer' to the thing that the self is. On the other hand, the view that the 'self' is a cultural construct invites questions as to its social function and political determinants; as to what legitimates its existence and explains its endurance in western culture; as to whether a less self-centred society may be a better one. The belief that the self can be localized on the brain is meaningless in this context for if the self is a cultural belief then it is stored together with other propositional attitudes and there is no reason to believe that it is privileged in any special way. If it is the case that beliefs are stored as both semantic and autobiographical memories, then the localization of the self in the brain should follow this rule. When it comes to historiography, supporters of this view will feel more comfortable treating the various theories of the self as parallel narratives, each addressing specific social and political needs (Bakhurst & Sypnowich, 1995; Rose, 1996). This chapter is written from this latter perspective and assumes that the 'psychological' concept of the self is a motivated narrative (in the sense of Neisser, 1993; Neisser & Fivush, 1994) which emerged during the nineteenth century to justify the 'scientific' study of the self, i.e. the application of manipulations, measurements and interpretations (Burns, 1979) to a concept that in earlier centuries would have passed it by (Mischel, 1977; Danziger, 1997a). For a superb analysis of the concept of self from the viewpoint of analytical philosophy see Lowe (1996). The use of the concept of self in immunology (Tauber, 1997) or psychoanalysis (Kogan, 1969; Strauss & Goethals, 1991; Modell, 1993) is metaphorical; broader still is the view taken by Taylor (1989), whose target seems to be the origins of the concept of 'modern identity'.

7. In this regard Morris (1972) has stated: 'Western individualism is far from expressing the common experience of community. Taking a world view, one might almost regard it as an eccentricity among cultures. Yet it is an eccentricity of great historical importance, because of the dominant role played by the West during the past five centuries' (p. 2).

8. Aristotle and followers discussed individuation within the wider frame of defining the soul and living things (Des Chene, 2000).

9. Stoicism refers to the philosophical views of a school of thought that lasted for about 600 years (third century BC to third century AD) and is divided into early, middle and later Stoa. The Stoics wrote on logic, physics and ethics and their unconventional views included rules of philosophical behaviour and a deontology for philosophers (Sandbach, 1994).

10. The Aristotelian concept of 'soul' is a crucial source for the notions of self and consciousness (Hartman, 1977; Des Chene, 2000).

11. 'it seems as if awareness exists and is produced when intellectual activity is reflexive and when that in the life of the soul which is active in thinking is in a way projected back, as happens with a mirror-reflection when there is a smooth, bright, untroubled surface . . . in the same way as regards to the soul, when that kind of thing in us which mirrors the images of thought and intellect is undisturbed, we see them and know them in a way parallel to sense-perception, along with the prior knowledge that it is intellect and thought that are active' (p. 199, Plotinus, 1966). The link between Plotinus and Bergson, and the latter's influence on early twentieth-century French psychiatry, requires exploration.

12. A similar argument was used 10 centuries later by the Reformers in their quarrel with Rome (McGrath, 1999). For example, Luther believed in the need for a psychological 'inner space' within which man and God could communicate without the help of intermediaries. Some have considered this view as the consolidation of the spatial metaphor of the self (Ginzo, 2000).

According to others (e.g. Arénilla, 2000), the same individualistic notion is at the basis of political liberalism which was to be converted by John Locke into the philosophical anthropology of capitalism.

13. Thus St Augustine (1991) writes: 'But where in my consciousness, Lord, do you dwell? Where in it do you make your home? What resting place have you made for yourself? What kind of sanctuary have you built for yourself?...I entered into the very seat of my mind, which is located in my memory, since the mind also remembers itself...For you are the Lord of the mind...But you remain immutable above all things, and yet have deigned to dwell in my memory' (pp. 200–1).

14. Historical evidence that Augustinian views directly influenced Descartes (Gouhier, 1978) provides the authors of this chapter with an adequate excuse to assume some continuity in regards to the history of the self and hence obviate dealing with the history in between the work of these two men (none the less, for views on the self before Descartes, see Burke, 1997).

15. Modern, revisionist readings of Descartes even suggest that, after all, he did not hold a naive dualist view (Baker & Morris, 1996) and that his model of consciousness was multidimensional (Sepper, 1996). For a full defence of the mind as an 'immaterial self', see Foster (1991).

16. Indeed, Cartesian dualism has even been blamed for the neglect by the neurosciences and medicine of the psychological and moral aspects of man (Gold, 1985).

17. 'existence itself; which determines a being of any sort to a particular time and place, incommunicable to two beings of the same kind. This, though it seems easier to conceive in simple substances or modes; yet, when reflected on, is not more difficult in compound ones, if care be taken to what it is applied' (II, xxvii, 4). Book II, chapter xxvii was added only to the 1694 (second) edition of the *Essay*. Consolidating the principle of individuation was part of the seventeenth century search for an image of man more fitting to the new science and economy than the one underlying the feudal system. The factors that might have operated in such a redefinition ranged from protestant ethics (Weber, 1958) to the body (Schoenfeldt, 1999), art (Sawday, 1997) and the concept of monster (Hanafi, 2000).

18. It has been argued that the weakest part of Locke's doctrine of the self is his overreliance on memory. For a history of the theories of the self after Locke, see Levin (1992).

19. On the role of the camera obscura as a metaphor in western thinking, see Kofman (1973).

20. Carried out by Pierre Coste, this translation appeared in 1700. Coste stayed for a time with Locke at the country residence of the Mashams (Oats, Essex) where the philosopher spent the final years of his life. By translating consciousness as *conscience*, Coste added a new meaning to the French term, freeing it from its earlier exclusive moralistic denotation (Davies, 1990; Yolton, 1991).

21. To the Cartesian view that the soul or mind appeared to the individual as a 'clear and distinct idea', Nicolas Malebranche (1638–1715) opposed the view that it was but a rather indistinct *sentiment intérieur* (term he preferred to *conscience*) (McCracken, 1983; Gueroult, 1987; Schmaltz, 1996).

22. These are the only two valid sources of knowledge in Lockean epistemology (Gibson, 1968).

23. 'as for our own existence, we perceive it so plainly and so certainly that it neither needs nor is capable of any proof... Experience then convinces us, that we have the intuitive knowledge of our own existence, and an internal infallible perception that we are'(IV, ix, 3).

24. There is no space here to deal with the important contribution of Diderot (Perkins, 1969), Mandeville & Fielding (Hundert, 1997), and Hölderlin & Novalis (Kneller, 1997). For a study of the self in France during this period, see Goldstein (2000).

25. Whilst developing his thought experiment about a statue that could come to life by dint of incremental perceptions, Condillac (1714–96) gave his views on the 'origin' of the self (Condillac, 1754 (reprinted 1984); Rousseau, 1986). Like Locke, Condillac (1984) believed that touch was the fundamental sense, and the first input into his statue was a tactile 'primordial feeling': 'Je l'appellerai *sentiment fondamental*; parce que c'est à ce jeu de la machine que commence la vie de l'animal: elle en dépend uniquement'. Somatic sensations modulate and finetune the *sentiment fondamental* (second part, chapter 1). As against Locke, Condillac believed that the *sentiment fondamental* was *innate* (rather than intuitive) and related to a 'feeling' elicited by the exercise of the function itself rather than by its content.

26. Influenced by Malebranche, Locke, Leibniz, Condillac and Hartley, Charles Bonnet (1720–93) proposed that the soul or mind was 'active' and that perceptions and movements only triggered the dormant innate ideas and sentiments it already possessed. This is the 'active' view of the mind that Maine de Biran (see below) was to develop at the beginning of the next century.

27. David Hartley (1705–57) tried to combine Lockean associationism with a personal interpretation of the Newtonian theory of 'vibrations' to the brain fibres. Nerve fibres responded to external stimuli by vibrating in specific ways and were associated with specific sensations which clustered up according to the law of association. Hartley was unclear as to how sensations and vibrations related or interacted and his views bordered on to Occasionalism. (Geulincx, a Cartesian philosopher, had proposed that on the *occasion* of each human volition, God produced a corresponding movement of the body; and on the *occasion* of each stimulus on the body, the corresponding idea in the mind of the recipient (McCracken, 1983).) On account of his doctrine of vibrations, claims have been made that Hartley started physiological psychology. Interestingly enough, Hartley himself felt that the doctrine of vibrations was dispensable and in the 1775 abridged edition of Hartley's *Observations*, Joseph Priestley (its editor) omitted most of the references to the theory of vibration. On Hartley and British associationism, see Hoeldtke (1967) and Allen (1999); for the view that during this period there was no real associationism in Britain, see Drever (1965).

28. Helvétius (1715–71) proposed a *reductio ad absurdum* of Lockean sensualism (which he had once followed) (Helvétius, 1771).

29. Rousseau (1712–78) was concerned about the question: what do I mean when I say 'myself' in the context of a narrative that includes memories and plans about me and others? This narrative could only make sense if there was a *deeper* self acting as a *sine qua non* for any and all experiences, which was the precondition for all thoughts that we have about ourselves (Hartle, 1983). Rousseau defined human nature in terms of interiority and *sens intime*. Ab initio, men were private islands and 'asocial' and the 'deep self' contained all the truths they needed. European trends, ranging from nineteenth-century Romanticism to twentieth-century Existentialism, have been influenced by Rousseau's view of the essential solitude of man. Technological advance had blunted man's capacity to find true definitions of goodness, rightness and nature in the depth of his very self where God had once deposited them (Perkins, 1969).

It was in this sense that society 'corrupted' man: like a siren song it prevented him from listening to the voice of his true self. The only path to truth was a return to interiority, to the self and to the subject within (Hartle, 1983). However, this solipsistic solution oscillates between emotions and thoughts and this renders it unstable. Followers had to choose: in the event, the Romantic movement chose emotions and Heidegger and Existentialism chose thinking as their path.

30. 'as memory alone acquaints us with the continuance and extent of this succession of perceptions, 'tis to be consider'd, upon that account chiefly, as the source of personal identity. Had we no memory, we never shou'd have any notion of causation, nor consequently of that chain of causes and effects, which constitutes our self or person ... [but] how few of our own past actions are there for which we have any memory? Who can tell me, for instance, what were his thoughts and actions on the first of January 1715, the 11th of March 1719, and the 3rd of August 1733? Or will he affirm, because he has entirely forgot the incidents of these days, that the present self is not the same person with the self of that time; and by that means overturn all the most establish'd notions of personal identity? In this view, therefore, memory does not so much produce as discover personal identity, by shewing us the relation of cause and effect among our different perceptions' (p. 262, Hume, 1967).
    For the view that Hume is just part of a wider process whereby the self was 'naturalized' at the end of the eighteenth century, thereby becoming susceptible to scientific management, see Martin & Barresi (1999).

31. On the value of the 'bundle theory', see Bricke (1980) and Biro (1993).

32. This complex concept is crucial to the understanding of post-Leibnitzian German philosophy in general and Kant's ideas in particular. Leibnitz coined the German term 'apperception' (based on the French *percevoir*) to refer to that form of acquisition of knowledge that resulted from reflection and not from intuition. Kant made apperception a central concept in his philosophy and divided it into empirical and transcendental. The former referred to knowledge gained by intuition, the latter to a more mysterious form of knowledge gained by 'understanding': examples of knowledge gained by transcendental apperception were the categories of thought and self or subject.

33. Kant's notion of the self, like others in his philosophy, is conceived of as 'self-generating'. In this regard, it has been claimed that it is a figurative application of the theory of 'self-generation', at the time rapidly replacing the older creationist view (Müller-Sievers, 1997).

34. It also created serious problems. For example, Schleiermacher predicted that it would lead to a nihilistic view of the concept of self (Thandeka, 1995).

35. A history of the self that does not include the contribution of Reinhold, Fichte and the Romantic movement would be incomplete. Sadly, there is no space in this chapter to deal with the work of these writers (for Fichte, see below).

36. The work of Johann Gottlieb Fichte (1762–1814) illustrates how the self had become part of the debate on the definition of the 'political person' and the foundations of human freedom. Ab initio, Fichte accepted Karl Reinhold's (1758–1823) foundationalist 'principle of consciousness' which the German philosopher had posited as the integrating and legitimating core for all the actions of the mind. Fichte then proceeded to replace Reinhold's principle by the 'self positing self or I' (Ameriks & Sturma, 1995) which, like Condillac's statue, could

gradually generate a picture of both itself and the world. This it did because the self was not a passive posit (*Tatsache*) but an act (*Tathandlung*). The world appears to the self as an obstacle or resistance, as governed by rules that the self cannot overcome (Breazeale, 1995). The self also defines itself in terms of other selves and this intersubjectivity becomes for Fichte the basis for all human freedom (Riobó, 1988; Neuhouser, 1990). A self-generating entity, Fichte's concept of self reflects well his voluntaristic and anticreationist views. Indeed, he believed the final choice of any belief depended upon personality (Suber, 1990). For all its interesting possibilities, Fichte's view of the self was not influential on German psychiatry; indeed, the philosopher Friedrich Heinrich Jacobi (father of the psychiatrist) in an open letter accused him of nihilism.

37. This definition was to be quoted soon enough by the grand Littré (1878): 'Le *moi*, la personne humaine en tant qu'elle a conscience d'elle-même, et qu'elle est à la fois le sujet et l'objet de la pensée. Le *moi* consiste dans ma pensée; donc *moi* qui pense n'aurais point été si ma mère eût été tuée avant que je fusse animé'.

38. For a detailed account of the concept of self in Royce, Bradley, Bosanquet, Ward, Car and other idealist philosophers of the end of the nineteenth century, see Tallon (1939).

39. The anatomoclinical model of disease encouraged the study of signs, i.e. of changes in behaviour or in regions of the body that could be detected by the five senses and measured.

40. During the nineteenth century, the concepts of self, consciousness and introspection provided each other epistemological support and are historically interdependent. Although the term introspection – as a means of accessing the self – seems to have been in occasional use as early as the seventeenth century, it only became a valid method of access to, and analysis of, 'psychological data' during the nineteenth and only for as long as Cartesianism and sensationalist psychologies were in vogue (Boring, 1953). None the less, it was occasionally challenged during this period. On this, see the debate between Comte and Mill (Wilson, 1991).

41. Johannes Müller (1801–58) proposed that each of the sense organs responded to stimuli in its own way, i.e. had its own 'specific energy'. The external world was thus perceived by the changes it produced in sensory systems. In his *On Imaginary Apparitions* (Müller, 1946) he proposed that the eye not only reacted to external optical stimuli but can also be excited by internal imaginary stimuli. This had an important impact on theories of visual hallucination.

42. *Commentatio De Caenesthesi*, doctoral thesis, 1794 (quoted in pp. 192–7, Pigeaud, 2001).

43. For some reason Ribot (1887) misinterprets Jouffroy, claiming that he 'held that we know not our own bodies save objectively, as an extended solid mass like all other bodies' (p. 7).

44. Ribot (1887) is a good example here.

45. The 'source' for the concepts and ideas for the main figures of nineteenth-century psychiatry remains unclear. For example, although ab initio Pinel had Lockean sympathies, in later work he abandoned some of them. Through his philosopher brother, Royer-Collard became interested in the Scottish Philosophy of Common Sense and this is an important source of concepts for nineteenth-century French psychiatry. Esquirol followed Condillac but 'indirectly', via the his 'teacher' Laromiguière. Griesinger was steeped in German materialism. Morel was influenced by Roman Catholic theology.

46. This area requires further research. Next to nothing has been written on the incorporation of the concepts of self, ego and person into nineteenth-century psychiatry.

47. 'There are cases where consciousness of personal psychic existence entirely disappears, and the patient looks upon himself as an object, and therefore speaks of himself in the third person. In such cases, along with the psychic transformation, there are profound disturbances of general sensibility, anesthesias (sic), which not only infrequently give rise to the delusion of being dead. Still more interesting are those cases in which, along with the abnormal ego, fragments of the former personality have been retained; or in which the latter has been broken up, as it were, into several personalities that are subject to the dominant circle of false ideas (multiple ego, division of the personality). In the latter case there still exists at least a continuity of consciousness which is only changed in content, there are not two persons, but it is the same individual having different circles of ideas. The various egoes (sic) are still necessarily held together by the unity of body-sensibility and the consciousness of the continuous series of the psychic phenomena in time. In some rare cases this connection is also wanting: episodically the patient is entirely a different personality. Owing to the fact that no rays of consciousness pass from the period of healthy mental life into the period of disease, and also owing to the fact that during the insane period no traces of memory are left behind, the patient lives a completely double existence, and presents two sharply differentiated personalities in time (double personality, alternating consciousness, double mental life). Such conditions are, for the most part, observed in females in connection with the development of puberty and as one of the symptoms of an hysterical neurosis. They are very closely related to spontaneous somnambulism' (pp. 97–8, von Krafft-Ebing, 1904).

48. p. 64, Reil (1803).

49. For a full analysis, see pp. 44–52, Viviani (1998).

50. Antoine-Athanase Royer-Collard (1768–1825) was professor of Legal Medicine at the Charenton and in 1819 was responsible for a course in mental medicine. His brother was the philosopher Pierre Paul Royer-Collard. The course in mental medicine was based on a document produced by A-A Royer-Collard in 1821 but published in 1843 by his son, Hippolyte Royer-Collard. A-A Royer-Collard drew on Maine de Biran's 1811 thesis to produce the document. And Maine de Biran provided comments to his questions and criticisms in the form of footnotes.

51. Maine de Biran (1766–1824) was a French royalist politician and philosopher who emphasized the value and autonomy of the inner life and of the will as the central elements in knowledge and in the formation of the true self. Although the latter already existed in an inchoate form in the animal, it only achieved its full form as an active, imaginative and free entity in the human (see Moore, 1970). In opposition to the sensationalism of Locke and Condillac, Maine de Biran had rejected the notion of the mind as a passive recipient of sensations and argued in favour of the existence of free will, an innate, active force (*activité libre*) which he linked intrinsically to existence itself. It was awareness of this free will that gave the person a 'concept of self'. In relation to disease, De Biran argued two points: firstly, in insanity the individual lost his sense of free will and with it his sense of self. Consequently, his 'behaviour' was governed only by the 'passive' faculties, which, in turn, were dependent on stimulation by internal and external impressions. Because the intellectual faculties were

under the control of the will and hence belonged to the self, then, for Maine de Biran, it was incompatible for the insane individual to be able to exercise these. Should even one such faculty be exercised by the individual, then he would have awareness of the self and would not be truly insane. To lose the self was to lose these faculties. Secondly, the passive faculties, because they were not subordinate to the self, could themselves be active without the self and hence act independently.

52. 'This active, free force [the will] of which man has awareness, is identical with the self' (Royer-Collard, 1843).

53. During this period Pinel's classification of mental disorders into mania, melancholia, idiocy and dementia predominated.

54. On the basis of his observations, Royer-Collard went on to make an important distinction in his conception of the self and disorder of the self in madness. Following Maine de Biran, he identified the sense of self with the awareness of an active force, the free will. However, whilst Maine de Biran considered these aspects as inseparable, Royer-Collard argued that a distinction could be made. He proposed that the self or will consisted of two components, namely freedom and awareness. The former could be lost but the latter was preserved and hence the self as a whole was only partially affected. In other words, where patients' awareness was preserved, their 'selves' were not lost, even though they were mad. Madness was not an absolute state but had infinite degrees. The self could be altered to greater and lesser degrees and was only lost completely in idiocy.

55. Sceptical voices criticizing the dissociation account can be heard from the beginning of the twentieth century (e.g. pp. 554–61, Blondel, 1924).

56. Based on the longitudinal observation of a case (Sally Beauchamp), Morton Prince (1854–1929), an American neurologist, developed a model of 'multiple personalities' that made use of mechanisms such as dissociation, synthesis and inhibition. He also provided a mechanism for the growth of the 'secondary' personality (Prince, 1929). *Conceptually*, there is little difference between his views and those propounded by Azam.

57. Hacking (1992) writes: 'these stories formed a canonical series of cases, but they were curiosities. They made no sense. There was no host culture to absorb them' (p. 20). Given his (understandable) eagerness to have a go at the construction of multiple personalities in and after Azam, Hacking is too dismissive of earlier contexts of analysis (Hacking, 1995). What makes earlier cases 'curiosities' is that we have not yet obtained sufficient information about them and their time! (For a history of cases before Azam, see Cutler & Reed, 1975; Coons, 1993.) For a balanced view on the historiography of multiple personality see Carlson, 1989.

58. '*Ich-Bewußtsein*' literally means 'I-consciousness' or 'ego-consciousness'.

59. This model of the self was used by Jaspers in the first edition of his *General Psychopathology*, although he does not quote Störring (see p. 56, Jaspers, 1913).

60. As mentioned above, the perceptual hypothesis on the origin of the self had its origin in French Condillacean sensualism and ultimately in Locke. H. Taine (quoted by Pick) was but a late follower of this tradition. On the other hand, the view that effort and volition played a role in the formation of the self had matured in the work of Cabanis, de Tracy, Maine de Biran and Laromiguière and survived under various guises right up to Wundt.

61. Thus Pick's 'disturbances of the self' included depersonalization, 'mental automatisms', awareness of alien control and passivity experiences.

62. For example, in France depersonalization was considered as an independent syndrome (Sierra & Berrios, 1997).

63. Traugott Konstantin Oesterrich (1880–1949) was a philosopher who taught at Tübingen and wrote on Kant, German philosophy in the second half of the nineteenth century and the history of the concept of possession (Oesterreich, 1954). He claimed to follow a phenomeno-logical line but this has been called into question (Spiegelberg, 1972).

64. Basically there are two issues here. One concerns the question of whether schizophrenia was always out there, hiding in nature, like a new species of spider or orchid in the forest ready to be discovered, or whether it is a construct like the notion of virtue, revolution or aesthetics. The latter view does not call into question the symptoms and signs that have since been included under the construct but the claim that the construct itself is a natural kind. For example, noses, eyes, cheeks, foreheads and lips have adequate anatomical and physiological reality and are natural kinds: the concept of face itself however is a construct (genetics and embryology no longer help at this cultural level of organization of knowledge) (Berrios, 2002). The second issue is whether the history of schizophrenia is the history of one object being gradually discovered and profiled by the toil of researchers or whether what Hecker, Kahlbaum, Kraepelin, Diem, Bleuler, Bumke, Mayer Gross, the Schneiders and others described were different notions pertaining to parallel research programmes, only that some earlier historians decided to see in this a linear, progressive and unitary research programme (Berrios, 2000).

65. Unless referenced against the two series of textbooks, claims that 'Kraepelin said' become meaningless. Whilst still training at Munich, he published the first edition of the *Compendium* (Kraepelin, 1883). The second edition, under a modified name, he published from Dorpat (Kraepelin, 1887) and new editions appeared in 1889, 1893, 1896 (the fifth and an important one), 1899, 1903–4, and 1909–15 (the eighth and the one everyone quotes, for parts of it were translated into English in Scotland). The second line of textbooks started in 1901 and they were called *Introduction to Clinical Psychiatry: 30 Lectures*; the second edition was in 1905 (with 32 lectures) in 1916, 1921 and 1927.

66. Interestingly, Berze (1987), a rather outspoken writer, criticized Bleuler on this account: 'His passage on the subject of consciousness takes up barely half a page in his otherwise wide-ranging book' (pp. 52–3).

67. An important nineteenth-century philosopher of mind, Franz Brentano's (1838–1917) influence on current psychology remains deep and wide. His emphasis on form, structure, intention and functioning (as opposed to analysis of psychological content in John Locke's fashion) is to be found behind phenomenology, some neuropsychological models, gestalt psychology, psychoanalysis and all the integrationist, meaning-related approaches found to this day in psychology and psychiatry. The views that influenced Berze are expounded in a book by Brentano entitled *Psychology from an Empirical Standpoint* (Brentano, 1973).

68. e.g. 'awareness could remain intact and the patient is able to say to himself: I am mad' (p. 62, Guislain, 1852); Similarly, Falret (p. 387, 1866) observed that many insane patients, 'have perfect awareness of their states, which is in great conflict with their ill behaviours'.

69. 'Because man, and such examples are not rare, can be hallucinated without being mad, for as long as he retains awareness, he is only suffering from a pathological state which he is able to judge and appreciate in the same manner as the physician himself' (p. 549, Baillarger, 1853).

70. Despine (1875) had expressed this explicitly, when he defined consciousness (*conscience personelle*) as knowledge of one's mental faculties, i.e. knowledge of what is perceived, remembered, reflected and felt.

71. 'it has been very difficult to persuade speculative psychologists who elaborate webs of philosophy out of their own consciousnesses that consciousness has nothing to do with the actual work of mental function; that it is the adjunct not the energy at work; not the agent in the process, but the light which lightens a small part of it . . . we may put consciousness aside then when we are considering the nature of the mechanism and the manner of its work' (p. 8, Maudsley, 1895).

72. 'each self thinks its own *thinks* or *things* – that is, thinks its own world; the true self, or what remains of it, perceives the world as it looks to sane persons, and the morbid self or double, perceives it as a strange and hostile world' (p. 304, Maudsley, 1895). In other words, he did not believe it was possible for an insane mind to make a rational judgement concerning its derangement. The madness was perceived as necessarily affecting the self because the self, in turn, was conceived as inherent within the operation of the mental faculties themselves. When these were disordered, then the 'self' relating to these faculties was likewise disordered and consciousness, in that regard, reflected the activity of the disordered self. It is a pity that these important observations were lost during the twentieth century when the simplistic view was taken that patients with schizophrenia could objectively report their *Ichstörungen* as if these extraordinary experiences did not distort the very structure of their 'reporting' self and of consciousness.

73. For example, Sartre used it in his novel *The Nausea*.

74. For a bibliography of basic science research into schizophrenia during the first 50 years of the twentieth century promising that the solution was 'just around the corner', see Lewis (1936); Bellak (1958).

2

The self in philosophy, neuroscience and psychiatry: an epistemic approach

Georg Northoff and Alexander Heinzel

Harvard University, Boston, MA, USA

Abstract

The self and self-consciousness are investigated in such different disciplines as neuroscience, psychiatry and philosophy. The resulting theories of these investigations are as different as are these three sciences. This often leads to the question which of the theories should be considered as the best theory or even as the true theory.

However in this chapter we hold the opinion that none of the different theories is comprehensive in a way that covers all the questions brought up by the other disciplines. We think that this is due to the fact that the three different sciences start from different perspectives, namely the first-person perspective, second-person perspective and third-person perspective. Consequently their resulting theories cannot be regarded as an absolute truth, but only as true in the scope of their perspective.

In this chapter the different perspectives are characterized according to their epistemic limitations and abilities. Furthermore it is shown how these perspectives lead to characteristic implications concerning the theories of the self in the different sciences.

Introduction

The self and self-consciousness have always been important problems in philosophy, especially dealt with in the philosophy of mind (Gloy, 1998). However the recent philosophy of mind often refers to Descartes' theory as its beginning (Seager, 1999). His special methodology and his theses have deeply influenced many of his successors. Descartes begins with our reflective consciousness, which questions anything. It results in a fundamental doubt towards everything except the fact that we think or doubt, e.g. the consciousness or the mind does not doubt its own existence. Descartes formulates this in his famous statement: 'I think, therefore I am' (*cogito ergo sum*).

His central thesis contains the premise of the epistemic privilege of judgements about our mind, our consciousness and our self-consciousness. This means that our own consciousness is better accessible to us than anything outside of it, which is normally called the external world. As Descartes puts it: 'For it may perhaps be the case that I judge that I am touching the earth even though the earth does not exist at all; but it cannot be that, when I make this judgement, my mind which is making the judgement does not exist' (Descartes, 1904, pp. 8–9).

This implies that we have a special perspective which allows us to get a certain knowledge about ourselves, i.e. our minds. This special perspective can be called the first-person perspective (FPP), because it presupposes a thinking *subject*. From the point of view of this subject, the philosophical investigation of consciousness, self-consciousness and of the external world starts. Such a philosophical conception leads to the problem how the thinking subject may be linked with the world. The answer of Descartes and many others is that it is directed to the world, which is called the 'intentionality or the aboutness of consciousness'.

Following Descartes the fundamental structure of the *cogito* and his thesis of epistemic privilege have become a starting point for many theories of consciousness and self-consciousness. Famous examples are German idealism, phenomenology and existentialism.

In contrast to these philosophical theories, the perspective underlying neuroscientific theories of the self is different. The neurosciences (like science in general) presuppose an objective world, which exists independently of human beings (i.e. independent of subjects and of consciousness). This world is characterized by its physical structure and its laws of nature. This perspective can be called the third-person perspective (TPP) because it aims to avoid completely every subjectivity linked with an individual standpoint, such as, for example, Descartes' *cogito*. A typical example is Melzack's theory of the body-self neuromatrix (Melzack, 1989). According to Melzack the neuromatrix is a complex neuronal network which generates a certain activation pattern (*neurosignature*). This activation pattern is continuously generated and accompanies each proprioceptive input. In this way the proprioceptive input has a special characteristic such that the input is attributed to the body itself. Moreover the neurosignature produces a particular quality of experience, which causes the feeling of a self.

Between these fundamentally different points of view in philosophy and neuroscience a rather intermediate perspective exists, which is attributed to psychiatry and psychotherapy (Northoff, 2000). According to Bollas (1997), patients in psychotherapy should take an intrasubjective relation to themselves, i.e. patients should have a relation to the self as an object. It is crucial for patients to achieve a certain distance to the self. From an epistemic point of view, this process can be described as a shift from the FPP to the second-person perspective (SPP). In this perspective patients may be able to consider their own mental state from new points of view proposed by the therapist.

The concept of the self in psychotherapy, and in particular in psychoanalysis, has two main sources: firstly, similar to philosophy, the direct experiences of sensations and of mental states, and secondly, the indirect experiences of mental states via introspection, i.e. the experience of one's own body and mind as an object (Jacobson, 1978).

In this chapter we do not want directly to contradict the different theories of the self. We rather want to contribute to a deeper understanding of their scope. It is the central thesis of this chapter that these theories of the self cannot be considered as a general truth, but only as true according to a certain perspective. To that end we will characterize the perspectives underlying the different theories of the self. Then we will try to show how the statements of the theories of the self are related to the perspectives from which they are generated, so that they can be considered as relative to a certain perspective.

Characteristics of the perspectives

Epistemic abilities and limitations
First-person perspective

The FPP is generally associated with the experience of mental states of one's own person; mental states of another person cannot be experienced in the FPP. Consequently, the experience of mental states in FPP is private and not accessible to the public, so that FPP provides *intrasubjective experience.*

In contrast to the experience of our own mental states within the FPP, we are unable to recognize mental states in general within FPP independently, whether they are our own ones or those of another person. Only in collaboration with the SPP is the FPP capable of recognizing mental states. Since the recognition of mental states is closely associated with their communicability the FPP itself is unable to communicate mental states to other persons.

If I eat sweet chocolate or drink my favourite wine I will have a certain (pleasant) experience about the taste of both. This experience is typically subjective. It is hard for me to describe the taste of my favourite wine to someone else. The only way for him to find out the taste of the wine seems to be to taste it himself. This means having an experience from the FPP.

Finally, in the FPP we are not able to experience and/or recognize neuronal or psychological states. For example, neuronal and/or psychological states presumably related to the taste of bitterness can neither be experienced nor recognized in FPP. Consequently, in the FPP we are completely 'blind' with regard to neuronal and psychological states.

Second-person perspective

In the SPP we are not able to experience mental states in general. However in the SPP we are able to recognize and judge mental states as experienced in the FPP which can be called 'phenomenal judgements' (Chalmers, 1996). The recognition of mental states in SPP is direct and not indirect via behaviour, as related to the respective mental state. SPP can be directly related to FPP such that the mental states experienced can be directly recognized. This *availability* (Shoemaker & Swinburne, 1984; Glover, 1988) of mental states in SPP concerns, similar to FPP, only our own mental states but not those of another person. The recognition of mental states in SPP is closely related to their communicability such that *phenomenal judgements* in SPP can be regarded as a kind of *nexus* between private experience (via FPP) and public communication (via TPP) – the SPP thus provides *intrasubjective communication* so that the person can communicate with him/herself.

For example, I can recognize directly my taste of the chocolate's sweetness but I am unable to recognize the taste of bitterness in another person other than via behaviour. Consequently the SPP can be directly linked to FPP only with regard to our own mental states but not in the case of mental states of another person. Furthermore the ability to recognize mental states in SPP is closely associated with their communicability. If SPP itself is disturbed although FPP is still functioning, as is the case in the neuropsychiatric disease of catatonia, the experience of mental states can no longer be recognized and communicated – the person no longer, speaks and moves as is indeed the case in catatonic patients (Northoff, 2000).

The SPP has no access to neuronal states at all, which are thus not *available* in SPP. Psychological states may however be experienced in SPP whereas they cannot be recognized as such – similar to FPP with regard to mental states, the experience of psychological states in SPP only concerns those of the individual person, but not those of another person (Varela, 1998).

Third-person perspective

In the TPP we can neither experience nor recognize mental states, such that mental states are not at all *available* for the TPP. In contrast to mental states, the TPP can recognize psychological and behavioural states from other persons, although those states of the individual person cannot be accounted for in TPP. Consequently the TPP, unlike FPP and SPP, does not concern private, i.e. intrasubjective, states but rather public states, such as intersubjectively accessible states (Davidson, 1984; Holly, 1986; Brennan, 1989/1990). The TPP thus provides *intersubjective communication*. Although not directly, as in SPP, the mental states of other persons can nevertheless be indirectly recognized in TPP via their psychological and behavioural manifestations.

For example, if I eat bitter chocolate my friend can see by my face my grimacing and other alterations in my gestures and my attention which accompany my experience of bitterness. Hence he has indirect access to my mental state via its accompanying behavioural and psychological alterations, whereas he has neither access to my experience of bitterness, as my FPP, nor is he able to recognize directly my mental state, as in SPP.

The importance of the TPP can be nicely demonstrated in the case of an isolated loss of TPP, as is the case in patients with autism. Autistic patients are no longer able to recognize psychological and behavioural manifestations or, even if they can recognize them, they are no longer able to interpret and relate them to the other person (Frith 1998). These patients are not able to lead an intersubjective communication, although they have *intrasubjective experiences*, as provided by FPP, as well as, *intrasubjective communication* via SPP, so these patients can be characterized by an isolated deficit in *social cognition*.

Properties of the experiences in different perspectives
First-person perspective

The mental states in FPP can be characterized by phenomenal qualia, transparency, presence and nonstructural homogeneity.

Phenomenal qualia refer to two properties, phenomenal and qualitative, which can be best described as a kind of 'raw feeling' (Metzinger, 1995, pp. 22–24). The term 'qualitative' denotes this feeling whereas the term 'phenomenal' circumscribes a pure experience without any other ingredients such as reflection or recognition, thus referring to the rawness of the feeling. This raw feeling, reflecting the appearance of mental states in FPP, has been described by Nagel (1984) as 'what it is like?' which can thus be reformulated as 'what kind of feeling is the raw (or pure) experience like?' For example, tasting the bitterness of chocolate can be described as raw feeling which has no other ingredients than the feeling or the experience itself such that we have pure experience or a raw feeling since there is no further experience (as related to FPP) and/or any kind of recognition (as related to SPP and/or TPP) involved.

Transparency of mental states in FPP refers to lucidity, immediateness, a feeling of direct contact, a feeling of completeness and *phenomenal certainty* (Metzinger, 1995, pp. 25–27). Lucidity describes the direct givenness of the content of the mental state such that one assumes that the content of the mental states is an (objective) part of the world. Tasting bitterness of the chocolate is directly related to the (objective) chocolate itself, but not to our own (subjective) abilities of tasting. Immediateness of mental states can be described by closeness of their contents without any kind of mediation. We do have the experience that the bitterness of the chocolate is directly given without any further experience or recognition. We feel that we are in direct contact with the bitterness itself, thus considering the bitterness as an objective part of the chocolate, i.e. world, which leads us to a *naive realism.* Moreover, we have the feeling of completeness without any possibility of deception as a kind of phenomenal certainty. We are convinced or phenomenally certain that we experience the bitterness not only itself but, in addition, completely, thus covering the whole range of bitterness in our experience in FPP.

Presence of mental states in FPP refers to their temporal dimension (Metzinger, 1995, p. 31). The contents of mental states in FPP appear as present without any further mediation by the past or the future. However the presenceness of the contents of mental states in FPP does not appear to be isolated from the past and the future. Rather, both dimensions, past and future, are included and integrated within presenceness, which by itself is extended such that the past and the future dimensions can flow into the state of presenceness. Inclusion of the past dimension within presenceness can be called *retention* and inclusion of the future *protention* (Husserl, 1966). Such an integration and inclusion of the past and future dimension generate a *subjective time* in the experience of mental states in FPP which can no longer be equated with *objective time* though, similar to naive realism in transparency (see above), we do often confound subjective and objective time if there is no clock available. For example, the bitterness of a chocolate is experienced in FPP as *eternal* or *timeless* since during the experience we are convinced that the bitterness can never change and will remain a property of the chocolate for ever, i.e. we experience an eternity of bitterness whereas past, present and future are included and integrated into each other such that, in contrast to objective time, they can no longer be distinguished from each other in subjective time. Only the fact that the bitterness of the chocolate will taste different on the next day will make us aware of temporal and therefore subjective temporal relativity of the taste of bitterness of the chocolate.

Nonstructural homogeneity of experience of mental states in FPP refers to appearance of *wholeness* of *system properties* which cannot be reduced to distinct structures, parts or elements (Gadenne, 1996, pp. 26–28). Consequently we do experience a wholeness and not distinct parts or elements which can be integrated within wholeness. For example, the bitterness of the chocolate is experienced as a whole and not by integration or inclusion of distinct parts or elements. If we try to reduce the wholeness to some parts or elements, the wholeness would vanish and the experience, i.e. the respective mental state, would disappear or dissolve. Once I try to figure out the distinct parts of the experience of bitterness of the chocolate, my experience of bitterness would disappear immediately.

Second-person perspective

The states as recognized in SPP no longer appear as phenomenal but still as qualitative. The feeling is no longer raw, i.e. there is no pure experience since other ingredients beside the feeling, such as recognition and reflection, are involved. However there is still a kind of feeling involved, though this feeling is partially transformed by the other ingredients. For example, if I recognize that my taste of the chocolate could be characterized by bitterness, I still have a feeling of bitterness but not as pure and clear as during the experience of bitterness in FPP itself. One may therefore characterize the feeling in SPP not by rawness but rather by *reflection* or *recognition*, so that one could speak of a recognized or reflected feeling. In addition one could therefore speak of *nonphenomenal qualia* and 'What kind of feeling is the recognition like?'

The recognized states in SPP may appear as semitransparent. Their appearance can still be characterized by lucidity and a feeling of direct contact, whereas there is no longer an immediateness and a feeling of completeness. The feeling of direct contact is lost because the states as obtained in SPP are no longer phenomenal since pure experience or rawness of feelings is lacking, so that the content can be accounted for only indirectly via mediation by recognition, i. e. reflection. Since the content of state is mediated by recognition and reflection, the feeling of completeness is lost. If the feeling of completeness is lost, there can no longer be any phenomenal certainty such as an absolute certainty about the content of the state. Consequently, a certain phenomenal uncertainty about the content in the states in SPP arises. For example, if we taste bitterness in FPP we are absolutely certain about the bitterness, but once we recognize this bitterness in SPP the *phenomenal certainty* from FPP becomes relativized and undermined by doubt, i.e. *phenomenal uncertainty*.

The states recognized in SPP appear as semipresent. There is still a presence of the content in the temporal dimension of the present whereas, in contrast to the states in FPP, this presence no longer includes and integrates the temporal dimensions of the past and the future, such that there is neither retention nor protention. The states in SPP are thus still grounded in the present, but they are isolated from past and future. For example, the taste of bitterness in FPP is eternal (see above), including and integrating all three dimensions such that these cannot be distinguished at all. The recognition of the taste of bitterness in SPP is still present in the immediate present, but it can neither be connected with the past nor with the future so that it no longer appears as eternal.

The states recognized in SPP can be characterized by an appearance of structural homogeneity. The states in SPP do still appear as one wholeness and therefore as homogeneous. However this wholeness can be dissected into distinct parts and elements without dissolving the state itself entirely, as was the case in FPP (see above). A certain structure appears in the states in SPP which Metzinger calls 'phenomenal structure' (Metzinger, 1993, 1995).

Third-person perspective

The states in TPP appear as nonphenomenal and nonqualitative since they are neither accompanied by pureness of experience or rawness of feeling, nor by any kind of feeling at all. For example, we have no experience of the taste of bitterness of the chocolate of other people; we know it but we do not experience or (directly) recognize their taste of bitterness. As a result intersubjective knowledge of other persons as obtained in TPP does not include intrasubjective experience/feeling of the individual person as related to FPP and SPP so that there are neither (phenomenal or nonphenomenal) qualia nor a 'what it is like?' in TPP.

States in TPP no longer appear transparent at all. They are neither lucid and immediate nor related to a feeling of direct contact and completeness. For example, the knowledge of the taste of bitterness in another person is only mediated by verbal and behavioural indicators as a kind of knowledge and thus indirectly to a degree of incompleteness concerning the 'what it is like', i.e. the pure experience. Thus we can never be entirely sure whether another person really tastes the bitterness of the chocolate. There is phenomenal uncertainty ('Is the person *really* tasting the bitterness?') coupled with *factual certainty* such as certainty about the fact of the taste of chocolate as reflected indirectly, i.e. verbal and behavioural indicators.

The states in TPP no longer appear as present. They are neither grounded in the present, as is the case in SPP (see above), nor do they integrate and include the past and future temporal dimension. Consequently the contents of the states in TPP appear as temporally isolated timeless facts neither belonging to the present nor to the past or future. We can apply objective time measures to them which gives us their external orientation in time. For example, we look at our clock and thus for physical, i.e. objective, time when somebody is tasting bitterness for hours in order to get temporal orientation, whereas we have no idea of subjective time in TPP.

The states in TPP appear as structural and heterogeneous. In contrast to states in FPP and SPP, there is no wholeness at all in states related to TPP since there are only parts and elements. Consequently states in TPP show a heterogeneous structure which can be dissolved and reintegrated in various ways so that they do not appear as monadic and atomic (Churchland, 1985; Dennett, 1988).

The different perspectives and the theories of the self

In this section we want to show how different theories of the self can be related to the different perspectives described above. The different perspectives with their different abilities and limitations lead to characteristic implications concerning the self.

First-person perspective

Mental states as experienced in FPP can be characterized by centralization such that they seem to presuppose a centre from which the experience is made. This centre can be described as a focus or as a standpoint (Metzinger, 1995, pp. 27–30; Northoff, 2000). If there is a centre as a standpoint one concludes that somebody must stand on this centre as a standpoint experiencing mental states. It is this person which is called *I* – this conclusion with an inference of a subject as an *I* is called 'centre intuition' by Metzinger (Metzinger, 1993, pp. 236–237). In the normal case we presuppose only one centre so that there is only one unified *I* which is related to the own person as a kind of *self-centralization*. For example, the experience of bitterness of chocolate is related to my own person, so that, unlike in psychosis (see below), I can say that *I* experience the bitterness.

However, in a state like depersonalization/derealization, experienced as *ego-disturbances* in psychosis, there is no longer any self-centralization since individual mental states are no longer related to the *I* of the individual person but rather to the *I* of another person as a kind of nonself or foreign centralization (Northoff, 2000). Or there may be a multiplication of *I* with several personalities and multiple centralizations, as seems to be the case in multiple-personality disorder (Metzinger, 1993, pp. 236–237; Northoff, 2000).

How can the possibility of *centralization* be further characterized? Firstly, central-ization can be described by a point of view. It is a particular standpoint from which *I* make the experience of the bitterness of the chocolate and it is this standpoint which can be distinguished from all other standpoints of other persons. It is this standpoint from which I experience the world so that my view of other persons is determined by my standpoint as my point of view. In the case of the experience of mental states in FPP the centre, i.e. the *I*, and the point of view are entirely identical so that, unlike in SPP (see below), both cannot be distinguished from each other, i.e. the point of view of the FPP is from the inside (and not from the outside as in SPP) of the centre of the *I*.

Secondly, centralization can be characterized by *intentionality*. The experience of a mental state is directed towards and related to a particular content. For example, a taste is directed towards and related to bitterness of a chocolate. This seems self-evident; however, while eating the chocolate it is not evident that I relate the taste to bitterness and then to the chocolate. Consequently the centralization goes along with certain *contents*, and this is called *intentionality* (Gadenne, 1996). Furthermore, this content as related to the point of view of the *I* can be distinguished from the context so that the question of the *content–context* relationship arises (Hurely, 1998).

Thirdly, the possibility of centralization seems to be closely related to the body, as the *lived body* (Merleau-Ponty, 1963; Northoff, 1995; Metzinger, 1997). The lived body is closely related to the possibility of the *action–perception cycle* (Hurely, 1998). If there is no longer any possibility of transforming perceptions into actions the generation of a standpoint as the point of view of the *I* is disturbed so that the centralization of the experience in FPP with an inference of an *I* is disturbed (Metzinger, 1997; Hurely, 1998). As a result the lived body, metaphorically speaking, seems to be the harbour where the *I* is anchored, i.e. the lived body seems to be a necessary condition for the possibility of centralization.

As shown above, centralization is closely related to the self of the person experiencing a mental state. The self of a person taking a FPP can be experienced, whereas it cannot be recognized as a self, since this is only possible in SPP. If there is pure experience the question of the classification of the underlying self as an attribution to a particular person cannot be raised – the impossibility of the attribution to another person makes the question itself impossible. Consequently, mental states in FPP are considered to be the pure manifestation of the *I* going along with a prereflexive self-confidence as a feeling of identity and an infinite closeness.

Secondly, is there empirical evidence for such a case with presence of phenomenal qualia and concomitant absence of self-centralization and prereflexive self-confidence? Considering identity disturbances in schizophrenic patients (Northoff, 2000) and drug-induced psychosis (mescalin, LSD, etc.; Metzinger, 1993) one can summarize that these persons do indeed experience noncentred phenomenal qualia without attributing them to one particular *I* as the centre. Consequently, empirically, phenomenal qualia and self-centralization are not necessarily tied together since both can dissociate from each other. However it remains unclear whether the inverse dissociation is possible as well, so that there is self-centralization without phenomenal qualia.

In contrast to SPP and TPP, there is no access to the states of other persons so that one can speak of a *self-transparency* without any kind of *nonself-transparency* (Metzinger, 1995, pp. 29–30). Mental states in FPP do thus generate an internal world with the *I* of that particular person as the centre of phenomenal structure of experiences. Since mental states as experienced in FPP do generate both a phenomenal space (see above) and an *I*, the *I* is located in that space within the person itself as an internal world on its own. This internal world is opposed to the external world as that of other peoples which is closely associated with the distinction between subjectivity and objectivity. The internal world as generated in the mental states of FPP is centred around the *I* of that particular person and thus does not include any point of view from other persons – mental states in FPP can therefore be characterized by pure subjectivity without any ingredients of intersubjectivity and/or objectivity (see below).

Second-person perspective

The states as recognized in SPP can still be characterized by centralization since they can be attributed to the own person as the *I*, i.e. there is still self-centralization. However, as shown above, there is no longer pure experience but recognition coupled with experience. It is the component of recognition which allows us the detection of the centre from which these experiences are made. In addition, in SPP it is possible to consider the subjective experiences of other persons which can be attributed to the self of these other persons. Consequently one can no longer speak of an exclusive self-centralization but rather of a self and other centralization. If the individual centre of experience becomes relativized by means of the possibility of further centres of experience, the standpoint can no longer be exclusively from the inside but rather from the outside (Northoff, 2000). The individual centre from which mental states are experienced in FPP is still visible in SPP but is no longer experienced by itself. Consequently in SPP I do take a look at my own mental states, so that I will be able to make phenomenal judgements.

In contrast to FPP, where the pure experience is dominated by the content, states in SPP can be characterized by drawing a relationship between content and context, i.e. the one centre of the individual self is put into the context of centres of other persons. It is this relativization of the own centre in SPP by means of introducing centres of other persons which establishes a connection between the centres of the own and other selves. As a result the own centre is no longer equated with the world itself so that states in SPP can no longer be characterized by intentionality. For, example, the recognition of the taste of bitterness of chocolate invokes the question of how other people taste the same chocolate, i.e. in contrast to FPP, bitterness and chocolate are no longer automatically equated in the SPP.

Similar to mental states, the body can be seen from the outside in SPP. If I recognize my own body I am able to localize my own body in the world and to compare it with bodies of other people. I may recognize that I experience my body as much larger than that of another person although, objectively, it is much smaller. As a result my subjective body as the *lived body* can be compared with the objective body as the body of other persons in SPP so that the SPP mediates between both kinds of bodies, i.e. the *lived* (subjective) and the *objective* body. With regard to the experience of the lived body in FPP, the recognition of my lived body in SPP is made from a point of view from outside the lived body, which thus can be considered as the nexus between the subjective and the objective body as the bodies of the individual and other persons. However it should be noted that, in contrast to our own body, we have no epistemic access to the lived body of other persons so that we recognize only their objective body in TPP (see below). Consequently it is clear for our own persons how perceptions are transformed into action such that both are experienced and recognized as a unity or as a *perception–action cycle*, whereas in other persons we can recognize action and perception only as separate functions which are not directly and intimately related to each other (Merleau-Ponty, 1963; Northoff, 1995; Hurely, 1998).

As described above, phenomenal judgements in SPP are no longer exclusively centralized around the *I* of that particular person. In contrast to FPP, the *I* of other persons can be recognized as well. Since both *Is*, the one of the individual person and the one of the other person, can be recognized, a distinction between *I* and *thou/you* is possible. One may argue that both *I* and *thou/you* are recognized from the outside so that the two *Is* cannot be distinguished from each other. This is indeed true, but both can be distinguished from each other with regard to their relationship to FPP: the *I* of the individual person is closely related to the experience of a phenomenal qualia whereas the *I* of the other person is not – I can recognize the other person but I cannot have its pure experiences so that any kind of raw feeling is related to my *I* and not to the one of the other person. On the level of recognition, as related to SPP, we therefore have access to other persons whereas on the level of experience, as related to FPP, there is no access to states of other persons. As a result, states in FPP remain intrasubjectively whereas states in SPP can be characterized by the possibility of *intersubjectivity*. The possibility of intersubjectivity in SPP is however related to a necessary (in an empirical sense) loss of phenomenal qualia so that in SPP the *I* of the own and other persons can be recognized only from the outside – the *I* or the subjective self, as presupposed in the pure experience in FPP, is transformed into an objective self (Nagel, 1986) in SPP.

In contrast to FPP, there are several selves in SPP, so that, due to the inclusion of the selves of other persons, the own self must be distinguished from the selves of the other persons. This distinction is made by the *relation of mineness* (Metzinger, 1993) which can be considered as a relation between the subjective self of the pure experience in FPP and the objective self of the recognition in SPP. The possibility of such a relation of mineness is necessarily (in an empirical and logical sense) related to the possibility of SPP: if there is only an FPP without any kind of SPP the question of the necessity of the distinction between the own and other selves would never be raised because in this case there would only be one self, i.e. the self of the own person. For example, in the case of identity disturbances in schizophrenia, this relation of mineness can no longer be generated: the subjective self of the pure experiences in FPP cannot be related to the objective self of recognition in SPP so that both kinds of selves no longer match each other. Consequently schizophrenic patients link their subjective self with a *wrong* objective self, thus attributing their own mental state in FPP with another person as recognized in SPP – the relation of mineness thus becomes transformed into a *relation of otherness* with resulting identity disturbances (Northoff, 2000). States in SPP can thus be characterized by intersubjectivity, thus taking an intermediate position between subjective states in FPP and objective states in TPP.

Third-person perspective

In contrast to FPP and SPP, TPP does not presuppose any kind of centre from which the own person other persons and/or the world are experienced or recognized. As a result there is no *I* or *self-centralization* in the state of TPP so that TPP has neither access to the self of the own person nor to that of other persons.

What kind of standpoint is presupposed in TPP? There is no point of view from the inside since there are no phenomenal-qualitative states in TPP. Furthermore, TPP is unable to make phenomenal judgements so that it has no access from the inside as is the case in SPP. Hence TPP does not seem to be anchored or grounded in the world as it is reflected in the absence of any kind of standpoint as a point of view.

Since the TPP does not presuppose any kind of standpoint, the question of intentionality remains superfluous. There are no states which are directed towards the world so that the problem of equation between content and world is no longer virulent. No equation between the contents of the states and the world is necessary since it is the world itself which appears in the states of TPP. Consequently the distinction between content and context as presupposed in both FPP and SPP is no longer necessary in TPP – content and context are identical in states of TPP.

If there is no centre, an anchorage in the body is not necessary. Therefore, unlike in FPP and SPP, states in TPP are independent of the body so that the lived body seems to have no importance at all for TPP. If states in TPP are not centred, the individual body can no longer be experienced or recognized as a lived body, i.e. the body is just an objective body similar to all other objects in the world, without any particular relationship to the person taking TPP. If there is no relationship between body and person in TPP, action and perception cannot be linked to each other and are thus considered as entirely separate function without any kind of feedback effects as a necessary presupposition for the generation of a perception–action cycle (Merleau-Ponty 1963; Hurely, 1998). Hence, focusing exclusively on TPP, any kind of phenomenological approaches to the body with the assumption of a lived body and a perception–action cycle would be superfluous and furthermore, one would never come up with such an idea.

If there is no centralization at all, there is neither an *I* nor a *you/thou* in TPP. Consequently states in TPP can be characterized neither by subjectivity nor by intersubjectivity but rather objectivity: if there is no *I*, states cannot be subjective and if there is no *you/thou*, states cannot account for intersubjectivity. States in TPP are therefore objective since, unlike in FPP and SPP, they are no longer related to any kind of person, either the own one or others. Thus persons in general can not be distinguished from objects or things so that there is no essential difference between person and things in TPP.

The TPP can be characterized by objective states apparently reflecting the external world as it is. There is neither an internal world as it is related to FPP nor a bridge between the different internal worlds as is the case in SPP. Consequently the relation between states and the external world is not questionable in TPP since both can be equated with each other, so that the TPP is closely related with an externalism.

Conclusions

Summing up, we draw the following conclusions. Firstly, distinct characteristics of experiences are related to different perspectives. As we tried to show above, neuroscience, philosophy and psychiatry execute their investigation from different perspectives. These different perspectives are responsible for the different kinds of experiences or facts which underlie the theories in philosophy, neuroscience and psychiatry. Therefore what might be called the *truth* of their theories should not be considered as an absolute truth, but as a truth relative to a certain point of view.

Secondly, the concept of self as it is mostly understood is closely related to any FPP. The properties we attribute generally to the self appear as necessary linked to the perspective of the first person.

Thirdly, if we consider the self from another perspective, it changes completely. For example, properties visible from the FPP can no longer be detected in TPP and vice versa. The self appears so different in the FPP, SPP and TPP that it may even be said that we are not talking about the same thing. Thus the question arises of who is talking about the *real* self. We believe that is one of the reasons why it is so difficult to combine and integrate the different sciences in transdisciplinary theories.

Fourthly, we propose avoiding such ontological questions. The concepts of self should be considered as relative to the respective perspective. This means that there is no superiority or inferiority among neuroscience, philosophy and psychiatry. All their theories of the self have a certain justification according to their perspective and also a certain limitation according to their perspective.

Fifthly, since the concept of self is relative to perspectives, philosophical accounts of the concept of the self should not only be based on ontological considerations, but should include epistemic considerations as well. Furthermore, instead of discussing ontological considerations, the discussion should rather focus on linkages and relations between different perspectives and thus the different meanings of self in order to provide an integrative transperspectival theory of the self allowing for transdisciplinarity.

Sixthly, epistemic relativity of the concept of self should be considered in both neuroscience and psychiatry where it may lead to new therapeutic and empirical approaches. Inclusion of self in different perspectives may lead to a broadened and better understanding of the relationship between brain function and subjective experience as it is central for both neuroscience and psychiatry. Furthermore, such a transperspectival account of the self may lead to new forms of diagnosis and therapies in neuropsychiatric disorders of the self as is, for example, the case in schizophrenia and personality disorders. (For further readings on the idea and the consequences of the different perspectives and a possible unifying principle, see Northoff (2001) and Northoff (2002).)

REFERENCES

Bollas, L. (1997). *Der Schatten des Objekts: Das ungedachte Bekannte. Zur Psychoanalyse der frühen Entwicklung.* Stuttgart: Klett-Cotta.

Brennan, A. (1989/90). Fragmented selves and the problem of ownership. *Proceedings of the Aristotelian Society*, **90**, 143–58.

Chalmers, D.J. (1996). *The Conscious Mind.* Oxford: Oxford University Press.

Churchland, P.M. (1985). Reduction, qualia and the direct introspection of brain states. *Journal of Philosophy*, **15**, 8–28.

Davidson, D. (1984). First-person authority. *Dialectica*, **17**, 101–11.

Dennett, D. (1988). Quining qualia. In Consciousness, ed. A. Marcel & E. Bisiach, pp. 42–77. Oxford: Oxford University Press.

Descartes, R. (1904). Principles of philosophy. In *Oeuvres de Descartes*, ed. C. Adams & P. Tannery, pp. 34–78. Paris: J. Vrin.

Frith, U. (1998). Literally changing the brain. *Brain*, **121**, 1011–12.

Gadenne, V. (1996). *Bewusstsein, Kognition und Gehirn, Einführung in die Psychologie des Bewusstseins.* Bern: Hans Huber.

Glover, P. (1988). *The Philosophy and Psychology of Personal Identity.* London: Penguin.

Gloy, K. (1998). Bewußtseinstheorien. Munich: Verlag Karl Alber.

Holly, W.J. (1986). On D. Davidson first person authority. *Dialectica*, **40**, 153–6.

Hurely, S.L. (1998). *Consciousness in Action.* Cambridge, MA: Harvard University Press.

Husserl, E. (1966). *Zur Phänomenologie des inneren Zeitbewußteins*, pp. 123–78. The Hague: Martinus Nijhoff.

Jacobson, E. (1978). *Das Selbst und die Welt der Objekte.* Frankfurt am Main: Suhrkamp.

Melzack, R. (1989). Phantom limbs, the self and the brain. *Canadian Psychology*, **30**, 1–16.

Merleau-Ponty, M. (1963). *Phänomenologie der Wahrnehmung.* Translated by R. Boehm. Berlin: De Gruyter.

Metzinger, T. (1993). *Subjekt und Selbstmodell.* Paderborn: Schöningh Press.

Metzinger, T. (1995). *Conscious Experience.* Thoverton: Imprint Academic.

Metzinger, T. (1997). Ich-Störungen als pathologische Formen mentaler Selbstmodellierung. In *Neuropsychiatrie und Neurophilosophie*, ed. G. Northoff, pp. 169–91. Paderborn: Schöningh Press.

Nagel, T. (1984). *Über das Leben, die Seele und den Tod.* Frankfurt am Main: Neurowissenschaftliche Bibliothek, Etteneum.

Nagel, T. (1986). *The View from Nowhere.* Oxford: Oxford University Press.

Northoff, G. (1995). *Neuropsychiatrische Phänomene und das Leib-Seele Problem: Qualia im Knotenpunkt zwischen Gehirn und Subjekt.* Essen: Die blaue Eule Verlag.

Northoff, G. (2000). Phänomenale, tiefenpsychologische und neurowissenschaftliche Perspektiven der Katatonie: eine epistemische Betrachtung. In *Depression, Manie und schizoaffektive Psychosen*, ed. H. Böker, pp. 34–67. Giessen: Psychological Publisher.

Northoff, G. (2001). 'Brain-paradox' and 'embedment' – do we need a 'philosophy of the brain'? *Brain and Mind*, **2**, 195–211.

Northoff, G. (2002). *Philosophy of the Brain. Hypothesis of 'Embedment'*. Amsterdam: John Benjamins.

Seager, W. (1999). *Theories of Consciousness*. Trowbridge, Wiltshire: Redwood Books.

Shoemaker, S. & Swinburne, R. (1984). *Personal Identity*. Oxford: Basil Blackwell.

Varela, F. (1998). Neurophenomenology: a methodological remedy for the hard problem. In *Explaining Consciousness – The Hard Problem*, ed. J. Shear, pp. 1–13. Cambridge, MA: MIT Press.

3

Phenomenology of self

Dan Zahavi

Danish National Research Foundation; Center for Subjectivity Research and University of Copenhagen, Copenhagen, Denmark

Abstract

Initially, three different philosophical concepts of self are distinguished: a Kantian, a hermeneutical, and a phenomenological concept. The phenomenological concept is then analysed in detail. The first step of the analysis consists in an investigation of the first-personal givenness of phenomenal consciousness; the second step involves a discussion of different concepts of self-consciousness, a discussion which culminates in a criticism of the so-called higher-order representation theory. In conclusion, the article provides some examples of how the phenomenological concept of self may be of use in empirical science (psychiatry and developmental psychology).

Introduction

In the following chapter, I wish to outline and discuss some of the reflections on self that can be found in phenomenology. But let me start with a cautionary remark. Phenomenology is not the name of a philosophical *position*. It is the name of a philosophical *tradition* inaugurated by Husserl (1859–1938), and comprising among its best-known champions philosophers like Scheler, Heidegger, Schutz, Gurwitsch, Fink, Merleau-Ponty, Sartre, Levinas, Ricoeur and Henry. Like any other philosophical tradition, the phenomenological tradition spans many differences. This also holds true for its treatment and analysis of the self. In short, there is not one single phenomenological account of the self, just as there is not one single account of the self to be found in analytical philosophy. There are a variety of different accounts. In what follows, I have consequently been forced to make a certain selection, and to focus on what I take to be one of the most promising proposals.

Different notions of self

It would be something of an exaggeration to claim that the concept of self is unequivocal and that there is a widespread consensus about what exactly it means to be a self. Quite to the contrary, the contemporary discussion is bursting with completing and competing notions of self. In a well-known article from 1988, Ulric Neisser distinguished five different selves: the ecological self, the interpersonal self, the extended self, the private self and the conceptual self (Neisser, 1988, p. 35). Eleven years later, Galen Strawson summed up a recent discussion on the self that had taken place in *Journal of Consciousness Studies* by enumerating no fewer than 21 concepts of self (Strawson, 1999, p. 484). Given this escalating abundance it is very easy to talk at cross-purposes, particularly in an interdisciplinary context. One cannot simply take it for granted that one's interlocutor understands the same by the term self as oneself.

Some kind of taxonomy is obviously called for, so let me start by contrasting the notion of self which I wish to present with two other paradigmatic ways of conceiving of the self.

A Kantian suggestion: the self as a pure identity-pole

This traditional view insists on distinguishing between the identical self on the one hand and the manifold changing experiences on the other. In turn, I can taste an icecream, smell a bunch of roses, admire a statue of Michelangelo and recollect a hike in the Alps. We are faced here with a number of different experiences, but they also have something in common: they all have the same subject, they are all lived through by one and the same self, namely myself. Whereas the experiences arise and perish in the stream of consciousness, the self remains as one and the same through time. More specifically, the self is taken to be a distinct *principle of identity* which stands apart from and above the stream of changing experiences, and which for that very reason is able to structure it, and give it unity and coherence (cf. Kant, 1956, pp. B132–B133).

The concept of self at play here is a very formal and abstract concept. Every experience is always lived through *by* a certain subject, it is always an experience *for* a certain subject. The self is consequently defined as the pure subject, or ego-pole, that any episode of experiencing necessarily refers back to. It is the subject of experience rather than the object of experience. Rather than being something which can itself be given as an object for experience, it is a necessary condition of the possibility for (coherent) experience. We can infer that it must exist, but it is not itself something that can be experienced. It is an elusive principle, a presupposition, rather than a datum, rather than something which is itself given. Were it given, it would be given for someone, i.e. it would be an object, and therefore no longer a self (cf. Natorp, 1912, pp. 8, 40). As Kant writes in *Kritik der reinen Vernunft*: 'It is ... very evident that I cannot know as an object that which I must presuppose to know any object' (Kant, 1956, p. A 402).

A hermeneutical suggestion: the self as a narrative construction

A quite different way of conceiving the self takes its point of departure in the fact that self-comprehension and self-knowledge, rather than being something that is given once and for all, is something that has to be appropriated, and which can be attained with varying degrees of success. As long as we live, we can become acquainted with new aspects of ourselves. Self-knowledge is consequently a dynamic and unending process. The same, however, can also be said for what it means to be a self. The self is not a thing; it is not something fixed and unchangeable, but rather something evolving, something that is realized through one's projects, and therefore something which cannot be understood independently of one's own self-interpretation. In short, one is not a self, in the same way one is a living organism. One does not have a self in the same way that one has a heart or a spleen (Taylor, 1989, p. 34).

According to this view, which has become increasingly popular lately, the self is taken to be a construction. It is the product of conceiving and organizing one's life in a certain way. When confronted with the question 'Who am I?' we will tell a certain story, emphasizing certain aspects that we deem to be of special significance, to be that which constitutes the *leitmotif* in our life, that which defines who we are, that which we present to others for recognition and approval (Ricoeur, 1985, pp. 442–443). I attain an insight into my character traits by situating them in a life story that traces their origin and development: a life story that tells where one is coming from, and where one is heading. This narrative, however, is not merely a way of gaining insight into the nature of an already existing self. On the contrary, the self is first constructed in and through the narration. Who we are depends upon the story we (and others) tell about ourselves. The story can be more or less coherent, and the same holds for our self-identity. The narrative self is consequently an open-ended construction, which is under constant revision. It is pinned on culturally relative narrative hooks, and organized around a set of aims, ideals and aspirations (Flanagan, 1992, p. 206). (One should notice that if this construction is regarded as some kind of fiction, as something that lacks any ontological significance, the narrative account turns out to be a variant of the no-self doctrine.) It is a construction of identity that starts in early childhood, continues for the rest of our life, and involves a complex social interaction. Who one is depends on the values, ideals and goals one has: it is a question of what has significance and meaning for one, and this, of course, is conditioned by the community of which one is part. Thus, it has often been claimed that one cannot be a self on one's own, but only together with others, as part of a linguistic community. As Charles Taylor puts it: 'There is no way we could be inducted into personhood except by being initiated into a language' (Taylor, 1989, p. 35).

The phenomenological suggestion: the self as an experiential dimension

The phenomenological alternative I now wish to consider can be seen as a replacement of the first notion of self, and as a necessary founding supplement for the second notion of self. The crucial idea is that an understanding of what it means to be a self calls for an examination of the structure of experience, and vice versa. To put it differently, the claim being made is that the investigations of self and experience have to be integrated if both are to be understood. More precisely, the self is claimed to have an experiential reality; it is taken to be closely linked to the first-person perspective, and is in fact identified with the very first-personal *givenness* of the experiential phenomena. As the French phenomenologist Michel Henry would put it: the most basic form of selfhood is constituted by the self-manifestation of experience (Henry, 1963, p. 581; Henry, 1965, p. 53). To be conscious of one*self* is not to capture a pure self that exists in separation from the stream of consciousness, rather it just entails being conscious of an experience in its first-personal mode of givenness, that is, from 'within'. The self referred to is consequently not something standing beyond or opposed to the experiences, but is rather a feature or function of their givenness. According to this view, the self is neither an ineffable transcendental precondition, nor is it a social construct that evolves through time; rather it is an integrated part of our conscious life, which has an immediate experiential reality.

This third concept of self is, just like the Kantian concept, a very formal and minimalist concept, and it is obvious that there are far more complex forms of self. But when this is said, the phenomenological notion nevertheless strikes me as being of pivotal significance. It is fundamental in the sense that nothing which lacks this dimension deserves to be called a self. Thus the experiential self could be characterized as the *core self*. Let me in the following try to articulate this view in slightly more detail.

First-personal givenness

Experiences are not something that one simply has, like coins in the pocket. On the contrary, experiences are normally taken to be characterized by having a subjective 'feel' to them, i.e. a certain (phenomenal) quality of 'what it is like' or what it 'feels' like to have them. Whereas we cannot ask what it feels like to be a piece of soap or a radiator, we can ask what it is like to be a chicken, an alligator or a human being, because we take them to be conscious, i.e. to have experiences. To undergo a conscious experience necessarily means that there is something it is like for the subject to have that experience (Nagel, 1974, p. 436; Searle, 1992, pp. 131–132). This is obviously true of bodily sensations like pain or nausea. But it is also the case for perceptual experiences, desires, feelings and moods. There is something it is like to taste an omelette, to touch an ice cube, to crave chocolate, to have stage fright, to feel envious, nervous, depressed or happy. However, it would be a mistake to limit the phenomenal dimension of experience to *sensory* or *emotional* states alone. There is also something it is like to entertain abstract beliefs; there is something it is like to believe that the square root of $9 = 3$, just as there is an experiential difference between accepting or denying that Hegel was the greatest of the German idealists, i.e. there is what one could call a qualitative feel to the different propositional attitudes. As Strawson writes: 'the apprehension and understanding of cognitive content, considered just as such and independently of any accompaniments in any of the sensory-modality-based modes of imagination or mental representation, is part of experience, part of the flesh or content of experience, and hence, trivially, part of the qualitative character of experience' (Strawson, 1994, p. 12; cf. Husserl, 1984, pp. 73, 667–676; Zahin, 2003).

Is it possible to elucidate this experiential quality in further detail? Whereas the object of A's perceptual experience is intersubjectively accessible in the sense that it can in principle be given to others in the same way that it is given to A, A's perceptual experience itself is only given directly to A. Whereas A and B can both perceive the numerically identical same cherry, they both have their own distinct perception of it, and can share these just as little as B can share A's bodily pain. B might certainly realize that A is in pain; he might even sympathize with A, but he cannot actually feel A's pain the same way A does. It is here customary to speak of an *epistemic asymmetry*, and to say that B has no access to the *first-personal givenness* of A's experience.

When one is directly and noninferentially conscious of one's own occurrent thoughts, perceptions or pains, they are characterized by a first-personal givenness, that immediately reveals them as one's own. This first-personal givenness of experiential phenomena is not something quite incidental to their being, a mere varnish that the experiences could lack without ceasing to be experiences. On the contrary, it is this first-personal givenness that makes the experiences *subjective*. To put it differently, with a slightly risky phrasing, their first-personal givenness entails a built-in self-reference, a primitive experiential self-referentiality. When I am aware of an occurrent pain, perception or thought from the first-person perspective, the experience in question is given immediately, noninferentially and noncriterially as *mine*. If I feel hunger or see a sunrise, I can neither be in doubt nor mistaken about who the subject of that experience is, and it is nonsensical to ask whether I am sure that I am the one who feels the hunger. But whether a certain experience is experienced as mine or not, does not, however, depend upon something apart from the experience, but precisely upon the givenness of the experience. If the experience is given in a first-personal mode of presentation, it is experienced as *my* experience, otherwise not.

Obviously, this form of egocentricity must be distinguished from any explicit I-consciousness. I am not (yet) confronted with a thematic or explicit awareness of the experience as being owned by or belonging to myself. Nevertheless, the particular primary presence or first-personal givenness of the experience makes it mine, and distinguishes it for me from whatever experiences others might have (Husserl, 1959, p. 175; Husserl, 1973, pp. 28, 56, 307, 443).

In the light of these considerations, it is tempting to equate the first-personal mode of givenness with a certain primitive form of selfhood. One does not need to conceive of the self as something standing apart from or above the experience, nor to conceive of the relation between self and experience as an external relation of ownership. It is also possible to describe the first-personal givenness of an experience itself, that is, its self-givenness or self-manifestation, as the most basic form of selfhood. It is precisely the primary presence or first-personal givenness of a group of experiences which constitutes their 'mineness' or *ipseity* (from the Latin, *ipse*, which means 'self' or 'himself'), i.e. makes them subjective, makes them belong to a particular subject. In this case the self would not be something standing opposed to the stream of consciousness, but an essential part of its structure. To have a self-experience would not entail the apprehension of a special self-object; it would not entail the existence of a special experience of self, alongside other experiences but different from them, but simply the acquaintance with an experience in its first-personal mode of presentation, that is, from 'within'. As Evans puts it: '[F]rom the fact that the self is not an object of experience it does not follow that it is non-experiential' (Evans, 1970, p. 145). Thus, when Hume in a famous passage in *A Treatise of Human Nature* declares that he cannot find a self when he investigates his own mental life, but only particular perceptions or feelings (Hume, 1888, p. 252), it seems natural to conclude that he overlooked something in his analysis, namely the specific givenness of his own experiences. He was looking for the self in the wrong place, so to speak.

One way to capture this point is by replacing the traditional phrase 'subject of experience' with the phrase 'subjectivity of experience'. Whereas the first phrasing might suggest that the self is something that exists apart from or above the experience, and for that reason something that might be encountered in separation from the experience and even something the experience might occasionally lack, the second phrasing excludes these types of misunderstanding. It makes no sense to say that the subjectivity of the experience is something that can be detached or isolated from the experience, nor for that matter that it is something the experience can lack. But to stress the subjectivity of experience is not an empty gesture. On the contrary, it is to insist upon the basic egocentricity of experiential phenomena.

How does the self as experiential dimension stand to the self as pure identity-pole, and to the self as narrative construction? As already mentioned, it replaces the first and complements the second. Thus, one advantage of the view just outlined is that it is capable of accounting for certain of the features normally associated with the pure identity-pole model, particularly its ability to account for the identity of the self through time, without actually having to posit the self as a separate entity over and above the stream of consciousness. After all, it is perfectly legitimate to insist on the *difference* between our singular and transitory acts and the abiding dimension of first-personal experiencing. Whereas we live through a number of different experiences, the first-personal experiencing itself remains as an unchanging dimension. Of course, this should not be misunderstood. Distinguishability is not the same as separability. We are not dealing with a pure or empty field of experiencing upon which the concrete experiences subsequently make their entry. The field of experiencing is nothing apart from the concrete experiences. Nevertheless, the moment we expand the focus to include more than a single experience it becomes not only legitimate but also highly appropriate to distinguish the strict singularity of the field of first-personal givenness from the plurality of changing experiences. To use a nice formulation by Klawonn, the latter are exposed in it (Klawonn, 1991, pp. 77, 128). It is their exposure in this field of first-personal givenness which makes them mine. Against that background, the self could be described as the invariant dimension of first-personal givenness in the multitude of changing experiences.

When it comes to the relation between the self as experiential dimension and the self as narrative construction, the case is also relatively straightforward. The two notions of self are so different that they can easily complement each other. In fact, on closer consideration it should be clear that the notion of self introduced by the narrative model is not only far more complex than, but also logically and ontologically dependent upon, the experiential self. Only a being with a first-person perspective could make sense of the ancient dictum 'know thyself'; only a being with a first-person perspective could consider her own aims, ideals and aspirations as her own, and tell a story about it.

To avoid unnecessary confusion, it may be appropriate to make a terminological distinction. When we are dealing with the experiential self, we should stick to the term 'self', since we are exactly dealing with a primitive form of self-givenness or self-referentiality. But when we are dealing with the narrative model, it would be better to speak not of the self, but of the *person* as a narrative construction. After all, what is being addressed by this model is exactly the nature of my personality or personal character: a personality that evolves through time, and which is shaped by the values I endorse, and by my moral and intellectual convictions and decisions.

Two forms of self-consciousness

Given that the phenomenological tradition approaches the question of self by focusing on its experiential givenness and by taking the first-person perspective seriously, it should not come as a surprise that the phenomenological discussion of self is often to be found in the context of an analysis of self-consciousness. Thus, like the German Idealists, the phenomenologists have typically taken an investigation of self-consciousness to be a key to an understanding of what it means to be a self. To put it differently, the phenomenologists would typically argue that no account of self that failed to explain the accessibility of the self to itself could be successful.

One prevalent conception to be found within phenomenology, for instance in Husserl and Sartre, is the idea that the experiential dimension is characterized by a pervasive prereflective self-consciousness. At first sight, this claim might seem preposterous, but let me try to explain what is meant by the terms 'self-consciousness' and 'prereflective'.

I cannot merely be aware of red roses, fresh coffee or the Brahms' Fourth Symphony, I can also be aware that these objects are seen, smelt and heard, that different perceptions are taking place, and that *I* am the one experiencing them, just as I may be aware that *I* am sad, curious or tired. The phenomenologists will typically insist that self-consciousness must be understood in a very broad sense. It is not merely something that only comes about the moment one scrutinizes one's experiences attentively (not to speak of it being something that only comes about the moment one recognizes one's own mirror image, or refers to oneself using the first-person pronoun, or is in possession of identifying knowledge of one's own life story). On the contrary, it is taken to be legitimate to speak of a primitive type of self-consciousness whenever I am acquainted with an experience in its first-personal mode of presentation. If the experience is given in a first-personal mode of presentation to me, it is (at least tacitly) given as *my* experience, and it can therefore count as a case of self-consciousness. That is, it is taken to be legitimate to speak of self-consciousness the moment I am no longer simply conscious of a foreign object, but of my experience of the object as well, for in this case my subjectivity reveals itself to me. Thus, the phenomenologists take the question of self-consciousness to be not primarily a question of how consciousness is aware of a *self*, but rather as a question of how it is aware of *itself*, that is, of how it can appear or manifest itself for itself.

Given this definition, the phenomenological discussion of self-consciousness has obvious affinities with the contemporary discussion of phenomenal consciousness. In fact, phenomenal consciousness is precisely interpreted as a primitive form of self-consciousness: whenever I am acquainted with an experience in its first-personal mode of givenness, that is, whenever there is a 'what it is like' involved with its inherent quality of 'mineness', we are dealing with a form of self-consciousness. This is why Sartre can write that it is just as necessary for an experience to exist self-consciously, as it is for an extended object to exist three-dimensionally. To use the standard example: a pain is necessarily painful. It can only exist consciously, that is, the pain and the feeling of pain cannot be separated – not even conceptually

(Sartre, 1943, pp. 20–21; Sartre, 1948, pp. 64–65). This reasoning, highly convincing as it is when it comes to feelings of pain or pleasure, holds true, Sartre insists, of all experiences: 'This self-consciousness we ought to consider not as a new consciousness, but as *the only mode of existence which is possible for a consciousness of something*' (Sartre, 1943, p. 20).

When speaking of self-consciousness as a permanent feature of our consciousness, however, neither Sartre nor Husserl is referring to what is known as *reflective* self-consciousness, since this is considered to be a derived type of self-consciousness. Reflection (or, to use more current names, 'introspection', 'internal monitoring' or 'higher-order representation') is generally understood as a process whereby consciousness directs its intentional 'gaze' at itself, thereby taking itself as its own object. But why is this type of self-consciousness derivative, and why is it necessary to posit the existence of a more fundamental form of self-consciousness? Why is it ultimately necessary to criticize the view that a mental state, be it a thought, a feeling or a perception, only becomes conscious, only manifests itself subjectively, when it is taken as an object by some kind of higher-order representation, by some kind of internal monitoring? Let me present this criticism in some detail, since – if valid – it should be of decisive significance. After all, the higher-order representation theory is still very popular and widespread, not only in analytical philosophy, but also in cognitive psychology. (Although the following criticism can already be found in the writings of the phenomenologists, it has been systematically articulated in the work of a group of German philosophers known as the *Heidelberg School*: Dieter-Henrich, Ulrich Pothast, Konrad Cramer and Manfred Frank.)

It is customary to distinguish between two uses of the term 'conscious', a transitive and an intransitive use. On the one hand, we can say of an experience that it is conscious *of x, y* or *z*. On the other hand, we can say of an experience that it is conscious *simpliciter* (rather than nonconscious). According to the higher-order representation theory, intransitive consciousness is not an intrinsic property but a relational property (Rosenthal, 1997, pp. 736–737), i.e. it is a property which the mental state only has in so far as it stands in a relevant relation to something else. For a mental state to be intransitively conscious is for it to be accompanied by a suitable higher-order representation, namely a higher-order thought or perception about that state. It is this higher-order representation that confers intransitive consciousness on the mental state it is about; in fact 'the mental state's being intransitively conscious simply consists in one's being transitively conscious of it' (Rosenthal, 1997, p. 739). One implication of this position is that creatures lacking the cognitive resources to entertain such higher-order beliefs also lack conscious mental states. Thus, in the view of one advocate of this approach, animals as well as infants under the age of 3 have no phenomenal consciousness and have no dimension of subjectivity (Carruthers, 1998, p. 216). They are blind to the existence of their own experiences; there is in fact nothing it is like for them to feel pain or pleasure. In my view, this implication by itself can serve as a *reductio ad absurdum* of the higher-order representation theory. But let me provide an additional argument by addressing the following fundamental questions: How can the interaction between two otherwise nonconscious processes cause one of them to become conscious? How can the fact of being the intentional object of an nonconscious second-order state confer first-personal givenness or 'mineness' on an otherwise nonconscious first-order mental state? Answers to these questions must be provided by the higher-order representation theory if it is to be convincing.

The higher-order representation theory claims that a certain mental state, in order to manifest itself phenomenally (and not merely remain *nonconscious*), must await its objectivation by a subsequent second-order thought or perception. However, it is not enough for the theory to explain how a certain state becomes conscious. It has to explain how the state comes to be given as *my* state. For, as already mentioned, when one is directly and noninferentially conscious of one's own occurrent thoughts, perceptions or pains, they are characterized by a first-personal givenness that immediately reveals them as one's own. And, as Bieri puts it, if one speaks of mental states and forgets to mention that these states feel like something for somebody, one does not merely leave *something* out, one leaves *everything* out (Bieri, 1982, p. 18). But in order for the perception to appear as *my* experience, as an experience or state that *I* am in, it is not sufficient that the perception in question A is grasped by a second-order thought or perception B. If A is to be given as *mine*, it is not enough that B is de facto about A. B must recognize itself in A. That is, the first-order experience must be grasped as being identical with the second-order state (and since a *numerical identity* is excluded, the identity in question must be that of belonging to the same subject or being part of the same stream of consciousness). This poses a difficulty, however, for what should enable the nonconscious second-order state to realize that the first-order experience belongs to the same subjectivity as itself? In order to identify something as oneself one has to hold something true of it that one already knows to be true of oneself. That is, if the second-order state is to encounter something as itself, if it is to recognize or identify something as itself, it obviously needs a prior acquaintance with itself (Cramer, 1974, p. 563). Consequently, the second-order mental state must await either a third-order mental state that can confer intransitive consciousness on it, in which case we are obviously confronted with a vicious infinite regress, or it must be admitted that the second-order mental state is itself already in possession of phenomenal consciousness from the very start, and that would of course involve us in a circular explanation, presupposing that which was meant to be explained, and implicitly rejecting the thesis of the higher-order representation theory: that all phenomenal consciousness is brought about by a process of higher-order representation (cf. Henrich, 1970, p. 268; Frank, 1991, pp. 498, 529; Zahavi, 1999, pp. 14–37).

Any convincing theory of consciousness has to account for the first-personal or egocentric givenness of our conscious states, and has to respect the difference between our consciousness of a foreign object and our consciousness of our own subjectivity. Any convincing theory of consciousness has to be able to explain the distinction between *intentionality*, which is characterized by a *difference* between the subject and the object of experience, and *self-consciousness*, which implies some form of *identity*. But this is exactly what the higher-order representation theory fails to do. Thus, it is highly questionable whether one can account for the givenness of phenomenal consciousness by sticking to a traditional model of object-consciousness and then simply replacing the external object with an internal one. When one is aware of one's occurrent thoughts, feelings, beliefs and desires, one is not confronted with objects of any sort, and this is exactly what the theory overlooks.

The general lesson to learn from this argument is that there are good reasons not to take intransitive consciousness as a *relational property*, since every relation, especially the subject–object relation, presupposes a *distinction* between two (or more) relations and this is exactly what generates the problem. That is, the first-personal givenness of experience (and, by implication, the core self) should not be taken as the product of a successful self-identification, higher-order representation, reflection, internal monitoring or introspection, but rather be treated as an *intrinsic feature* of experience.

The criticism directed against the attempt to understand the basic self-referentiality of phenomenal consciousness as the result of a higher-order representation is not meant to imply that such a higher-order representation is impossible, but merely that it always presupposes the existence of a prior unthematic, nonobjectifying, prereflective self-consciousness as its condition of possibility. This primitive prereflective self-consciousness is not due to a secondary act or reflex but is a constitutive aspect of the experience itself. The experience is conscious of itself at the time of its occurrence. (The classical elaboration of this can be found in Husserl's famous lectures on inner time-consciousness. (cf. Husserl, 1966; Zahavi, 1999, pp. 63–90.) The first-order mental state must already be tacitly self-conscious, since it is the fact of it being already mine, already being given in the first-personal mode of presentation, that allows me to thematize it. And the second-order mental state must also already be prereflective self-conscious, since it is this that permits it to recognize the first-order state as belonging to the same subjectivity as it*self* (Henry, 1965, pp. 76, 153). In short, it is necessary to distinguish *prereflective* self-consciousness, which is an immediate, implicit and irrelational, nonobjectifying and nonpropositional self-acquaintance, from *reflective* self-consciousness which, at least in certain forms, is an explicit, conceptual and objectifying thematization of consciousness. Whereas the higher-order representation theory might throw light upon *explicit* self-experience, it cannot explain the origin of self-consciousness as such, it cannot account for the first-person perspective as such.

However, and this must be emphasized, to speak of prereflective self-consciousness is not to speak of a thematic self-consciousness (Sartre, 1936, pp. 23–24, 66; Sartre, 1943, p. 19). Thus, the self-consciousness in question may very well be accompanied by a fundamental ignorance. Although I cannot be unconscious of my present experience, I may very well ignore it in favour of its object, and this is of course the natural attitude. In my everyday life, I am absorbed by and preoccupied with projects and objects in the world, and do not single out my experiential life for special attention. Thus pervasive prereflective self-consciousness is definitely not to be understood as total self-comprehension, but is rather to be likened to a precomprehension that allows for subsequent reflection and thematization. One can argue in favour of a pervasive self-consciousness and still accept the existence of the unconscious in the sense of subjective components which remain ambiguous, obscure and resist comprehension. That is, one should distinguish between the claim that our consciousness is characterized by an immediate self-givenness and the claim that consciousness is characterized by total self-transparency. One can easily accept the first and reject the latter, i.e. one can argue in favour of the existence of a pervasive self-consciousness and still take self-comprehension to be an infinite task (Ricoeur, 1950, pp. 354–355).

Implications

Although it may be thought that a discussion of different notions of self and different types of self-consciousness is a rather academic exercise with no real impact, this is far from true. Quite the contrary, the account of self and self-consciousness presented above has a number of interesting implications. Let me mention a few.

Self and schizophrenia

Schizophrenia is often taken to involve disorders of self and self-experience. Fundamental alterations in the sense of possession and control of one's own thoughts, actions, sensations or emotions figure among the most prominent symptoms in the advanced stages of the disease. According to one very popular model, these symptoms can be explained as the result of a defect in the process of internal monitoring. Thus the model assumes that we recognize thoughts, emotions and movements as our own due to such a process of self-monitoring. It is this mechanism that, so to speak, labels the thoughts as 'mine', and if this labelling process goes wrong, the thoughts will be perceived as alien (Frith, 1992, p. 80). This is exactly what is supposed to happen in schizophrenia. The process breaks down, and since the patient's mental states are not accompanied by an internal monitoring, they are not recognized as his or her own.

This entire set-up has an obvious, but unargued presupposition. It is assumed that the 'mineness' of experience comes about as the result of a higher-order representation, but if this model is wrong, as I have suggested above, if the 'mineness' is an integral part of normal experience, the explanation offered by this prominent model cannot be right (cf. Zahavi, 1999, pp. 153–156; Gallagher, 2000).

This is not to say that schizophrenia does not involve self-disorders but they will have to be understood differently. Perhaps it is even debatable whether such passivity phenomena as thought insertion do in fact confront us with experiential phenomena that lack the usual quality of 'mineness'. Obviously there is nothing wrong in thinking that foreign thoughts occur in foreign minds. It is only the belief that foreign thoughts occur in one's *own* mind that is pathological and dreadful. But since the afflicted subject is aware that it is he himself rather than somebody else who is experiencing these foreign thoughts, since the subject does not confuse thoughts occurring in foreign minds with foreign thoughts occurring in his own mind, it is debatable whether these 'foreign' thoughts really lack the quality of 'mineness', whether they really lack the first-personal mode of givenness. Since one remains the subject of the alien thought, it is doubtful whether the foreignness of the experience is due to a lack of *ownership* in the formal sense. Sass has suggested that the feeling of depersonalization may ultimately be due to an exacerbation of self-consciousness, a kind of ultrareflection, rather than due to a lack or loss of self-consciousness. The subject is so obsessively preoccupied with his or her experiences that they are gradually transformed and substantialized into objectlike entities, which are then experienced as alien, intrusive, involuntary and independent (Sass, 1994, pp. 12, 38, 91, 95). Just as our movements may become inhibited if we pay too much attention to them, something similar can happen with our mental life. Due to the continual self-observation and compulsive self-analysis, the normal integrated whole of our experiences is split apart. Although the experiences are continuously accessible 'from the inside', they now appear as alienated fragments.

Nonconceptual self-consciousness

Some philosophers who are inclined to take selfhood and self-consciousness to be intrinsically linked to the issue of self-reference would argue that the latter presupposes the possession of a first-person *concept*. One is only self-conscious the moment one can *conceive* of oneself *as* oneself, and has the linguistic ability to use the first-person pronoun to refer to oneself (Baker, 2000, p. 68; cf. Lowe, 2000, p. 264). In contrast to Carruthers, Baker doesn't deny that animals and infants are subjects of experience, and that they experience things consciously from their own egocentric perspective, but according to her, they lack first-person concepts of themselves, and are consequently not self-conscious (Baker, 2000, pp. 60–66, 69).

This view obviously takes self-consciousness to be something that emerges in the course of a developmental process, and to depend upon the eventual acquisition of concepts and language. But does it actually match recent findings in the psychology of perception and developmental psychology (cf. such authors as Gibson, Stern, Butterworth and Neisser), or does it not rather adopt a far too cognitive and conceptual take on self-consciousness?

In a recent book entitled *The Paradox of Self-Consciousness* Bermúdez has taken a number of these empirical findings seriously, and he argues that it is necessary to accept the existence of a variety of nonconceptual forms of self-consciousness that are 'logically and ontogenetically more primitive than the higher forms of self-consciousness that are usually the focus of philosophical debate' (Bermúdez, 1998, p. 274). Bermúdez even claims that there are primitive forms of self-consciousness already in place from birth. These forms obviously precede the mastery of language and the ability to form full-blown rational judgements and propositional attitudes, but they can serve as a foundation for more advanced types of self-consciousness. Drawing on Gibson's ecological approach, which argues that the very flow pattern of optical information provides us with an awareness of our own movement and posture and that all perception consequently involves a kind of self-sensitivity, a coperception of self and of environment (Gibson, 1986, pp. 111–126), Bermúdez writes: 'If the pick-up of self-specifying information starts at the very beginning of life, then there ceases to be so much of a problem about how entry into the first-person perspective is achieved. In a very important sense, infants are born into the first-person perspective. It is not something that they have to acquire ab initio' (Bermúdez, 1998, p. 128).

It should be obvious that there are affinities between Bermúdez' position and the phenomenological approach I have outlined above. (For a more extensive discussion of these similarities, cf. Zahavi, 2002.) Not only can the phenomenological perspective on self accommodate the existence of prelinguistic and nonconceptual forms of self-experience. Through its targeted criticism of the higher-order representation theory it can also provide additional arguments for their existence. In fact, to show that phenomenal consciousness as such entails a primitive form of self-consciousness is to make the strongest case possible for the existence of prelinguistic and nonconceptual forms of self-consciousness. Thus, like Bermúdez, I would readily acknowledge that there are more advanced forms of self-consciousness, which do in fact presuppose the use of language, but the primitive self-consciousness that is part and parcel of phenomenal consciousness is independent of such conceptual sophistication. To put it very simply: the newborn does not have to master the words and concepts 'pain', 'hunger', 'frustration' and 'mine' in order to feel the pain, the hunger and the frustration from a first-person perspective. Even prelinguistically, an infant can be aware of itself, for this self-acquaintance does not require any thematic or conceptual identification – in fact, no *identification* at all is involved – but merely that the acquaintance has the requisite first-person form. Even prior to any conceptual discrimination between self and world or between self and other, the child is self-conscious due to the unique first-personal givenness of its experiences. Self-consciousness does not arise thanks to a conceptual discrimination between self and world, but is the condition of possibility for any such discrimination.

Further work

According to the phenomenologists, it is a decisive mistake to take the problem of consciousness to be first and foremost a question of how to relate consciousness to the brain, first and foremost a question of how to reduce consciousness to mind- and meaningless matter. Not only do they take this enterprise to be futile for various conceptual reasons, but they would also argue that such a take completely overlooks the urgent need for a thorough investigation of the first-person perspective on its own terms. To put it differently, although the phenomenologists have typically conceived of the experiential dimension as being so fundamental that no noncircular explanation of it is possible, they would deny that such an outlook puts a hold on further analysis. After all, there is much more to the question of phenomenal consciousness than a mere recognition of its irreducibility. A thorough elucidation of its structures requires investigations into the connection between self, ego, person, first-personal givenness, intentionality, thematic and marginal consciousness, reflective and prereflective self-consciousness, time-consciousness and body awareness. It would exceed the limits of this chapter to account in more detail for these issues, but let me at least mention a few of the questions that have typically been addressed by the phenomenologists in the course of their investigation. (For a full-scale presentation and discussion of the theories of self-consciousness found in recent analytical philosophy of mind (Castañeda, Shoemaker, Rosenthal, etc.), in the Heidelberg School (Henrich, Frank) and in phenomenology (Husserl, Sartre, Merleau-Ponty, Henry, etc.), cf. Zahavi, 1999.)

The methodological problem

To what extent is it possible to investigate the self? If the self as experiential dimension is basically to be equated with the *subjectivity* of experience, if rather than being an object that we can encounter in the world it is the very perspective that permits any such encounter, to what extent can it then be made accessible for direct examination? Will any examination not necessarily take the self as an *object* of experience, and thereby transform it beyond recognition?

The problem of temporality

My own experiences are present to me in a way that the experiences of others cannot be. This presence also has a temporal connotation. My current experiences are present rather than past or future. To put it differently, it is not possible to account for such a basic phenomenon as the first-personal givenness of phenomenal consciousness without taking temporality into consideration. Moreover, any convincing theory of self-consciousness should not only be able to account for the prereflective self-consciousness of a current experience, but should also be able to explain how it is possible to be self-conscious across temporal distance, and recall a past experience as one's own.

The problem of the body

The difference between a first-person and a third-person perspective does not coincide with the traditional difference between mind and body. As an analysis of *proprioception* reveals, the body itself can appear in a first-person perspective, and the investigation of the different modes of bodily appearance is indispensable for a more comprehensive analysis of what it means to be a self. This is especially the case if one wishes to understand the relation between one's awareness of oneself as an elusive subjective dimension, i.e. something that is neither a mental nor a worldly *object*, and one's awareness of oneself as an intersubjectively accessible entity in the world.

The problem of intersubjectivity

Not only can I be aware of myself, I can also be aware of other selves, and an analysis of selfhood must consequently deal with the problem of *intersubjectivity*. It must do so not because every type of self-consciousness is intersubjectively mediated, but because a theory of what it means to be a self must avoid conceiving of the self as an exclusive first-person phenomenon, as something that only exists in the form of an immediate and unique inwardness. Had this been the case, I would only know of one case of it – my own – and would never get to know any other. That is, one has to be very careful not to conceive of self in such a way that intersubjectivity becomes an impossibility. Let me quote Merleau-Ponty's concise diagnosis of the problem:

If the sole experience of the subject is the one which I gain by coinciding with it, if the mind, by definition, eludes 'the outside spectator' and can be recognized only from within, my *cogito* is necessarily unique, and cannot be 'shared in' by another. Perhaps we can say that it is 'transferable' to others. But then how could such a transfer ever be brought about? What spectacle can ever validly induce me to posit outside myself that mode of existence the whole significance of which demands that it be grasped from within? Unless I learn within myself to recognize the junction of the *for itself* and the *in itself*, none of those mechanisms called other bodies will ever be able to come to life; unless I have an exterior others have no interior. The plurality of consciousness is impossible if I have an absolute consciousness of myself (Merleau-Ponty, 1945, pp. 427–428).

Conclusion

In the previous sections I have characterized the *first-personal givenness* of phenomenal consciousness as a primitive type of self-consciousness. To undergo a conscious experience (to taste coffee, to feel pain, to recollect a trip on the Rhine) necessarily means that there is something it is like for the subject to have that experience. But in so far as there is something it is like for the subject to have experiences, there must be some consciousness of these experiences themselves; in short, there must be self-consciousness. As Flanagan puts it: 'all subjective experience is self-conscious in the weak sense that there is something it is like for the subject to have that experience. This involves a sense that the experience is the subject's experience, that it happens to her, occurs in her stream' (Flanagan, 1992, p. 194). But whenever there is self-consciousness, whenever there is a 'what it is like' involved with its inherent quality of 'mineness', there is also a primitive form of selfhood involved. Needless to say, if this is true, there are rather obvious consequences for the attribution of both self and self-consciousness to animals. As for the question of where to draw the line, i.e. as for the question of whether it also makes sense to ascribe phenomenal consciousness to lower organisms such as birds, amphibians, fish, beetles and worms, this is a question that I will leave for others to decide. All I can say is, that *if* a certain organism is in possession of phenomenal consciousness, *then* it must also be in possession of both a primitive form of self-consciousness and a core self. (For an interesting discussion of different types of self-consciousness in animals, cf. Mitchell, 1994 and Sheets-Johnstone, 1999.)

Thus, my conclusion is that experiential self-consciousness, or to put it differently, the self as an experiential dimension, is an integrated part of consciousness as such.

REFERENCES

Baker, L.R. (2000). *Persons and Bodies*. Cambridge: Cambridge University Press.

Bermúdez, J.L. (1998). *The Paradox of Self-Consciousness*. Cambridge, MA: MIT Press.

Bieri, P. (1982). Nominalismus und innere Erfahrung. *Zeitschrift für philosophische Forschung*, **36**, 3–24.

Carruthers, P. (1998). Natural theories of consciousness. *European Journal of Philosophy*, **6**, 203–22.

Cramer, K. (1974). 'Erlebnis'. Thesen zu Hegels Theorie des Selbstbewußtseins mit Rücksicht auf die Aporien eines Grundbegriffs nachhegelscher Philosophie. In *Stuttgarter Hegel-Tage 1970*, vol. 11, ed. H.-G. Gadamer, pp. 537–603. Bonn: Hegel-Studien.

Evans, C.O. (1970). *The Subject of Consciousness*. London: George Allen & Unwin.

Flanagan, O. (1992). *Consciousness Reconsidered*. Cambridge, MA: MIT Press.

Frank, M. (1991). Fragmente einer Geschichte der Selbstbewußtseins-Theorie von Kant bis Sartre. In *Selbstbewußtseinstheorien von Fichte bis Sartre*, ed. M. Frank, pp. 413–599. Frankfurt am Main: Suhrkamp.

Frith, C. (1992). *The Cognitive Neuropsychology of Schizophrenia*. Hillsdale, NJ: Lawrence Erlbaum.

Gallagher, S. (2000). Self-reference and schizophrenia: a cognitive model of immunity to error through misidentification. In *Exploring the Self*, ed. D. Zahavi, pp. 203–39. Amsterdam: John Benjamins.

Gibson, J.J. (1986). *The Ecological Approach to Visual Perception*. Hillsdale, NJ: Lawrence Erlbaum.

Henrich, D. (1970). Selbstbewußtsein, kritische Einleitung in eine Theorie. In *Hermeneutik und Dialektik*, ed. R. Bubner, K. Cramer & R. Wiehl, pp. 257–284. Tübingen: Mohr.

Henry, M. (1963). *L'Essence de la Manifestation*. Paris: PUF.

Henry, M. (1965). *Philosophie et Phénoménologie du Corps*. Paris: PUF.

Hume, D. (1888). *A Treatise of Human Nature*. Oxford: Clarendon Press.

Husserl, E. (1959). *Erste Philosophie II (1923–4)*. Husserliana VIII. Den Haag: Martinus Nijhoff.

Husserl, E. (1966). *Zur Phänomenologie des inneren Zeitbewußtseins (1893–1917)*. Husserliana X. The Hague: Martinus Nijhoff.

Husserl, E. (1973). *Zur Phänomenologie der Intersubjektivität I*. Husserliana XIII. The Hague: Martinus Nijhoff.

Husserl, E. (1984). *Logische Untersuchungen II*. Husserliana XIX/1–2. The Hague: Martinus Nijhoff.

Kant, I. (1956). *Kritik der reinen Vernunft*. Hamburg: Felix Meiner.

Klawonn, E. (1991). *Jeg'ets Ontologi.* Odense: Odense Universitetsforlag.

Lowe, E.J. (2000). *An Introduction to the Philosophy of Mind.* Cambridge: Cambridge University Press.

Merleau-Ponty, M. (1945). *Phénoménologie de la Perception.* Paris: Éditions Gallimard.

Merleau-Ponty, M. (1964). *Sense and Non-Sense.* Evanston, IL: Northwestern University Press.

Mitchell, R.W. (1994). Multiplicities of self. In *Self-awareness in Animals and Humans*, ed. S.T. Paker, R.W. Mitchell & M.L. Boccia, pp. 81–107. Cambridge: Cambridge University Press.

Nagel, T. (1974). What is it like to be a bat? *Philosophical Review*, **83**, 435–50.

Natorp, P. (1912). *Allgemeine Psychologie.* Tübingen: J.C.B. Mohr.

Neisser, U. (1988). Five kinds of self-knowledge. *Philosophical Psychology*, **1**, 35–59.

Ricoeur, P. (1950). *Philosophie de la Volonté I. Le Volontaire et l'Involontaire.* Paris: Aubier.

Ricoeur, P. (1985). *Temps et Récit III: Le Temps Raconté.* Paris: Éditions du Seuil.

Rosenthal, D.M. (1997). A theory of consciousness. In *The Nature of Consciousness*, ed. N. Block, O. Flanagan & G. Güzeldere, pp. 729–53. Cambridge, MA: MIT Press.

Sartre, J.-P. (1936). *La Transcendance de l'Ego.* Paris: Vrin.

Sartre, J.-P. (1943). *L'Être et le Néant.* Paris: Gallimard.

Sartre, J.-P. (1948). Conscience de soi et connaissance de soi. *Bulletin de la Société Française de Philosophie*, **XLII**, 49–91.

Sass, L.A. (1994). *The Paradoxes of Delusion.* London: Cornell University Press.

Scheler, M. (1973). *Wesen und Formen der Sympathie.* Bern: Francke Verlag.

Searle, J.R. (1992). *The Rediscovery of the Mind.* Cambridge, MA: MIT Press.

Sheets-Johnstone, M. (1999). *The Primacy of Movement.* Amsterdam: Benjamins.

Strawson, G. (1994). *Mental Reality.* Cambridge, MA: MIT Press.

Strawson, G. (1999). The self and the SESMET. In *Models of the Self*, ed. S. Gallagher & J. Shear, pp. 483–518. Thorverton: Imprint Academic.

Taylor, C. (1989). *Sources of the Self.* Cambridge, MA: Harvard University Press.

Zahavi, D. (1998a). The fracture in self-awareness. In *Self-awareness, Temporality, and Alterity*, ed. D. Zahavi, pp. 21–40. Dordrecht: Kluwer Academic Publishers.

Zahavi, D. (1998b). Brentano & Husserl on self-awareness. *Études Phénoménologiques*, **27–28**, 127–68.

Zahavi, D. (1999). *Self-awareness and Alterity. A Phenomenological Investigation.* Evanston: Northwestern University Press.

Zahavi, D. (2000). Self and consciousness. In *Exploring the Self*, ed. D. Zahavi, pp. 55–74. Amsterdam: John Benjamins.

Zahavi, D. (2001). Beyond empathy: phenomenological approaches to intersubjectivity. *Journal of Consciousness Studies*, **8**, 151–67.

Zahavi, D. (2002). First-person thoughts and embodied self-awareness. Some reflections on the relation between recent analytical philosophy and phenomenology. *Phenomenology and the Cognitive Sciences* **1**, 7–26.

(2003). Intentionality and phenomenality. A phenomenological take on the hard problem. *Canadian Journal of Philosophy* (in press).

Zahavi, D. & Parnas, J. (1998). Phenomenal consciousness and self-awareness: a phenomenological critique of representational theory. *Journal of Consciousness Studies*, **5**, 687–705.

4

Language and self-consciousness: modes of self-presentation in language structure

Maxim I. Stamenov

Georg-August-Universität Göttingen, Germany and Bulgarian Academy of Sciences, Sofia, Bulgaria

Abstract

One of the most prominent diagnostic symptoms of schizophrenia amounts to hearing an inner voice that is not attributed to the self. A proper explanation of the nature of the schizophrenic condition requires, correspondingly, an orientation of the relations between language faculty and self-consciousness – both in norm and in pathology. The aim of this chapter is to offer an overview of some basic aspects of this relationship. The presentation will be by necessity brief and selective, as the problem area is wide and there is virtually no literature explicitly dealing with it from a linguistic perspective.

In the first part of the chapter the point is made that speech, inner speech in particular, serves as the subtlest (and, in a sense, the ultimate) vehicle of online maintained self-awareness. The experience of voice here and now provides the self with the means of making itself 'visible' during language performance. In inner speech the loop between perception cum motor behaviour cum perception is the shortest one and is enacted with the highest possible time resolution. Thus, inner speech forms the most compact perceptual–motor loop (the shortest 'specious present') capable of supporting self-awareness online. In the very same time, it serves as a phenomenal correlate of very complex cognitive processes implementing human thinking. If this is the case, the estrangement from one's voice is indicative of a foundational disturbance in self-awareness.

In the second part of the chapter it is shown than an act of self-consciousness requires much more than the capacity to monitor online one's own behaviour, as is the case with self-awareness. The latter is deictic, unique for each single successive act of cognition and without effective means to track its own identity outside the bounds of the specious present. Self-consciousness, on the other hand, requires symbolic means by which the self can represent itself as a component of an explicit cognitive representation at any time as 'the same self'. Here language becomes indispensable for the development and maintenance online of self-consciousness in the individual. The foundational symbolic means for self-representation in language is the first-person personal pronoun *I*. This *I* is the most unusual symbol humans have at their disposal. The uniqueness of its function is due to the specificity of its reference, meaning and capacity for coreference.

The peculiarity of the first two aspects of *I*'s function is as follows: there is no possibility of linking on a regular basis the reference and the meaning of the self without the mediation of the linguistic sign of *I*. To serve its function, the *I* must refer in one direction – toward the implicit central executive, while it gets its meaning from another world, the world of current explicit cognitive representation. In order to face these two incommensurable requirements (the first negating the possibility of having representational content, the other requiring it) put by its reference and meaning, the linguistic *I* acquires the characteristics of nonspecularity – it becomes part of the explicit linguistic content without being capable of being visualized (in the way one can visualize a chair).

But this is not the end of the capacities of the linguistic *I*. Being a pronoun, it can corefer to an antecedent from a previous clause. The chain of coreference can be made not only between a noun and a pronoun or two explicit pronouns, as in the popular William Jamesian example *I am the same I I was yesterday*, it could also be between an explicit pronoun and a trace (a pronoun invisible at the surface structure of the corresponding sentence). Thus it becomes possible to have a representation of the self that is invisible not only in the mental image of the situation we describe with the means of language, but also invisible in the language structure, too, i.e. doubly invisible – an absent nonspecular self capable of supporting an explicit act of self-consciousness.

It is this finely tuned scaffolding of an ever-evolving invisible, unique and identical self supported by a vast orchestra of language-driven cognitive processes that becomes shattered with the advent of schizophrenia.

The levels of language structure and the possibilities for self-presentation

From a linguistic point of view, it seems feasible to consider three levels of the implementation of the self and corresponding possibilities for actualizing an act of self-consciousness supported by language structure:

1. at the level of speech, i.e. as an inner or outer voice (where we tend to believe that we can apparently unmistakably (actually incorrigibly; cf. Brook & DeVidi, 2001, for discussion) differentiate 'Am I talking now or somebody else?');
2. at the level of symbolic (sign-like, word-like) representation of the self. Here the primary means appear to be the forms of the first-person personal pronoun – *I* (in the position of the subject of the corresponding sentence), *me* (in the position of the direct object) and, e.g., *to me* (in the position of indirect object); and
3. at the level of a cognitive act capable of actualizing a state of self-consciousness. The minimal explicit cognitive representation of the self, I will argue below, is equivalent to a simple sentence.

I will discuss the problem of language-specific self-consciousness along the following two main venues. I will claim that the execution of speech and its experience in the mind as inner voice form the subtlest layer of *self-awareness*. *Self-consciousness*, on the other hand, requires for its implementation the minimal pattern of simple sentence (clause) with its associated syntactic, semantic and pragmatic characteristics. Some of these characteristics are activated ready-made from the long-term memory (LTM), others serve as scaffolding for the construction online of the current version of the self.

The experience of inner voice and self-awareness

The subtlety of the relation between perception and execution of speech and self-consciousness was acknowledged by William James when he pointed out that:

> the 'Self of selves', when carefully examined, is found to consist mainly of a collection of those peculiar motions [described before this passage as 'different movements of e.g., jaw-muscles, brow, glottis, etc.'; my addition: MS] in the head or between the head and the throat (James, 1890, p. 288)

The final source of self-awareness appears to be the mapping between the experience of voice (as the qualitative correlate of one's cogitating acts as a thinker) and some 'inner movements' between one's own head and throat.

One possible interpretation of William James' idea could be the following one (in line with the current understanding of how mind and brain function). A necessary requirement for the realization of an act of self-awareness here and now (online) is the causal matching between two streams of events – in the motor behaviour of the organism on the one hand, and in the field of perception on the other hand. When they become correlated in a causal relation, i.e. each motor action leading to a predictable change in the perceptual field, I automatically have the feeling that it is I who contribute the change. The establishment of this correlation evokes the gut feeling of agency and the possibility of realizing an explicit act of self-awareness through appropriately tuned monitoring.

In inner speech the loop between perception cum motor behaviour cum perception is the shortest one and is enacted with the highest possible time resolution. Thus, the inner speech forms the most compact perceptual–motor loop (the shortest 'specious present') capable of supporting self-awareness online. In the very same time, it serves as the phenomenal correlate of very complex cognitive processes implementing human thinking. The next two sections will provide some evidence for this claim.

Some aspects of human voice processing online

Compared to other perceptual, motor and cognitive processes, speech (both inner and outer) possesses some unique characteristics unlike all other stimuli to which we are exposed or behaviours we perform. Firstly, it is enacted at extremely rapid rates, bearing in mind the complexity of motor commands to be performed by the speaker or the speed of recognition and analysis during the decoding of speech signals on the side of the hearer. The rate of fluent speech is estimated to be between 15 and 25 phonetic segments (approximated by the letters of the alphabet) per second. This is much faster than the processing of all other types of stimuli in the mind which can proceed at the rate of seven to nine segments (chunks) per second according to Miller (1956). This speed-up is due to the development in the brain during human phylogenesis of a specialized processor for articulate speech which is different from the processors dealing with all other sorts of sounds and noises around us. Speech encoding and decoding by format frequency transitions, integrated spectral onset cues and other related cues serve as the basis for speeded vocal communication. On the motor side, the speed-up becomes possible due to the specificity of the human supralaryngeal vocal tract and the capacity to control its performance. The fast performance apparently also helps to maintain in the specialized echoic memory longer stretches of sounds per time unit, thus further broadening the potential for speech processing in the working memory (WM) (cf. Lieberman, 1991, pp. 37–38, 59, 106 for further discussion).

Another change in the brain's circuitry during phylogenesis was instrumental in allowing voluntary control of vocalization and the capacity to monitor one's own speech (its experiential correlate is hearing one's voice in one's head even when one does not talk or intend to talk overtly). In the last years experimental psycholinguistic investigations, e.g. of the team of Willem Levelt, show that in adults inner and outer speech processes are supported online by dual-feedback cognitive architecture. Two brain circuits provide the opportunity for monitoring one's own speech performance which serve apparently different purposes. One monitors outer speech for errors like slips of the tongue, incorrect pronunciation or inappropriate intonation patterns. The other monitors inner speech more on the level of what one intends to say on the conceptual–intentional level (both in the case when one plans afterwards to utter behaviourally or when one thinks for himself/herself; cf. Levelt, 1989, pp. 460–463; Levelt et al., 1999; Postma, 2000).

Levelt (1989, p. 470), correspondingly distinguishes in his model an internal loop and an external loop in monitoring of speech. In external speech two more modules are enacted – those performing actual articulation and actual audition – which are not needed in the case of performance of internal speech (execution of phonetic plans for speech). Recent experimental data of Wheeldon & Levelt (1995) and Levelt et al. (1998) indicate that the phonological word representations which form the basis for self-monitoring of inner speech are accessed about 200 ms before the actual execution of the motor speech articulation, thus confirming the theoretical prediction. This split route between the conscious access to phonetic plans and their actual motor execution helps to control what is to be uttered online or to comprehend speech pronounced at a speed several times faster compared to the usual tempo (cf. Mehler et al., 1993). In other words, outer and especially inner speech are the most complex and fastest completely interiorized motor behaviour of which humans are capable on a regular basis. Due to this quite peculiar cognitive architecture, one can monitor one's speech for the sake of planning and intentions, as well as for slips of the tongue and correctness of pronunciation. This is achieved, most probably, by learning how to oscillate one's voluntary attention between the two monitoring mechanisms.

The ontogenetic basis of voice processing

Language capacity and its performance are entrenched in our minds much deeper than we tend to expect, not only during online processing, but also ontogenetically. Psycholinguistic studies show that for every human individual the exposure to human voice starts during the fetus stage of ontogenetic development. The first stimuli coming on a regular basis from the outside environment amount to hearing one's mother's voice in the womb. According to many researchers (DeCasper & Spence, 1986; Spence & DeCasper, 1987; cf. Mehler & Dupoux, 1994, p. 155 for discussion), the fetus has already started to learn, particularly in regard to its mother's voice, whose vibrations are transmitted to the amniotic fluid in the womb, especially sounds of low frequencies. The fetus's auditory system develops around the 30th week of gestation. The amniotic fluid, however, significantly distorts the voice of the mother (Mehler & Dupoux, 1994, p. 163). What the fetus can apparently discern is what one can hear from a conversation, e.g. in a bathroom, with a head submerged in a bathtub. Still, one can hear melodic contours, rhythms and accentuation which differ from language to language. This exposure may have a triggering effect for the formation of proper neural mechanisms in the language-dominant left hemisphere during the ongoing process of brain maturation. Thus, it may be the case that the brain structures specialized for acquiring language are in action before birth and support the establishment of a preference for speech sounds compared to all other noises and sounds. This preference appears to rest on spectral parameters unique to speech, but does not involve basic acoustic parameters the speech shares with other sounds and noises (Mehler & Dupoux, 1994, p. 155).

The intrauterine exposure to the human voice may serve as a point of departure for the formation of brain mechanisms responsible for speech processing in the left hemisphere, as well as for fitting to them vocal gestures by one's own mechanisms controlling speech production (according to the motor theory of speech perception; cf. Liberman & Mattingly, 1985). The possibility for intrauterine calibration of perceptual–motor loop supporting speech is at least partly corroborated by the data from the laboratory of Jacques Mehler. It was found, for example, that even bilinguals who appear to be perfect in perception and production of two languages like French and Japanese process prosodic information according to the strategy of one of the languages: this strategy remains the same independently of the fact that it may not completely fit the phonetic structure of the other language (cf. Cutler et al., 1992). Still, it is appropriate to notice that the calibration (setting the parameters for the perceptual–motor loop in processing the human voice) may be not for a particular language, e.g. French exclusively, but for a particular type of language, e.g. accent- versus syllable- versus mora-based language (cf. Nazzi et al., 1998; Ramus et al., 2000). In our example, if the fetus hears French in the womb s/he will 'attune' for syllable-based languages like French, Italian and Spanish, but not specifically for French. If the latter conjecture is considered plausible, this means that the matching between hearing and enacting the speech with one's own vocal apparatus is established some time after the 30th week of gestation, i.e. in utero. Correspondingly, a malfunction in the link between them and the correlative experience of the voice in the head as not belonging to 'me' may be due to some factors of brain intrauterine maturation.

It is important to emphasize that the hypothetical calibration affects not perception of speech as such but the interface between what one hears and what one can do with one's own motor apparatus, because speaking is a capacity not only to hear, but also to produce sounds of language fitting to what one hears. This fitting can be achieved by an innate input–output matching mirror neuron system specialized for this purpose (for a discussion of mirror neurons, cf. Stamenov & Gallese, 2002). It is at this level (the matching between heard characteristics of voice and limiting the potential for one's own possible vocal gestures) that the 'attunement' may act, more specifically and definitively. Otherwise, newborns and very young infants appear to react to change in the type of language – syllable-based versus mora-based versus accent-based – i.e. they perceive the differences between them after birth (cf. Nazzi et al., 1998). This result means that the hypothetical calibration did not affect the mechanism for speech perception *per se*, at this age. If these data are interpreted as a proof against the intrauterine calibration, then a different mechanism for attunement to voice experience should be inferred – of learning through forgetting. Even if the infant at birth can distinguish different classes of languages, this capacity becomes attenuated by the age 10–12 months. At this age babies stop distinguishing the contrasts in sounds that do not belong to their own native language (Mehler & Dupoux 1994, p. 168). Thus, the other alternative – learning by forgetting effect in matching to each other the capacities for perception and motor action of speech into a loop – is limited by that age. (For further discussion of the problems of the ontogenetic development of aspects of implicit and implicit memory, cf. Rovee-Collier et al., 2000.)

The estrangement from one's inner voice and the pathology of self-awareness

The schizophrenic condition comes to corroborate the idea that there is a subtle and intimate link between inner voice and the very roots of self-awareness and self-identity. It is remarkable to acknowledge that auditory hallucination should be considered so characteristic of this illness that 'a person with true auditory hallucinations should be assumed to have schizophrenia until proven otherwise' (Torey, 1988, p. 48). This point is also reiterated in the *Diagnostic and Statistical Manual of Mental Disorders* (DSM-IV) diagnostic battery where the criterion of voice hallucination appears to be the most robust and well-defined one:

Note: Only one Criterion A symptom [the Diagnostic Criteria A of schizophrenia are: (1) delusions; (2) hallucinations; (3) disorganized speech; (4) grossly disorganized or catatonic behavior; and (5) negative symptoms: my addition: MS] is required if delusions are bizarre or hallucinations consist of a voice keeping up a running commentary on the person's behavior or thoughts, or two or more voices conversing with each other (American Psychiatric Association, 1994, p. 285)

Alienation from one's inner voice and bizarre delusions seem to form the most specific aspects of schizophrenic experience. Bizarre delusions may also be due to the incapacity to maintain a permanent and secure link both with the self and with the external reality in the inner colloquy (a function supported by explicit and implicit language-specific cognitive processing; cf. also Crow, 2000). This once again seems to point to the special status of speech in establishing and maintaining secure self-awareness and self-identity online.

It remains to be explored exactly which aspects of the perceptual–motor speech mechanism come under attack in schizophrenia resulting in the experienced estrangement from one's inner voice. The causal malfunctions contributing to it could be potentially traced to genetic factors guiding brain maturation as early as the 30th week of an individual's intrauterine development or up to the end of the first year of life. On the other hand, it may be the case that the voice estrangement is due to a general failure in the mechanism of voluntary attention *per se*, making it unable to track and coordinate online the parallel performance of the loops for inner and outer speech control. The latter is the explanation which finds wider support of the professionals in the medical circles. The problem with it is exactly its generality: it does not provide an explanation for the strong preference to estrangement from an inner voice in schizophrenia compared to the other possible forms of modality-specific (e.g. taste, smell, touch) hallucinations and delusions.

The self as a sign – the personal pronoun *I* and the deictic here and now

An act of self-consciousness requires symbolic means by which the self can represent oneself as a component of an explicit cognitive representation. The basic means for symbolic representation of the self in language structure is the first-person singular personal pronoun *I*. It is important to note that the *I* is quite unlike other symbols (signs) of language. If we assume that the signs are words and word-like units which are saved in the LTM on a permanent basis as phonetic and graphic form (e.g. *chair*), semantic content (what is the meaning associated in English with the graphic form *chair*) and the set of referents to which this form–content pair can apply, we immediately become aware that the *I* (and the other first- and second-person personal pronouns) possesses some peculiarities. For example, it is difficult to ascribe to it any semantic (representational) content whatsoever outside the context of the current (here-and-now) use.

The *I* is a quite peculiar linguistic sign, probably the most unusual symbol in general, on several counts:

1. It is supposed to refer in a communicative situation to the current speaker. When somebody else starts to speak, the *I* immediately becomes appropriated by the next speaker.

2. At the same time, it evokes (for every speaker) the correlative concept of implicit or explicit *you*, the addressee of the current utterance inherent in any communicative situation. In other words, the *I* can refer to the subject of consciousness only in juxtaposition to an alter ego, another subject of consciousness. There is no *I* outside a communicative situation. The use of *I* signals not only self-consciousness on the side of the user, but opens an intersubjective dimension to consciousness. The *I*, strictly speaking, signifies one of the poles of the binary differentiation between the current speaker and the audience here and now.

3. The *I*, as a member of the class of personal pronouns, is also supposed to corefer, i.e. anaphorically to find its reference in a lexical entry from a previous sentence in a stretch of a coherent written text or spoken discourse.

The anaphorical function of *I* is related, strictly speaking (as we will see below in more detail), to the possibility of linking the *I* to any third-person speaker, as in:

(1)   a *Barry$_i$ said: 'I$_i$ am hungry'.*
      b *Barry$_i$ said that he$_i$ is hungry.*

Everybody would agree that *I* in (1)a (under certain conventions representing the communicative behaviour of others) refers not to *Maxim* (the person who happened to write this sentence) but to *Barry*. Linguists would, however, also insist that *I* corefers anaphorically in the same way *he* does in (1)b.

Unlike the third-person personal pronouns like *he, she* or *it* which can only corefer (except in the case of the dummy subject *it*; cf. section 'Every sentence must have a self' below for further discussion), the *I* can also refer. From the first-person perspective, the *I* refers to me here and now. This is not as self-evident a claim as it may look at first sight. For example, when I utter now:

(2)   a *Ten years ago I had a better memory.*
      b *I am the same I I was yesterday.*

to whom is the *I* in (2)a–b supposed to refer? It seems reasonable to claim that this *I* refers not to me here and now, but to me from yesterday or from 10 years ago. This is, however, not the case. As we will see below, the *I* must refer to the present implicit (executive) self here and now. Only via the establishment of a link with the current self in charge can one reach the self from yesterday or from 10 years ago. This is achieved through projection of the present-time implicit (*nonspecular*) self into the reconstructed situation how it looked like *yesterday* or *10 years ago*. The *I* always has a referent here and now, but a nonspecular one, i.e. one with no representational content associated with it on a permanent basis. This is an important claim which requires some further elucidation and illustration.

The *I* is nonspecular, because it refers here and now (deictically) to the current implicit executive self. It is a pointer to an invisible referent. Thus, there is no context-free concept (or meaning) attachable to the sign of the self on a permanent basis. If the opposite was the case, this concept should have been saved in LTM and activated from there each time I use my *I* (and only in the cases when I use 'my *I*', but not when you use 'your *I*'). This concept, then, could serve as a basis for a 'permanent self-same self (homunculus)'. But there is no such concept which can be attached to the *I* in the way the concept of 'chair' is attached to the word form *chair*.

The nonspecularity of the *I*'s referent introduces an important asymmetry in the explicit structure of episodic experience compared to verbalization of this same experience. For example, when I narrate what happened to me, e.g.:

(3)   *I saw a yellow Jaguar on New Oxford Street yesterday.*

I may indeed imagine the car, as it passed by yesterday when I walked down New Oxford Street in London. I do not recollect myself as seeing the car, i.e. I do not see myself seeing the car. I just imagine the car in my reconstructed experience. When I verbalize my past experience, however, I *have to* introduce myself into the explicit language structure. In language the self as the subject of experience (as agent, experiencer or beneficiary) must be explicated. It is language that puts upon me this obligation. In remembering past experience, on the other hand, my self remains implicit; it leaks through the requirement to see the car from a certain perspective, from the perspective I saw it (it seems to me now) yesterday. This asymmetry shows what the nonspecularity of the self is about and poses a problem to the proper definition of 'self-conscious mental state'. If we accept that the state of consciousness of remembering a past experience is 'self-conscious' but not only 'object-conscious' (in 3, the yellow Jaguar), then all the states of consciousness requiring an access to episodic LTM will be simultaneously states of self-consciousness, too. The same would also apply to all verbal descriptions of my current perceptual experiences, as in *I see a banana now*, as much as they can be put into words.

I think that the problem with the *I* absent in experience and present in its verbalization could be solved along the lines already glimpsed above. There is no representational content associable with the position of *I* in (3). The *I* in any language-specific representation serves as a place-holder, i.e. allocates a virtual position for the self, a perspective-marker in sentence structure. This place could be occupied by the understanding self if it generates a correlate of the language structure in the module of spatial cognition, reconstructing the experience in question. The 'place-holder' serves as the position where the implicit self was or will be during the next cognition. Every time the self explicates itself in language structure it projects in the subjective past or future a place-holder for itself, a *réservé* position. Thus a specific chain of coreference is established between the implicit self and the *I*. From the point of view of the implicit self, the position of the *I* is one it can project itself into during the very next cognition. On the other hand, the *I* finds its referent and the source of continuity and stability in the implicit self from where it started its projection. This oscillating loop of mutual determination during each successive act of verbal consciousness forms an important aspect of its specificity. I will further deal with this topic after representing some defining features of sentence structure.

If the referred-to implicit self has no representational content whatsoever attached to it on a permanent basis, from where comes the meaning which always seems to be associated with the acts of becoming self-conscious? It comes with the syntactic and semantic structure of the sentence in which the *I* inevitably becomes embedded. This is the reason why the analysis of sentence structure (the content of which could be about distant future or past) is important for the proper comprehension of the structure of the self-representations. By the act of projection into the stage of the sentence, the self can become dissociated from the current here and now and moved to any virtual world.

Due to the peculiarity of its functioning, the process of learning how to use the *I* also has a specificity of its own. Early during their first-language acquisition children quite commonly mistake the use of first-person pronoun and third-person pronouns and personal names in referring to themselves, as in *Peter wants a cookie* or *He wants a cookie*, having in mind *I want a cookie*, as noticed and quite extensively studied by Georgov (1905) in his pioneering monograph dealing with the ontogenesis of self-consciousness and language (for discussion, cf. Stamenov, 1999). What is important to acknowledge is that children seldom, if ever, mistake, in this way, the reference of *I* with *you* in face-to-face interaction, i.e. they do not tend to make the mistake of uttering *You want a cookie*, having in mind *I want a cookie*.

In schizophrenia, the pathology of self-experience may include a linguistically signalled alienation from oneself via the anomalous preference for being addressed in face-to-face interaction not with a correlative to *I–you* but in third-person, e.g. with one's personal name (cf. Torey 1988, p. 53), as in (4)b versus (4)a:

(4)   a *Renée do this.*
      b *You do this.*

The very nonspecularity of the *I* coupled with the loss of the link to the referred to implicit self may cause the schizophrenic to feel insecure in referring to oneself with it and being referred to by the correlative *you*. This estrangement from oneself and corresponding insecurity is, consequently, signalled by the demand to be referred to with the 'unique' proper name one possesses.

Word and sentence as vehicles of consciousness and self-consciousness

There are two first-order candidates for being the basic units of language in both the comprehension and production of language structure. These are word and sentence. The words are elements that are saved on a permanent basis in the long-term semantic memory. Their meaning and phonetic form must be, correspondingly, learnt by rote in order to be saved in LTM. The association between their meaning and form is basically arbitrary, as is the case of the prototypical linguistic sign – the noun. Concrete nouns like *chair* or *penguin* are the best candidates for being 'good' signs. The use of some word automatically activates its meaning from the memory. Apes and dolphins are capable of mastering symbols of this kind. There are, however, linguistic signs which have symbolic characteristics quite unlike the 'good' nouns. Examples of these classes of words are pronouns and verbs. Pronouns refer, unlike nouns. Verbs not only refer but also bind other referring words into clauses and sentences.

Sentences, on the other hand, are not to be found in LTM in order to be reactivated ready-made. Instead, they are constructed online, always anew on each occasion from the building material of words (there are exceptions – sentences reproducible by rote as a whole, e.g. *How do you do?*). Each sentence construction means realization of at least two different cognitive events online in two different central processors of the mind – the ones responsible for processing syntactic structure and for meaning. Both these events are triggered by aspects of the verb's structure. Verbs thus serve as a link or bridge between the two basic units of language – word and sentence. In coming to sentence structure in this way, we want to find out aspects of structure and meaning conferred to the self as a component of language-specific cognitive representation.

The verb, its structure and meaning

Every time we say something we need a finite verb form to express our thought. The activation of the lexical entry of some verb from the LTM triggers two events in the mind:

1. the operations in the syntactic processor of the mind necessary and sufficient for constructing a well-formed clause;
2. the operations necessary and sufficient for forming a semantic (representational) correlate of the lexical meaning of that verb in the form of spatial-like mental image or an abstract semantic relation, e.g. for *to cut* 'what it is like to cut something'.

The important thing to keep in mind is that the verb has this Janus-like capacity – to trigger in a coordinated way at least one representational and one computational event in two different central systems in the WM. This split action potential may seem to have nothing to do specifically with self and consciousness. Actually it is, most probably, the crucial one for the formation and functioning of the conscious verbal mind as a two-in-one stream. This is the case because our successive verbal thoughts are minimally constituted by sentences. And every sentence has an explicit (actually uttered) or implicit (not uttered but reconstructible from the other explicit constituents of the current utterance) finite verb. The chaining of verbs means maintenance of two-in-one stream of thought – one specular (if enacted in the format of mental imagery), the other nonspecular (syntactic).

The two events in question – the syntactic and the semantic one – cooccur on a regular basis. When we enact the one, the other follows automatically; still, these are two different events, which happen in two *different* central processors – language-specific syntactic organ and the multimodal integrative spatial–cognition system. And every time there is a cooccurrence of events in the two processors, we have a case of language-mediated meaningful event in consciousness. The cooccurrence is made synchronous by the act of activation and processing of verb-specific information. The two events do not follow each other as a conditioned reflex or as a logical inference; they cooccur, they coincide, they enact each other in a reversible way – from meaning to form or from form to meaning. They implement a new way of interaction and exchange of information in cognition, an interaction which is only possible in the minds of humans using language. The coordinated action online of the syntactic and semantic processor supports the functioning of the nonspecular self (cf. the section on 'the self as a sign', above); the syntactic processor further supports the identity tracking of the absent nonspecular self (cf. section on 'complex sentence structure and the case for absent nonspecular represented self', below).

The best fit between the verb as a word from the LTM and its syntactic and semantic potential can be found in *self-initiated* behavioural actions, like *eat, push* or *give*. These are the verbs that are learned first by small children on entering language. They are easy to imagine, easy to name, seeing the action performed and easy to comprehend. Correspondingly, in the very structure of these verbs there is always a slot, a place-holder for the self: *I eat a fruit, John pushed me, Paul gave a book to me*, etc.

Types of structure and meaning associated with the verb

The verb has three different aspects of meaning and structure associated with it on a permanent basis. The first aspect is that of the lexically specified representational content. The latter is quite abstract. It is aptly conceptualized, from a point of view fitting our orientation, by Lyons (1977) in the following way:

1. A static situation or a *state* is one that is conceived of as existing, rather than happening, and as being homogeneous, continuous and unchanging throughout its duration.
2. A dynamic situation that is extended in time is a *process*.
3. A dynamic situation which is momentary is an *event*.
4. A dynamic situation that is under the control of an agent is called an *action*:
   (a) A *process* that is under the control of an agent is called an *activity*.
   (b) An *event* that is under the control of an agent is an *act* (Lyons, 1977, p. 483).
5. An additional set is formed by verbs like *be* and *have*, which serve the establishment of identity or class attribution, or equivalence of two concepts, e.g. as in *I am Napoleon Bonaparte*, of feature or property ascription, e.g. *I am good*, of possession, e.g. *I have a banana*, and the like.

According to this taxonomy, the explicated in an act of self-reflection self can be the patient or experiencer of a state, process or event. The self can be an agent of an activity or act. The self can make attributions about her/his own qualities and characteristics using the verbs for existence, identity and possession.

The verb also possesses on a permanent basis an argument structure consisting of obligatory for explication and optional for explication arguments. Without the explication of the obligatory arguments the sentence, including the verb form in question, will not achieve the status of semantic well-formedness. The interesting thing is that the upper limit of the argument structure of the verb is quite low (having in mind the overall capacities of LTM to remember information). There are only five types of verbs, in this respect:

1. Zero-argument verbs: *It rains*, *It snows*, etc.
2. One-argument verbs:
   (a) Unaccusative verbs: *I fell*.
   (b) Unergative verbs: *I laughed*.
3. Two-argument verbs: *I killed Bill*.
4. Three-argument verbs: *carry, bring, give, send, move*.
5. Four-argument verbs: *exchange, sell, buy, trade*.

The three- and four-argument structures in their majority denote dynamic situations which are executed by human agents, suffered by human experiencers (patients) or done for the benefit of human individuals. Each of these argument positions could be occupied, correspondingly, by the verbal representation of the self. The verbs denoting actions within the free-market economy in point 5 appear to form the upper limit of the verb capacity to have an argument structure associated in a permanent way with it. The upper limit of representability, from this point of view, amounts to the explicit four-argument representation of the following two complementary types:

(5)   a [*I bought* [*a car for $500*]*from you.*]
          $S^1 \rightarrow [S^2 \rightarrow [O^1 - O^2] \leftarrow S^3]$
      b [*You sold* [*a car for $500*]*to me.*]
          $[S^2 \rightarrow [O^1 - O^2] \leftarrow S^3] \leftarrow S^1$

The simple sentence patterns in (5)a–b show the upper limit of the cognitive potential of a single discrete structure of consciousness (from the point of view of the actors–arguments associable on a permanent basis with it).

The argument structure of the verb could be aptly conceptualized as the common denominator or interface between two different structural specifications coming along with the activation of the corresponding verb from the LTM – the semantic (or theta) grid and the syntactic subcategorization frame. The latter two are not only commensurable to each other, but also deviate systematically. Thus they should be kept apart.

The language-specific semantic roles of the self

The description of the semantic structure of language can also be given at a quite high level of abstraction. The most detailed taxonomies include a list of 12–15 semantic (theta) roles. These roles are supposed to generalize over everything that can happen (as a static or dynamic situation) in the individual, society and in the universe. The main theta roles the self can occupy are the following ones:

• *Agent:* the participant in an event that causes things to happen (the instigator of action), e.g. *I am talking to my dog,* where some *I* initiates and enacts the act of talking;
• *Patient:* the participant that undergoes the outcome of some action (seen from the third-person perspective). This is the object or person who undergoes the result of the action named by the verb, as in *Peter is beating John* or *Peter is rolling the rock.* I can apparently represent myself in this role as, e.g. in *Jill is pushing me out of the room;*
• *Possessor:* a person possessing an object or characteristics, e.g. *a pencil of mine;*
• *Experiencer:* a person who consciously, i.e. first-person, undergoes some mental process or state, e.g. *I tremble;*
• *Beneficiary:* the person who will benefit from the action denoted by the verb, e.g. *Mary bought a rose for me.*

The roles mentioned are as a rule associable on a permanent basis with the meaning of the corresponding verb. Projecting the self into one of them means automatically its explication in the overt syntactic and semantic structure. Please note the problem with the roles of patient versus experiencer when I insert myself in the position of a direct object of a transitive verb. The problem becomes evident in the case of *Peter is beating me* where *me* seems definitely better to interpret as an experiencer, while in the case of *Peter is beating John*, *John* is a straightforward patient of the action.

The syntactic subcategorization frame of the verb

The syntactic subcategorization frame associable with a verb is not identical to its theta-role grid. The syntactic structure forms an independent (modular) tier of language-specific representation. Thus, the three sentences in (6) all have the same syntactic two-argument structure consisting of subject and direct object of the corresponding verbs. The syntactic subject position may be occupied, however, by arguments with different semantic roles:

(6)   a   *I am beating Jimmy.*
      b   *I fear spiders.*
      c   *I received a letter.*

In (6)a the subject position is occupied by an agent. In (6)b this position is occupied by an experiencer. In (6)c the same position is occupied by the beneficiary of the action signified by the verb. If this is the case, we have no other choice but to maintain the thesis about the independence of syntactic structure and semantic structure. If they match each other and deviate from each other, they can serve as a perfect vehicle for implementing specular and nonspecular versions of the self in the asymmetric oscillating way (as described in the section on 'the self as a sign', above) on a moment-to-moment basis.

Every sentence is a small drama: about the representational potential of verbal mind

In the first approximation, the sentence consists of a verb with its argument positions filled with appropriate referring expressions. Prototypically, a sentence formulates and expresses some cognitive event with its actors and circumstances. For example:

(7)   *I married last month.*

signals a momentous event in the drama of somebody's autobiography, the drama signposted in our society by births, graduations, jobs, weddings and funerals.

   The small dramas staged by the cognitive content of each sentence could be either elaborated according to a subordinate scenario, i.e. the way a typical wedding is enacted, or according to a superordinate scenario – the place of wedding in sketching the path of some individual through life. This is supposed to mean that the episodic knowledge can be represented, elaborated and compressed recursively at different levels by sentential expression. This episodic knowledge is mediated to a very significant degree by the semantic structure of language (while not equated to it). It is saved as episodic memory in the LTM of each individual and codes the cultural component of the human form of life. The culture-specific component of this knowledge is due to the acquisition of strategic skills of how to link together different small dramas into larger-scale ones, or, vice versa, how to elaborate some scenario first sketched as a single event, as in (7) above. These strategies of elaboration and/or compression are very complex (for an orientation and an illustrative example, please consult van Dijk, 1997) and go a long way above and away from the consideration of language structure proper. They are, at least partially, under the control of the self. S/he can choose on which aspect of the current cognitive representation to concentrate (to focus on it) and make an attempt to elaborate further. This is one of the reasons why the way of wording of experience matters. (For the psychopathology of discourse processing, cf. Abu-Akeel, 1999; Gernsbacher et al., 1999; for discussion of the correlative psychopathology of experience, cf. Zahavi, 2000.)

If we concentrate on the outcome of the unificational action of the verb and its arguments (but also adjuncts and other additional structure I have no place to deal with), the first characteristic of the resulting sentence, quite appropriate to the current discussion, is that as a rule it consists of more than one proposition. Even very simple-looking sentences of natural language represent the outcome of complex analytical and integrational procedures realized by processes of implicit cognition. If we linearize analytically the mental content expressed in verbal thought according to its propositional structure (function + argument), as language gives us the opportunity to do that too, we will get sequences like the following one, not unlike the way a Universal Turing machine performs or Forrest Gump from the Hollywood movie:

(8)   *I am a girl. The girl is small. The girl carries a bag. The girl wears shoes. The girl wears a skirt. The skirt is yellow. The shoes are black.*

Please note that in (8), with a strictly serial way of information processing, we are quite limited in the possibilities of developing our thought. There is also no rule-governed way to refer back to an entity mentioned in previous sentences.

The same mental content can be expressed nonproblematically within a single clause sentence:

(9)   *I am a small girl with a black bag and a yellow skirt.*

One of the problems this compression helps optimize is that of coreference (establishment of identity of reference in more than one cognitive action). In the seven sentences in (8) the referents of *I*, *girl*, *shoes* and *skirt* must again and again be identified as 'the same ones', while in the single-clause frame of (9) we do not need to take care of that. Cognitively, this means a radical optimization in the way of coordination in the performance of WM, i.e. of the processors in charge of syntax, spatial cognition and abstract thought. This also means, please note, their *binding together* via a mechanism of interprocessorial coreference. This is done by actualizing a cognitive representation of simple sentence format representing a dynamic situation. Correspondingly, the self can become staged in fairly complicated cognitive scenes with multiple possibilities of tracking referential identity and attributions of features, qualities and characteristics.

The basic emergent characteristics constitutive of sentence structure

The filling of the argument positions of a verb with appropriate noun phrases with corresponding theta roles is a constructive action, but this action is not enough to create a sentence pattern. Traditionally, two further features of the sentence are mentioned as emergent and constitutive of its structure, unlike the structure of words (including verbs) and phrases (i.e. units of the intermediate level of language structure serving as components forming sentence as a higher-level unit). These are the predicative relation (predication) and the modality. Each of them, as we will shortly see, contributes in a specific way to our capacity of becoming self-conscious.

In the current context of language studies, predication is reinterpreted more technically as implemented in two functional projections constituting the syntactic core of sentence structure – these are formulated as tense and agreement functional projections. (There are more technically specified syntactic conditions imposed on predication, e.g. c-command, control, binding, interactions with theta roles, coordination, but I will not deal with them here; cf. Haegeman & Guéron, 1999, for further orientation.)

The basic distinction to be made in the grammatical category of tense is the distinction between present and nonpresent. The present is the time of the current speech event. Nonpresent refers to future or past events. The present tense is the tense of be-here-now. It is remarkable, in this respect, that the unmarked present tense is used quite rarely in communicative situations. There are not very many everyday occasions where I can keep a running commentary of what happens to me as experience or in the world around me. Thus the schizophrenic condition strikes the observer as communicatively bizarre on several counts – the content of the inner-voice messages is a third-person commentary about one's own behaviour and/or second-person verbal reactions to one's thoughts to be heard by oneself as a second-person addressee or as a third-person being around (in the mind).

The nonpresent tense (past or future) dissociates from the here and now and signals the requirement to start to generate or to maintain a coherent virtual mental model of some past or future situation. Thus we exchange the current flow of perceptual input and motor output with a mental image of something which is presently not available. This is an act of cognitive dissociation between the content of the explicit mental representation and the perceptual world given in its immediacy here and now. The dissociation, however, is a specific one. The link to the present speaking situation is always kept intact, but with the means of modality (cf. below) signalling the current propositional attitude of the speaking self. This propositional attitude can also become explicated by lexical means, e.g. by adverbials like *possibly*, *necessarily*, *probably*, etc.

The point is that when we speak about nonpresent events, we always do so on the basis of the present speech situation. If I am now talking to some addressee about the possibility of finding life on Mars, this is related, in one or other way, to my present intentions, motivations, beliefs and expectations. The category of tense, while signalling (in the majority of cases) the dissociation from the perceptual world, always maintains a link to the present communicative situation, explicitly or implicitly, and the position and perspective on it of the self. Thus, whenever we talk we automatically constitute ourselves as selves. One of the foundational means for establishing this implicit or explicit self-consciousness is imposed via the requirement to use tensed verb forms in order to construct well-formed sentences.

The other requirement for sentence formation associable with predication is that of agreement. It amounts to a rule to mark formally in an agreement pattern the subject with the verb, as is overtly done in English only in the third-person singular but not in the other two persons:

(10)   a *Peter loves Mary.*
      b *I love Mary.*
      c *You love Mary.*

Other languages, however, mark on a regular basis all the persons in singular and plural for obligatory agreement with the subject of the corresponding sentence. Such languages include German, Bulgarian, Spanish and Italian.

At first sight, agreement looks less capable of being meaningfully interpreted, although it must be functional, i.e. it must serve a purpose. Without going into details and controversies, I will make the claim that the psychological underpinning of the formal requirement for agreement in sentence structure is to mark by syntactic means the *online binding* of at least two separate mental contents coming from LTM and/or other modules in WM. The grammar overtly signals this emergent sentence characteristics by the feature of agreement of the subject with the verb, as in *John loves Mary.* Agreement goes with *John*, not with *Mary*. It will go with *Mary* in the sentence *Mary loves John* (which means something different).

The second emergent grammatical category constitutive of sentence is modality. It provides the basic grammatical means by which the speaker *must* express his/her attitude towards the status of the event represented by the content of the corresponding sentence. This means that modality binds the self to the explicit semantic content of the current utterance via an attitude to it generated and maintained here and now, i.e. independently of the time expressed in the explicit cognitive content (which could be about present, future or past events).

In contemporary linguistic theory usually two different types of modality are distinguished. The first is called epistemic modality and indicates judgement of certainty/uncertainty about the reality of the event described by linguistic means. The second type of modality is called deontic and indicates volition toward the event. Both help constitute the implicit and capable of being explicated self either as a cognizing or as a volitional agent (with emotions, attitudes, beliefs and motivations), as in:

(11)   *I want to become a billionaire.*
(12)   *The train may arrive in several minutes at Victoria station.*
(13)   *The earth is flat.*
(14)   *I know that the earth is round.*

In (11) I express deontic modality. In (12) I express epistemic modality related to my being aware that I am not certain that some event will happen some time in the near future. In (13) I assert that the earth is flat. In (14) I make a statement I am certain it is true. In each of these cases, modality is an indispensable component constitutive of the corresponding cognitive happening. When there are no overt linguistic markers of it, as in (13), it is set as 'unmarked', i.e. as assertive. The unmarked modality of language-specific representation is that of certainty, of factuality and truthfulness of the representative content of the corresponding sentence. This certainty forms the root modal link of the self to the verbal object of consciousness. It makes the explicit mental representation incorrigible (cf. Brook & DeVidi, 2001). It is important to realize the by-default value of this relationship, as it is this relation of by-default certainty that becomes shattered in schizophrenia.

Thus, predication and modality establish the most prominent emergent characteristics pertaining to verbal consciousness. On the one hand, the cognitive content of every sentence has the capacity and the possibility to dissociate itself from the previous one and from the current external context. On the other hand, the dissociated cognitive representation remains integrated here and now to the implicit executive self via the modality link. The bond between the implicit self and the cognitive content of the sentence is nonpredicative. This is important to reiterate.

In this way, the mind avoids the trap of infinite regress in relating the self to the mental contents to which it has access.

Every sentence must have a self

A slogan credited to Chomsky formulates the following axiom of generative grammar: 'every sentence must have a subject'. This is a strictly formal requirement concerning the position of syntactic subject in the sentence. The justification for it is to be found in the language-immanent computational and/or functional specificity of the well-formed sentence (including infinitive constructions and small clauses; cf. Haegeman & Guéron, 1999, for further orientation). Basically, it concerns the necessity to fill out the argument positions of the finite verb form of the corresponding sentence. This axiom is not supposed to have a meaningful correlate in experience. Just the opposite, as we saw above, the position of the grammatical subject can be occupied by entities with different theta roles.

This slogan can be taken to have two possible replicas in our context:
1. Every sentence must have a subject = Every sentence must have an implicit self.
2. Every sentence can have an explicit self = In every sentence there must be a position reserved for potential inclusion of the self.

The second thesis could be easily proven: every sentence, e.g. *The earth is flat*, can get an explicit self, as in e.g. *I think that the earth is flat* or *I believe that the earth is flat*. This is achieved via relativization. Thus the implicit self can always become explicated.

It may appear that, with the simple proof provided above, we also find support for the plausibility of (1). This is not necessarily the case, because what is supposed to be proven is that specifically the position of the grammatical subject (but not that of direct object or indirect object) is the linguistic replica of the position of implicit self in the structure of consciousness. As one can see from the discussion thus far, this is not the case. The self can also occupy the position of object and indirect object in the corresponding sentence. Interestingly enough, it cannot get into an adjunct position, i.e. it can only be inserted in an argument position of some finite verb form. There is, still, some analogy between the place-holding function of *I* in (15)a and the place-filling position of *it* in (15)b:

(15)   a *I am afraid.*
       b *It is raining.*

In the former case, there is no context-free representational content associable with the *I*, the *I* is nonspecular. In the latter example, there is no argument position and semantic role associable with the event of raining. The *it* serves as an empty place-holder for the position of grammatical subject, a 'dummy grammatical subject', a syntactic place-holder. Unlike *I*, however, it is also devoid of any semantic content whatsoever within the sentence perspective. It just serves as a filler of empty obligatory syntactic position in order for the sentence to achieve grammatical well-formedness. It remains to be investigated how far one can get in relating the two cases to each other – the semantic place-holder *I* and the syntactic place-holder *it* – and justifying which of them is the causally efficient 'original' and which is the 'replica'.

Every sentence can have an explicit self, but no more than one, please – the complementary function of pronominals and anaphors

It may well be the case that it is language that insinuates to us the intuition about the uniqueness of the self. Language structure itself blocks the possibility of multiple explicit appearances of the self in one and the same mental representation (given as a clause in natural language) where the self is staged as *both* grammatical subject and object of some mental event, as in (16)a:

(16)   a   *I_i see me$_i$.
        b I_i see myself$_i$.

(16)a is an anomalous English sentence. In order to express the identity of the reference of subject and object of the verb *to see*, the language uses not two personal pronouns but a personal pronoun for the subject and a member of another specific class of pronouns – reflexive pronouns, e.g. *myself* in (16)b – for expression of the idea that the object and the subject corefer to one and the same entity, forming a coindexed chain with it. In order to explain the difference between (16)a and (16)b we should briefly discuss the mechanism of linguistic anaphora.

Anaphora (as a general term) encompasses the phenomena of pronominal reference and various kinds of ellipsis. To my knowledge, such phenomena are absent even in a rudimentary form from the systems of communication of other species. For example, there seems to be no equivalents of the personal, reflexive or possessive pronouns in the communicative systems of bees, ants, apes and dolphins. The personal pronouns, for example, cannot be equated to the pointing gestures toward the speaker as *I* or the hearer as *you*. The system of anaphora is much more complex. The common denominator of all sorts of anaphora appears to be that an element or construction is dependent for its interpretation on being associated in a rule-governed way to some other linguistic element in the context of current conversation. It is the binding theory within the government-and-binding version of generative grammar that provided the most influential account of the possible relationships between anaphoric elements and their antecedents (cf. Haegeman & Guéron, 1999). Within this theory, two classes of anaphora are distinguished from the point of view of their scope of antecedent binding – pronominals and anaphors.

An anaphor signals that what is distinguished in language structure as 'two entities' in occupying syntactic positions which can be taken by two nouns referring to two distinct objects in the world is, as a matter of fact, one and the same entity in some cognitive structure. An anaphor, even if it appears in an argument position in the same clause, requires for its interpretation a link to another argument within its governing category (in the majority of the cases the corresponding clause), e.g.:

(17)   a *Helen hates herself.*

Anaphors like reflexive pronouns (like *myself*) and reciprocals (like *each other*) must be locally bound, i.e. bound within the same clause, as in (18)a:

(18)   a *I$_i$ entertained myself$_i$.*
        b **I$_i$ remember that you entertained myself$_i$.*
        c *I$_i$ remember that I$_i$ entertained myself$_i$.*

(18)b is not a well-formed sentence, because *myself* must find its antecedent within the same clause, and *you* cannot serve that purpose. In (18)c, on the other hand, there is a fitting candidate for an antecedent, the *I* of the subordinate clause. (For further information about the origin and diachronic development of personal and reflexive pronouns in English and the possibilities of representing with them a unified versus an alienated [further dissociated from itself] self, cf. Haiman, 1998, pp. 67–79.)

A pronominal expression, on the other hand, is in complementary distribution with anaphor and must be free in its governing category. This means that in:

(17)   b *Helen hates her.*

her must be interpreted as somebody who is not identical with *Helen,* but must find its antecedent on a distance longer that the current clause. The same rule applies for:

(17)   c *She$_i$ hates her$_j$.*

In (17)c *she* and *her* must trace their antecedents to two different referring expressions from the previous sentences of the same utterance. Each of them, by itself, remains uninterpretable.

In linguistic theory, first- and second-person pronominals are treated like the third-person pronominals. At first sight, their behaviour appears to be the same, i.e. the antecedent of a first-person as well as a third-person pronoun cannot be too close, i.e. within the same clause:

(18)   d **I$_i$ saw me$_i$.*
        e **They$_i$ saw them$_i$.*

There are, however, important differences between them. A third-person pronoun cannot occupy sentence initial position (without a previous context). Thus, while (18)f is an interpretable sentence with the pronoun *I* in the sentence-initial position, (18)g is a ill-formed sentence – *they* must look for a coreferent from the context before, not after, its own appearance, thus it cannot corefer with *dancers*:

(18)   f I_i *forgot that the dancers saw me$_i$.*
        g **They$_i$ forgot that I saw dancers$_i$.*
        h *The dancers$_i$ forgot that I saw them$_i$.*

(18)h is a well-formed sentence, because the coreferent of *them* is available in the clause immediately preceding the one where *them* appears. Thus, it turns out that the *I*, unlike the third-person pronouns, can refer (but not only to corefer).

Which is, then, the primary function of *I* – to refer to the nonspecular self, or to corefer anaphorically in the way the other personal pronouns do? The possibility of finding a definitive answer to this question may look hopeless to a cognitive psychologist. What sort of experiment could definitively prove a case like this one? The problem, however, is quite easy to decide strictly on linguistic grounds. We can extract the subordinate clauses from (18)f and (18)h and see they can stand up and be interpretable independently (i.e. without the possibility of coreferring):

(18)   i *The dancers saw me.*
        j **I saw them$_i$.*

(18)i can be interpreted as a separate independent sentence without invoking an antecedent from the context from a previous sentence. This means that *me* can refer directly, i.e. it does not need to be bound to *I* in (18)f in order to become interpretable. (18)j, however, is *per se* uninterpretable. *them* requires the activation of a noun from a previous sentence.

Thus we have shown that two *explicit* distinct forms of the first-person personal pronoun do not necessarily form a chain of coreference with each other. Both *I* and *me* in (18)f can refer directly. Thus we have quite simple proof about the priority of reference to coreference which is applicable to self-consciousness, but not to third-person object-bound consciousness. While the first-person pronouns can corefer, they do not need to function like that in order to perform their function successfully. What matters in the final resort is the referential link of the explicit pronoun to the implicit executive self here and now.

The coreferential chain becomes, however, essential in the case the nonspecular place-holder *I* (or *me*) itself becomes an absentee from the explicit syntactic structure of the corresponding sentence. This feat (dual presence-in-absence – both of form and meaning – of the sign representing the self) also becomes possible with the exclusive support of language structure. For achieving dual absence, we need the context of a complex sentence (or a correlate of a complex sentence, including an infinitive construction or a small clause).

Complex sentence structure and the case for absent nonspecular represented self

I made the point above that the *I* is a place-holder with no explicit context-free representational content. During each new act of sentence processing, the link between the implicit executive self and the explicated *I* must be reestablished. Thus in (19)a we have twice to link the *I* to the implicit self of the current speaker. What we are missing (or need to infer in order to make these two sentences coherent) is the causal relation between them. This causal relation is explicated in (19)b, and, lo, the self vanished along with the verb for volition *want*. Actually it vanished not once but twice! Once as the agent of the act of volition, and the second time as the agent of talking. The place of the agent doing the talking remains, however, 'marked' by a gap, this time a literal absence of any linguistic form from the surface structure of the sentence. The *I* which is the agent of *talking* must be there, but it is not visible at all – either in meaning or in form. The gap is there according to the axiom 'Every sentence must have a subject'. It also applies to infinitive constructions. We find out who is supposed to talk due to the establishment of the coreference chain between the 'gap', called trace **t**, and its antecedent in the matrix clause (as coindexed in 19b):

(19) a *I am too stubborn. I won't talk to Mary.*
     b *I_i am too stubborn t_i to talk to Mary.*
        'Because I_i am too stubborn, I_i do not want to talk to Mary'
     c *People do not want to talk to me. I am too stubborn.*
     d *I_i am too stubborn **e** to talk to t_i.*
        (i) 'Because I_i am too stubborn, **people** do not want to talk to **me$_i$**'.
        (ii) *'Because I_i am too stubborn, I_i do not want to talk to **people**'.

In (19)c we have once again a chain of two sentences. We should expect that if we attempt an operation of unification analogous to that from (19)a to (19)b, we will achieve a comparable result. The result is, however, once again a surprise – this time two entities vanish from the surface structure of the previous two sentences – *people* and *me* – as one can see in (19)d. The gaps in the latter example are marked as **e** (empty category) and t_i (trace), i.e. here we have two different types of empty slots locating the position of the subject and/or the object of the verb *to talk*. t_i is identical to the self (the I_i in the main sentence with whom it is correspondingly coindexed). It was effaced (deleted) from the overt syntactic structure by a language-specific operation. **e** was never there; it was inserted as a last-resort operation in an attempt to achieve a well-formed sentence structure from the available explicitly syntactic pattern (for a discussion of examples of this type but in the third person, cf. Chomsky, 1993, pp. 23–25; Chomsky, 2000, p. 35; for the concepts of empty category and trace, cf. Haegeman & Guéron, 1999).

Coreference tracking is an unconscious syntax-specific cognitive operation. It can serve the function of keeping intact the identity of the self within the horizon of a complex sentence without the latter being visible both in the format of spatial cognition and at the level of the surface syntactic form. This is an example of *absent nonspecular self*, and a self which must still be there in order for the sentence to achieve well-formedness and be capable of being correctly interpreted. Thus we may claim that we have here a lacuna, a gap, but an explicit gap, as this position is language-specific but not that of the executive implicit right-hemisphere self (cf. Vogeley et al., 1999). The rule on how to fill gaps like these is available to all speakers of English. No one would make the mistake of interpreting (19)d as (19)d(ii); all interpret it unanimously as (19)d(i).

The problems just presented are the subject matter of quite technical treatments in contemporary theory of grammar. The general point should still be clear – syntactic processing offers different possibilities to efface, to delete a component of the overt structure of the sentence and still be capable of keeping track of its identity via the means of anaphora. The gaps in the overt language structure continue to matter. These gaps can help hide the self while supporting its identity on a scale larger than the current clause in a rule-governed way. The formal rules for establishing such long-distance dependencies provide the scaffolding for maintenance of self-consciousness with specific linguistic means. In the case of absent nonspecular self, the only way to track it is coreference. This is achieved by a different mechanism from the one tracking the reference of the *I*. It remains to be investigated whether each of them can break down independently, leading to different syndromes of the self.

The representational potential of complex sentence and the scope of self-consciousness

If the clause is the minimal cognitive environment for representing the self, what is the upper limit, then, of maintaining a coherent single self-conscious representation with the means of language structure? Complex sentences appear to be the exclusive means offering this extra service to self-consciousness. They provide the structural grid capable of explicit implementation of the intersubjective (ego–alter ego) mind. They establish the structural–functional basis for the development of discursive consciousness – of self-and-other consciousness in interpreting ongoing conversation. The foundational structural basis is established by sentences consisting of two clauses. They provide the grid for explicit interpersonal binding on an oscillatory *I–you* basis as in:

(20)   *I see that you see me.*

The two-clause sentence gives the mind the opportunity to bind two separate and separable cognitive events which otherwise cannot be reliably concatenated by the ad hoc laws of sequence in psychological association. Language-specific for the concatenation of the two cognitive events in (20) is not only the explicit use of *I* and *you* (signalling the change of perspective which can be enacted in two separate sentences which are not structurally bound to each other in a language-specific way) but also the inclusion in a recursive way of the clause *that you see me* in the direct-object position of the matrix verb *see* in the main (higher-order) clause.

A three-clause sentence provides the mind with the possibility of closing the loop between implicit computation and explicit representation in implementing the intersubjective mind (i.e. this is the upper limit of explicit self-and-other representation; for further discussion, cf. Stamenov, 1997):

(21)   *I see that you see that I see you.*

This loop of mutual bonds is impossible to achieve with a chain of simple sentences. The simple sentence still does not make us self-conscious the way we can and are. With chains of simple sentences we will look like Forrest Gump. It is the complex sentence that makes the difference for the implementation of self-consciousness, as we know it today – capable apparently ad infinitum of oscillatory splits and loops. Complex sentence is the scaffolding helping to plan and control the dynamics of self-evolution during online cognitive processing. It creates and maintains the links online between three different place-holders of the executive self – its present implicit executive one, one potential explicit one, and one for the other interlocutor's (*you*) theory of mind.

The examples provided above can also help us become aware that what is basically lost in schizophrenia, apparently, is not (or at least not primarily) the high-level capacity for coreference with oneself, but the 'direct' reference to the implicit self online during any single successive cognitive act of becoming aware of some mental contents. If the schizophrenic loses reliable access to the implicit self as a reference point (cf. Langacker 1987, 1997) for each explicit sign representing him/her, the only mechanism for self-reference tracking s/he can possibly rely on would be coreference. But the language-specific anaphoric self-tracking is as fragile as one can imagine. Without the possibility of anchoring oneself online to the current executive implicit ego, the maintenance of the ego's identity is in constant danger of undergoing an unpredictable dissociation with the end of the current complex sentence. It is this permanent fear of impending breakdown which features prominently in the descriptions of schizophrenic experience (cf. Torey, 1988). Outside the horizon of a single sentence pattern self-identity may oscillate hectically down (or up) 'the indefinite spiral of reflexivity' of Dennett (1991, p. 310) and one may end up identifying oneself proverbially with Napoleon Bonaparte or Cleopatra (as one can rely only on narratives for establishing coherence in one's mental functioning).

Conclusion

There are four language-specific ways of identifying and tracking the self in conscious experience through: (1) inner-voice monitoring; (2) outer-voice monitoring; (3) reference to the nonspecular self; and (4) anaphoric binding to an absent nonspecular self. These four ways of referring to and binding the self operate at the level of up to sentence structure formation. Discourse- and narrative-specific strategies for maintaining the continuity in self-identity add further complexity and sophistication to self-consciousness.

Self-awareness is supported by a whole set of feedback-based sensorimotor loops in different sensory modalities and kinaesthesia. Thus, it is impossible to make the case for the exclusive relationship between language capacity and self-awareness. The execution of inner speech, however, seems to form the subtlest level of it.

With self-consciousness the situation is rather different. Having in mind the specific online relationship between the implicit self, the explicit mental content and the possibility for the implicit self always to be projected at the stage of consciousness, it is quite difficult to imagine how self-consciousness, as we know it from first-person experience, could function without the implicit and explicit support of language structure but only on the basis of spatial cognition (mental imagery) format. The nonspecular self and the absent nonspecular self become possible only with the means of language. It is language that provides the symbolic means for continuous tracking of the self and empowers it with specific syntactic and semantic features. At the same time, it always keeps updated the deictic (pragmatic) here-and-now link to the executive functions of mind via pronominal reference and modality, providing the self with a sense of integrity and uniqueness. Thus, language radically broadens the potential of self-awareness to a coherent and extended-in-time singular self-consciousness. It is this finely tuned cognitive orchestra that becomes shattered in schizophrenia as an illness of the self.

REFERENCES

Abu-Akeel, A. (1999). Impaired theory of mind in schizophrenia. *Pragmatics and Cognition*, 7, 247–82.

American Psychiatric Association. (1994). *Diagnostic and Statistical Manual of Mental Disorders*, 4th edn. Washington: APA.

Brook, A. & DeVidi, R. (eds) (2001). *Self-awareness and Self-reference.* Amsterdam: John Benjamins.

Chomsky, N. (1993). *Language and Thought.* Wakefield, RI: Moyer Bell.

Chomsky, N. (2000). *New Horizons in the Study of Language.* Cambridge: Cambridge University Press.

Crow, T.J. (2000). Schizophrenia as the price the *Homo sapiens* pays for language: a resolution of the central paradox in the origin of the species. *Brain Research Reviews,* **31,** 118–29.

Cutler, A., Mehler, J., Norris, D. & Segui, J. (1992). The monolingual nature of speech segmentation in bilinguals. *Cognitive Psychology,* **24,** 381–410.

DeCasper, A.J. & Spence, M.J. (1986). Prenatal maternal speech influences newborns' perception of speech sounds. *Infant Behavior and Development,* **9,** 133–50.

Dennett, D. (1991). *Consciousness Explained.* Boston: Little, Brown.

Georgov, I. (1905). Die ersten Anfänge des sprachlichen Ausdrucks für das Selbstbewusstsein bei Kindern. *Archiv für die gesamte Psychologie,* **5,** 329–404.

Gernsbacher, M., Tallent, K.A. & Bolliger, C.M. (1999). Disordered discourse in schizophrenia described by the structure building framework. *Discourse Studies,* **1,** 355–72.

Haegeman, L. & Guéron, J. (1999). *English Grammar: A Generative Perspective.* Oxford: Blackwell.

Haiman, J. (1998). *Talk is Cheap: Sarcasm, Alienation, and the Evolution of Language.* New York: Oxford University Press.

James, W. (1890). *Principles of Psychology,* vols I–II. New York: Henry Holt.

Langacker, R.W. (1987). *Foundations of Cognitive Grammar,* vol. 1: *Theoretical Prerequisites.* Stanford: Stanford University Press.

Langacker, R.W. (1997). Consciousness, construal, and subjectivity. In *Language Structure, Discourse and the Access to Consciousness,* ed. M. Stamenov, pp. 49–75. Amsterdam: John Benjamins.

Levelt, W.J.M. (1989). *Speaking: From Intention to Articulation.* Cambridge, MA: MIT Press.

Levelt, W.J.M., Praamstra, P., Meyer, A.S., Helenius, P. & Salmelin, R. (1998). A MEG study of picture naming. *Journal of Cognitive Neuroscience,* **10,** 553–67.

Levelt, W.J.M., Roelofs, A. & Meyer, A.S. (1999). A theory of lexical access in speech production. *Behavioral and Brain Sciences,* **22,** 1–75.

Liberman, A.M. & Mattingly, I.G. (1985). The motor theory of speech perception revised. *Cognition,* **21,** 1–36.

Lieberman, P. (1991). *Uniquely Human: The Evolution of Speech, Thought, and Selfless Behavior.* Cambridge, MA: Harvard University Press.

Lyons, J. (1977). *Semantics,* vols I–II. Cambridge: Cambridge University Press.

Mehler, J. & Dupoux, E. (1994). *What Infants Know: The New Cognitive Science of Early Development.* Cambridge: Blackwell.

Mehler, J., Sebastian, N., Altmann, G. et al. (1993). Understanding compressed sentences: the role of rhythm and meaning. In *Temporal Information Processing in the Nervous System,* ed. P. Tallal, A.M. Galaburda, R. Llinas & C. von Euler. *Annals of the New York Academy of Sciences,* **682,** 272–282.

Miller, G. (1956). The magic number 7 plus minus two: some limits in our capacity for processing information. *Psychological Review,* **50,** 135–47.

Nazzi, T., Bertoncini, J. & Mehler, J. (1998). Language discrimination by newborns: towards an understanding of the role of rhythm. *Journal of Experimental Psychology: Human Perception and Performance*, **24**, 756–66.

Postma, A. (2000). Detection of errors during speech production: a review of speech monitoring models. *Cognition*, **77**, 97–131.

Ramus, F., Hauser, M.D., Miller, C., Morris, D. & Mehler, J. (2000). Language discrimination by human newborns and by cotton-top tamarin monkeys. *Science*, **288**, 349–51.

Rovee-Collier, C., Hayne, H. & Colombo, M. (2000). *The Development of Implicit and Explicit Memory*. *Advances in Consciousness Research*, vol. 24. Amsterdam: John Benjamins.

Spence, M.J. & DeCasper, A.J. (1987). Prenatal experience with low-frequency maternal-voice sounds influences neonatal perception of maternal voice samples. *Infant Behavior and Development*, **10**, 133–42.

Stamenov, M.I. (1997). Grammar, meaning and consciousness: what sentence structure can tell us about the structure of consciousness. In *Language Structure, Discourse and the Access to Consciousness*, ed. M. Stamenov, pp. 277–342. Amsterdam: John Benjamins.

Stamenov, M.I. (1999). First language acquisition and the ontogenetic development of self-consciousness in the work of Ivan Georgov. In *The Emergence of Modern Language Sciences: Studies on the Transition from Historical-comparative to Structural Linguistics in Honor of E.F. Konrad Koerner*, ed. S. Embleton, J.E. Joseph & H.J. Niederehe, pp. 91–106. Amsterdam: John Benjamins.

Stamenov, M.I. & Gallese, V. (eds) (2002). *Mirror Neurons and the Evolution of Brain and Language*. Amsterdam: John Benjamins.

Torey, E.F. (1988). *Surviving Schizophrenia: A Family Manual*. New York: Harper & Row.

van Dijk, T.A. (1997). Cognitive context models and discourse. In *Language Structure, Discourse and the Access to Consciousness*, ed. M. Stamenov, pp. 189–226. Amsterdam: John Benjamins.

Vogeley, K., Kurthen, M., Falkai, P. & Maier, W. (1999). Essential functions of the human self model are implemented in the prefrontal cortex. *Consciousness and Cognition*, **8**, 343–63.

Wheeldon, L.R. & Levelt, W.J.M. (1995). Monitoring the time course of phonological encoding. *Journal of Memory and Language*, **34**, 311–34.

Wheeler, M.A. (2000). Varieties of consciousness and memory in the developing child. In *Memory, Consciousness, and the Brain: The Tallinn Conference*, ed. E. Tulving, pp. 188–99. Philadelphia: Psychology Press.

Zahavi, D. (ed.) (2000). *Exploring the Self: Philosophical and Psychopathological Perspectives on Self-experience*. *Advances in Consciousness Research*, vol. 23. Amsterdam: John Benjamins.

Part II

Cognitive and neurosciences

5

The multiplicity of consciousness and the emergence of the self

Gerard O'Brien and Jonathan Opie

Department of Philosophy, University of Adelaide, South Australia, Australia

Abstract

One of the most striking manifestations of schizophrenia is thought insertion. People suffering from this delusion believe they are not the author of thoughts which they nevertheless own as experiences. It seems that a person's sense of agency and sense of the boundary between mind and world can come apart. Schizophrenia thus vividly demonstrates that self-awareness is a complex construction of the brain. This point is widely appreciated. What is not so widely appreciated is how radically schizophrenia challenges our assumptions about the nature of the self. Most theorists endorse the traditional doctrine of the *unity of consciousness*, according to which a normal human brain generates a *single* consciousness at any instant in time. In this chapter we argue that phenomenal consciousness at each instant is actually a *multiplicity*: an aggregate of phenomenal elements, each of which is the product of a distinct consciousness-making mechanism in the brain. We then consider how certain aspects of self might emerge from this manifold substrate, and speculate about the origin of thought insertion.

Introduction

Schizophrenia is a complex and heterogeneous disease, incorporating at least three distinct subsyndromes: *psychomotor poverty* (poverty of speech, lack of spontaneous movement, blunting of affect), *disorganization* (inappropriate affect, disturbances of the form of thought) and *reality distortion* (Liddle, 1987; Johnstone, 1991). The reality distortion syndrome encompasses the so-called 'positive' symptoms of schizophrenia, which include auditory hallucinations, delusions of persecution and delusions of reference. Of these, thought insertion is arguably the most bizarre. People suffering from this delusion believe that some of the thoughts they experience are not their own:

I look out the window and I think that the garden looks nice and the grass looks cool, but the thoughts of Eammon Andrews come into my mind . . . He treats my mind like a screen and flashes his thoughts onto it like you flash a picture (reported by Mellors, 1970, p. 17).

To get a feel for how bizarre this is, contrast thought insertion with the experience of hearing voices. The standard explanation of such auditory hallucinations is that the voice the schizophrenic 'hears' is actually inner speech which has been misidentified as emanating from someone else. The error, in this case, is comprehensible: we've all had the experience of being uncertain whether the noise we just heard was real or imagined. (There is evidence, however, that many of the delusions classified as verbal hallucinations are much closer in their phenomenology to thought insertion. See Graham & Stephens, 1994, pp. 94–97.) Thought insertion, on the other hand, is not a case of mistaking an introspection for a perception. Those who suffer with this delusion are quite aware that the thought has arisen *in their own minds*. But despite this recognition they still disown it: the thought doesn't have any 'mineness' attached to it.

Given this symptomatology, it is not surprising that the working presupposition of most current research in this area is that schizophrenia is, at least in its delusional form, a disease of the self. Despite this focus, what has not been sufficiently appreciated is how radically schizophrenia challenges our assumptions about the nature of the self. Crucial to being a human self is the possession of a certain sort of inner life, one which encompasses a distinction between one's own thoughts, feelings and actions, and the world in which one is embedded. Conventional wisdom has it that this kind of self-consciousness is a unitary faculty, and, moreover, one that is of a piece with phenomenal consciousness in general. However, by demonstrating that it is possible to be aware of the boundaries of one's mind without acknowledging that all of the thoughts contained therein are one's own, the delusion of thought insertion suggests that this traditional conception of self-consciousness actually conflates two quite distinct capacities.

The first is the brain's capacity to distinguish its mind from the rest of the world. This capacity produces a *sense of subjectivity*: an awareness that certain thoughts, perceptions and feelings comprise the mental life of a single psychological subject. The second is the brain's capacity to distinguish between self-initiated thoughts and actions and mental occurrences of which it is merely the passive recipient (e.g. perceptions). This capacity produces a *sense of agency*: the brain's awareness of itself as the source of the thoughts and imaginings that occur within its boundaries. (The distinction between *subjectivity* and *agency* is nicely developed by Graham & Stephens, 1994.) Thought insertion demonstrates that these two capacities can come apart: schizophrenics afflicted with this delusion believe that they are not the agents of some of the thoughts contained within their own minds. From this perspective, schizophrenia would seem to be a disease that undermines a person's sense of agency, while leaving his or her sense of subjectivity intact.

The distinction between these two kinds of self-awareness, and the fact that they can be selectively impaired, means that it is no longer possible to talk of our experience of self as though it were a single, monolithic entity, and hence assume that there must be a single, all-encompassing explanation which does it justice. For example, the facts that explain the brain's capacity to draw a distinction between its mind and the world must be different from those which explain its capacity to represent itself as a cognitive agent. Furthermore, because subjects can experience certain thoughts and yet disown any agency in respect of them, the different aspects of selfhood would appear to be achievements over and above the brain's capacity to manufacture individual conscious experiences. In schizophrenia, in other words, we have a vivid demonstration that the self is a complex construction of the brain that is to some degree independent of its capacity to generate consciousness.

We would go further. We believe that schizophrenia offers a unique window on the cognitive operation of the brain. It reveals a relationship between the structure of consciousness and the brain's cognitive machinery that is very different from the conception which has dominated our thinking for centuries. Most theorists in this area, either explicitly or implicitly, endorse the traditional doctrine of the *unity of consciousness*, according to which a normal (intact) human brain generates a *single* consciousness at any instant in time (rather than several distinct consciousnesses), and hence a single *stream* of consciousness over time (rather than parallel tributaries). However, what we know of schizophrenia suggests that, far from being a unity, phenomenal consciousness at each instant is actually a *multiplicity*: an aggregate of phenomenal elements, each of which is the product of a distinct consciousness-making mechanism in the brain. We will call this, for reasons to be explained shortly, the *multitrack* model of consciousness, by contrast with the *single-track* model that is implicit in the doctrine of the unity of consciousness.

Our aim in this chapter is to make good on these claims. We begin by introducing the multitrack model of consciousness, partly by contrasting it with its more conventional (single-track) counterpart, before considering the evidence for this model. We go on to consider how some aspects of self might emerge from the distributed and manifold substrate of consciousness, and enter into some speculations as to how the failure of this emergence gives rise to the symptoms of schizophrenia.

The multiplicity of consciousness

Many, if not most, contemporary theorists working in the field of consciousness studies endorse the doctrine of the unity of consciousness. According to this doctrine, the intact human brain produces a single consciousness at each instant, as opposed to several distinct consciousnesses. Here we argue that this doctrine is mistaken: far from being a unity, phenomenal consciousness is actually a multiplicity. Before proceeding, however, we must provide a clearer picture of what the supposed unity of consciousness entails about the way the brain makes consciousness.

What does the unity of consciousness entail?

At the outset let us quickly dispense with a naive, albeit influential, understanding of the unity of consciousness. Some would have it that consciousness is a unity because it is a serial stream comprising a single informational content at each moment (see, for example, Penrose, 1989, p. 399). Like a solo chorister, who, by virtue of the limitations of the human vocal folds, can only produce one note at a time, consciousness is taken to be single-voiced or *monophonic*. This reading of the unity of consciousness can hardly be sustained. Even the most casual inspection of instantaneous conscious experience shows it to contain contents drawn from a number of different modalities. Sound and vision, for example, don't compete for a place in awareness; both are simultaneously present. You may not be able simultaneously to react to, or focus on, disparate sources of experience, but the phenomenology they generate can certainly cooccur.

If we suppose that consciousness incorporates a number of distinct content-ful elements at each instant, then it is best likened to *polyphonic* choral music. Musical polyphony involves two or more simultaneously active voices, such that at any moment there are a number of different notes being sounded. We think it is safe to say that most theorists regard moment-by-moment consciousness as informationally polyphonic. However, a question immediately arises for an advocate of the unity of consciousness: if consciousness is polyphonic, in what sense is it a unity? The unity on offer can't be the unity of an undifferentiated whole, because, by assumption, experience is actually a *composite* structure: it is assembled from numerous contentful elements that have been fused together in some way. The polyphony of consciousness entails, therefore, that any proponent of the traditional doctrine of the unity of consciousness is committed to there being a *single consciousness-making mechanism or process* in the brain, whose task it is to bind these different contents together into a unity. On the one hand, the task of combining multiple representational contents in a single experience must be performed by some physical mechanism or process. And on the other, if we suppose that the brain implements more than one such mechanism or process, then it must be capable of simultaneously generating more than one experience, contrary to the unity doctrine.

Given this constraint, there appear to be only two roads open to the advocate of a polyphonic, but unitary consciousness: (1) treat conscious experience as the product of a single, central neural *system* where informational contents must be re-presented to be made conscious, or (2) opt for a somehow unitary consciousness-making *process* that acts simultaneously on the brain's many distinct information-processing sites.

A representative example of the former approach is Baars' 'global workspace' model of consciousness (1988, 1997). Baars begins with the premise that the brain contains a multitude of distributed, unconscious processors all operating in parallel, each highly specialized, and all competing for access to a global workspace – a kind of central information exchange for the interaction, coordination and control of the specialists. Such coordination and control is partly a result of restrictions on access to the global workspace. At any one time only a limited number of specialists can broadcast global messages (via the workspace), since different messages may often be contradictory. Those contents are conscious which gain access to the global workspace (perhaps as a result of a number of specialists forming a coalition and ousting their rivals) and are subsequently broadcast throughout the brain (Baars, 1988, pp. 73–118).

In support of this model, Baars claims there is a brain structure suited to the role of workspace, namely the extended-reticular-thalamic-activating system (ERTAS), which includes the reticular formation, the thalamus, and the 'diffuse thalamic projection system' (p. 124). The ERTAS is particularly suited to the role of 'global broadcaster', given the bidirectional projection system that it incorporates. Moreover, there is 'evidence of a feedback flow from cortical modules *to* the ERTAS' and of global information feeding 'back into its own input sources'. Baars suggests that '[both] kinds of feedback may serve to strengthen and stabilize a coalition of systems that work to keep a certain content on the global workspace'. That is, given the competitive nature of access to consciousness, 'a circulating flow of information may be necessary to keep some contents in consciousness' (p. 134).

This kind of model provides an explanation for the unity of consciousness, because the ERTAS acts as an executive *composer* and *broadcaster*. Its role is to combine a number of distinct contents hailing from different sense modalities into a single work, which it then broadcasts polyphonically. The unity of consciousness, on this story, is not imposed by the *seriality* of the stream of contents broadcast (as would be the case with a monophonic executive), but by virtue of there being a *single* broadcasting mechanism.

As to the second route available to the advocate of the unity of consciousness in the face of its manifest polyphony, a number of neuroscientists have suggested that distributed time-locked neural oscillations might fit the bill. Consider, for example, Damasio's proposal:

The integration of multiple aspects of reality, external as well as internal, in perceptual or recalled experiences, both within each modality and across modalities, depends on the time-locked co-activation of geographically separate sites of neural activity within sensory and motor cortices, rather than on a neural transfer and integration of different representations towards rostral integration sites. The conscious experience of these co-activations depends on their simultaneous, but temporary, enhancement ... against the background activity on which other activations are being played out (Damasio, 1989, p. 39).

Damasio here explicitly repudiates the central theatre model, and builds his account around the known parcellation and distribution of information processing in the brain. What brings content-bearing activity to consciousness is its temporary enhancement as a result of time-locked coactivation with contents coded elsewhere in the brain. Time-locking 'integrates' contents coded at 'geographically separate sites', which are then capable of simultaneously entering consciousness. *Time-locked enhancement* is thus a candidate for a single consciousness-making process. This putative process occurs simultaneously at many separate sites, and is unitary in virtue of being phase-locked, or falling within a single well-defined temporal window of some kind.

Single-track versus multitrack models of consciousness

It is reasonable to ask whether such approaches to consciousness are the only option. Once it is acknowledged that instantaneous consciousness is polyphonic, and once this fact is considered in the light of the parcellation of information processing in the brain, an alternative way of thinking about the relationship between the structure of consciousness and brain activity clamours for attention. Instead of requiring that the multiple contents of moment-by-moment experience be re-presented in some central system, or that they be integrated in a single global process, why not suppose that these contents contribute to instantaneous experience via *multiple* mechanisms of consciousness-making scattered across the brain?

We can't resist employing another musical metaphor here to clarify this alternative polyphonic model of consciousness and to distinguish it from its more orthodox counterpart (O'Brien & Opie, 1998). Before the advent of modern studios the only way to record music was to get all the musicians in a room together, place a microphone in their midst, and start up the band. The signal from the microphone would then go through a limited amount of processing before leaving a groove on a wax disc, or more recently, a magnetic trace on a tape. Such a recording is said to be *single-track*, since there is no way to separate out the individual contributions of the musicians – they are packaged into a single structure. By contrast, on a *multitrack* recording one or more separate tracks is devoted to each musical instrument. As a result, while all the musical parts combine to make up the total sound during playback, *at the level of the recording* one can distinguish between them.

The polyphonic models surveyed thus far are all single-track theories of consciousness. Whether one treats conscious experience as the product of a single, central neural *system* where informational contents must be re-presented to be made conscious, as in Baars' account, or whether one opts for a unitary consciousness-making *process* that acts simultaneously on the brain's many distinct information-processing sites, as in Damasio's story, one assumes that *at the level at which it is made* by the brain, instantaneous consciousness is a single thing. When it comes to consciousness-making, the normal brain has just one track. By contrast, a multi-track theory of consciousness regards instantaneous consciousness as being made up of a number of parallel tracks: a collection of phenomenal elements, each generated by a distinct mechanism in the brain.

It might be objected that information in one sensory modality sometimes *influences* the content of experience in another. A salient example is the McGurk effect, whereby what subjects report *hearing* is partly determined by what they *see*. (See McGurk & MacDonald (1976). We owe this example to Tim Bayne. For Bayne's critique of the multitrack model, and our reply, see Bayne (2000) and O'Brien & Opie (2000), respectively.) This looks problematic for a multitrack account because the various parts of the polyphonic mix don't appear to be truly independent of one another. But the multitrack account is committed only to the claim that the various parts of experience are generated locally, at the very sites where their information contents are fixed. This does not require content-fixations to be completely causally independent of one another. At any given moment there are presumably all sorts of influences, both intrasensory and intersensory, criss-crossing the brain, such that conscious contents not only co occur, but mutually influence and shape one another. Such causal links are perfectly consistent with the multitrack model, so long as the consciousness-making mechanisms themselves are manifold and localized.

The distinction between single-track and multitrack approaches to consciousness is not well-appreciated in the literature. (The only other place we have seen this distinction explicitly drawn is in a recent discussion of consciousness by Searle (2000). Searle distinguishes between what he calls the unified field approach (single-track model) and the building block approach (multitrack model). Having said that, Damasio shows himself to be alive to the possibility of a multitrack theory (see Damasio, 1999, especially pp. 123–124 and pp. 165–166).) Because of their unquestioning allegiance to the traditional doctrine of the unity of consciousness, most theorists don't even entertain the possibility of a multitrack theory. As a result they overlook what we think is a more parsimonious account of consciousness, one that is more consistent with both our moment-by-moment phenomenal experience and our neuroscientific understanding of the mechanisms subserving cognition. In the next subsection we examine the evidence, both phenomenological and neuroscientific, in favour of this alternative approach to explaining how the brain makes consciousness.

Evidence for the multitrack model of consciousness

Consider, first, the phenomenological evidence. Close attention to instantaneous experience reveals it to be a complex *aggregate* of many elements. Right now, for example, as you concentrate on these sentences, your phenomenal experience is very rich, comprising visual experiences (the shapes, textures and colours of these sentences, together with other objects in the room), auditory experiences (noises from outside the room), tactile experiences (the chair pressing against your body), proprioceptive experiences (the position of your limbs) and understanding experiences (what these words and sentences mean), to name a few. These parts are relatively independent, because they can be altered or lost without substantially affecting the others (try closing your eyes for a moment); like the parallel tracks on a multitrack recording, the loss of any one mode of consciousness merely reduces the total 'sound'.

This independence among the parts of experience is even evident, to some extent, *within* modalities. Consider Figure 5.1. It can be seen as a flight of stairs in normal orientation, with rear wall uppermost; as an inverted flight of stairs, with front wall uppermost; or even as a flat line drawing, with no perspective. And whichever of these interpretations one adopts, the details of line and colour remain the same. That is, our experience here incorporates not only lines and regions, but also some abstract phenomenology (a sense of perspective) which is subject to a degree of voluntary control. What is striking here is the looseness of fit between the more abstract and the more concrete parts of experience. It seems that, like a sound engineer, we have some capacity to control which parts go into the mix, and how they will sound.

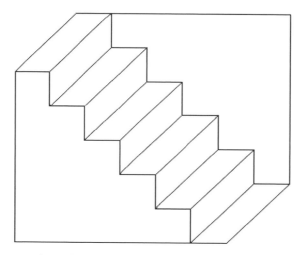

Figure 5.1   Inverting stairs.

Although this evidence is suggestive of the multitrack model, it is strictly speaking equivocal where the single-track/multitrack distinction is concerned. The case for multitrack polyphony starts to look quite compelling, however, when these phenomenological data are combined with a range of neuroscientific findings. Neurologists have long studied the experiential consequences of brain injury. They observe complicated patterns of ablation and sparing, both across and within modalities. It is possible, for example, to lose the capacity visually to detect (or experience) motion, while retaining other aspects of visual experience (Zeki, 1993, p. 82), or to lose colour sensations while retaining visual form and motion experiences (Sacks, 1995, pp. 1–38). Phenomenal deficits of this kind are now known to be the result of lesions in specific parts of the brain. Lesion studies have, in fact, been instrumental in establishing the degree and kinds of functional specialization and localization in the brain. The picture that is emerging is of a brain which divides and conquers, with broad divisions among modalities and task domains reflected in large-scale anatomical divisions (e.g. primary visual processing in occipital cortex, auditory processing in temporal cortex, planning and working memory in frontal cortex), while more fine-grained functional distinctions are reflected in correspondingly restricted anatomical divisions and loci (e.g. visual motion detection in area V5, colour processing in V4). Other kinds of studies, such as functional magnetic resonance imaging (fMRI), position emission tomography (PET), microelectrode and event-related potential (ERP), which are effective over a wide range of spatial and temporal scales, have lately confirmed and enriched this picture with regard to both normal and abnormal function.

The following picture emerges: pathological *losses* of phenomenology are associated with brain lesions at specific sites, while transient but related *alterations* in experience (caused by changes in input or task demands) are found to covary with activity at these same sites. Thus, variations in conscious experience appear to march in lock-step with reproducible, physically localized variations in brain activity, variations, moreover, at brain sites where the relevant informational contents are thought to be encoded. From here it is a short step to the following conclusion: the brain sites that code for particular informational contents are the very sites where those contents are made conscious. Since the contents and associated brain loci are multiple, phenomenal consciousness is multitrack.

A further, tantalizing, piece of evidence for the multitrack model has recently been discovered by Zeki and Bartels. They discuss experimental work on visual processing that suggests that when the different attributes of a visual scene are presented simultaneously, these attributes are not perceived at the same time. It appears that colour is perceived before orientation, which in turn is perceived before motion, the difference between colour and motion being about 60–80 ms (Bartels & Zeki 1998, p. 2329). Experiments in which subjects are asked to pair two rapidly alternating states of two attributes (e.g. a bar with two possible orientations and two possible colours) reveal systematic misbinding of attributes relative to their actual time of occurrence (Zeki & Bartels 1998, p. 1583). This suggests to Zeki & Bartels that there are 'multiple visual micro-consciousnesses which are asynchronous with respect to each other' (p. 1584), which in turns leads them to advocate a multitrack theory: 'consciousness is not a unitary faculty, but . . . consists of many micro-consciousnesses' (Bartels & Zeki 1998, p. 2327).

The upshot of all this is that the multitrack model of phenomenal consciousness has to be taken quite seriously. It is consistent with the phenomenological and neuroscientific evidence, and doesn't succumb to any obvious a priori objections. Rather, this model appears a viable alternative to current single-track orthodoxy.

The emergence of the self

One area where abandoning the traditional doctrine of the unity of consciousness has major ramifications is in our understanding of the self. Single-track theorists typically explain how the brain constructs a self by deploying exactly the same resources they use to explain the generation of conscious experience. From this perspective, the self and its experiences represent a package deal: the very existence of the latter presupposes the existence of the former (see, for example, Damasio, 1999). This is part of the 'conventional wisdom' to which we alluded in the introduction. But it is wisdom that is put under pressure by the symptoms of schizophrenia. Schizophrenia, in its delusional variant, is a condition that impairs some aspects of self-consciousness while leaving others intact. In particular, sense of agency can come apart from sense of subjectivity. This suggests that the self, when all is well, is a complex entity constructed out of independently conscious parts – a multiplicity, not a unity.

In this section we briefly discuss these implications of the multitrack model of consciousness for the nature of the self, and examine some recent speculations about the neurological basis of schizophrenia which support this perspective.

According to the multitrack model, conscious experience is not unitary; it is a complex amalgam of coconscious elements, each generated by a distinct conscious-ness-making mechanism somewhere in the brain. If one adopts this perspective then it is no longer possible to regard *self*-consciousness as the product of a cen-tralized workspace, or of a single global process such as time-locked coactivation. Consciousness ceases to be a package deal as far as its neural realization is con-cerned – there are as many independent physical loci of consciousness as there are distinct information-processing paths in the brain. This means, of course, that our conjectures about the degree of parcellation of self-directed experience are answer-able to the neurocomputational facts. But the symptoms of schizophrenia already offer some grounds for expecting there *not* to be a single neural locus of self and self-consciousness. At a first pass, then, we ought to be wary of the view that the conscious self is physically unitary in the strong sense implied by the doctrine of the unity of consciousness.

As it happens, current conjectures about the neural basis of schizophrenia provide a good deal of support for this multitrack perspective on the self. It is widely held that the positive symptoms of schizophrenia are a pathology of agency, involving changes in the consciousness of action (Frith et al. 1998, Georgieff & Jeannerod, 1999). The leading hypothesis about the physical basis of the disease is that it results from a breakdown in communication among a number of brain regions, including frontal, temporal and cingulate cortices, and various subcortical structures. This lack of integration is thought to be a kind of temporal disconnection syndrome caused by the desynchronization of numerous widely distributed neural systems (Cleghorn & Albert, 1990; Vogeley, 1999). Hand in hand with this hypothesis goes a view about the neural basis of self, namely, that it depends on many distinct centres of self-representation within the brain; from cortical regions associated with somatotopic body mapping and action mapping, through regions that function to distinguish between self-initiated and externally caused events (Georgieff & Jeannerod, 1998), up to regions such as prefrontal cortex that play a crucial role in organizing behaviour. Georgieff & Jeannerod conclude that:

> functions like agency or self-consciousness cannot be mapped on a single localization, even if the involved area seems to fulfil criteria for such a function, in terms of multimodal coding, spatial and temporal integration, etc. The solution to this problem would be to continue further in the direction of fractionating such broad entities as self-construct into more operational elements, and then to relate these elements to specific cortical functions (Georgieff & Jeannerod, 1999, Sect. 2.2).

On a view like this, self-consciousness clearly comes out as multitrack, and the changes in sense of agency associated with schizophrenia as failures of integration among distinct self-representing regions, probably caused by their temporal disconnection.

But if phenomenal consciousness, and self-consciousness in particular, are multitrack, what is one to make of the impression most of us have of being a single, integrated subject? Or, to put it more tendentiously: how does a self emerge from the multiplicity of consciousness? This is a difficult question, largely because there are several senses in which one might claim to be a 'single subject'. Without entering into that murky territory here, we can offer one relatively straightforward answer that is consistent with the multitrack model of consciousness: a self emerges when the multiple tracks of self-directed experience produced by the brain are sufficiently *representationally coherent*. (We use the word 'sufficiently' in this characterization advisedly, since it renders selfhood a matter of degree. We regard this as a strength of the proposal.) Representational coherence concerns the way the various contents of experience relate to each other. In normal circumstances we don't experience a 'blooming, buzzing confusion', but a structured world of discrete objects arrayed in space, a world in which events unfold in a regular, law-like way, and in which informational contents fall into meaningful spatiotemporal patterns. This registration of contents, which is both intramodal (e.g. colour and form) and intermodal (e.g. the registration of proprioceptive, auditory and visual contents as one types on a keyboard), also occurs at the level of specifically self-directed representations. Thus, I typically recognize an action as mine *as* I perform it, am aware of how it fits with my plans, and discover how it affects things about me (and vice versa), all in a real-time, rapidly updated feedback cycle.

Representational coherence is not an invariable feature of conscious experience – it is a hard-won computational achievement, as demonstrated by the many cases (often the result of trauma) in which the brain fails to produce an integrated model of the world. To take a single example, subjects recovering from damage to striate cortex sometimes have quite peculiar visual phenomenology as the visual elements that are normally bound individually 'reappear':

At first the patient will see pure motion (usually rotary) without any form or colour. Then brightness perception returns as a pure Ganzfield – a uniform brightness covering the whole visual field. When colours develop they do so in the form of 'space' or 'film' colours not attached to objects. The latter develop as fragments which join together and eventually the colours enter their objects to complete the construction of the phenomenal object (Smythies, 1994, p. 313).

Normal integration of colour and form to produce coherent objects is initially absent here. Schizophrenia likewise results from an inability to integrate distinct informational contents, but at the level of self-consciousness, such that self-initiated actions or thoughts fail to be recognized as one's own.

The emergence of a self therefore presumably depends on some mechanism that acts to bring the multiple, locally generated contents of conscious experience into register with one another. In particular, such a mechanism must render coherent the multiple streams of self-representation upon which so much of our behaviour depends. A promising manoeuvre for the multitrack theorist is to appropriate one of the neural mechanisms/processes that single-track theorists deploy to explain the production of consciousness, and redeploy it in the new role of explaining the brain's construction of a self. For example, the multitrack theorist might focus on the ERTAS as a neural structure likely to be involved in global communication and integration, as does Baars, but treat it as a *self-maker*, rather than a consciousness-maker.

If we adopt this proposal then it is possible to regard instantaneous consciousness as a multiplicity, rather than a unity, and yet still claim that it is 'unified'. The sense in which consciousness is 'unified' is not a matter of *oneness*, but a matter of representational coherence. Such coherence, perhaps courtesy of the ERTAS (corticocortical circuits may play a role too), goes some way towards explaining how a self emerges from the multiple strands of representational activity in the brain. This proposal is attractive in the current context because it is reasonable to conjecture that schizophrenia is a disease which impairs the capacity of consciousness-making mechanisms to produce a coherent set of experiences. Instead, possibly as a result of desynchronization, these mechanisms operate in an autonomous fashion, producing experiences whose contents are disconnected and discontinuous with one another. This gives rise to the familiar symptoms of schizophrenia. In the case of delusions of thought insertion, for example, it is precisely because one part of the brain generates a thought that is representationally discontinuous with mental contents being produced elsewhere that the patient judges it to be alien, and hence disowns it. What we see here is a partial disintegration of the self, but not in the sense of the self failing to be a single thing – on the multitrack view it was never that in the first place – rather, in the sense that the many self-directed representations produced by the brain no longer hang together as a coherent system.

We finish with a word of caution. Although representational coherence may play a pivotal role in the emergence of our sense of agency, it is not clear that it can account for what we earlier termed our 'sense of subjectivity'. Schizophrenics and others who suffer quite radical breakdowns in the connectedness and continuity of their experience generally have no doubt that these anomalous experiences belong to them (see above). The representational incoherence of the parts of experience doesn't appear to undermine the phenomenal 'togetherness' that characterizes a single subject of experience. A multitrack theorist must therefore appeal to a different set of resources to account for this feature of consciousness. One possibility is that such *subject unity* depends on some feature of brain organization more basic than that which is responsible for representational coherence. For example, the very causal connectedness of the brain as a whole, which is such that a signal can pass from any part of the brain to any other via no more than half a dozen synapses, might be the physical basis of subject unity – even under conditions where representational coherence has broken down. The detailed working-out of this proposal is, however, a task we must leave for another time.

REFERENCES

Baars, B.J. (1988). *A Cognitive Theory of Consciousness.* Cambridge: Cambridge University Press.
Baars, B.J. (1997). *In the Theater of Consciousness: The Workspace of the Mind.* New York: Oxford University Press.

Bartels, A. & Zeki, S. (1998). The theory of multi-stage integration in the visual brain. *Proceedings of the Royal Society of London. B*, **265**, 2327–32.

Bayne, T. (2000). The unity of consciousness: clarification and defence. *Australasian Journal of Philosophy*, **78**, 248–54.

Cleghorn, J.M. & Albert, M.L. (1990). Modular disjunction in schizophrenia: a framework for a pathological psychophysiology. In *Recent Advances in Schizophrenia*, ed. A. Kales, C.N. Stefanis & J. Talbot, pp. 59–80. New York: Springer Verlag.

Damasio, A. (1989). Time-locked multiregional retroactivation: a systems-level proposal for the neural substrate of recall and recognition. *Cognition*, **33**, 25–62.

Damasio, A. (1999). *The Feeling of What Happens: Body and Emotion in the Making of Consciousness*. New York: Harcourt Brace.

Frith, C., Rees, G. & Friston, K. (1998). Psychosis and the experience of self. *Annals of the New York Academy of Sciences*, **843**, 170–8.

Georgieff, N. & Jeannerod, M. (1998). Beyond consciousness of external reality: a "who" system for consciousness of action and self-consciousness. *Consciousness and Cognition*, 7, 465–77.

Georgieff, N. & Jeannerod, M. (1999). Deconstruction of self-consciousness in schizophrenia. Contribution to the ASSC e-seminar *The Human Self Construct and Prefrontal Cortex in Schizophrenia*. http://www.phil.vt.edu/ASSC/vogeley/georgieff1.html

Graham, G. & Stephens, G.L. (1994). Mind and mine. In *Philosophical Psychopathology*, ed. G. Graham & G.L. Stephens, pp. 91–109. Cambridge, MA: MIT Press.

Johnstone, E.C. (1991). Defining characteristic of schizophrenia. *British Journal of Psychiatry*, suppl. **13**, 5–6.

Liddle, P.F. (1987). The symptoms of chronic schizophrenia: a re-examination of the positive–negative dichotomy. *British Journal of Psychiatry*, **151**, 145–51.

McGurk, H. & MacDonald, J. (1976). Hearing lips and seeing voices. *Nature*, **264**, 746–8.

Mellors, C.S. (1970). First-rank symptoms of schizophrenia. *British Journal of Psychiatry*, **117**, 15–23.

O'Brien, G. & Opie, J. (1998). The disunity of consciousness. *Australasian Journal of Philosophy*, **76**, 378–95.

O'Brien, G. & Opie, J. (2000). Disunity defended: a reply to Bayne. *Australasian Journal of Philosophy*, **78**, 255–63.

Penrose, R. (1989). *The Emperor's New Mind*. New York: Oxford University Press.

Sacks, O. (1995). *An Anthropologist On Mars*. Sydney: Picador.

Searle, J. (2000). Consciousness. *Annual Review of Neuroscience*, **23**, 557–78.

Smythies, J.R. (1994). Requiem for the identity theory. *Inquiry*, **37**, 311–29.

Vogeley, K. (1999). Cortico-cortical and subcortical implementation of the self construct. Contribution to the ASSC e-seminar *The Human Self Construct and Prefrontal Cortex in Schizophrenia*. http://www.phil.vt.edu/ASSC/vogeley/vogeley9.html

Zeki, S. (1993). *A Vision of the Brain*. Oxford: Blackwell.

Zeki, S. & Bartels, A. (1998). The asynchrony of consciousness. *Proceedings of the Royal Society of London. B*, **265**, 1583–5.

6

Asynchrony, implicational meaning and the experience of self in schizophrenia

Philip J. Barnard

MRC Cognition and Brain Sciences Unit, Cambridge, UK

Abstract

This chapter opens by outlining the basic architecture of interacting cognitive subsystems (Barnard, 1985, 1999) and then briefly summarizes its application to depression (Barnard & Teasdale, 1991; Teasdale & Barnard, 1993). The account of depression relies on the idea that cognitive-affective processes involve two distinct kinds of meaning: propositional meaning and implicational meaning. Propositional meaning is referentially specific while implicational meaning is more abstract and generic in nature. Affect and ideation are linked up in schematic models encoded as implicational meanings. Among other things, these schematic models represent our sense of *self*. In a context where negative self-schematic models dominate mental processing, feedback from propositional and body state representations acts to regenerate negative self-models and, in doing so, sustains depression.

The chapter then considers how the mechanisms underlying processing exchanges between two types of meaning can be extended to develop accounts of the *core* symptoms of a broader range of psychopathologies and the individual variation so often seen in symptom expression. The extension postulates four underlying sources of variation that constrain the dynamic processing of *meaning*. They are: (1) variation in the content of semantic representations; (2) variation in the rate of change in the content of mental images; (3) variation in the *mode* in which mental processes operate; and (4) variation in the synchronization of the processes that generate meaning. All four sources of variation are needed to account for variation in symptom expression across and within types of psychopathology.

In schizophrenia, it is hypothesized that the processing exchanges between the two kinds of meaning become desynchronized. This results in the generation of semantic images in the mind in which components of implicational meaning come together in patterns that lie outside the bounds of prior 'normal' variation in the content of semantic representations. The mechanism adapts to reshape its *schematic models* of experiences of self and others. It may also alter the characteristic modes in which processes operate. Just as depression may see a *reduced* sense of self-agency associated with negative affect, so experience in schizophrenia may result in the remodelling of self- and other agency in terms of generic, implicational dimensions such as control, causality and change. It may also alter how affect, or the lack of it, is related to them. Properties of the processing of implicational meaning, and its configural consequences for activity in the wider interacting cognitive subsystems architecture are used to derive an account of both the positive and the negative symptoms of schizophrenia.

The published literature on the biological and cognitive-affective underpinnings of schizophrenic experience contains a huge range of specific theories. The account offered here draws on several prior theoretical proposals concerning the underpinnings of such psychopathologies. They include problems with perception, attention and multimodal integration; problems with meta-representation; problems in the autoregulation of mentation in the presence of significant discrepancies in self-representation as well as claims that affect itself lies at the heart of the disorder. The chapter concludes by considering how the concept of implicational meaning, and processing activity that depends upon it, can help to unify several strands of theoretical reasoning about schizophrenia. Implicational meaning is constructed by integrating the first-order products of visual, acoustic and bodily sensation with the products of processing *propositional* meaning. The schematic models embodied at an implicational level of representation then function both to control the generation of new propositions and to control visceral and somatic responses like facial expression. Implicational meaning provides a theoretically grounded means of unifying facets of schizophrenic experience that have been addressed by otherwise distinct theories. Since asynchronous processing is central to the account offered, there are potentially very direct links between an information-processing analysis and potential dysfunctions in the underlying neurological architecture that might, for example, arise from problems associated with network structure, interhemispheric communication or with the operation neurotransmitter systems.

Introduction

In schizophrenia, personal experience and understanding of self are significantly disrupted in complex and subtle ways. Such disruptions have posed a difficult and enduring challenge for theory development. Firstly, schizophrenic experiences are often hard to capture and convey in words (Hurlburt, 1990; Frith, 1992). Secondly, the self has multiple facets. Strawson (1999), for example, listed no less than 25 different ways of qualifying the term and extensive interdisciplinary debate has provided little consensus of thought concerning the self and its properties (Gallagher & Shear, 1999). Thirdly, when we seek accounts of schizophrenia in computer models of the mind, or in terms of brain mechanisms, we run the risk of reducing self-experience and self-representations to mere labels for constructs in a box diagram or neural network. In clinical contexts, such theories are justifiably found wanting.

Following the path pioneered by Frith (1992), this chapter considers what cognitive theory can contribute to debates about self-representations, our subjective experience of them, and how both can be disrupted in psychopathologies. The arguments are all based on an architecture for the mind called interacting cognitive subsystems, or ICS (Barnard, 1985, 1999). It is a modular architecture of nine subsystems, each specialized to process representations of information in different

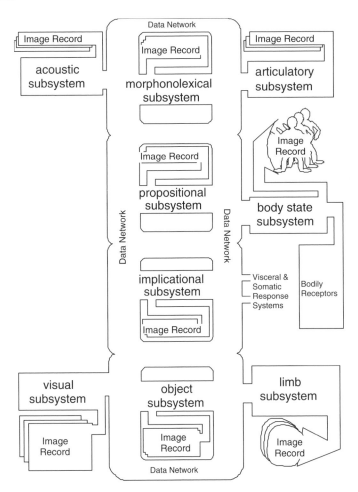

Figure 6.1   An overview of the interactive cognitive subsystems architecture.

domains of mental life (Figure 6.1). Some deal with auditory–verbal representations (acoustic, morphonolexical (MPL) and articulatory). Others handle representations involved in the visuospatial control of action (visual, object and limb). Two deal with representations of meaning (propositional and implicational) and another with body state representations. Each subsystem has its own 'memory', called an image record.

Like other multilevel theories (e.g. see Teasdale, 1999a), ICS assumes that the processing of meaning, including self-related material, is based upon interactions between levels of mental representation. ICS postulates two qualitatively distinct levels of meaning. Propositional meaning is referentially specific. It is the sort of meaning we express in sentences. Implicational meaning is more abstract. It is latent meaning rather than articulated meaning. It integrates over sensory, bodily and ideational dimensions to create, among other things, elaborate schematic models of the self as construed in ideation, in a body state and in an environmental context. It supports generic senses of knowing or intuitions. Implicational meaning can be affectively charged, and equates with a sense of 'knowing with the heart'. Propositional meaning equates more to 'knowing with the head'. Processing exchanges between these two levels of meaning are the 'central engine' of mental life (Teasdale & Barnard, 1993). These exchanges drive the thematic evolution of ideation over time and its affective correlates.

ICS has been used to formulate a theory of unipolar depression (Barnard & Teasdale, 1991; Teasdale & Barnard, 1993; Teasdale, 1999b). In depressed states, the central engine readily enters a form of dynamic interlock. Schematic models at an implicational level generate negative propositions about the self and its inability to control situations, to cause things to happen or to bring about change. These negative propositions are then used to generate feedback to the implicational subsystem. The result is that the same negative schematic model is regenerated. Figure 6.2 depicts this interaction as the black flow pattern. It illustrates another

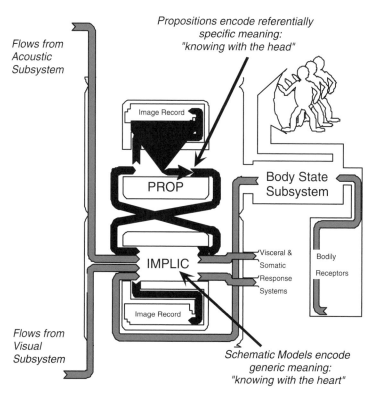

Figure 6.2   The processing loops in interactive cognitive subsystems model that can enter interlock and maintain a depressed state. Prop, propositional subsystem; Implic, implicational subsystem.

feedback loop between implicational and body state representations. This loop, along with inputs from processing acoustic and visual patterns, contributes to the regeneration and maintenance of negative self-modelling at the implicational level.

This account has many properties in common with other theories. It incorporates the idea that variation in self-representation, derived from experience, contributes to vulnerability (e.g. Beck, 1976). It also relies on the widely held view that discrepant meanings play an important role in processing and in the operation of feedback loops (Higgins, 1987; Carver & Scheier, 1998). ICS also has a number of distinctive features. The contrasting properties of propositional and implicational meaning are one such feature. Another is the idea that mental processes can work together in different modes, and that the mode adopted relates to our phenomenological awareness of what is on the mental landscape. A process can be configured to transform information as it arrives; it can reconfigure to use representations recently copied into the memory record in a mode called *buffered processing*; or it can reconfigure to look at the longer-term regularities preserved in its memory record. Of these modes, only the buffered state results in focal awareness. The black triangular structure (Figure 6.2) illustrates the buffered processing of an extended propositional representation and some 'rational' aspect of referentially specific meaning would thus be in focal awareness (Teasdale & Barnard, 1993; Teasdale, 1999b).

In the evolving ICS account of depression, self-representations, the modes in which they are processed and rates of change in their content are three key sources of variation. These sources help us to characterize differences in the mental activity of those likely to experience anxious, depressed or elated moods at the extremes of normal variation and those able to remain within the normal range. In depression, for example, there will be some variation in the specific propositions being generated, but a depressogenic model of the self is continually regenerated at the implicational level. This implies a *low rate of change* in information at this level of self-representation. In contrast, a flight of ideas in mania (Goodwin & Jamison, 1990) would be associated with processing positive or mixed-valence schematic models and *high rates of change* in implicational representations, with pressure of speech a potential consequence of rapid ideation.

The theory predicts that depression will remit, not when specific negative meanings are less accessible, but when there is a qualitative shift in the generically encoded schematic model of self at the heart of mental life (Teasdale et al., 1995). It also implies that the mode entered can be systematically related to rates of change. A short-term discrepancy or change may attract the buffered mode, and bring the content of that discrepancy into focal awareness. A stable pattern, including enduring self-related discrepancies, may not attract the buffered mode and these discrepancies would then be out of focal awareness. Depression, with a low rate of change in implicational meaning, may be typified by a pattern of mental activity in which the dominant configuration, as in Figure 6.2, involves the buffered mode operating on propositional representations (Teasdale, 1999b). In mania, implicational meaning and its more generic content are more likely to attract and sustain the buffered mode. If this configuration were to dominate, then the 'specifics' of propositional meaning would remain largely unevaluated in extended ideation and would tend to remain outside focal awareness. Both are features that might help account for why manic states are associated with impulsive behaviours, like spending sprees (Goodwin & Jamison, 1990).

Figure 6.2 also illustrates how information arriving from sensory sources, perhaps an angered tone of voice, a critical facial expression and a lethargic body state, are integrated with products of processing propositional meaning and thus contribute to the formation of implicational representations. This figure suggests a fourth source of variation. For information from distinct sources to integrate in a normal pattern, bits and pieces of information must all arrive at the right time. If the timing of the exchanges between propositional and implicational levels were to become desynchronized, then patterns of meaning would be discrepant with previously established patterns. Representations would be created in the mind whose nature and use lie outside the range that typify normal processing, and which would have profound consequences for ideation, affect, our experience of them and how we adapt to them.

This chapter has three aims. The first is to provide outline accounts of the core signs and symptoms of schizophrenia based upon the hypothesis that they all arise as consequences of asynchronous processing between two levels of meaning. Variations in representations, modes of processing, rates of change and asynchronies will all contribute to variation in symptom expression over time and over individuals. A secondary aim is to illustrate how these sources of variability provide a theoretically motivated basis for understanding why certain symptoms overlap with those expressed in other diagnostic categories of psychopathology. The third aim is to illustrate how thinking in terms of sources of variation might help to bridge the gulf between theoretical descriptions and clinical realities.

Theoretical foundations for variation in representations, modes of processing and rates of change

All subsystems work in exactly the same way. They differ only in the *mental code* used to build representations (Teasdale & Barnard, 1993). From very simple principles concerning the construction and use of representations, properties of more complex

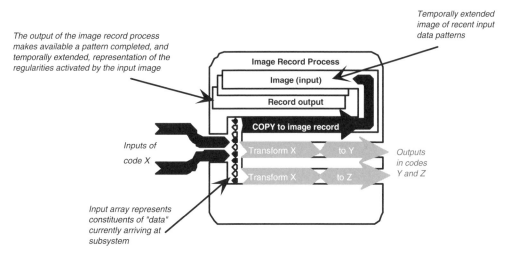

Figure 6.3   The copy and image record processes of an interactive cognitive subsystems subsystem.

interactions across the entire architecture can be inferred and specified. These relate to the *images* constructed in each subsystem and the configural flows between subsystems that give rise to their formation or follow on from their formation.

Each subsystem is composed of three kinds of processes (Figure 6.3): a copy process, a record process and processes that transform mental representations. Inputs arriving at a subsystem are mapped into an input array. This contains the information pattern arriving at the subsystem *now*. The copy process transfers this pattern to the image record. The input to the image record creates a temporally extended trace, or image, of recently arrived inputs. It is a dynamic representation of a sequence of information patterns and this reflects *rates of change* in input. It is that subsystem's short-term memory.

The record is depicted as three overlapping layers – the image (input) layer, an intervening layer and a record output layer. As with many other approaches, in-formation is viewed as hierarchically structured. As constituents arrive, those that go together are structured into basic units. The record then abstracts superordi-nate organizations of basic units that arrive over time. It preserves the invariants that underlie experience, be they sensory, perceptual, semantic or motoric regular-ities. It is a subsystem's long-term memory. The image records are the theoretical foundation for *representational variability*, be it related to the particular language we acquire (auditory-verbal records) or related to conceptual knowledge and self-representation (propositional and implicational records).

The image record is not a passive repository. It is a process. Its dynamic input constantly generates an output. This third layer of the record provides record output

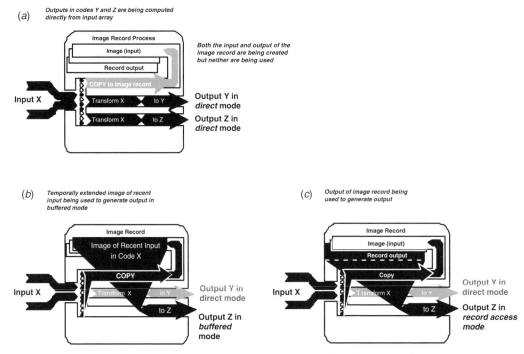

Figure 6.4   Three modes of process operation: (a) direct; (b) buffered; (c) record access.

(Figures 6.3 and 6.4). The middle layer supports the mapping from record input to record output. The output contains a temporally organized trace of superordinate regularities that have recently been activated by input. Like a pattern recognition mechanism, an incomplete image on input can have missing components computed from past regularities. Retrieval is not like searching indices in a library for a book, finding it on the shelves and then opening it. The record process responds to its input by automatically opening relevant books on the right pages on the output layer. A process can simply reconfigure for record access, look at these pages and then transform what is found (Figure 6.4c).

The third type of process carries out these transformations. In direct mode (Figure 6.4a), a process reacts to moment-to-moment changes in information patterns as they arrive. This mode supports fast and automatic processing. When the moment-to-moment changes are hard to transform in real time, the process can reconfigure to look at the input image. This creates a mechanism for the *buffered* use of extended representations of recent input (Figure 6.4b). Operating in one of three modes, processes generate intricate configurations of flow between subsystems (Figure 6.5).

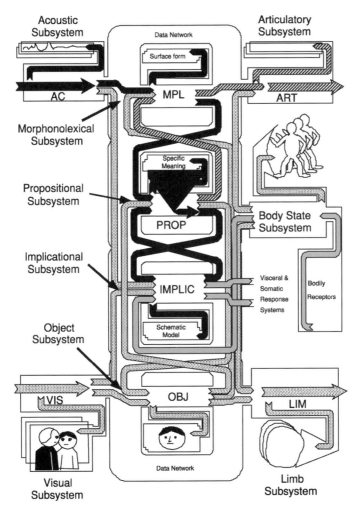

Figure 6.5   A dynamic patterning of information flow among subsystems. See Figure 6.1 for definition of abbreviations.

Images, awareness, flow and self-representation

As information flows among subsystems, images are constantly created at each level of representation. In ICS, the copy processes provide the foundations for awareness. Distributed over the nine subsystems they create dynamic, short-lived images in the mind. As a collective, and through their construction of representations, they support our diffuse sense of the products of mental activity across the entire architecture. So, the images in the visual and auditory subsystems are what we 'see' and 'hear' in the world, while the body-state image is what we 'feel' in the body.

Those in the MPL and object subsystems support our experiences of verbal and visual imagery 'in the head'. The articulatory and limb subsystems create images of subvocal speech and intended movements. The propositional image supports experiences of *knowing that* 'I am 52 years old, balding, with a job, wife and two volatile teenage sons'. It represents the cold facts, the self-as-object, or something akin to William James' (1890/1983) 'me-self'. The implicational image supports our experience of the wider schematic context in which the *knowing that . . .* is embedded. Here it is combined with other knowledge of family and career and where it is linked to 'senses' of satisfaction or disappointment, to looking forward to the future or being apprehensive about it. It represents self-as-subject or something akin to James' 'I-self'. Although representations of self and others are of central importance in psychopathologies, propositional and implicational representations cover all domains of human knowledge.

It is important to think of ICS as a *dynamic* system. Figure 6.5 is not a wiring diagram. Nor, like the earliest forms of box models (Waugh & Norman, 1965), are processing stages strictly ordered. Flows intersect and interact in configurations. The information in images, and that available from record outputs, is constantly changing. Processes also continually alter their modes of operation in a collective effort to sustain processing efficiency and adaptive behaviour. There is no homunculus controlling activity. The functions of a 'central executive' are fulfilled by interchanges between propositional and implicational meanings (Barnard, 1999).

For example, the configuration for language understanding is highlighted in black in Figure 6.5. Speech waveforms (AC) are transformed into words and phrases (MPL), and their referential meaning is mapped into the propositional image. Here, word meanings can be linked up with meaning arriving from current visuospatial processing, such as a pointing gesture accompanying a request like 'Please pass *that* cup'. Propositional meaning is used to generate implicational constituents which come together in the implicational image with constituents derived from current sensory patterns such as tone of voice, facial expression and bodily feelings to yield an implicational model. Such models can concurrently generate additional material that is fed back to the propositional subsystem where it can constrain or extend the interpretation of the incoming linguistic stream, and create new propositions online that form the basis for any verbal responses. Reciprocal cycles of processing activity between the two levels of meaning support the thematic evolution of ideational content and allied constructs like evaluation, appraisal, generalization, inference and any affective experiences associated with them.

The modes adopted by processes are determined by information states. When asked a question like 'When did you last see your father?' the modes within the central engine might adjust several times in a few hundred milliseconds. The process transforming propositions into implicational meanings might switch from buffered mode to access current output of the propositional record. If the 'answer' were not there, then processes would automatically reconfigure to access relevant models in the implicational record to generate fresh input to the propositional image. Successive mode changes and record access at both levels might be required until a referentially specific answer, like 'last Sunday', is resolved and evaluated as appropriate in that context. At which point the buffer might again shift to the propositional process that generates the exact wording (MPL) for speech output (see Figure 6.10, below).

A process transforming a representation can only deal with one stream of information at a time, and can only work in one mode at a time (Barnard, 1985). Direct processing and record access occur out of awareness. Only the buffered mode mediates focal awareness, and only one process in a wider configuration can be buffered at a given time. Focal awareness is therefore selective in two ways. We are focally aware of the *qualitative* properties of the mental image whose content is being buffered, and we are also focally aware of the content of the particular stream of information being selected from that image for onward transformation (Teasdale & Barnard, 1993). Subjective experience and theoretical functions are now closely coupled. The point where the buffer resides is the implicit locus of control for activity throughout a configuration. It determines both the rate of flow through the configuration and what is selected to flow through it. The buffer will move to a point in that configuration where it is best placed to deal with significant changes in image content; to resolve uncertainties or discrepancies in those images; or to coordinate use of relevant image records.

If things go seriously wrong in one part of the architecture, such as asynchronous exchanges between levels of meaning, then image content will be affected. Configural patterns of information flow will be perturbed, and changes in the way buffered processing is characteristically used to coordinate mental activity will be reflected in altered states of awareness. Schizophrenic experiences of self, others and the world will be attributed to the formation, in the implicational image, of schematic models that lie outside the normal range. Certain signs and symptoms will follow as effects of central asynchronies propagate across the architecture. Other signs and symptoms will appear as the implicational record degrades, and as the architecture increasingly comes to rely on its other resources to sustain and coordinate its activities.

As the other half of the central engine partnership, the propositional subsystem plays a key role in propagating the effects of abnormal formations of implicational meaning and in compensating for their consequences. The propositional subsystem accepts three inputs that combine to produce referentially specific meanings (Figure 6.6). In addition to input from the implicational subsystem, it receives inputs from the MPL and object subsystems. It also generates output to each of these subsystems. An internal feedback loop between the propositional and MPL

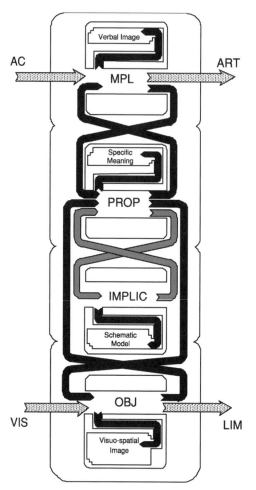

Figure 6.6   Flow patterns into, and out of, the propositional subsystem. See Figure 6.1 for definition of abbreviations.

subsystems can be active even when no output is directed through to overt articulation. In the MPL image, thoughts have verbal form 'in the head', that are open to interpretation as 'voices' by patients, and occasionally others (Leudar & Thomas, 2000), and their meaning can once again be fed back for further propositional and implicational processing. On the visuospatial side, the propositional subsystem can create object-level representations. The object image can be used to guide visual attention to objects in perceptual search or, when products are passed to the limb subsystem, to coordinate sequences of actions in the world. When operating solely as an internal feedback loop, exchanges between propositional and object subsystems are what enable us to form and use abstract visuospatial images in the mind (imagine your own coffee mug . . .).

The propositional subsystem is viewed as a resource unique to the human mind. Its presence means that the thematic evolution of human ideation can occur concurrently with the online conceptual control of actions in the world. It enters into one reciprocal loop with the MPL subsystem, which is what enables us to coordinate speaking and listening. It enters into another with the object subsystem, which is what enables us to coordinate movements in a changing visual world. The exchanges between propositional and implicational meaning endow us with the extra processing power to think abstractly about what we are doing while conversing and walking. Its presence also endows us with the potential for unique psychopathologies in the processing of meaning.

The theoretical foundation of asynchrononous processing of image content

Two things follow from the arrangement of processes in ICS. Firstly, the conceptual products of propositional processing of external inputs will always arrive in the implicational image *later than* the immediate products of sensory processing linked to the same inputs. Some products of sensory patterns, like tone of voice and facial expression, are fed direct to the implicational subsystem (Figure 6.2). Other components of implicational meanings are established by processing MPL or object structures and propositional meaning. These longer routes inevitably take more time (Figure 6.5). Secondly, when propositional processes interact with implicational processes, any feedback received by the implicational subsystem will be copied back into its image *with a characteristic lag* on the content of that image to which the feedback relates.

The buffered mode enables a subsystem to identify, be aware of and associate invariant patterns of information when their parts are offset in time. The processes that transform subsystem inputs into outputs will have *learned* to react to patterns in the image that originated from external and internal sources but are separated by *characteristic* lags. Figure 6.7 shows a more elaborate rendering of the buffered processing of the implicational image. The input array is expanded to show separate patterns coming from the acoustic, visual, body state and propositional flows. The implicational image is expanded to show 11 time slices of the input that has recently been copied into it. The record process is not shown in this figure.

It needs to be remembered that this is a dynamic image. Information is continually flowing along its extent, from right to left, as new patterns arrive. The small symbols are the constituents of implicational meanings. Groupings of circles and squares are marked with large ovals. These are basic units of implicational representation. An implicational model is an organized structure of these units. The figure shows propositions being generated in buffered mode from some hypothetical schematic model B. This model links one basic unit in the three sensory channels

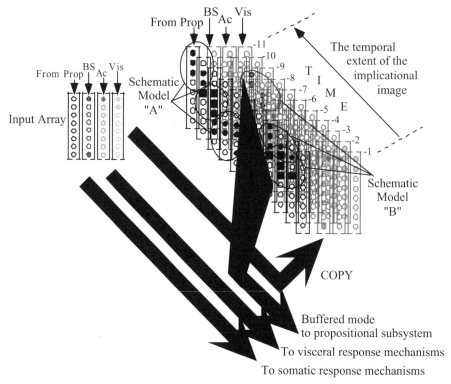

Figure 6.7   An illustration of how propositions are generated in buffered mode, from normal formations of basic units of implicational representations. See Figure 6.1 for definition of abbreviations.

that arrived first, to two other basic units, in the propositional channel. One is a pattern of black circles, the other a pattern of black squares. The black squares lag the circles. The squares represent material that has been fed back into the implicational image as a result of a central engine exchange with the propositional subsystem. A similar pattern is shown for schematic model A, processed a few moments earlier.

If there were disruption in the production of a neurotransmitter such as dopamine, or some other problem with network connectivity, then the feedback (squares) from propositional processes might deviate from its characteristic offsets from the material (circles) to which it relates. Theoretically, offsets can be constant and small or constant and large. Alternatively, offsets could *vary* from one time to another. Rather like a faulty distributor in a car ignition system, the feedback could be 'advanced' or 'retarded' relative to some ideal value. In all cases, the result would be abnormal formations of implicational meanings. In Figure 6.8, the black squares have been delayed by one time slice. The expected pattern is now marked with white squares. The discrepant positions between known and actual contain question marks. These

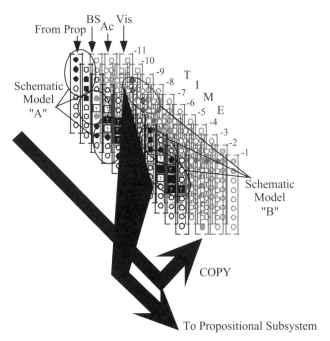

Figure 6.8   An illustration of how propositions are generated in buffered mode from abnormal formations of ill-formed individual basic units in the implicational image. See Figure 6.1 for
definition of abbreviations.

discrepancies are concentrated in the same general areas for models A and B to apply,
but the constituents of adjacent basic units are now intermingled. In Figure 6.9,
the feedback has been delayed by three time slices. In those areas where basic
units of feedback should be, there is no pattern. These areas contain large question
marks. The feedback actually appears in two other quite distinct regions of the
image, that can be processed, not as part of models A and B, but as parts of a third
model, C.

The disruptive effects of varying the delay in auditory feedback of one's own voice
are well known. With a short extra delay, speech production is significantly disrupted
(Flanagan, 1951). With longer delays, smooth production is resumed. It seems that
the feedback stream can be isolated and 'streamed out' at its characteristic offset
and with longer artificial delays. However, in between these bounds, the feedback
stream is difficult to separate from a stream carrying the intended vocal output.
Figures 6.8 and 6.9 demonstrate that exactly the same kind of argument can be
applied to the processing of two levels of meaning.

When exchanges between two levels of meaning become asynchronous, the immediate products of sensory and body state processing are also going to be misaligned with ideational and affective correlates in the feedback stream. Bleuler's

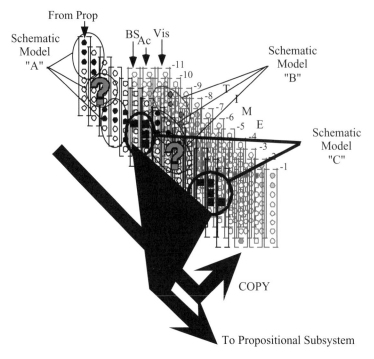

Figure 6.9   The generation of propositions, in buffered mode, from abnormal organizations of relatively well-formed basic units in the implicational image. Purely for the purposes of illustration, the temporal extent of the propositional channel has been extended beyond its assumed limit. See Figure 6.1 for definition of abbreviations.

(1911/1950) original conception that different mental faculties undergo some form of separation is realized in this theoretical framework by stream separation within the implicational image.

Symptom expression

Acute signs and symptoms

Implicational representations lack the referential specificity of propositions. Just as the precise wording of a sentence is lost when creating a representation of its propositional meaning, so the precise details of propositions are summarized when sent to the implicational subsystem. When asynchronous exchanges initially develop, implicational images are discrepant with prior regularities in experience and the architecture would automatically attempt to model these new patterns. In doing so, it would make use of internally generated exchanges with the propositional subsystem and access record content in an effort to interpret, resolve and 'explain' these new states. Frith (1992) cites Ruocchio's (1991) personal account: 'There are things that happened to me that I have never found words for, some lost now, some of which I still search desperately to explain ...'.

Such observations dovetail neatly with the hypothesis that such experiences relate to the processing of abnormal formations of generic, rather than specific meaning. The correlates of buffering ill-formed implicational images might include 'auras' or generic 'senses' of unfamiliarity and strangeness. Misaligned sensory patterns might be felt to have special significance (Hemsley, 1992). The experiences would be difficult to express in words and to resolve, since asynchronous feedback results in generic meanings that do not fit in where they should. The negative affective correlates of discrepancy might include discomfort, apprehension or terror. Positive correlates might occur if some discrepant pattern resolves into an apparently meaningful pattern, perhaps leading to a sense of insight or revelation.

The ordering of propositions is vital for the formation of schematic models. 'I took a drink and vomited' means something quite different from 'I vomited and took a drink'. At an implicational level, the drink would typically be modelled as a causal influence in the former, but as a restorative measure in the latter. In cycles of central engine activity, constituents of implicational meaning, the stuff from which specific propositions are computed, get mixed up. While small offsets would still permit propositions to be generated, the products of central engine activity would be disorganized and many kinds of association, be they causal attributions or otherwise, could be derived. As with the effects of delayed auditory feedback, the smooth interoperation of the dynamic exchanges between levels of meaning would be disrupted.

Were the system to reconfigure to buffer processing of propositional images for language production (Figure 6.10), then the underlying implicational image would be out of focal awareness. When configured in this mode *knowing that* ... some specific meaning held would be in focal awareness. If the propositions were now passed through to overt articulation, they would be realized as incoherent speech. Being intermingled at their source in the implicational image, propositions would not necessarily follow one from another and this would result in signs such as illogicality, tangentiality, derailment or loss of goal (Frith, 1992). Out of awareness, the asynchronous feedback into the implicational image would be contributing to distorted image content and, through this, the potential for continued incoherent thought.

Since the products of sensory and body state processes are concurrently fed into the implicational image, conditions exist where sensory properties, like tone of voice, facial expressions and changes in body state, would also be misaligned with their ideational correlates (Figure 6.8). These, in turn, create conditions for disruptions to the normal receptive dynamics of voice or face recognition, as well as in their expression (Cutting, 1985; Murphy & Cutting, 1990; Braun et al., 1991). The

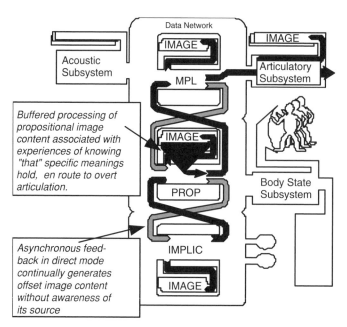

Figure 6.10   Language production under conditions of asynchronous processing in the central engine. See Figure 6.1 for definition of abbreviations.

implicational subsystem (Figure 6.2) contains separate processes for mapping to somatic and visceral responses. This would make it possible for the somatic correlates of flattened expressive affect to be in evidence while affect was none the less being *felt* as a result of visceral and ideational feedback to the implicational image (Neale et al., 1998). Asynchronously constructed implicational image content, and the configurations associated with its use, can thus account for disorganized ideation, misinterpretation of generic properties of sensation as well as the expression of incongruous or flattened affect.

When temporal offsets are greater (Figure 6.9), the feedback generates a stream of separated basic units. These have the potential to be processed as a distinct implicational model (C in Figure 6.9). Buffered processing would bring into focal awareness a generic sense of relatively well-formed units unconnected to the models that had actually led to their formation. If the content of these units were to propagate through to morphonolexical realisation, then verbal images of this separate stream would be made available (Figure 6.11a). These would cooccur in a mental context where sensory patterns are also out of alignment in the implicational image. Together, these images provide conditions for auditory hallucinations to occur. If the system dynamically alternates between the buffering of implicational (Figure 6.11a) and MPL images (Figure 6.11b), then the experience would be of a verbal stream *not associated with* self-as-agent. Reciprocal cycles of activity between the two levels

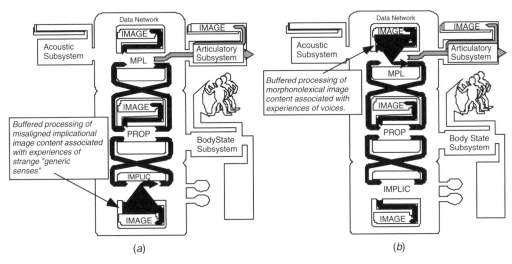

Figure 6.11   Processing of abnormal formations of meaning in (a) a configuration where implicational meanings are buffered and (b) where verbal images of the products of central engine activity are buffered and being fed back for semantic interpretation. See Figure 6.1 for definition of abbreviations.

of meaning would then evaluate, appraise, generalize and draw inferences about these information states. Any shifts in buffered processing to some propositional resolution (Figure 6.10) would correspond to *knowing that* these thoughts were in some way linked to some other agent or force, perhaps being inserted or spoken by them, or being taken by or broadcast to them. If similar products of central engine ideation propagated to processing coordinated in the visuospatial domain (Figure 6.6), then equivalent experiences would relate to actions controlled by some external agent or force.

Longer-term adaptations

Different offsets, or worse still, offsets that themselves vary over time, provide points of departure for many patterns of symptoms and illness trajectories. These will depend upon how the system adjusts its representations and the modes characteristically adopted in their processing. Here, just a few examples will be used to illustrate the theoretical reasoning associated with interactions between the extent of asynchronies, representational variation, rates of change and modes of processing.

Faced with image content outside the range of prior experiences, record processes would automatically attempt to remodel any new regularities within both levels of meaning. Major remodelling of systems of self-, other- and world representation occurs in the course of normal cognitive development. When significant transitions occur in either infancy or adolescence, they are often accompanied by phases of oversimplified or 'black-and-white' thinking as well as emotional volatility (Harter, 1999). Adaptation to new organizations of basic units arising from large and consistent offsets should follow a similar course. Variation across individuals would lie in the exact form of implicational models derived to accommodate the ideational and affective attributes of these new organizations. This would not be a matter of some faulty mental logic (Bentall et al., 1991), nor a failure in self-monitoring *per se* (Frith, 1992). It would be more a matter of establishing new statistical regularities in the cooccurrences of basic units and modelling the causal origins of their presence. The precise trajectory into delusional systems, such as paranoia, would obviously depend on the particular generic models of self, and the social and physical world that held before the condition developed. The trajectory would also depend on any black-and-white or egocentric thinking that might occur during exchanges between levels of meaning as the remodelling progresses.

With short offsets in the implicational image, the remodelling of representational systems would be expected to follow very different trajectories. Where constituents of adjacent basic units are intermingled, the record process would need to abstract new basic units as well as modelling their organization. If successive cycles of internally generated ideation, with its derailed and incoherent sequences, were to persist for months, statistically reliable 'generic' patterns might prove hard to establish. Were the short lags to be continuously *variable*, conditions might even exist where *few, if any* meaningful regularities arise in internally generated ideation. In either case, the record process in the implicational subsystem would itself undergo varying degrees of degradation. The remodelling would result in significant weakening of past associations as new ones are sought. To return to the analogy of the record process as a library, when the image record is accessed and used, some 'books' predating the onset of the condition might automatically have been opened but in the wrong context, or on the wrong page. They might well be interspersed with other incoherent books written after onset. Such an extensive breakdown in the substrates of ideation would come to be realized in negative signs. Internally generated willed action and coherent social interaction would become increasingly difficult to sustain as a result of degradation and incoherent organization within the stock of schematic models.

The flow patterns permitted in ICS (Figure 6.5) mean that the effects of asynchronous exchanges on the systems of propositional and implicational meaning would not be symmetric. Some of the stock of propositional regularities could be sustained by inputs to the propositional subsystem that arise in the course of dialogues with others, via the flows from acoustic through MPL levels. Other propositional regularities can be sustained through interactions with the physical and social worlds via flows from the visual and object subsystems. Peripheral processes for handling the surface form of language and for coordinating visuospatial action would not necessarily be badly impaired by the problems associated with implicational synthesis. The wider system could still be configured to control speech and action. None the less, if significant degradations of implicational models do occur, then exchanges between the two levels of meaning would no longer drive the normal thematic evolution, elaboration and evaluation of thought content. When mapped to effector subsystems controlling speech or movement, the inevitable result would be two further negative signs: poverty of speech and poverty of action.

The modes characteristically adopted to control and coordinate activity across configurations would also adapt to the new circumstances. With persistently discrepant content, mental activity could not easily be coordinated by extensive buffered processing of the implicational image. As this record process degrades, any accessing of its output would also tend to yield less and less in the way of useful products. The wider system would adapt to coordinate use of its residual capabilities by preferentially buffering the content of images in other subsystems and accessing their records.

In phases of mental activity where discrepant meanings predominate at the implicational level, processing activity might tend to adopt a configuration coordinated from the propositional image. When implicational models no longer provide a systematic modulating influence, conditions can exist where feedback from either the MPL subsystem or the object subsystem to the propositional level can enter interlock. In both cases, the same propositional content would then tend to perseverate in focal awareness. This would be directly analogous to the kind of interlock that Teasdale & Barnard (1993) argue sustains depression, but now operating between different levels of representation.

Indeed, stereotyped behaviours can all be regarded as resulting from interlocked feedback loops. With more extreme degradations of the implicational record process, little in the way of internally generated material would be fed into the propositional image. Coupled with a lowered likelihood, via social communication or real-world action, of externally generated input, there would be low rates of usable change in either propositional or implicational representations. These provide conditions where the wider system would need to reconfigure again and buffer more peripheral images. In these images, there would at least be some rate of systematic change linked to input flows from environmental or bodily sources. In these phases of mental activity, the buffer might 'retire' to coordinate the residually active configurations from the MPL image, the object image or the body state image. In the latter case, interlocked loops can develop between body state and limb subsystems, or between body states and any residual sensory streams represented in the implicational image. These would be an entirely plausible theoretical foundation for stereotypies involving repetitive simple movements such as rocking, nodding or grimacing (Wing et al., 1974). Repetitive speech or repeated, apparently pointless, action sequences could arise when buffering at either the MPL image or the object image is used to control effector processes. In normal conditions, the central engine provides inputs to these images that function to redirect the course of processing on the basis of ideation. With a substantially lowered likelihood of such top-down control, a variety of interlocked peripheral configurations can be sustained via bottom-up feedback from sensory flows, and access to peripheral records of their recent course, or access to the implicational record and its residual representations of sensory streams.

Conclusions

This chapter had three aims. The first was to provide an account of the core signs and symptoms of schizophrenia. All were hypothesized to arise as consequences of asynchronous processing exchanges between two levels of meaning. Asynchronous feedback creates abnormal formations of meaning in the implicational image. These result both in configural adjustments of mental processing activity and in the remodelling of implicational records. Patterns of symptoms were explained on the basis of four theoretically grounded and intercoupled dimensions of variation: in representations; in rates of change; in modes of processing; and in departures from synchronous processing.

The second aim was to illustrate how these dimensions might help explain why certain symptoms exhibited across the schizophrenic spectrum can overlap with those expressed in other categories of psychopathology. To this end, the introduction included brief theoretical accounts of unipolar depression and bipolar affective disorder. The former was associated primarily with the influence of the representational dimension, through vulnerability, on modes adopted and rates of change. The latter was linked primarily to the influence of rates of change in image content and its effects on modes and representations. In this chapter the schizophrenic spectrum has now been linked to the influence of departures from synchrony on the other three dimensions. Since each dimension influences the others, specific diagnostic categories can be viewed as occupying potentially overlapping ranges in a space defined by coordinates on the four dimensions. Covariation along the representational, mode and rate dimensions would enable us to understand why around a third of schizophrenics also experience depression (Creer & Wing, 1975). The delusions associated with mania are also often hard to distinguish from those of the schizophrenic spectrum (Bentall & Kinderman, 1999). How this might come about can serve as a slightly more detailed example of the application of the theoretical reasoning.

The theory predicts that very fast rates of processing in mania could create the same kinds of states in the implicational image as asynchronous feedback. In successive cycles of central engine operation, the process transforming implicational models into propositions would only be able to pick out a subset of the basic units in each model as they 'fly by' in the image. As a result only partial products of processing successive models would be represented in the feedback to the implicational image. The partial products of processing two models A then B could then reappear in that image as candidates for the formation of a new schematic model, C, in much the same way as the longer lags of asynchronous processing (Figure 6.9). When operating close to the uppermost extremes of rates of change, novel combinations might underpin highly imaginative thinking, often associated with mania (e.g. Jamison, 1993), or it might precipitate delusional ideation. The underlying brain mechanisms that give rise to rapid or asynchronous processing might prove to be very different. However, at the level of mental architecture, abnormal organizations of basic units of implicational representation would be the common casual factor underlying delusional ideation in both schizophrenia and mania.

This dimensional analysis suggests other conjectures about common causes. The differences between autism and Asperger's syndrome (Frith, 1991; Happe, 1994) might also follow from variations in feedback into the implicational image. Longer stream offsets result in well-formed basic units (Figure 6.9) and hence would be linked to the higher-functioning end of this spectrum. Shorter or variable offsets would lead to intermingled constituents (Figure 6.8) and to lower levels of functioning. Exactly the same kind of theoretical logic as that used here could then be applied to their similarities and differences. Similarities and differences with the strereotypies, communicative difficulties and social functioning observed in schizophrenia would again be explored along the other dimensions. Adaptation to stream offsets in schizophrenia typically occurs only *after* a stock of adolescent implicational models is in place. Similar offsets in infancy would affect the developmental trajectory of that entire stock, rather than the remodelling of a well-established stock.

The third aim was to illustrate how this kind of analysis might help bridge the gulfs that can exist between theoretical description and clinical realities. The attempt to place symptom variation within a diagnostic category, and overlaps between categories, on firm theoretical foundations, represents one route to narrowing these gulfs. It is also a route favoured by other theorists (e.g. Bentall, 1990). Day-to-day clinical endeavour is all about the management of symptom variation within and among individuals. This in turn depends on interviews and interventions delivered to guide mental activity back into some 'normal' range.

Two distinctive features of ICS, noted in the introduction, were the proposed properties of implicational and propositional meanings, and the coupling of modes of processing with subjective awareness. Both played a role in framing a new intervention for major depression (Teasdale, 1999b) which is proving effective in preventing relapse (Teasdale et al., 2000). Implicational meaning is not simply 'a node' in network, nor is it just a label for a 'box' in a flow diagram of the mind. It is a complex coding system that brings the roots of ideation, sensation and bodily representation together in intricate patterns that are subjectively experienced. It makes general contact with subjective reports about knowing one set of things about the self 'with the head', and a different set of things 'with the heart'. It also provides a possible means of characterizing properties of an individual patient's schematic models (Gumley et al., 1999) and work is underway to explore how an analysis based upon ICS might help shape interventions for preventing relapse in schizophrenia (Gumley & Power, 2000).

REFERENCES

Barnard, P.J. (1985). Interacting cognitive subsystems: a psycholinguistic approach to short term memory. In *Progress in the Psychology of Language*, vol. 2, ed. A. Ellis, pp. 197–258. London: Lawrence Erlbaum.

Barnard, P. (1999). Interacting cognitive subsystems: modeling working memory phenomena within a multi-processor architecture. In *Models of Working Memory: Mechanisms of Active Maintenance and Executive Control*, ed. A. Miyake & P. Shah, pp. 298–339. New York: Cambridge University Press.

Barnard, P.J. & Teasdale, J.D. (1991). Interacting cognitive subsystems: a systemic approach to cognitive-affective interaction and change. *Cognition and Emotion*, **5**, 1–39.

Beck, A.T. (1976). *Cognitive Therapy and the Emotional Disorders*. New York: International Universities Press.

Bentall, R.P. (1990). The syndromes and symptoms of psychosis: or why you can't play 20 questions with the concept of schizophrenia and hope to win. In *Reconstructing Schizophrenia*, ed. R.P. Bentall, pp. 23–60. London: Routledge.

Bentall, R.P. & Kinderman, P. (1999). Self-regulation, affect and psychosis: the role of social cognition in paranoia and mania. In *Handbook of Cognition and Emotion*, ed. T. Dalgleish & M. Power, pp. 354–81. Chichester: Wiley.

Bentall, R.P., Kaney, S. & Dewey, M.E. (1991). Paranoia and social reasoning: an attribution theory analysis. *British Journal of Clinical Psychology*, **30**, 13–23.

Bleuler, E. (1911/50). *Dementia Praecox or the Group of Schizophrenias*. Translated by E. Zinkin. New York: International Universities Press.

Braun, C., Bernier, S., Proulx, R. & Cohen, H. (1991). A deficit of primary facial expression independent of bucco-facial apraxia in chronic schizophrenia. *Cognition and Emotion*, **5**, 147–59.

Carver, C.S. & Scheier, M.F. (1998). *On the Self-regulation of Behaviour*. Cambridge, UK: Cambridge University Press.

Creer, C. & Wing, J.K. (1975). Living with a schizophrenic patient. *British Journal of Hospital Medicine*, **14**, 73–82.

Cutting, J. (1985). *The Psychology of Schizophrenia*. Edinburgh: Churchill Livingstone.

Flanagan, J.L. (1951). Effect of delay distortion upon the intelligibility of speech. *Journal of the Acoustical Society of America*, **23**, 303.

Frith, U. (ed.) (1991). *Autism and Asperger's Syndrome*. Cambridge, UK: Cambridge University Press.

Frith, C.D. (1992). *The Cognitive Neuropsychology of Schizophrenia*. Hove: Lawrence Erlbaum.

Gallagher, S. & Shear, J. (1999). Editor's introduction. In *Models of the Self*, ed. S. Gallagher & J. Shear, pp. ix–xviii. Thorverton, UK: Imprint Academic.

Goodwin, F.K. & Jamison, K.R. (1990). *Manic Depressive Illness*. Oxford: Oxford University Press.

Gumley, A. & Power, K. (2000). Is targeting cognitive therapy during relapse in psychosis feasible? *Behavioural and Cognitive Psychotherapy*, **28**, 161–74.

Gumley, A., White, C.A. & Power, K. (1999). An interacting cognitive subsystems model of relapse and the course of psychosis. *Clinical Psychology and Psychotherapy*, **6**, 261–79.

Happe, F. (1994). *Autism: An Introduction to Psychological Theory*. London: UCL Press.

Harter, S. (1999). *The Construction of the Self: A Developmental Perspective*. New York: Guilford Press.

Hemsley, D.R. (1992). Disorders of perception and cognition in schizophrenia. *Revue Europeenne de Psychologie Applique*, **42**, 105–14.

Higgins, E.T. (1987). Self-discrepancy: a theory relating self and affect. *Psychological Review*, **94**, 319–40.

Hurlburt, R.T. (1990). *Sampling Normal and Schizophrenic Inner Experience*. New York: Plenum Press.

James, W. (1890/1983). *Principles of Psychology*. Harvard: Harvard University Press.

Jamison, K.R. (1993). *Touched with Fire: Manic-depression and the Artistic Temperament*. New York: Free Press Paperbacks.

Leudar, I. & Thomas, P. (2000). *Voices of Reason, Voices of Insanity*. London: Routledge.

Murphy, D. & Cutting, J. (1990). Prosodic comprehension and expression in schizophrenia. *Journal of Neurology, Neurosurgery and Psychiatry*, **53**, 727–30.

Neale, J.M., Blanchard, J.J., Kerr, S., Krin, A.M. & Smith, D.A. (1998). Flat affect in schizophrenia. In *Emotions in Psychopathology*, ed. W.F. Flack & J.D. Laird, pp. 353–64. Oxford: Oxford University Press.

Ruocchio, P.J. (1991). First person account: the schizophrenic inside, *Schizophrenia Bulletin*, **17**, 357–9.

Strawson, G. (1999). The self and the sesmet. In *Models of the Self*, ed. S. Gallagher & J. Shear, pp. 483–518. Thorverton, UK: Imprint Academic.

Teasdale, J.D. (1999a). Multilevel theories of emotion. In *Handbook of Cognition and Emotion*, ed. T. Dalgleish & M. Power, pp. 665–81. Chichester: Wiley.

Teasdale, J.D. (1999b). Emotional processing, three modes of mind, and the prevention of relapse in depression. *Behaviour Research and Therapy*, **37**, S53–S77.

Teasdale, J.D. & Barnard, P.J. (1993). *Affect Cognition and Change: Re-modelling Depressive Thought*. Hove: Lawrence Erlbaum.

Teasdale, J.D., Taylor, M.J., Cooper, Z., Hayhurst, H. & Paykel, E.S. (1995). Depressive thinking: shifts in construct accessibility or in schematic mental models. *Journal of Abnormal Psychology*, **104**, 500–7.

Teasdale, J.D., Segal, Z.V., Williams, J.M.G. *et al.* (2000). Prevention of relapse/recurrence in major depression by mindfulness-based cognitive therapy. *Journal of Consulting and Clincial Psychology,* **68**, 615–23.

Waugh, N.C. & Norman, D.A. (1965). Primary memory. *Psychological Review,* **72**, 89–104.

Wing, J.K., Cooper, J.E. & Sartorius, N. (1974). *Description and Classification of Psychiatric Symptoms.* Cambridge: Cambridge University Press.

7

Self-awareness, social intelligence and schizophrenia

Gordon G. Gallup, Jr,[1] James R. Anderson[2] and Steven M. Platek[3]

[1] Department of Psychology, State University of New York at Albany, Albany, NY, USA
[2] Department of Psychology, University of Stirling, Scotland
[3] Department of Psychology, Drexel University, Philadelphia, PA, USA

Abstract

The purpose of this chapter is to review the evidence concerning mirror self-recognition as a measure of self-awareness and examine its applicability to schizophrenia. The evidence suggests that the ability to identify yourself correctly in a mirror is not only related to the capacity to conceive of yourself, but may also be related to your ability to take into account what other individuals may know, want or intend to do. This ability to make accurate inferences about mental states in others (known as mental state attribution, theory of mind or social intelligence) begins to emerge during childhood at the same point in time as mirror self-recognition. Species that fail to recognize themselves in mirrors fail to show any evidence that they can infer mental states in one another. Also consistent with the proposition that these phenomena go hand in hand, recent neuropsychological evidence shows that self-awareness and mental state attribution in humans appear to be a byproduct of brain activity that is related to the frontal cortex. As detailed here and elsewhere in this volume, there is growing evidence that both self-awareness and mental state attribution is impaired in schizophrenic patients and that schizophrenia may be related to frontal lobe dysfunction.

Mirror self-recognition

Mirrors have a number of unique psychological properties. In principle, mirrors represent a means of seeing yourself as you are seen by others. In front of a mirror you are literally an audience to your own behaviour. Contrary to the way humans typically respond to themselves in mirrors, most animals react as if they were seeing other animals, and even after periods of extended exposure seem incapable of realizing that their behaviour is the source of the behaviour being depicted in the reflection (Gallup, 1968). Based on a method developed a number of years ago (Gallup, 1970), it turns out that the ability to recognize yourself in a mirror is subject to a number of constraints that apply both within and between species. The method consists of the unobtrusive application of facial marks that can only be seen in a mirror. In the original study, a number of socially housed chimpanzees were given several days of exposure to themselves in a mirror. Initially they reacted as if they were seeing another chimpanzee and engaged in a variety of species-typical social responses directed toward the reflection. After a couple of days, however, they began to use the mirror to respond to themselves, such as grooming and investigating parts of their bodies they had not seen before. In an attempt to demonstrate that the chimpanzees had learned that their behaviour was the source of the behaviour depicted in the mirror (i.e. self-recognition), the mirror was removed and each animal was anaesthetized. Once unconscious, they were removed from their cages and a bright red, odourless, nonirritating alcohol dye was applied to the uppermost portion of an eyebrow ridge and the top half of the opposite ear. The chimpanzees were then returned to their cages and allowed to recover from the effects of anaesthesia in the absence of the mirror. There are three special properties to this procedure. First, since the marks were applied to chimpanzees' faces while they were unconscious they would have no information about the application of these marks. Second, the dye was carefully chosen to be free from any residual tactile and/or olfactory cues. And finally, the marks were strategically placed at predetermined points on their faces so that they could not be seen without a mirror.

Once the animals had fully recovered from the anaesthesia, they were fed and given water, and their behaviour was monitored for a 30-min period to determine the number of times they might accidentally contact these facial marks prior to seeing themselves in a mirror. At the conclusion of this pretest phase, the mirror was then brought back into the room as an explicit test of self-recognition. Upon seeing their reflection in the mirror the chimpanzees reached up and began to touch and investigate these marks on their faces. They also occasionally looked at and smelled their fingers after having made direct contact with the marks that could only be seen in the mirror.

Self-recognition research: phylogenetic and ontogenetic trends

Chimpanzees are not the only nonhuman primates capable of correctly interpreting their reflection in a mirror. Spontaneous mirror-guided self-exploration and investigation of normally invisible marks have been reported in other great apes: orangutans and bonobos (Lethmate & Ducker, 1973; Suarez & Gallup, 1981; Westergaard & Hyatt, 1994; Walraven et al., 1995). The evidence regarding the fourth great ape, the gorilla, is mostly negative (Gallup & Suarez, 1981, Ledbetter & Basen, 1982, Shillito et al., 1999; but see Patterson & Cohn, 1994). The observed distribution of self-recognition among the great apes suggests that the protohominid precursor to great apes and humans was self-aware, and that the ancestors of modern gorillas were self-aware but later lost the capacity (see Gallup, 1998, for details). Even within species there is considerable variability in the expression of self-recognition (Povinelli et al., 1993).

More striking than any differences within and between the great apes is an apparent phylogenetic gap in self-recognition between great apes and all other nonhuman primates. In the original study (Gallup, 1970) macaque monkeys were also tested using the same procedures as with chimpanzees, but no evidence was found of self-recognition either in the monkeys' spontaneous reactions to their reflection or in response to being marked on facial areas that were not visible without a mirror. Instead, the monkeys showed only social reactions and some habituation to the strange conspecific in the mirror. This species difference led to the hypothesis that, among primates, the capacity for self-recognition might be limited to humans and great apes. Since then many researchers have set out to find evidence for self-recognition in monkeys, but in spite of some highly original and tenacious campaigns their endeavours have been in vain (for reviews of this literature see Anderson, 1984a, 1994; Gallup, 1988; Anderson & Gallup, 1999).

To summarize the phylogenetic picture regarding self-recognition: when first confronted with their reflection in a mirror, most nonhuman primates respond as if they were in the presence of another animal. They typically display species-specific postures and facial expressions and emit vocalizations that normally occur in social situations. Over time social responses diminish as the animal habituates to the reflection. In some great apes, social responding gives way to appropriate use of the mirror for self-exploration as self-recognition emerges. In monkeys, however, the transition from other- to self-oriented responding does not occur. Self-recognition has been demonstrated in other domains and with other forms of self-representational stimuli, including reflections in water, shadows, photographs and video, but no monkey (i.e. no primate other than a human or a great ape) has shown convincing reproducible evidence of self-recognition when presented with any of these stimuli (Anderson, 1999).

In the case of humans, much effort has gone into tracing the development of self-recognition in infancy (for reviews see Lewis & Brooks-Gunn, 1979; Anderson, 1984b, Rochat, 1995). Up to the age of 12 months an infant will typically respond to its reflection as if in the presence of another infant, with attempts to contact the image, while often smiling and vocalizing. In the second year of life social responses decrease while more sober examination of the reflection, coyness and even avoidance may start to predominate. If a version of the mark test is conducted (usually involving the decoy procedure of pretending to wipe the child's nose), most infants by the age of 24 months respond appropriately by locating the mark once they see it in the mirror. The youngest infant to pass the mark test was 15 months of age. It is interesting that in chimpanzees the ontogeny or emergence of self-recognition appears to be developmentally delayed relative to humans. Most chimpanzees do not show compelling evidence of self-recognition until they reach early adolescence – 5–7 years of age (Povinelli et al., 1993) – although some are more precocious.

Self-awareness and mental state attribution

One of us has theorized that organisms that can conceive of themselves, as evidenced by their ability to recognize themselves in mirrors, ought also to be capable of engaging in mental state attribution (Gallup, 1982). In other words, self-recognition and social intelligence may be a reflection of a common underlying process, namely the ability to conceive of yourself in the first place. According to the model, if you are self-aware (i.e. you can become the object of your own attention, you are aware of being aware, you are aware of your own existence) then, in principle, you ought to be in a position to use your experience to infer the existence of comparable experiences in others. While it may be true that no two people ever experience the same event in exactly the same way, as members of the same species we share pretty much the same receptor systems and underlying neurological hardware. Therefore, there is bound to be considerable overlap between my experience and yours. For example, if you know what it is like to swing a hammer to drive a nail only to miss and hit your finger, then you have a means of modelling that experience in others and empathizing should the same thing happen to them. Not only can you use your experience to map different features of experience in others, but given a knowledge of your own mental and emotional states and their relationship to various external events you have a means of modelling mental states in others as well. In other words, knowledge of self paves the way for an inferential knowledge of others. Inferring mental states in others is a consequence of being able to represent mental states in yourself, i.e., knowledge of mental states in others builds on your personal knowledge of your own mental states. This ability to infer and take into account what other people may or may not know, want or intend to do is referred to in the literature as mental state attribution, theory of mind or social intelligence. Humans routinely try to take into account how other people feel and make inferences and attributions about what they may have in mind, what they want, what bothers them or what they plan to do.

There are several ways to illustrate this capacity (Gallup, 1998). One involves what happens in an interpersonal exchange when this ability fails to be activated, or what can be called a 'mindless conversation'. Have you ever had the experience of someone approaching you and initiating a conversation in midstream, as though you had been privileged to their prior thoughts? That is, they come up to you out of the clear blue and say 'Gee, that really makes me mad!' or 'What do you think we ought to do about it?' You say, of course, 'What makes you mad?' or

'Do about what?' In each instance, it's a clear failure on the part of the person who started the conversation to take into account what the listener knows or does not know. In order to have a meaningful conversation both participants have to provide sufficient background information in order for the message to be meaningful. Another example involves what might happen if your dog returns home with his nose full of quills following an encounter with a porcupine. With a concern for your pet's well-being you would either have to take him to a veterinarian to have the barbed quills removed, or you could get a pair of pliers and attempt to extract them yourself. If you were to opt for the latter, it would probably be an excruciating ordeal. It is not that you would experience any pain as a consequence, but given your prior experience with pain it would prove virtually impossible not to empathize with what you assume to be going on inside the dog's head as you extract the quills and witness his reaction. It is not necessary that you have ever been quilled, but only that you have had prior experience with pain. That is, you would use your previous experience with pain to generalize and infer the existence of a comparable experience on the part of your dog. For you or I, it probably would not matter whether the victim of the porcupine encounter was a dog, a rabbit, an elephant or a pig. It would not matter who the victim was, it would be unpleasant to participate in or even watch the extraction process. However, how do you think another unrelated dog would react to your dog as the quills were removed? Any veterinarian can tell you that dogs are generally oblivious to pain and suffering in other dogs. It's not that dogs are incapable of experiencing pain. Indeed, we suspect that the experience of pain in dogs shares much in common with that of humans. But a major difference is that, unlike people, dogs cannot conceive of themselves and therefore fail to use their experience of pain to model or infer painful experiences in other creatures, whether they are other dogs or other species. Consistent with these observations, Anil et al. (1997) examined the reaction of pigs to the slaughter of other pigs. In addition to measuring heart rate and taking blood assays to monitor stress, behavioural observations were also made. Although there was evidence of stress due to handling, they report that giving pigs the opportunity to witness other pigs being killed produced no signs of apparent distress or concern.

Testable implications of the model

It is possible to test the theoretical connection between self-awareness and mental state attribution in at least four separate domains. According to the model, species that fail to recognize themselves in mirrors should, as the previous example suggests, fail to show evidence of being able to represent mental states in other animals. Likewise, children that are too young to realize that it is their behaviour that represents the source of the behaviour being depicted in a mirror should be incapable of taking into account what other people perceive, want or know. Similarly, according to the model, both mental patients who respond inappropriately to themselves in mirrors and others with neurological conditions that interfere with self-awareness should also show evidence of impaired mental state attribution.

Mental state attribution in animals

According to the model, species that are incapable of recognizing themselves in mirrors should fail to show evidence of being able to engage in a variety of introspectively based social strategies (e.g. attribution, deception, empathy, gratitude, grudging, role playing) because of their inability to represent mental states in others. Despite a number of attempts, there is no evidence among primates that monkeys that fail to recognize themselves in mirrors can take into account what other monkeys know, want or intend to do (Povinelli et al., 1991). Indeed, the evidence suggests that monkeys may not even know what they know, in the sense that they cannot represent mental states in themselves (Cheney & Seyfarth, 1990).

In the case of chimpanzees and orangutans, the evidence for mental state attribution is mixed and as a consequence the jury is still out. The question of whether chimpanzees can make inferences about mental states has become quite a contentious issue (Heyes, 1998). Although numerous studies have been conducted, the question often boils down to whether results might be due to learning rather than mental state attribution. Whereas Hare et al. (2000) have recently reported that chimpanzees are capable of taking into account what other chimpanzees can or cannot see, the evidence suggests that they fail to make accurate inferences about what humans can or cannot see (Povinelli & Eddy, 1996).

Mental state attribution in children

Between 18 and 24 months of age, which is the same time that young children learn to recognize themselves in mirrors, children begin to show evidence of making primitive inferences about mental states in others. This is not to say that a mature and highly sophisticated theory of mind suddenly emerges at the same point in development as self-recognition. Rather, the ability to take into account the existence of mental and emotional states in others progresses through a series of increasingly more sophisticated stages that begin at about a year and a half to 2 years of age. By the time children are 4 years old they can not only infer what other people know, but they can take into account false beliefs, i.e. they can represent mental states in others which are at variance with what they know to be true.

Prior to learning to recognize themselves in mirrors, when children witness other children crying and in distress they typically begin to cry themselves. However, in what has been described as an explosion of prosocial behaviour (Zahn-Waxler & Radke-Yarrow, 1982), once they reach about 18 months of age their behaviour undergoes a striking change. Rather than cry when they see other children crying, they respond by trying to provide toys and food as solace and will often attempt to solicit aid from adults. It is as if once children have developed the ability to conceive of themselves they begin to use their prior experience with distress to model and infer comparable experiences in others and make attempts at social intervention. With the emergence of self-recognition children begin to show many other precursors to a mature theory of mind. Between 18 and 36 months of age children start to explain and predict what other people do by inferring their desires and intentions (Schultz & Wells, 1985; Dunn, 1991; Lewis & Mitchell, 1994; Carruthers & Smith, 1996). They are able to direct the attention of others by pointing (Butterworth, 1994), and they can even follow the attentional focus of others to objects outside their own visual field (Butterworth & Jarret, 1991). At this point in development, children are also able to understand the perceptual states of others by inferring what other people can or cannot see (Lempers et al., 1977; Flavell et al., 1981).

Neurological underpinnings of self-awareness: the frontal cortex

In support of the theory that the ability to conceive of oneself is what paves the way for making inferences about mental states in others (Gallup, 1982), there is growing evidence that self-awareness and mental state attribution are localized in roughly the same or at least very similar areas of the human brain. More specifically, it appears that the frontal cortex (often the right prefrontal cortex) is involved in self-recognition, autobiographical (episodic) memories and the ability to take into account what other people may or may not know, want or intend to do (mental state attribution).

Starting with an example of evidence implicating hemispheric lateralization of self-recognition, consider a study by Keenan et al. (1999). In response to seeing facial images presented on a computer screen, human subjects were asked to press a particular key as soon as they could; one key if it was their own face, another if it was a friend, and still another key if it was a stranger. Whereas there were no differences in reaction time to the different faces when they used their right hand to press the keys, subjects identified their own faces significantly faster with their left hand than faces of other people. This left-hand advantage for self-face recognition was true of faces presented both upright and inverted. As a consequence of contralateral hemispheric dominance, the left-hand advantage for identifying self-faces implies that self-recognition is related to activity in the right hemisphere.

In a recent study of patients undergoing intracarotid amobarbital inactivation of the right hemisphere, Meador et al. (2000) found that many patients experienced asomatognosia, or the inability to recognize their own hand. Out of 62 patients undergoing WADA preoperative evaluation for surgery, 82% could not recognize their own hand at some point during inactivation of the right hemisphere. Among the patients who experienced right hemisphere deactivation and failed to recognize their own hand, the authors report that the patients 'uniformly thought it was someone else's hand'. There is a striking parallel between these results and an earlier study of the ability of nonhuman primates to engage in mirror-guided reaching behaviour as a means of locating hidden objects. Menzel et al. (1985) devised a task that required primates to reach through a hole in an opaque barrier to find incentives positioned at different locations on the other side. While the subjects could not directly see where the incentives were hidden, there was a mirror placed overhead that they could use to locate the incentive and to monitor the position and movement of their hand relative to where it was. Menzel et al. tested both chimpanzees and rhesus monkeys with extensive prior experience with mirrors for their ability to solve this problem. Whereas chimpanzees solved the problem almost immediately, rhesus monkeys were completely incapable of locating the incentives by watching the movement of their own hand in the mirror. Indeed, Menzel et al. report that during the testing procedure many of the rhesus monkeys would vocalize and threaten the image in the mirror when they saw their hand move toward the food, as if it represented the hand of another monkey! The parallel between the behaviour of patients undergoing right hemisphere deactivation and rhesus monkeys who consistently fail to show evidence of self-recognition suggests that there is something in the right side of the human brain that is missing in the rhesus monkey brain. These results also demonstrate that self-recognition not only applies to facial features but to other body parts as well.

In a series of recent studies using functional magnetic resonance imaging, Kircher and his colleagues (Kircher et al., 2001) found evidence of brain activation in the left prefrontal cortex when subjects viewed their own faces, but not when they saw other faces. Activation of the frontal cortex also occurred when people were presented with adjectives that described their own attributes as compared with those that were not self-relevant. In some instances, damage to the frontal cortex can lead to the loss of mirror self-recognition. Breen and her colleagues (Breen et al., 2000, 2001) describe a number of cases of mirrored-self misidentification, in which patients with damage to the right frontal cortex identify other people appropriately but react to themselves in mirrors as though they were seeing someone else.

Other studies also implicate the right prefrontal cortex as critical for self-recognition. Using positron emission tomography, Fink et al. (1996) found activation in the right frontal cortex when subjects were presented with personal statements concerning themselves, but not when presented with comparable statements about others. As measured by both functional magnetic resonance imaging and event-related potentials, Keenan et al. (2001) have also shown that the presentation of self-faces selectively activates areas in the right prefrontal cortex. Likewise, patients who are incapable of identifying their own faces but show no prosopognosia or severe dementia often have damage to the right prefrontal cortex (Spangenberg et al., 1998).

As further evidence that self-related activities may be controlled by the frontal cortex, Nyberg et al. (1996) have shown that during retrieval of autobiographical words there is activation in the right frontal cortex. There are also a number of case studies of patients with damage to the right prefrontal cortex who show focal retrograde amnesia for autobiographical information, but exhibit no deficits in their ability to retrieve and recall other information (Markowitsch & Ewald, 1997; see also chapter 9). Similar studies implicating the right frontal cortex as being involved in autobiographical (autonoetic) memory are reviewed by Wheeler et al. (1997), and recent overviews of attempts to localize self-awareness in the brain are provided by Keenan et al. (2000) and in chapter 8 (this volume).

It is also interesting in this context that the emergence of an autobiographical memory in children does not occur until 18–24 months of age (Howe & Courage, 1993), which is the same time that infants begin to show evidence of mirror self-recognition. At a year and a half and 2 years of age the frontal cortex in infants is growing more rapidly than any other part of the brain (Milner, 1967). Finally, in the context of the fact that gorillas fail to recognize themselves in mirrors, it is important to note that the frontal cortex is smaller and less well developed in gorillas than in other great apes (Semendeferi, 1999).

Mental state attribution and the frontal cortex

A number of studies also implicate the same areas of the brain that are related to self-awareness as being involved in making inferences about what other people are thinking. For instance, Happe et al. (1999) compared right hemisphere-damaged patients with those who had left hemisphere damage along with normal controls on a number of different theory of mind tasks. Not only were patients with damage to the right hemisphere poorer than the other groups in their interpretation of mental state attribution narratives, but they were worse at identifying the point of a joke when the humour required an understanding of the mental state of the characters. Similarly, Stone et al. (1998) report that patients with damage to the right frontal cortex had difficulty representing false beliefs or states of mind in other people that were contrary to what they knew to be true. Other data implicating a relationship between damage to the right hemisphere and deficits in mental state attribution are provided by Siegal et al. (1996) and Stone et al. (1998).

In normal subjects, Baron-Cohen et al. (1994) found increases in right orbitofrontal activity using single-emission computed tomography when subjects read mental state terms, as compared to nonmental state descriptors. A problem, however, with imaging studies is that, while they suggest the involvement of different brain areas in mental state attribution, they fail to isolate which areas are necessary. To address this issue, a recent study by Stuss et al. (2001) examined two different types of mental state attribution in brain-damaged humans with focal lesions in frontal and nonfrontal parts of the brain. Patients with different focal brain lesions, along with appropriate controls, were tested for visual perspective taking and for their ability to detect instances of deception. Patients with lesions specific to the right frontal lobe were impaired for both forms of mental state attribution. On the other hand, lesions elsewhere in the brain (including the left frontal lobe) did not affect patients' ability to take into account what other people were seeing or the ability to infer that they were being misled. Thus, as is true for self-awareness, the integrity of the right frontal cortex appears not only to be correlated with, but an important condition for, mental state attribution.

Is self-recognition an indicator of self-awareness?

Is the ability to recognize yourself in a mirror evidence for an underlying capacity to conceive of yourself, or, as some people have argued (Swartz, 1998), is self-recognition simply an isolated anomaly without any important cognitive implications? The recent neurological evidence is consistent with the proposition that mirror self-recognition is indeed a robust and valid indicator of a fundamental sense of self. The fact that the neurological basis for self-recognition appears to be located in the same part of the brain as self-evaluation and episodic memories strongly suggests that these capacities are tapping into a common self-representational system located in the frontal cortex. Moreover, in support of the proposal made over 20 years ago (Gallup, 1982), theory of mind or mental state attribution also appears to be localized in the right frontal lobe. Thus, on the basis of the current neuropsychological evidence, self-recognition, self-awareness and mental state attribution would appear to be related to a common underlying process.

Implications of the model for schizophrenia

Self-recognition

It is not uncommon for schizophrenics to react to themselves in mirrors as though the image represented that of another person. A characteristic feature of the response to one's own mirror image in schizophrenia is a feeling of alienation from the reflected face, which may be perceived as independently alive, sinister or distorted

(Harrington et al., 1989). Treating the image as though it were someone else is not infrequent, with patients talking to and laughing at their reflection (Rosenzweig & Shakow, 1937). In extreme cases there may be *negative autoscopy*, in which the individual claims to see no image at all in the mirror (Frith, 1992). Many schizophrenics also show an unusual fascination with mirrors – an effect that appears to hold up across cultures (Hsia & Tsai, 1981). It has even been suggested that early signs of preoccupation with mirrors may be a precursor to the subsequent onset of full-blown schizophrenic symptoms (Abley, 1930). In a now classic series of studies, Traub & Orbach (Traub & Orbach, 1964; Orbach et al., 1966) devised an adjustable distorting mirror for use in evaluating schizophrenic patients. When presented with a distorted image of themselves, normal subjects were able to make the appropriate adjustments, by activating a series of motors, to achieve an undistorted reflection of themselves. Schizophrenics, however, often seemed incapable of adjusting the mirror to remove the distortions from their own reflection. As a control for possible psychophysical differences, Traub & Orbach also presented both schizophrenics and normal people with the distorted image of a door and discovered there were no differences between the two groups in their ability to adjust the mirror surface to achieve an undistorted image of the door.

In an attempt to assess further the possibility that schizophrenics may be impaired in their ability to conceive of themselves, we (Platek & Gallup, 2002) recently attempted to replicate and extend the Keenan et al. (1999) study of hemispheric lateralization of self-recognition. College students were given the Schizotypal Personality Questionnaire (SPQ) as a means of measuring individual differences in premorbid schizophrenic tendencies. Relatives of schizophrenics score higher on the SPQ (Kremen et al., 1998), suggesting that schizophrenic traits exist on an underlying continuum within the population at large. Recall that Keenan et al. found that subjects identify their own faces faster when responding with their left hand. While we also found that students with low SPQ scores identified pictures of themselves faster with their left hand, those with high SPQ scores showed just the opposite effect. Individuals with schizotypal traits took longer to respond to their own faces with their left hand than they did with their right. Such evidence of compromised self-face recognition (i.e. the shift from a left-hand advantage to a left-hand disadvantage as a function of SPQ scores) implicates underlying differences in right hemisphere function.

It would be interesting to test schizophrenics on the task devised by Menzel et al. (1985) where the subject is required to reach through an opening in an opaque partition and use a mirror placed overhead to locate hidden incentives. Because of the evidence for their loss of self-awareness you might predict that schizophrenics would respond just as WADA patients and rhesus monkeys, and treat the displaced image of their own hand as if it was the hand of someone else.

Consistent with this prediction, Daprati et al. (1997) report that schizophrenics have difficulty distinguishing between their own hand and the hand of someone else when the image of the hands is presented on a television monitor in real time. In light of the way schizophrenics react to themselves in pictures and mirrors, it is not surprising that other studies have shown that self-monitoring is seriously defective in schizophrenia, often to the extent that patients fail to recognize that activities such as speech are self-initiated (Frith, 1992; Blakemore et al., 2000).

Mental state attribution

There is growing evidence that schizophrenics show theory of mind deficits, i.e. they are impaired in their ability to take into account what other people are thinking or how they feel (e.g. Frith & Corcoran, 1996; Corcoran et al., 1997). Not only do schizophrenics perform poorly on traditional theory of mind tests, but their ability to appreciate humour that requires making certain assumptions about mental states in others is also impaired (Corcoran et al., 1997). It is interesting that non-schizophrenic patients who sustain damage to the right frontal cortex also show a diminished ability to appreciate humour (Shammi & Stuss, 1999). As would be expected, young children also have difficulty comprehending humour based on inferences about mental states (Dunn, 1994). Such findings are consistent with a growing body of evidence that implicates the frontal cortex as playing an important role in mental state attribution and further suggest frontal cortical involvement in schizophrenia. In the context of their impaired/delayed ability to recognize themselves in mirrors, it is interesting to note that autistic children also show theory of mind deficits (Baron-Cohen et al., 1993).

The role of the frontal cortex

There is mounting evidence that schizophrenia may be associated with frontal lobe dysfunction. Schizophrenics are often deficient on a variety of clinical neuropsychological tests used to diagnose patients with frontal lobe damage. For example, the Wisconsin Card Sorting Test has been shown to be a reliable means of diagnosing people with damage to the frontal lobes (Milner, 1997), and schizophrenics are often deficient in their performance on this test (Van der Does & Van der Bosch, 1992; Potterat et al., 1997). Similarly, patients with dorsolateral prefrontal cortical lesions have difficulty inhibiting reflexive glances to peripheral visual cues (Pierrot-Deseilligny et al., 1997) and schizophrenics show comparable deficiencies on the antisaccade task (McDowell & Clementz, 1997). Consistent with the possibility of frontal lobe involvement in schizophrenia, there is also evidence of frontal cortex pathology (Frith, 1997; Goldman-Rakic & Selemon, 1997) as well as structural abnormalities in the prefrontal cortex (Buchanan et al., 1998) of some schizophrenic patients.

Thus, schizophrenic patients appear not only to show impairment in their sense of self and in their ability to take into account what other people have on their mind, but they show evidence for frontal lobe dysfunction as well. These data derived from schizophrenics map surprisingly well on to the proposition (Gallup, 1982) that mental state attribution is an extension of the capacity to conceive of yourself, and the corollary neuropsychological evidence which shows that both self-awareness and mental state attribution are a byproduct of brain activity that appears to be related to the frontal cortex.

Implications for autism

Although the data are incomplete, the evidence suggests that, in contrast with normal children, self-recognition among autistic children appears later in life and may be absent in 20–30% of cases. Whereas Neuman & Hill (1978) found self-recognition in six out of seven autistic boys with a mean age of 8.9 years, others have typically obtained smaller proportions of positive instances. Using 15 autistic children with a mean age of 7.9 years, Ferrari & Matthews (1983) reported self-recognition in just over 50%. Dawson & McKissick (1984) found evidence of self-recognition in 11 out of 15 autistic children with a mean age of 5.6 years. In the largest study to date of a group of 52 autistic children, Spiker & Ricks (1984) report evidence of mirror self-recognition in just under 70% of the sample. Thus, since self-recognition may be developmentally delayed and even absent in some autistic children, according to the model one would expect to find evidence of faulty or impaired mental state attribution among children with autism. Baron-Cohen (2000) provides a recent review of the growing body of evidence that shows that autistic children are impaired in their ability to track mental states in others.

Implications for senile dementia

In a series of studies by Biringer et al. (Biringer et al., 1988; Biringer & Anderson, 1992, 1993) it has been found that, as the dementia progresses, Alzheimer's patients often reach a point at which they lose the capacity to recognize themselves in mirrors. Using the Global Deterioration Scale (GDS) as a measure of dementia, Biringer et al. report that most patients scoring 5 on the GDS show self-recognition, whereas only about half of patients at GDS 6 and none at GDS 7 recognize themselves in mirrors. It is important to note that the loss of self-recognition among senile patients appears to occur prior to the onset of prosopagnosia or the inability to recognize familiar faces. Biringer & Anderson (1992) tested patients for their ability to recognize familiar faces on video, and found that three out of four of those who failed to show signs of self-recognition were able to recognize faces of familiar others.

Another interesting and testable implication of the model would be to determine when Alzheimer's patients begin to experience mental state attribution deficits. Although self-recognition and mental state attribution emerge at about the same point in time during infancy, mental state attribution in children undergoes a series of developmental steps over several years and becomes progressively more sophisticated. Therefore, we would predict that mental state attribution deficits among Alzheimer's patients should appear in reverse order, i.e. impairment in the most sophisticated forms of social intelligence would be expected to become evident prior to the loss of self-recognition. But with the loss of self-recognition the ability to track experiences and mental states in others should disappear.

In the context of dementia, it is also interesting to note that the more primitive/basic social stimulus properties of mirrors have been used to manage wandering in institutionalized elderly patients, by reducing unauthorized exits from the ward (Mayer & Darby, 1991). By placing a full-length mirror on the door to the ward, contact with the door was substantially reduced. The authors speculated that the mirror was an effective deterrent to wandering because patients who walked toward the door were surprised by the approach of an apparent stranger in the mirror.

Acknowledgements

The authors thank the following individuals for helpful suggestions and comments on earlier versions of this chapter: Donald T. Stuss, Jack D. Maser, Glenn Sanders, Jesse M. Bering, Rebecca L. Burch and Daniel J. Shillito.

REFERENCES

Abley, P. (1930). Le signe du miroir dans les psychoses et plus specialement dans la demence precoce. *Annales Medico-Psychologiques*, **88**, 28–36.

Anderson, J.R. (1984a). Monkeys with mirrors: some questions for primate psychology. *International Journal of Primatology*, **5**, 81–98.

Anderson, J.R. (1994). The monkey in the mirror: the strange conspecific. In *Self-awareness in Animals and Humans: Developmental Perspectives*, ed. S.T. Parker, R.W. Mitchell & M.L. Boccia, pp. 315–29. New York: Cambridge University Press.

Anderson, J.R. (1984b). The development of self-recognition: a review. *Developmental Psychobiology*, **17**, 35–49.

Anderson, J.R. (1999). Primates and representations of self. *Current Psychology of Cognition*, **18**, 1005–29.

Anderson, J.R. & Gallup, G.G. Jr (1999). Self-recognition in nonhuman primates: past and future challenges. In *Animal Models of Human Emotion and Cognition*, ed. M. Haug & R.E. Whalen, pp. 175–94. Washington, DC: American Psychological Association.

Anil, M.H., McKinstrey, J.L., Field, M. & Rodway, R.G. (1997). Lack of evidence for stress being caused to pigs by witnessing the slaughter of conspecifics. *Animal Welfare*, **6**, 3–8.

Baron-Cohen, S. (2000). The cognitive neuroscience of autism: evolutionary approaches. In *The New Cognitive Neurosciences*, 2nd edn, ed. M. Gazzaniga, pp. 1249–57. Cambridge, MA: MIT Press.

Baron-Cohen, S., Tager-Flusberg, H. & Cohen, D. (1993). *Understanding Other Minds: Perspective from Autism*. Oxford: Oxford University Press.

Baron-Cohen, S., Ring, H., Moriarty, J. et al. (1994). Recognition of mental state terms: a clinical study of autism and a functional neuroimaging study of normal adults. *British Journal of Psychiatry*, **165**, 640–9.

Biringer, F. & Anderson, J.R. (1992). Self-recognition in Alzheimer's disease: a mirror and video study. *Journal of Gerontology: Psychological Science*, **47**, 385–8.

Biringer, F. & Anderson, J.R. (1993). Self-recognition in Alzheimer's disease: use of mirror and video techniques and enrichment. In *Recent Advances in Aging Science*, vol. 1, ed. E. Beregi, I.A. Gergely & K. Rajczi, pp. 697–705. Bologna: Monduzzi Editore.

Biringer, F., Anderson, J.R. & Strubel, D. (1988). Self-recognition in senile dementia. *Experimental Aging Research*, **14**, 177–80.

Blakemore, S.J., Smith, J., Steel, R., Johnstone, E.C. & Frith, C. (2000). The perception of self-produced sensory stimuli in patients with auditory hallucinations and passivity experiences: evidence for a breakdown in self-monitoring. *Psychological Medicine*, **30**, 1131–9.

Breen, N., Caine, D., Coltheart, M., Hendy, J. & Roberts, C. (2000). Towards an understanding of delusions of misidentification: four case studies. *Mind and Language*, **15**, 74–110.

Breen, N., Caine, D. & Coltheart, M. (2001). Mirrored-self misidentification: two cases of focal onset dementia. *Neurocase*, **7**, 239–54.

Buchanan, R.W., Vladar, K., Barta, P.E. & Pearlson, G.D. (1998). Structural evaluation of the prefrontal cortex in schizophrenia. *American Journal of Psychiatry*, **155**, 121–7.

Butterworth, G. (1994). Theory of mind and the facts of embodiment. In *Children's Early Understanding of Mind: Origins and Development*, ed. C. Lewis & P. Mitchell, pp. 115–32. Hove, UK: Erlbaum.

Butterworth, G. & Jarret, N.L.M. (1991). What minds have in common space: spatial preverbal communication in human infancy. In *Attention and Performance*, ed. M. Jeannerod, pp. 605–24. Hillsdale, NJ: Erlbaum.

Carruthers, P. & Smith, P.K. (1996). *Theories of Theories of Mind*. Cambridge: Cambridge University Press.

Cheney, D.L. & Seyfarth, R.W. (1990). *How Monkeys see the World: Inside the Mind of Another Species*. Chicago: University of Chicago Press.

Corcoran, R., Cahill, C. & Frith, C.D. (1997). The appreciation of visual jokes in people with schizophrenia: a study of 'mentalizing' ability. *Schizophrenia Research*, **24**, 319–27.

Daprati, E., Frank, N., Georgieff, N. et al. (1997). Looking for the agent: an investigation into consciousness of action and self-consciousness in schizophrenic patients. *Cognition*, **65**, 71–86.

Dawson, G. & McKissick, F.C. (1984). Self-recognition in autistic children. *Journal of Autism and Developmental Disorders*, **17**, 383–94.

Dunn, J. (1994). Changing minds and changing relationships. In *Children's Early Understanding of Mind: Origins and Development*, ed. C. Lewis & P. Mitchell, pp. 297–310. Hove, UK: Erlbaum.

Ferrari, M. & Matthews, W.S. (1983). Self-recognition deficits in autism: syndrome-specific or general developmental delay? *Journal of Autism and Developmental Disorders*, **13**, 317–24.

Fink, G.R., Markowitsch, H.J., Reinkemeier, M. et al. (1996). Cerebral representations of one's own past: neural networks in autobiographical memory. *Journal of Neuroscience*, **16**, 4257–82.

Flavell, J.H., Everett, B.A., Croft, K. & Flavell, E.R. (1981). Young children's knowledge about visual perception: further evidence for the Level 1–Level 2 distinction. *Developmental Psychology*, **17**, 99–103.

Frith, C.D. (1992). *The Cognitive Neuropsychology of Schizophrenia*. Hillsdale, NJ: Lawrence Erlbaum.

Frith, C.D. (1997). Functional brain imaging and the neuropathology of schizophrenia. *Schizophrenia Bulletin*, **23**, 525–7.

Frith, C.D. & Corcoran, R. (1996). Exploring 'theory of mind' in people with schizophrenia. *Psychological Medicine*, **26**, 521–30.

Gallup, G.G. Jr (1968). Mirror-image stimulation. *Psychological Bulletin*, **70**, 782–93.

Gallup, G.G. Jr (1970). Chimpanzees: self-recognition. *Science*, **167**, 86–7.

Gallup, G.G. Jr (1982). Self-awareness and the emergence of theory of mind in primates. *American Journal of Primatology*, **2**, 237–48.

Gallup, G.G. Jr (1988). Towards a taxonomy of mind in primates. *Behavioral and Brain Sciences*, **11**, 255–6.

Gallup, G.G. Jr (1998). Self-awareness and the evolution of social intelligence. *Behavior Processes*, **42**, 239–47.

Goldman-Rakic, P.S. & Selemon, L.D. (1997). Functional and anatomical aspects of prefrontal pathology in schizophrenia. *Schizophrenia Bulletin*, **23**, 437–58.

Happe, F.G., Brownell, H. & Winner, E. (1999). Acquired 'theory of mind' impairments following stroke. *Cognition*, **70**, 211–40.

Hare, B., Call, J., Agnetta, B. & Tomasello, M. (2000). Chimpanzees know what conspecific's do and do not see. *Animal Behavior*, **59**, 771–85.

Harrington, A., Oepen, G. & Manfred, S. (1989). Disordered recognition and perception of human faces in acute schizophrenia and experimental psychosis. *Comprehensive Psychiatry*, **30**, 376–84.

Heyes, C.M. (1998). Theory of mind in non-human primates. *Behavioral and Brain Sciences*, **21**, 101–48.

Howe, M.L. & Courage, M.L. (1993). On resolving the enigma of infantile amnesia. *Psychological Bulletin*, **113**, 305–26.

Hsai, Y.F. & Tsai, N. (1981). Transcultural investigation of recent symptomatology of schizophrenia in China. *American Journal of Psychiatry*, **138**, 1484–6.

Keenan, J.P., McCutcheon, N.B., Freund, S. et al. (1999). Left hand advantage in a self-face recognition task. *Neuropsychologia*, **37**, 1421–5.

Keenan, J.P., Wheeler, M.A., Gallup, G.G. Jr & Pascual-Leone, A. (2000). Self-recognition and the right prefrontal cortex. *Trends in Cognitive Science*, **4**, 338–44.

Keenan, J.P., McCutcheon, N.B. & Pascual-Leone, A. (2001). Functional magnetic resonance imaging and event related potentials suggest right prefrontal activation for self-related processing. *Brain and Cognition*, **47**, 87–91.

Kircher, T.T.J., Senior, C., Phillips, M.L. et al. (2000). Towards a functional neuroanatomy of self-processing: effects of faces and words. *Cognitive Brain Research*, **10**, 133–44.

Kircher, T.T.J., Senior, C., Phillips, M.L. et al. (2001). Recognizing one's own face. *Cognition*, **78**, B1–B15.

Kremen, W.S., Faraone, S.V., Toomey, R., Seidman, L.J. & Tsuang, M.T. (1998). Sex differences in self-reported schizotypal traits in relatives of schizophrenic probands. *Schizophrenia Research*, **34**, 27–37.

Ledbetter, D.H. & Basen, J. (1982). Failure to demonstrate self-recognition in gorillas. *American Journal of Primatology*, **2**, 307–10.

Lempers, J.D., Flavell, E.R. & Flavell, J.H. (1977). The development in very young children of tacit knowledge concerning visual perception. *Genetic Psychology Monographs*, **95**, 3–53.

Lethmate, J. & Ducker, G. (1973). Untersuchungen zum Selbsterkennen im Spiegel bei Orang-utans and eingen anderen Affenarten. *Zeitschrift fur Tierpsychologie*, **33**, 248–69.

Lewis, M. & Brooks-Gunn, J. (1979). *Social Cognition and the Acquisition of Self.* New York: Plenum Press.

Lewis, M. & Mitchell, P. (eds) (1994). *Children's Early Understanding of Mind: Origins and Development.* Hove, UK: Erlbaum.

Markowitsch, H.J. & Ewald, K. (1997). Right-hemispheric fronto-temporal injury leading to severe autobiographical retrograde and moderate anterograde episodic amnesia. *Neurology, Psychiatry and Brain Sciences*, **5**, 71–8.

Mayer, R. & Darby, S.J. (1991). Does a mirror deter wandering in demented older people? *International Journal of Geriatric Psychiatry*, **6**, 607–9.

McDowell, J.E. & Clementz, B.A. (1997). The effect of fixation condition manipulations on anti-saccade performance in schizophrenics: studies of diagnostic specificity. *Experimental Brain Research*, **115**, 333–44.

Meador, K.J., Loring, D.W., Feinberg, T.E., Lee, G.P. & Nichols, M.E. (2000). Anosognosia and asomatognosia during intracarotid amobarbital inactivation. *Neurology*, **55**, 816–20.

Menzel, E.W., Savage-Rumbaugh, E.S. & Lawson, J. (1985). Chimpanzee (*Pan troglodytes*) spatial problem solving with the use of mirrors and televised equivalent mirrors. *Journal of Comparative Psychology*, **99**, 211–17.

Milner, D. (1997). *Human Neural and Behavioral Development.* Springfield, IL: Charles C. Thomas.

Neuman, C.J. & Hill, S.D. (1978). Self-recognition and stimulus preference in autistic children. *Developmental Psychobiology*, **11**, 571–8.

Nyberg, L., McIntosh, A.R., Cabeza, R. et al. (1996). Network analysis of positron emission tomography regional cerebral blood flow data: ensemble inhibition during episodic memory retrieval. *Journal of Neuroscience*, **16**, 3753–9.

Orbach, J., Traub, A.C. & Olson, R. (1966). Psychological studies of body-image II: normative data on the adjustable body-distorting mirror. *Archives of General Psychiatry*, **14**, 41–7.

Patterson, F.G.P. & Cohn, R.H. (1994). Self-recognition and self-awareness in lowland gorillas. In *Self-awareness in Animals and Humans: Developmental Perspectives*, ed. S.T. Parker, R.W. Mitchell & M.L. Boccia, pp. 273–90. Cambridge: Cambridge University Press.

Pierrot-Deseilligny, C., Gaymard, B., Muri, R. & Rivaud, S. (1997). Cerebral ocular motor signs. *Journal of Neurology*, **244**, 65–70.

Platek, S.M. & Gallup, G.G. Jr (2002). Self-face recognition is affected by schizoptypal personality traits. *Schizophrenia Research*, **57**, 311–15.

Potterat, E., Perry, W. & Braff, D.L. (1997). Measuring the density of executive functioning in schizophrenic patients. *Biological Psychiatry*, **41**, 86S.

Povinelli, D.J. & Eddy, T.J. (1996). Factors influencing young chimpanzees' (*Pan troglodytes*) recognition of attention. *Journal of Comparative Psychology*, **110**, 336–45.

Povinelli, D.J., Parks, K.A. & Novak, M.A. (1991). Do rhesus monkeys (*Macaca mulatta*) attribute knowledge and ignorance to others? *Journal of Comparative Psychology*, **105**, 318–25.

Povinelli, D.J., Rulf, A.B., Landau, K.R. & Bierschwale, D.T. (1993). Self-recognition in chimpanzees (*Pan troglodytes*): distribution, ontogeny, and patterns of emergence. *Journal of Comparative Psychology*, **107**, 347–72.

Rochat, P. (1995). Perceived reachability for self and others by 3–5-year-old children and adults. *Journal of Experimental Child Psychology*, **59**, 317–33.

Rosenzweig, S. & Shakow, D. (1937). Mirror behavior in schizophrenic and normal individuals. *Journal of Nervous and Mental Disease*, **86**, 166–74.

Schultz, T.R. & Wells, D. (1985). Judging the intentionality of action-outcomes. *Developmental Psychology*, **21**, 83–9.

Semendeferi, K. (1999). The frontal lobes of the great apes with a focus on the gorilla and the orangutan. In *The Mentalities of Gorillas and Orangutans*, ed. S. Parker, R. Mitchell & H. Miles, pp. 70–95. Cambridge: Cambridge University Press.

Shammi, P. & Stuss, D.T. (1999). Humor appreciation: a role of the right frontal lobe. *Brain*, **122**, 657–66.

Shillito, D.J., Gallup, G.G. Jr. & Beck, B.B. (1999). Factors effecting mirror behavior in western lowland gorillas, *Gorilla gorilla*. *Animal Behavior*, **57**, 999–1004.

Siegal, M., Carrington, J. & Radel, M. (1996). Theory of mind and pragmatic understanding following right hemisphere damage. *Brain and Language*, **53**, 40–50.

Spangenberg, K., Wagner, M.T. & Bachman, D.L. (1998). Neuropsychological analysis of a case of abrupt onset following a hypotensive crisis in a patient with vascular dementia. *Neurocase*, **4**, 149–54.

Spiker, D. & Ricks, M. (1984). Visual self-recognition in autistic children: developmental relationships. *Child Development*, **55**, 214–25.

Stone, V.E., Baron-Cohen, S. & Knight, R.T. (1998). Frontal lobe contributions to theory of mind. *Journal of Cognitive Neuroscience*, **10**, 640–56.

Stuss, D.T., Gallup, G.G. Jr & Alexander, M.P. (2001). The frontal lobes are necessary for theory of mind. *Brain*, **124**, 279–86.

Suarez, S.D. & Gallup, G.G. Jr (1981). Self-recognition in chimpanzees and orangutans, but not gorillas. *Journal of Human Evolution*, **10**, 175–88.

Swartz, K.B. (1998). Self-recognition in nonhuman primates. In *Comparative Psychology: A Handbook*, ed. G. Greenberg & M. Haraway, pp. 849–55. New York: Garland.

Traub, A.C. & Orbach, J. (1964). Psychophysical studies of body image I: The adjustable body-distorting mirror. *Archives of General Psychiatry*, **11**, 53–66.

Van der Does, A.W. & Van der Bosch, R.J. (1992). What determines Wisconsin Card Sorting Test performance in schizophrenics? *Clinical Psychology Review*, **12**, 567–83.

Walraven, V., van Elsacker, L. & Verheyen, R. (1995). Reactions of a group of pygmy chimpanzees (*Pan paniscus*) to their mirror images: evidence for self-recognition. *Primates*, **36**, 145–50.

Westergaard, G.C. & Hyatt, C.W. (1994). The responses of bonobos (*Pan paniscus*) to their mirror images: evidence of self-recognition. *Human Evolution*, **9**, 323–9.

Wheeler, M.A., Stuss, D. & Tulving, E. (1997). Toward a theory of episodic memory: the frontal lobes and autonoetic consciousness. *Psychological Bulletin*, **121**, 331–54.

Zahn-Waxler, C. & Radke-Yarrow, M. (1982). The development of altruism: alternative research strategies. In *The Development of Prosocial Behavior*, ed. N. Eisenberg, pp. 107–30. New York: Academic Press.

8

The neural correlates of self-awareness and self-recognition

Julian Paul Keenan,[1] Mark A. Wheeler[2] and Michael Ewers[2]

[1] Department of Psychology, Montclair State University, Upper Montclair, NJ, USA
[2] Department of Psychology, Temple University, Philadelphia, PA, USA

Abstract
Attempts to elucidate the brain correlates of self-awareness have existed for centuries. However, only now is a clear picture emerging. Based on case studies and modern neuroimaging, it appears that the right hemisphere and the prefrontal cortex, probably the right prefrontal cortex, is dominant for self-related processing. Studies implicating the right hemisphere/prefrontal cortex have focused on self-recognition, self-face recognition, autobiographical episodic memory and autonoetic consciousness. We present this evidence and argue that the right hemisphere/prefrontal cortex may be dominant for the self.

Introduction

This chapter attempts to integrate a number of experimental findings pertaining to the neural correlates of the self and self-related processing. In this context, we have previously suggested that the brain be viewed as an Alexander Calder mobile, delicate and balanced, with a certain interdependence amongst the elements (Keenan, 2001). Calder's mobiles are fragile, with wire or string holding together elements typically made of metal in such a manner that perfect balance is achieved across the entire creation. These elements, which on some levels can be described as discrete units, are never wholly independent, and their actions shift as the environment changes. Destruction of a single unit often affects the entire brain, even if the change across distant regions is subtle. Further, different environmental conditions, analogous to different cognitive demands, often involve numerous elements, and the same element is often involved under numerous tasks.

Employing the mobile as a model, it appears that when the self is engaged in certain cognitive tasks, common elements or structures appear to be involved. However, these regions and networks are implicated in other cognitive and noncognitive performances and a true single module for the *centre of self* is highly improbable.

However, as the mobile tends towards certain postures under similar wind conditions, it appears that the demands on self-related processing across different paradigms and methods may engage similar structures. Yet, the removal of a single unit of the mobile is unlikely completely to disrupt any complex task for which that unit is normally a component. Acts of self-evaluation, self-recognition or self-knowing are not devastated by minor injuries in the neural networks that mediate self-related processing, but these acts are compromised by such injuries. A rapidly expanding literature attests to the existence of neocortical regions that participate in self-related processing.

In the investigation of self-related processing, it is important to isolate the neurocognitive components of self in order to consider them separately from other components of the task. For example, suppose it had been discovered that older children outperformed younger children on tasks requiring them to make decisions about themselves. Even if this capacity does increase throughout childhood, there is no way to know how the finding should be interpreted. While there may be a developmental increase in the ability to reflect upon one's self, it is also possible that differences in general cognitive and decision-making skills are sufficient to account for the difference between age groups. To draw conclusions about the self confidently, it is critical to select adequate control measures. For example, if younger and older children did not differ in their abilities to make decisions about other people, but still showed age differences when making self-related decisions, then it would be reasonable to hypothesize that there might be age-related changes in the mental representation of the self that exist independently of other maturational changes. Not surprisingly, in many cases it can be difficult to control rigorously for all possible competing explanations.

Still, we believe that a scientific investigation of the neural correlates of *self* and *self-related processing* is possible, and can encompass evidence from a diverse variety of approaches, including functional neuroimaging, developmental and comparative psychology, neuropsychology and psychopathology. After reviewing the evidence from several different areas, we have come to a few conclusions.

1. Involvement of the human prefrontal cortex is necessary for a number of sophisticated cognitive acts involving self-recognition and self-evaluation.
2. The right prefrontal cortex may play a stronger role than the left in such processes.
3. Self-recognition bears a *family resemblance* to other complex neurocognitive abilities that may require self-referential processing, such as episodic remembering, introspection and theory of mind.
4. Disruption of the self-related networks is a critical feature of many psychiatric disorders, including the anxiety disorders and schizophrenia.

Self-recognition

The ability to recognize others develops relatively early, both phylogenetically and ontogenetically. All mammals, as well as human infants above the age of about 8 months, have little difficulty recognizing other organisms with which they have interacted in the past. Yet, while general person recognition is evident, the ability for self-recognition appears to be a much more difficult task. At face value, this is surprising since organisms that are regularly exposed to mirrors should have had ample opportunity to discover the correspondence between their actions and the reflected image.

The measurement of self-recognition in animals and young humans has been formalized via the mirror test (Gallup, 1970; Lewis & Brooks-Gunn, 1979). Successful performance requires the subject to recognize the mirror reflection as an image of oneself. In the initial critical demonstration, Gallup exposed a group of chimpanzees in front of a mirror for 10 days to establish a baseline of behaviour, and to familiarize the animals with the mirror. After the tenth day, the chimpanzees were anaesthetized and a mark of odourless dye was applied in an unobtrusive location above the eyebrow, so that it could not be directly seen by the animal. When the mirror was reintroduced, all the chimpanzees immediately directed touches towards the mark on their forehead, indicating that they understood the correspondence between the mirror and themselves. Successful performance on the mirror test has been demonstrated by both chimpanzees and orangutans (Kitchen et al., 1996; Povinelli et al., 1997). However, both gorillas (Suarez & Gallup, 1981; Shillito et al., 1999) and monkeys (Gallup, 1977; Suarez & Gallup, 1986) appear to fail the test, though there is counterevidence in the gorillas, indicating that they may in fact pass the test (Patterson, 1984). Gallup has implied that self-recognition indicated via this test is an indicator of self-awareness, that is, the ability to model one's own mental state (Gallup, 1970). Successful performance also implies that an organism can withdraw attention from the environment and direct such attention towards his/her self.

Similarly, young children cannot recognize themselves in mirrors. When an infant below the age of approximately 14–18 months is exposed to a mirror, he or she may demonstrate knowledge that the mirror image represents a reflection of objects placed in front of it. Still, most children cannot pass the self-recognition test until the age of approximately 18 months (Lewis & Brooks-Gunn, 1979). This performance implies an interesting dissociation with respect to self and nonself behaviours. Although children below the age of 18 months can (1) recognize others, (2) understand the reflective properties of mirrors and (3) learn the correlation between their movements and the movements of the reflection, they cannot use a mirror to direct attention to themselves. We suggest that this dissociation implies the later development of some neurocognitive representation of the self that allows its possessors to think about themselves independently of their current environment.

Evidence for this proposition comes from an experiment by Lewis and colleagues Lewis et al., 1989). Children ranging in age from 9 to 24 months were given the opportunity to show self-directed behaviour in the mark test, and were also observed in two different situations that could potentially elicit fear or embarrassment, respectively. Results showed that self-referential behaviour in the mirror task appears to be a requirement for self-conscious emotions like embarrassment, but not for the more primitive emotion of fear. Only the children who passed the mirror self-directed behaviour task were capable of showing embarrassment in potentially embarrassing situations. There was no similar relation with fear – children were equally likely to be afraid of the stranger whether or not they could use the mirror to attend to themselves. A nice feature of the study was that the general findings were true not only across ages, but also within particular age groups. For example, the 18- and 21-month-olds that had not yet achieved self-recognition could not become embarrassed. The authors argued that embarrassment is not only a more sophisticated emotion, but it is more self-evaluative. It requires the child to feel conspicuous, and to monitor his or her behaviour, before evaluating the behaviour with respect to social norms.

Similar to embarrassment, the correct use of personal pronouns such as 'I', 'me', and 'you' follows self-recognition in the mirror task (Miller et al., 1990). Howe and colleagues (Howe & Courage, 1997) have pointed out that correct use of these pronouns requires an inversion of the normal point of view, one that reflects an awareness of themselves as both a subject and an object in the world, and their appreciation between the distinction between self and other. The mirror task appears to be tapping into a relatively advanced variety of self-awareness that is a requirement for further self-evaluative thoughts.

In terms of brain correlates of self-recognition, it is difficult to isolate a single cortical region that underlies self-recognition, yet the ventromedial regions of the right prefrontal cortex would appear to be the strongest candidates. Two converging bits of evidence support this belief. One is the fact that the ventromedial prefrontal cortex shows the largest increase in volume in species ascending from primates to humans. Similarly, it is one of the last regions to mature in the developing human infant, suggesting that any function dependent upon the integrity of ventromedial cortices may show delayed development.

Also, there are a number of reports of adult patients with organic brain injuries that demonstrate failures of self-recognition. Examining these issues, Todd Feinberg has been involved in a series of studies regarding the recognition of own-body parts. He describes *asomatognosia*, or neglect for own-body movement or identification.

First, in a series of right hemisphere-damaged patients, he found that the incidence of asomatognosia was increased and related to damage in the supramarginal gyrus (Feinberg et al., 1990). Patients with damage to this region were unable to identify their own hand. This study was originally intended to include left hemisphere patients, but it was reported that asomatognosia never occurred following left hemisphere damage.

In a recent study, employing WADA, (a method in which anaesthesia is applied selectively to each of the hemispheres) a similar result was found. When the right hemisphere was anaesthetized in 32 patients, only eight correctly identified that their own hand was in fact theirs. In the other 24 cases they identified their own hand as someone else's (Meador et al., 2000). Put simply, the investigators were able to induce self-recognition deficits or asomatognosia in their patients by inactivating the right hemisphere.

Self-face recognition

An increasing body of literature implies that face recognition is mediated by cortical regions outside those responsible for object recognition, with numerous investigations implicating the fusiform gyrus as a major locus for face recognition (Kanwisher et al., 1997, 1999). Prosopagnosia (a selective deficit in face recognition) has been consistently found to be associated with damage to this and neighbouring brain areas (Sergent & Poncet, 1990; Sergent & Gross, 1992). Neuroimaging studies have revealed that face recognition produces activation within the inferior temporal lobe, often within the fusiform gyrus (Kanwisher et al., 1997, 1998, 1999).

Although less attention has been paid to self-face recognition, converging lines of evidence suggest that a different neural circuit is involved in recognition of one's own face when compared to other face recognition. The prefrontal cortex, especially in the right hemisphere, appears to play some critical role in the recognition of one's own face. We have run a number of small studies employing functional magnetic resonance imaging (fMRI). In one study (Keenan et al., 2001a), we compared the subject's own face with the face of Bill Clinton. Underlying each of the faces was a series of descriptor phrases such as 'He thinks' or 'I think'. The idea was to focus attention either on the self or away from the self during viewing of a face. The results of the self-condition were compared to that of the Bill Clinton-condition. It was found that there was increased activation within the right inferior frontal gyrus on the border of the medial frontal gyrus when subjects viewed their own face compared to the famous face (Figure 8.1).

These data were followed up with another two subjects, along with our colleagues Mark George, Diana Vincent and Donna Roberts at the Medical University of South

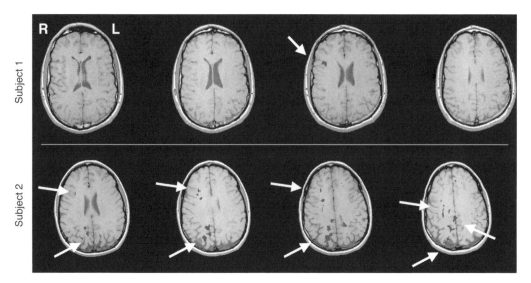

Figure 8.1   In one series of trials, two participants were shown their own face with a short list of descriptors underneath such as 'I think' or 'I feel'. This was contrasted with another series of trials in which participants were shown Bill Clinton's face with similar descriptors (e.g. 'He thinks'). Shown are four slices for each participant from ventral to dorsal employing functional magnetic resonance imaging. Displayed are regions of activation employing t-test ($P < 0.05$) for the self-famous condition; arrows point to increases.

Carolina (MUSC). Here subjects were presented with either their own face or the face of Albert Einstein. In a second series of scans, the subjects heard their own voice, which was contrasted with control, nonself phrases. In both subjects and in both conditions there was right ventral prefrontal activation when the self-condition was compared to the nonself-condition (Figure 8.2). It is of interest to note that in both the Albany and MUSC comparisons, significant striate and dorsal parietal activations were also found, perhaps suggesting that self-conditions engage differences in this region as well, which may be interpreted as differences in imagery demands between self and nonself tasks. Kircher et al. (2001) reported that the right limbic system and the left prefrontal cortex may be important for the viewing of the own face. Employing fMRI, they found these regions to be active during a version of a self-task that included morphing.

Lesion studies provide further evidence for the contribution of the right hemisphere to self-face recognition. Breen et al. (2001) report two cases with patients who had right hemisphere dysfunction based on neuropsychological testing. The patients were able to identify others via use of a mirror but insisted that their own image was not their own. Spangenberg et al. (1998) described a female patient who suffered from damage to the right hemisphere, including parietal, frontal and occipital regions, who was unable to recognize her own face. In both of these cases, a

Self-face - Famous-face   Self-voice - Control-voice

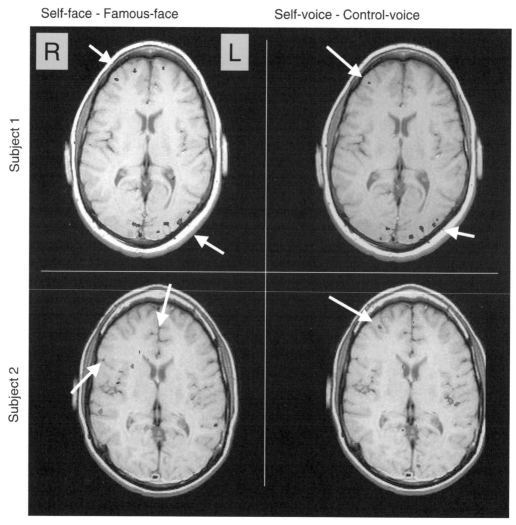

Figure 8.2   In another functional magnetic resonance imaging experiment, another two participants were presented with their own face in comparison with the face of Albert Einstein. Participants also heard their own voice in contrast to the voice of the experimenter. Arrows show regions of increased activity ($P < 0.05$) employing t-tests for the self–other conditions. This experiment was performed at the Medical University of South Carolina with the assistance of Mark George, Diana Vincent and Donna Roberts.

severe loss of self-recognition, particularly in terms of viewing the self in the mirror, occurred. While this phenomenon (loss of self-recognition) is not particularly rare, it is very uncommon that loss of self-identification occurs without prosopognosia or severe dementia. In these cases, both prosopognosia and dementia were limited. A final case, also with right hemisphere damage, has also been reported

(Feinberg & Shapiro, 1989). This patient, similar to the others, misidentified the own-face in the mirror.

Using transcranial magnetic stimulation (TMS), we have induced virtual brain lesions in healthy, human subjects. TMS allows for the temporary inactivation of a circumscribed brain region that is potentially responsible for the behaviour of interest. Here, subjects were presented with pictures of their own-face as well as the face of another person. It was found that TMS applied to the right and not the left prefrontal cortex resulted in impairment of self-identification. Similar results were obtained when faces were controlled for familiarity (from stranger to spouse/significant other) and emotionality (from Adolf Hitler to Albert Einstein).

While there are a number of ways to interpret these dissociations between face recognition and self-face recognition, we prefer the idea that a number of neocortical, probably prefrontal regions are highly involved in the performance of tasks involving the representation of self-related processing. For example, it is known that both hemispheres are capable of self-face recognition (Sperry et al., 1979), as examined in split-brain patients. However, it has also been found that right hemisphere presentation of the own-face (compared to familiar faces presented to the right hemisphere or left hemisphere presentations) leads to a significant increase in galvanic skin resistance (Preilowski, 1977). Further, when self-famous morphs are presented to patients undergoing WADA, a large discrepancy between the hemispheres emerges. When the right hemisphere is intact, the patients recall the self–famous morph as being self, whereas when the left hemisphere is intact, the self–famous morph is recalled as being famous (Keenan et al., 2001b). In terms of the prefrontal cortex, it is noted that a right hemisphere biasing emerges following the application of TMS, and that at least in one patient, right prefrontal lesioning is sufficient to cause a severe loss of self-recognition.

However, in terms of TMS, we have yet to induce a *self-face* agnosia in any of the subjects stimulated, and the differences observed (between self and other) are generally reaction time differences in which right prefrontal TMS leads to longer latencies in self-face recognition when compared to left prefrontal TMS. Further, case studies with exclusive loss of self-face recognition are rare. Finally, it appears that the left hemisphere generally has self-recognition capabilities. Thus while much evidence supports a right prefrontal/hemisphere hypothesis for the recognition of self, it is unlikely that the right prefrontal cortex exists as a *self-centre*.

Autonoetic awareness

Some recent theorists have argued that there are different levels of conscious awareness in the human adult. Autonoetic (or self-knowing) consciousness is the capacity that allows adult humans to represent mentally and to become aware of their protracted existence across subjective time – past, present and future. When autonoetically aware, an individual can focus attention directly on his or her own subjective experiences. This is distinct from *noetic awareness* which is experienced when one thinks objectively about something that one knows. More extensive discussions of these two varieties of consciousness can be found elsewhere (Tulving, 1987; Wheeler et al., 1997).

Evidence from lesion studies suggest that autonoetic consciousness relies upon the prefrontal cortex. There is now a rich body of evidence from both experimental and clinical reports of patients with frontal lobe damage, demonstrating deficits in the recollection of the past and the introspection of the present, as well as the anticipation of the future. After reviewing a number of case studies, Luria et al. (1964) concluded that most patients with large prefrontal lesions had a disturbed critical attitude toward themselves and were unable or unwilling to identify and address their deficits adequately. The same patients could notice those identical deficits in someone else if they were led to believe that the mistakes were committed by another person (Luria et al., 1964). Other observations imply that affected patients had difficulty in relating information to themselves. Ackerley & Benton (1947) noticed that their patients with frontal damage seemed unable to self-reflect and lacked the ability or desire to daydream or to engage in introspection. Some psychosurgery patients accepted the existence of their cognitive deficits yet did not appear concerned or resentful about their problems and often discussed their situation as if they were a casual observer (Ackerley & Benton, 1947). These conditions have been interpreted as disruptions in the fully developed autonoetic consciousness (Wheeler et al., 1997), which manifest themselves as a lack of awareness of the personal present. Affected patients cannot reflect about themselves and, similarly, cannot reflect on the knowledge that pertains to themselves in a meaningful way. Such disruptions tend to be associated with frontal lobe damage.

Perhaps the largest single source of prefrontal lobe patients came as a result of the prefrontal leucotomy procedure, a psychosurgery that was popular in the early and middle decades of the twentieth century (Moniz, 1936). With the goal of relieving various psychiatric symptoms, the technique involved severing the connections between the prefrontal cortex and the thalamus, thereby disconnecting the most anterior brain regions from the more posterior areas and rendering the frontal lobes essentially useless. Freeman & Watts (1950) published a comprehensive review, describing hundreds of individual cases of leucotomies. Although Freeman & Watts mentioned a diverse range of postsurgical symptoms, the authors concluded that the single outstanding cognitive deficit was the awareness of the self as an entity across time. They wrote that the patients lack 'an awareness of being in some sort the person one was yesterday and will be tomorrow, a sense (not often clearly conscious) of one's own self-continuity, of the duration of one's essential identity through changing experiences' (p. 316).

A recurrent theme throughout the literature is that frontal leucotomies change patients so that they are no longer interested in the sorts of past, present and future problems that were so absorbing before the operations. Although the patients knew all of the personal facts about their lives (noetic awareness) that they had known before, they had a detached attitude towards their problems.

Similar ideas have appeared more recently. The healthy adult's conscious states have been attributed to the brain's ability to access, somehow simultaneously, information concerning the personal past, present and future (Ingvar, 1985). This idea holds that the prefrontal cortex is specifically responsible for foresight, initiative and 'memories of the future'. Also, Stuss & Benson (1986) remarked that the highest level of self-awareness is the ability to reflect upon one's own essence, and is dependent upon the full operations of the prefrontal cortex.

Episodic memory

Perhaps the most common expression of autonoetic awareness is episodic memory, or the conscious recollection of a past event. Episodic recollection is a form of 'mental time travel' allowing an individual to reexperience a prior experience. It is distinct from the kind of memory carried by noetic consciousness. Memory of facts, not accompanied by the qualia of subjective experience, is called semantic memory. Thus, episodic memory is not merely an objective account of what has happened or of what has been perceived; rather, its contents are infused with the idiosyncratic perspectives, emotions and thoughts of the person doing the remembering. Episodic memory is fundamentally tied to the self, in that it allows for the awareness of facts and events that are fused with the self's past and that provide guidance to the self's future.

A growing body of evidence is emerging demonstrating impairments of episodic but not semantic memory due to damage to the prefrontal cortex. Wheeler et al. (1997) reviewed the lesion work since 1984 assessing the relation between frontal injuries and performance on a number of common laboratory tests of memory, such as free and cued recall, recognition and source memory. One major finding was that frontal-lobe patients are impaired on tasks to the extent that the tasks require episodic recollection. The act of recognizing a previously presented item, for example, can often be performed without recollection of the past. A number of experiments have demonstrated that participants do not only consciously recollect words from a studied list, relying upon episodic memory, but can also simply 'know' that the items were on the list, in the absence of recollection (Gardiner & Java, 1990). Also, compared to recognition, free recall and memory for source deteriorated much more than recognition in the frontal lobe patients. This asymmetry between impairment on recognition tests, when compared to tests of recall/source, can be attributed to the possibility that semantic memory may partially contribute to recognition performance. In contrast, lacking the availability of strong retrieval cues as provided by a recognition test, a free-recall test requires the subject to reconstruct the learning episode and thus taps the ability of autonoetic awareness. In other words, frontal lobe damage causes impairment of performance on a memory test to the degree that autonoetic awareness is required for a successful completion of the memory task.

There have been several patients described in whom episodic *personal–autobiographical* memory is disrupted in the absence of other cognitive deficits, including other memory processes (Markowitsch et al., 1993; Markowitsch, 1995; Calabrese et al., 1996). In these cases, damage to a network involving the right dorsolateral prefrontal cortex, possibly the right polar prefrontal cortex and the anterior temporal regions, may lead to impaired autobiographical retrograde retrieval. Further, damage to analogous regions on the left side appears to impair semantic memory while sparing retrograde autobiographical memory (Markowitsch et al., 1999). Brian Levine has recently reported a similar case in which a patient sustained damage to the right ventral prefrontal region with damage also to the uncinate fasciculus, a band of fibres leading from the prefrontal cortex to anterior temporal regions (Levine et al., 1998). This patient exhibited severe autobiographical retrieval deficits. These data map well on to the patients described by Stuss & Benson (1986), in whom right prefrontal damage appears to affect personal memories.

Neuroimaging studies with healthy populations appear to support these findings. In a positron emission tomography experiment, Fink and colleagues (1996) compared the consideration of autobiographical memories with 'impersonal memories'. Participants were scanned while listening to autobiographical memories, including phrases describing the subject's past, such as, 'When you were 15, you took part in a swimming marathon and succeeded in swimming 10 miles'. On comparing these sentences with impersonal statements (i.e. similar biographical statements from another person), it was found that there was significant activation in the cingulate and prefrontal regions, as well as the right temporal poles.

In summary, several lines of research converge on the finding that the prefrontal cortex serves the ability to become autonoetically aware of past events, i.e. intact episodic memory. No similar relation exists between the prefrontal cortex and semantic memory, implying that the self-components of episodic memory may be mediated by networks in these anterior regions.

Given these findings, we still do not believe that there is enough evidence for a discrete module in the neocortex that represents the self. However, there is now compelling, converging evidence from several independent sources that self-related processing may be partly independent from similar cognitive processes that do not focus upon the self. Further, the right prefrontal cortex may be a critical locus for self-related processing, though some have suggested that the right limbic system may also be highly involved (Kircher et al., 2001). By viewing the brain as a mobile, we must understand that it is rare that a single unit or module will be adequate to explain any given phenomenon–in particular, one as complicated as self-awareness. Yet the evidence appears to indicate that the right frontal cortex may provide a dominance or assist in providing a sustaining feeling of self-awareness.

REFERENCES

Ackerley, S.S. & Benton, A.L. (1947). Report of a case of bilateral frontal lobe defect. *Research Publications: Association for Research in Nervous and Mental Disease*, **27**, 479–504.

Breen, N., Caine, D. & Coltheart, M. (2001). Mirrored-self misidentification: two cases of focal onset dementia. *Neurocase*, **7**, 239–54.

Calabrese, P., Markowitsch, H.J., Durwen, H.F. et al. (1996). Right temporofrontal cortex as critical locus for the ecphory of old episodic memories. *Journal of Neurology, Neurosurgery, and Psychiatry*, **61**, 304–10.

Feinberg, T. & Shapiro, R. (1989). Misidentification-reduplication and the right hemisphere. *Neuropsychiatry, Neuropsychology, and Behavioral Neurology*, **2**, 39–48.

Feinberg, T.E., Haber, L.D. & Leeds, N.E. (1990). Verbal asomatognosia. *Neurology*, **40**, 1391–4.

Fink, G.R., Markowitsch, H.J., Reinkemeier, M. et al. (1996). Cerebral representation of one's own past: neural networks involved in autobiographical memory. *Journal of Neuroscience*, **16**, 4275–82.

Freeman, W. & Watts, J.W. (1950). *Psychosurgery*, 2nd edn. Springfield, IL: Charles S. Thomas.

Gallup, G.G. (1970). Chimpanzees: self-recognition. *Science*, **167**, 86–7.

Gallup, G.G. Jr (1977). Absence of self-recognition in a monkey (*Macaca fascicularis*) following prolonged exposure to a mirror. *Developmental Psychobiology*, **10**, 281–4.

Gardiner, J.M. & Java, R.I. (1990). Recollective experience in word and nonword recognition. *Memory and Cognition*, **18**, 23–30.

Howe, M.L. & Courage, M.L. (1997). The emergence and early development of autobiographical memory. *Psychological Review*, **104**, 499–523.

Ingvar, D.H. (1985). 'Memory of the future': an essay on the temporal organization of conscious awareness. *Human Neurobiology*, **4**, 127–56.

Kanwisher, N., McDermott, J. & Chun, M.M. (1997). The fusiform face area: a module in human extrastriate cortex specialized for face perception. *Journal of Neuroscience*, **17**, 4302–11.

Kanwisher, N., Tong, F. & Nakayama, K. (1998). The effect of face inversion on the human fusiform face area. *Cognition*, **68**, B1–11.

Kanwisher, N., Stanley, D. & Harris, A. (1999). The fusiform face area is selective for faces not animals. *Neuroreport*, **10**, 183–7.

Keenan, J.P. (2001). A thing done well: a reply to Dr Antti Revonsuo's 'Can functional brain imaging discover consciousness in the brain?' *Journal of Consciousness Studies*, **8**, 31–3.

Keenan, J.P., McCutcheon, N.B. & Pascual-Leone, A. (2001a). Functional magnetic resonance imaging and event related potentials suggest right prefrontal activation for self-related processing. *Brain and Cognition*, **47**, 87–91.

Keenan, J.P., Nelson, A., O'Connor, M. & Pascual-Leone, A. (2001b). Self-recognition and the right hemisphere. *Nature*, **409**, 305.

Kircher, T.T., Senior, C., Phillips, M.L. et al. (2001). Recognizing one's own face. *Cognition*, **78**, B1–15.

Kitchen, A., Denton, D. & Brent, L. (1996). Self-recognition and abstraction abilities in the common chimpanzee studied with distorting mirrors. *Proceedings of the National Academy of Sciences of the USA*, **93**, 7405–8.

Levine, B., Black, S.E., Cabeza, R. et al. (1998). Episodic memory and the self in a case of isolated retrograde amnesia. *Brain*, **121**, 1951–73.

Lewis, M. & Brooks-Gunn, J. (1979). *Social Cognition and Acquisition of Self*. New York, NY: Plenum.

Lewis, M., Sullivan, M.W., Stanger, C. & Weiss, M. (1989). Self development and self-conscious emotions. *Child Development*, **60**, 146–56.

Luria, A.R., Pribram, K.H. & Homskaya, E.D. (1964). An experimental analysis of the behavioral disturbance produced by a left frontal arachnoidal endothelioma. *Neuropsychologia*, **2**, 257–80.

Markowitsch, H.J. (1995). Which brain regions are critically involved in the retrieval of old episodic memory? *Brain Research and Brain Research Reviews*, **21**, 117–27.

Markowitsch, H.J., Calabrese, P., Haupts, M. et al. (1993). Searching for the anatomical basis of retrograde amnesia. *Journal of Clinical and Experimental Neuropsychology*, **15**, 947–67.

Markowitsch, H.J., Calabrese, P., Neufeld, H., Gehlen, W. & Durwen, H.F. (1999). Retrograde amnesia for world knowledge and preserved memory for autobiographic events. A case report. *Cortex*, **35**, 243–52.

Meador, K.J., Loring, D.W., Feinberg, T.E., Lee, G.P. & Nichols, M.E. (2000). Anosognosia and asomatognosia during intracarotid amobarbital inactivation. *Neurology*, **55**, 816–20.

Miller, P.J., Potts, R., Fung, H. & Hoogstra, L. (1990). Narrative practices and the social construction of self in childhood. *American Ethnologist*, **17**, 292–311.

Moniz, E. (1936). *Tentatives Operatoires dans le Traitement de Certaines Psychoses*. Paris: Mason.

Patterson, F. (1984). Self-recognition by gorilla *Gorilla gorilla*. *Gorilla*, **7**, 2–3.

Povinelli, D.J., Gallup, G.G. Jr, Eddy, T.J. & Bierschwale, D.T. (1997). Chimpanzees recognize themselves in mirrors. *Animal Behaviour*, **53**, 1083–8.

Preilowski, B. (1977). Self-recognition as a test of consciousness in left and right hemisphere of 'split-brain' patients. *Acta Nervous Super (Praha)*, **19**(suppl. 2), 343–4.

Sergent, J. & Gross, C. (1992). Face recognition. *Current Opinion in Neurobiology*, **2**, 156–61.

Sergent, J. & Poncet, M. (1990). From covert to overt recognition of faces in a prosopagnosic patient. *Brain*, **113**, 989–1004.

Shillito, D.J., Gallup, G.G. Jr, & Beck, B.B. (1999). Factors affecting mirror behaviour in western lowland gorillas, *Gorilla gorilla*. *Animal Behaviour*, **57**, 999–1004.

Spangenberg, K., Wagner, M. & Bachman, D. (1998). Neuropsychological analysis of a case of abrupt onset following a hypotensive crisis in a patient with vascular dementia. *Neurocase*, **4**, 149–54.

Sperry, R., Zaidel, E. & Zaidel, D. (1979). Self recognition and social awareness in the deconnected minor hemisphere. *Neuropsychologia*, **17**, 153–66.

Stuss, D. & Benson, F. (1986). The frontal lobes and control of cognition and memory. In *The Frontal Lobes Revisited*, ed. E. Perceman, pp. 141–54. Hillside, NJ: Lawrence Erlbaum.

Suarez, S. & Gallup, G. (1981). Self- recognition in chimpanzees and orangutans, but not gorillas. *Journal of Human Evolution*, **10**, 175–88.

Suarez, S.D. & Gallup, G.G. (1986). Social responding to mirrors in rhesus macaques (*Macaca mulatta*): effects of changing mirror location. *American Journal of Primatology*, **11**, 239–44.

Tulving, E. (1987). Multiple memory systems and consciousness. *Human Neurobiology*, **6**, 67–80.

Wheeler, M.A., Stuss, D.T. & Tulving, E. (1997). Toward a theory of episodic memory: the frontal lobes and autonoetic consciousness. *Psychological Bulletin*, **121**, 331–54.

9

Autonoetic consciousness

Hans. J. Markowitsch

University of Bielefeld, Bielefeld, Germany

Abstract

The term 'consciousness' and its possible cerebral representation are discussed in this chapter. A direct relation between consciousness, especially autonoetic consciousness, and memory – the episodic memory system – is outlined. Episodic memory is defined as the context-embedded memory system which allows mental travelling in time – into both the future and the past. The development and lifelong stability of a controlled, self-generated and self-reflected mental framework which allows us to evaluate past episodes and to anticipate the framework of ones happening in the future constitutes the basis for an integrated – autonoetically conscious – personality. Evidence for the importance of certain brain structures – particularly of the right hemispheric prefrontal and anterior temporal cortex – in processing autonoetic consciousness is provided and patients with impaired consciousness and impaired episodic memory (including patients with schizophrenia) are described, both neuropsychologically and with respect to their neural metabolism, as measured by functional imaging techniques. Stress and trauma situations with which the individual is insufficiently able to cope, but also conditions of psychic or physical deprivation or alteration (sleep deprivation, drug abuse, hormonal changes) influence the neural system and may thereby weaken the episodic memory system and affect autonoetic consciousness. It is speculated that especially portions of the inferior prefrontal and the anterior temporal cortex (predominantly of the right hemisphere) control autonoetic consciousness.

The term 'consciousness'

Consciousness is an iridescent term which defies a uniform definition (Wilkes, 1988). Moscovitch (2000) has recently tried to provide what he called an example for a serviceable definition of consciousness by stating that 'consciousness is a mental state that permits one to have a phenomenological awareness of one's experience'. Many other authors, such as Spittler (1992) and Giacino (1997), distinguished between several forms of consciousness, and Bisiach (1988) even wrote of the 'modularity of consciousness'. Spittler (1992) and Giacino (1997) argued that there are numerous disciplines engaged in studying consciousness and consequently there is a range from the normal waking state through awareness, personal identity and mutual knowledge to double consciousness (which can even be used for individuals with a dissociative disorder and to refer to several states of consciousness). Block (1995) made the distinction between *phenomenological consciousness* and *access consciousness*, Damasio (1998) categorized *core consciousness* and *extended consciousness* and Tulving repeatedly (Wheeler et al., 1997) distinguished three forms of consciousness: anoetic, noetic and autonoetic consciousness: 'Autonoetic (self-knowing) consciousness is the capacity that allows adult humans to mentally represent to become aware of their protracted existence across subjective time'. Noetic consciousness (knowing) refers to the awareness of symbolic representations of the world, and anoetic consciousness means the simple awareness of external stimuli.

Related to this view, which speaks for different degrees of complexity within the use of the term 'consciousness' is whether, and if so, to what degree, consciousness can be found throughout the animal kingdom or only in normal humans above a certain age. In Damasio's (1998) opinion, core consciousness (awareness) exists in many nonhuman species. Similarly, Mesulam (2000) wrote that '[f]rom a strictly behavioral point of view, the existence of consciousness might be inferred when a living organism responds to environmental events in an adaptive way that is not entirely automatic' (p. 93). On the other hand, he argued that species with more complex nervous systems will also have more complex forms of consciousness. Mesulam's argument implies that, due to the large-scale networks inherent in the human nervous system, the possibilities for an asynchronous action are also increased, especially under conditions of brain damage or dysfunction.

The possible representation of consciousness in the brain

The controversy between monism and dualism has recently regained weight due to the radical views of scientists such as Sheldrake (1988), Hameroff (1998) and Romijn (1997). Romijn proposed that 'the storage of declarative memories does not physically occur in the synaptic networks of the material brain but at a deeper, submanifest level' (p. 181). Scientists adhering to more conventional views usually assume that consciousness is represented in widespread neural networks from the reticular formation of the brain to the cerebral cortex (Tononi & Edelman, 1998; Markowitsch, 1999a; Young and Pigott, 1999) – an opinion already held a century ago (Markowitsch, 1995). Raichle (2000) held a similar view, but used the analogy of a symphony orchestra, stating that 'no one region (system) necessarily specifies the content of consciousness under all circumstances' (p. 1316).

There are, however, numerous shadings of this idea. Koch & Crick (1999) introduced the hypothesis that there are special sets of *consciousness neurons* and emphasized networks of the cerebral cortex, the thalamus and the basal ganglia as relevant for conscious representation. Other workers favoured the thalamocortical system (Bogen, 1997; Tononi & Edelman, 1998) or within the thalamus the intralaminar nuclei as the region inducing consciousness (Bogen, 1997) or the brainstem with the pedunculopontine and lateral dorsal tegmental nuclei (Smythies, 1999).

Aside from specific cortical or nuclear regions, a particular transmitter system, namely the cholinergic one, has been suggested as the relevant neural correlate of consciousness (Woolf, 1997; Perry et al., 1999). Acetylcholine is mainly produced in the basal forebrain region of the frontal lobes and these have a long-standing relation with higher and more complex aspects of consciousness such as self-awareness and autonoetic consciousness (Wheeler et al., 1997; Levine et al., 1998; Levine, 2000; Wheeler, 2000).

The frontal lobes as a major hub for conscious information processing

The frontal lobes have been a very special brain area since the beginning of modern brain research. Since the nineteenth century they have been regarded as the seat of the highest brain functions, including consciousness (Markowitsch, 1992, 1995). This view was lost over much of the twentieth century, but was reestablished recently in a more moderate version, especially on the basis of results from functional neuroimaging (Fink et al., 1996; Markowitsch et al., 1997b; Courtney et al., 1998).

The frontal lobes constitute a major portion of the cerebral cortex and consequently can be subdivided both anatomically and functionally. The crudest division is between a dorsal or dorsolateral and a ventral (inferior, orbitofrontal) part; sometimes a medial portion is added as a third one. From a clinical perspective, these portions stand for different functions as well: the dorsolateral particularly for impetus, willed actions and intentions; the orbitofrontal part regulates social behaviour (personality dimensions). Medial damage, especially if including the posteriorly adjacent cingulate cortex, may lead to akinetic mutism. The dichotomy between a dorsal and ventral partition is also found in schizophrenia, where the negative symptoms are related to the dorsal and the positive ones to the orbital aspects of the frontal lobes. Catatonic schizophrenia may be related to the mutism described after medial frontal damage. Nevertheless, functional overlaps between prefrontal regions can be detected as well, as Eslinger (1998) pointed out for the neural control of empathy.

One of the brain's functions, which earns the label 'highest' in the sense used by the old researchers (Bolton, 1903; Donath, 1923) is memory. Hering (known for his colour theory) more than 130 years ago stated: 'Memory connects innumerable single phenomena into a whole, and just as the body would be scattered like dust in countless atoms if the attraction of matter did not hold it together so consciousness – without the connecting power of memory – would fall apart in as many fragments as it contains moments' (translated in Hering, 1895).

While patients with damage restricted to the prefrontal cortex are never amnesic, nevertheless memory disturbances, such as a reduced free recall (compared to normal cued recall or recognition memory), can be found (Jetter et al., 1986). The appearance of functional neuroimaging techniques resulted in a number of studies demonstrating an engagement of prefrontal regions during various phases of memory processing. The findings of Tulving and coworkers (1994) led them to formulate what they termed the 'HERA-model', standing for hemispheric encoding retrieval asymmetry. The prefrontal cortex lies in the centre of this model, which states that portions of the left prefrontal cortex are engaged in the encoding of episodic (and semantic) memories, while portions of the right one are relevant for episodic memory retrieval.

As is evident from this last sentence, Tulving (as well as most other current memory theorists) assumes that memory is not a unitary function, but needs to be divided into several systems, of which the episodic and the semantic (declarative) memory systems are the most relevant ones for the discussion herein. Semantic memory is defined as declarable information, propositional, symbolically describable information – knowledge of facts such as that Madrid is the capital of Spain. Episodic memory, on the other hand, is seen as context-embedded and as requiring mental time travelling. It is accompanied by *autonoetic* consciousness and allows us to remember, while declarative memory allows us to know only. Episodic memory is considered to be embedded in semantic memory (Figure 9.1). Furthermore, episodic memory is considered to require prefrontal regions much more than does semantic memory.

The episodic memory system makes up the phylogenetically most advanced and hierarchically highest memory system which develops in childhood hand in hand with the construction and establishment of an integrated personality (Vargha-Khadem et al., 1997; Tulving & Markowitsch, 1998). This system depends conceptually on a number of intellectual capacities. It can be altered by stress and trauma situations with which the individual is insufficiently able to cope (Markowitsch, 1999b, 2000). Conditions of psychic or physical deprivation or alteration (sleep deprivation, drug abuse, hormonal changes) influence the neural system and may thereby weaken the episodic memory system and influence autonoetic consciousness.

Additional features, reasons for the above, and a more complete description and differentiation of the two memory systems can be found in Tulving & Markowitsch

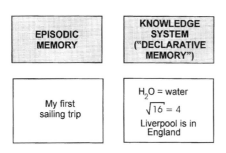

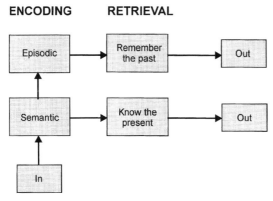

Figure 9.1   Principal features of the episodic and semantic (or declarative) memory systems and of their interdependence (after Tulving & Markowitsch, 1998).

(1998). For a somewhat differing approach to autobiographical memories, see Conway & Pleydell-Pearce (2000).

The findings of a prefrontal engagement in episodic memory processing have been documented in dozens of articles. However, there seems to be an anatomically more complex arrangement for retrieving old episodic (autobiographic) memories: for most of these, it can be assumed that they are strongly affect-laden and have been retrieved several times. We have found that their retrieval is dependent on the (ventral) prefrontal cortex, but additionally, on other structures, of which the temporopolar cortex stands out clearest (Fink et al., 1996). We have studied the retrieval of autobiographical information with various paradigms, all of which point to a right frontal or frontotemporal engagement during the retrieval of old personal memories (Fink et al., 1996; Markowitsch et al., 1997b, 2000c). Fink et al. (1996) compared brain activations when recollecting old personal episodes with recollecting episodes of someone else, unknown to the tested individual. Imaging one's own history resulted predominantly in a right temporofrontal activation pattern. In the study of Markowitsch et al. (2000c), brain activation during the retrieval of autobiographical episodes was compared with that during the retrieval of fictitious information which – to the outsider – had a content indistinguishable from that of the truly experienced episodes. Both kinds of information activated the frontotemporal cortex, but the truly experienced episodes showed a more marked right hemispheric frontotemporal activation pattern than did the retrieval of fictitious content.

In a third study, a paradigm corresponding to that of Fink et al. (1996) was used to study a patient with psychogenic amnesia (fugue) (Markowitsch et al., 1997b). The patient had lost access to his own biography. He agreed to participate in a functional activation paradigm during which we presented him with episodes of his past which we had collected from his wife and other close relatives. Contrary to the normals of Fink et al., the patient showed a central to left-hemispheric activation of his frontal lobes, suggesting that he more likely processed his biographic information as something neutral, not engaging him personally.

These findings stress the importance of the orbitofrontal cortex for affect-laden information processing and the existence of distinct neural nets for the reactivation of positively and negatively viewed autobiographic episodes. Seen together, they strongly revive the importance of especially the right frontal lobe for the processing of autonoetic memories.

The right prefrontal cortex and consciousness

As is evident from the above, especially portions of the right prefrontal cortex seem to be engaged in guiding the conscious representation of stored episodes, that is, in contextual reconstruction (Schacter, 1996; Schacter et al., 1996). Based on an extensive analysis of a patient with a strong tendency of false recognition after right prefrontal damage, Schacter (1996) argued that the 'right prefrontal cortex may be involved in setting up contextual representations that guide retrieval by allowing one to focus in on a target episode and filter extraneous activity' (p. 13530). Older people rather than younger people seem to have more problems in distinguishing feelings of familiarity or recollection for items which are similar to related ones which indeed have been perceived (Schacter et al., 1997). Furthermore, older people as well as patients with prefrontal damage have deficits in source memory (Janowsky et al., 1989; Craik et al., 1990; Henkel et al., 1998), that is, they fail to memorize where an item stems from or to what it is related to. Functional imaging results confirm the link between the prefrontal cortex and source memory (Rugg et al., 1999).

A particularly clear case of lost autobiographical consciousness after right hemispheric damage, disconnecting the inferior prefrontal from the anterior temporal lobe and therefore the proposed junction area for autonoetic memory retrieval

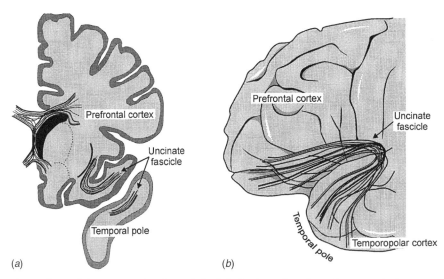

Figure 9.2   The regions of the temporal pole and the inferior lateral prefrontal cortex which are interconnected via the uncinate fascicle. This regional constellation of the right hemisphere is
assumed to control the retrieval of episodic memories, and the left-sided one that of the
knowledge system.

(Markowitsch, 1995; Fink et al., 1996), was given by Levine et al. (1998). These
authors described a patient, aged 36 years, who had sustained severe traumatic brain
injury when he was struck by a car while cycling. The patient's brain damage was
apparently restricted to the right ventral frontal cortex and underlying white matter,
including the uncinate fascicle. This fibre system, especially its ventral branch, has
been described as the crucial link between those portions of the prefrontal and
temporal cortex which are engaged in autonoetic memory retrieval (Markowitsch,
1995, 2000) (Figure 9.2).

The patient failed to recollect personal experiences predating brain injury while
being able to acquire new information long-term. In this way, he corresponds to a
number of patients with similar right-hemispheric frontotemporal injury who also
demonstrated this cognitive pattern (Kapur et al., 1992; Markowitsch et al., 1993a;
Kroll et al., 1997).

A very important contribution to the understanding of the brain's engagement in
self-recognition was provided by Keenan et al. (2000) (see chapter 8 in this book).
These authors reviewed their own work, done with functional imaging and repetitive transcranial magnetic stimulation, and that of others in order to demonstrate
that the self-processes of self-evaluation and autobiographical memory preferentially activate right-hemispheric frontotemporal networks.

Together, these data underline the crucial importance of the right frontotemporal region in autonoetic consciousness. While this junction area is certainly not the seat of consciousness, its activation seems nevertheless obligatory in order to obtain access to one's own past and therefore in order to defeat the splitting of memory into 'innumerable single phenomena' (Hering, 1895) or to become an automatically acting robot.

Schizophrenia, consciousness, memory and the frontal lobes

There are numerous diseases – both neurological and psychiatric ones – which may dissolve the integrated self which characterizes a healthy, alert individual. Sometimes, tiny brain lesions in strategic bottleneck regions of the diencephalon may permanently disrupt conscious reflection of one's own standing in the world (Markowitsch et al., 1993b); sometimes only facets of the past are blurred (Markowitsch et al., 1997c), or there is a temporary limited disruption of an otherwise continuous stream of information flow (Markowitsch, 2000).

Among the psychiatric diseases affecting consciousness, schizophrenia usually comes to mind first. The reasons are manifold: schizophrenia in itself is a nonunitary disease (but see Goldberg and Weinberger, 1995) which nevertheless is usually accompanied by attentional dysfunctions and a reduced processing speed (Carter et al., 1997; Brébion et al., 2000), frequently by hallucinations (Silbersweig et al., 1995; McGuire et al., 1996), by reduced insight (Collins et al., 1997; Lysaker et al., 1998) and by problems with memory processing (dementia praecox). All these deficits or behavioural changes are related to the prefrontal cortex, and indeed, schizophrenia has been closely related to the prefrontal cortex (Abbruzzese et al., 1997), with the 'dopamine hypothesis of schizophrenia' (Farde, 1997; Byne & Davis, 1999) and the finding of structural abnormalities in the prefrontal cortex of schizophrenics (Buchanan et al., 1998) being the most well-known features.

A metaanalysis on 70 studies that reported measures of long-term and short-term memory in patients with schizophrenia revealed a stable association between schizophrenia and memory impairment (Aleman et al., 1999). As in patients with prefrontal damage (Jetter et al., 1986), the deficits were more pronounced under free recall than under recognition conditions. Interestingly, the impairment was stable and not substantially affected by potential moderating factors such as illness duration and severity of psychopathology.

As mentioned above, the prefrontal cortex – and especially its right-hemispheric portion – is engaged in several aspects of conscious memory processing from sustained attention (Rueckert & Grafman, 1996) over working (or online) memory

(Courtney et al., 1998; MacLeod et al., 1998) and source monitoring (MacLeod et al., 1998; Henson et al., 1999) to the binding of all the original components of an experience. Even humour appreciation has been related to the right prefrontal cortex (Shammi & Stuss, 1999) and provides a link to the dimension affect (Cimino et al., 1991; Stuss & Alexander, 2000). The inferior prefrontal cortex has a major role in autobiographical memory processing (Fink et al., 1996; Markowitsch et al., 1997a, b; Markowitsch, 2000), a function severely impaired in schizophrenia (Feinstein et al., 1998).

Danion et al. (1999) showed particularly clearly that patients with schizophrenia have major problems in binding the separate aspects of events into a cohesive, memorable and distinctive whole. Using Tulving's 'remember–know' distinction (i.e. autonoetic vs. noetic consciousness), these authors demonstrated that schizophrenic patients had major deficits in source attribution, that is, in relational binding processes. Using a very different paradigm from that of Danion and coworkers, Daprati et al. (1997) nevertheless came to quite similar conclusions regarding conscious information processing in patients with schizophrenia. These authors required their patients to execute finger and wrist movements without direct visual control of their hand and by presenting them TV-screen images of their own or of an alien hand. Hallucinating or deluded patients had major problems in this source-monitoring task, confirming again the deficits of schizophrenic patients in relating their self to the environment.

Andreasen (2000) attempted to provide a model for the various findings of impaired action control, reduced levels of consciousness, intrusions, memory and attention disorders observed in patients with schizophrenia. She suggested the existence of a 'misconnected' circuit in schizophrenia which leads to what she termed 'cognitive dysmetria' or 'poor mental coordination' and which may be seen as equivalent to reduced consciousness. A crucial component of this cortical–cerebellar–thalamic–cortical circuit is the prefrontal cortex.

A related concept was introduced by Tononi & Edelman (1998) who pointed to the importance of the thalamocortical system for conscious experience and proposed the existence of a dynamic neural core which likewise typically includes posterior corticothalamic regions which interact with anterior cortical regions. They predicted that 'certain disorders of consciousness, notably dissociative disorders and schizophrenia, should be reflected in abnormalities of the dynamic core' (p. 1850). Furthermore, they predicted that the complexity of the dynamic core would correlate with the conscious state of the subject, and that the neural complexity would be higher during waking and during rapid-eye-movement (REM) sleep than during the deep stages of slow-wave sleep. (Similarly to Tononi & Edelman, Perry et al. (1999) related REM abnormalities to disturbed cholinergic pathways and to reduced consciousness, and Bogen (1997) stressed the interaction of the (nonspecific) thalamus with the cortex in the generation of consciousness – a view closely related to Dercum's (1925).)

All these ideas emphasize that consciousness is bound to synchronized or controlled activation patterns in neural circuits, the components of which can be determined and most likely include prefrontal areas which nevertheless have to interact with allocortical (limbic) and subcortical (thalamic, reticular and possibly also cerebellar) regions. Specific transmitter systems (dopaminergic, cholinergic) have to be added (Hasselmo, 1999; Perry et al., 1999) to complete this scenario which controls and regulates the contemplative power an individual can gain in order to evaluate and become aware of his or her standing in society and the world in general.

Most interestingly, lack of awareness of illness seems to be a powerful predictor of poor outcome in schizophrenia (Rossi et al., 2000).

Autonoetic consciousness and autonoetic memory

There are a number of conditions which lead to altered states of consciousness. Among them are focal and widespread brain lesions and numerous forms of psychiatric disturbances. Even temporary changes in body and brain metabolism caused, for example, by sleep deprivation, drug abuse or hormonal changes, influence the neural system and weaken the memory processing and autonoetic consciousness.

Psychiatric illnesses are no longer seen as distinct from neurological disorders (Markowitsch, 1996). In fact, the similarity between some psychiatric syndromes and neurological diseases has long been recognized. Capgras syndrome and reduplicative paramnesia are examples (Alexander & Stuss, 1998; Markowitsch, 1999c). Modern functional neuroimaging has especially demonstrated that many forms of psychiatric illnesses lead to altered brain metabolism. We have demonstrated that patients without access to their autobiographical past have a reduced metabolism in the right frontotemporal junction area, irrespective of whether the impairment was caused by psychic trauma or brain damage (Markowitsch, 1999b) (Figure 9.3).

Similarly, we found a direct correlation between memory and autobiographic awareness and brain metabolism in a patient with a psychic trauma condition: directly after the trauma, he had reduced self-awareness (e.g. acting 17 years old instead of 23 years old) and grossly impaired memory and a significantly reduced cerebral glucose metabolism compared to matched control subjects (Markowitsch et al., 1998). Furthermore the patient was depressed (which is not uncommon in

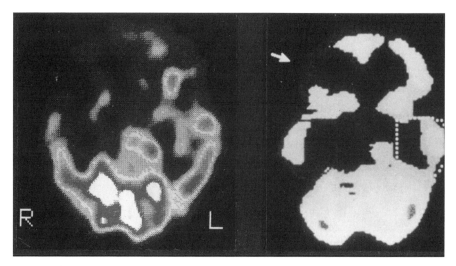

Figure 9.3   Horizontal single-photon emission computed tomography (SPECT) images through the brains of two patients with selective retrograde amnesia for autobiographical information. The section on the left is from a patient with a probable organically based amnesia (herpes simplex encephalitis; Calabrese et al., 1996). It was done 3 years postinfection and demonstrates the area of hypoperfusion in the right temporofrontal region. The section on the right shows the brain of a patient with probable psychogenic amnesia (Markowitsch et al., 1997a). Again, a significant metabolic reduction is visible in the right temporofrontal junction zone. (After Calabrese et al., 1996, and Markowitsch et al., 1997a.)

such patients; cf. Markowitsch et al., 1999). He was very hesitant to respond in any way and appeared fixed, inflexible and timid in his behaviour. His diagnosis was that of 'dissociative amnesia'. He received various forms of treatment: first tranquillizers, then tricyclic antidepressants. After 1 year of (frequently interrupted) therapy he regained memory and consciousness and his brain metabolism returned to normal levels (Markowitsch et al., 2000b) (Figure 9.4). Similarly, he became less shy and less depressed over time.

These examples demonstrate that modern brain research is able to find brain correlates for distinct psychic states and that in the near future it may even be possible to infer from an individual's brain metabolism about his or her awareness, consciousness and memory access.

An integrated self is dependent on autonoetic memory and consciousness. This was evident to an earlier generation of scientists; Ewald Hering's formulation, given above, is an excellent example. Further old as well as recent data come from individuals with identity disorders whose prominent negative symptoms are amnesia and depersonalization and whose main positive symptoms are multiple identities, fugues and false memories.

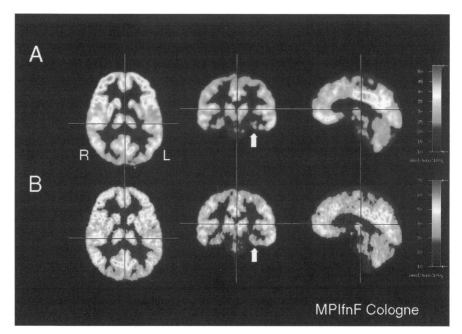

Figure 9.4   ^{18}F-2-fluoro-2-deoxy-D-glucose (FDG)-positron emission tomographic scans of a patient with trauma-based memory disorders and recovery after long-term therapy (Markowitsch et al., 1998, 2000b). (A) Horizontal, coronal and sagittal sections of the patient's brain 2 months after the trauma condition, showing a significantly reduced glucose metabolism all over the cerebrum and in particular in thalamic (cross-hair) and medial temporal regions. (B) Corresponding sections 12 months after the trauma condition and after various forms of therapeutic interventions, leading to significant behavioural recovery. Note that his cerebral metabolism is much stronger than initially (principally normal), which becomes clearer when noting the different scales shown on the right. (Courtesy of Dr Gerald Weber-Luxenburger, Cologne Max Planck Institute for Neurological Research.)

While the appearance of sensory and motor deficits (including those of language) usually leaves the self as it was prior to their occurrence, deficits in the domain of autonoetic memory and autonoetic consciousness are much more deleterious. They change the self – usually for the duration of illness, but sometimes even permanently. Patients with dementing illnesses – even when occurring at a young age (Markowitsch et al., 2000a) – and several types of patients with damage to bottleneck structures of memory processing (Markowitsch, 2000) or to areas within the ventral prefrontal/orbitofrontal cortex (Düzel et al., 1997; Levine et al., 1998; Keenan et al., 2000) belong to this category. Finally, it should be noted that the development of the self during childhood parallels the development of autonoetic consciousness and autonoetic memory (Perner & Ruffman, 1995). Autonoetic consciousness is consequently one of the most precious attributes of human beings.

REFERENCES

Abbruzzese, M., Ferri, S. & Scarone, S. (1997). The selective breakdown of frontal functions in patients with obsessive-compulsive disorder and in patients with schizophrenia: a double dissociation experimental finding. *Neuropsychologia*, **35**, 907–12.

Aleman, A., Hijman, R., de Haan, E.H.F. & Kahn, R.S. (1999). Memory impairment in schizophrenia: a meta-analysis. *American Journal of Psychiatry*, **156**, 1358–66.

Alexander, M.P. & Stuss, D.R. (1998). On: Capgras syndrome: a reduplicative phenomenon. *Journal of Psychomatic Research*, **44**, 637–9.

Andreasen, N.C. (2000). Is schizophrenia a disorder of memory or consciousness? In *Memory, Consciousness, and the Brain*, ed. E. Tulving, pp. 243–61. Philadelphia, PA: Psychology Press.

Bisiach, E. (1988). The (haunted) brain and consciousness. In *Consciousness in Contemporary Science*, ed. A.J. Marcel & E. Bisiach, pp. 101–20. Oxford: Clarendon Press.

Block, N. (1995). On a confusion about a function of consciousness. *Behavioral and Brain Sciences*, **18**, 227–47.

Bogen, J.E. (1997). Some neurophysiologic aspects of consciousness. *Seminars in Neurology*, **17**, 95–104.

Bolton, J.S. (1903). The functions of the frontal lobes. *Brain*, **26**, 215–41.

Brébion, G., Smith, M.J., Gorman, J.M. et al. (2000). Memory and schizophrenia: differential link of processing speed and selective attention with two levels of encoding. *Journal of Psychiatric Research*, **34**, 121–7.

Buchanan, R.W., Vladar, K., Barta, P.E. & Pearlson, G.D. (1998). Structural evaluation of the prefrontal cortex in schizophrenia. *American Journal of Psychiatry*, **155**, 1049–55.

Byne, W. & Davis, K.-L. (1999). The role of prefrontal cortex in the dopaminergic dysregulation of schizophrenia. *Biological Psychiatry*, **45**, 657–9.

Calabrese, P., Markowitsch, H.J. et al. (1996). Right temporofrontal cortex as critical locus for the ecphory of old episodic memories. *Journal of Neurology, Neurosurgery, and Psychiatry*, **61**, 304–10.

Carter, C.S., Mintun, M., Nichols, T. & Cohen, J.D. (1997). Anterior cingulate gyrus dysfunction and selective attention deficits in schizophrenia: [^{15}O]H$_2$O PET study during single-trial Stroop task performance. *American Journal of Psychiatry*, **154**, 1670–5.

Cimino, C.R., Verfaellie, M., Bowers, D. & Heilman, K.M. (1991). Autobiographical memory: influence of right hemisphere damage on emotionality and specificity. *Brain and Cognition*, **15**, 106–18.

Collins, A.A., Remington, G.J., Coulter, K. & Birkett, K. (1997). Insight, neurocognitive function and symptom clusters in chronic schizophrenia. *Schizophrenia Research*, **27**, 37–44.

Conway, M.A. & Pleydell-Pearce, C.W. (2000). The construction of autobiographical memories in the self-memory system. *Psychological Review*, **107**, 261–88.

Courtney, S.M., Petit, L., Haxby, J.V. & Ungerleider, L.G. (1998). The role of prefrontal cortex in working memory: examining the contents of consciousness. *Philosophical Transactions of the Royal Society of London B*, **353**, 1819–28.

Craik, F.I.M., Morris, L.W., Morris, R.G. & Loewen, E.R. (1990). Relations between source amnesia and frontal lobe functioning in older adults. *Psychology and Aging*, **5**, 148–51.

Damasio, A.R. (1998). Investigating the biology of consciousness. *Philosophical Transactions of the Royal Society of London B*, **353**, 1879–82.

Danion, J.M., Rizzo, L. & Bruant, A. (1999). Functional mechanisms underlying impaired recognition memory and conscious awareness in patients with schizophrenia. *Archives of General Psychiatry*, **56**, 639–44.

Daprati, E., Franck, N., Georgieff, N. et al. (1997). Looking for the agent: an investigation into consciousness of action and self-consciousness in schizophrenic patients. *Cognition*, **65**, 71–86.

Dercum, F.X. (1925). The thalamus in the physiology and pathology of the mind. *A.M.A. Archives of Neurology and Psychiatry*, **14**, 289–302.

Donath, J. (1923). Die Bedeutung des Stirnhirns für die höheren seelischen Leistungen [The importance of the frontal lobe for higher psychic processes]. *Deutsche Zeitschrift für Nervenheilkunde*, **23**, 282–306.

Düzel, E., Yonelinas, A.P., Mangun, G.R., Heinze, H.-J. & Tulving, E. (1997). Event-related brain potential correlates of two states of conscious awareness in memory. *Proceedings of the National Academy of Sciences of the USA*, **94**, 5973–8.

Eslinger, P.J. (1998). Neurological and neuropsychological bases of empathy. *European Neurology*, **39**, 193–9.

Farde, L. (1997). Brain imaging of schizophrenia – the dopamine hypothesis. *Schizophrenia Research*, **28**, 157–62.

Feinstein, A., Goldberg, T.E., Nowlin, B. & Weinberger, D.R. (1998). Types and characteristics of remote memory impairment in schizophrenia. *Schizophrenia Research*, **30**, 155–63.

Fink, G.R., Markowitsch, H.J., Reinkemeier, M. et al. (1996). Cerebral representation of one's own past: neural networks involved in autobiographical memory. *Journal of Neuroscience*, **16**, 4275–82.

Giacino, J.T. (1997). Disorders of consciousness: differential diagnosis and neuropathologic features. *Seminars in Neurology*, **17**, 105–12.

Goldberg, T.E. & Weinberger, D.R. (1995). A case against subtyping in schizophrenia. *Schizophrenia Research*, **17**, 147–52.

Hameroff, S.R. (1998). 'Funda-mentality': is the conscious mind subtly linked to a basic level of the universe? *Trends in Cognitive Sciences*, **2**, 119–27.

Hasselmo, M.E. (1999). Neuromodulation: acetylcholine and memory consolidation. *Trends in Cognitive Sciences*, **3**, 351–9.

Henkel, L.A., Johnson, M.K. & de Leonardis, D.M. (1998). Aging and source monitoring: cognitive processes and neuropsychological correlates. *Journal of Experimental Psychology: General*, **127**, 251–68.

Henson, R.N.A., Shallice, T. & Dolan, R.J. (1999). Right prefrontal cortex and episodic memory retrieval: a functional MRI test of the monitoring hypothesis. *Brain*, **122**, 1367–81.

Hering, E. (1895). *Memory as a General Function of Organized Matter*. Chicago: Open Court.

Janowsky, J., Shimamura, A.P. & Squire, L.R. (1989). Source memory impairment in patients with frontal lobe lesions. *Neuropsychologia*, **7**, 1043–56.

Jetter, J., Poser, U., Freeman, R.B. Jr & Markowitsch, H.J. (1986). A verbal long term memory deficit in frontal lobe damaged patients. *Cortex*, **22**, 229–42.

Kapur, N., Ellison, D., Smith, M.P., McLellan, D.L. & Burrows, E.H. (1992). Focal retrograde amnesia following bilateral temporal lobe pathology. *Brain*, **115**, 73–85.

Keenan, J.P., Wheeler, M., Gallup, G.G. Jr & Pascual-Leone, A. (2000). Self-recognition and the right prefrontal cortex. *Trends in Cognitive Sciences*, **4**, 338–44.

Koch, C. & Crick, F. (1999). Consciousness, neurobiology of. In *The MIT Encyclopedia of the Cognitive Sciences*, ed. R. Wilson & F. Keil, pp. 193–5. Cambridge, MA: MIT Press.

Kroll, N., Markowitsch, H.J., Knight, R. & von Cramon, D.Y. (1997). Retrieval of old memories – the temporo-frontal hypothesis. *Brain*, **120**, 1377–99.

Levine, B. (2000). Self-regulation and autonoetic consciousness. In *Memory, Consciousness, and the Brain*, ed. E. Tulving, pp. 200–14. Philadelphia, PA: Psychology Press.

Levine, B., Black, S.E., Cabeza, R. et al. (1998). Episodic memory and the self in a case of isolated retrograde amnesia. *Brain*, **121**, 1951–73.

Lysaker, P.H., Bell, M.D., Bryson, G. & Kaplan, E. (1998). Neurocognitive function and insight in schizophrenia: support for an association with impairments in executive function but not with impairments in global function. *Acta Psychiatrica Scandinavica*, **97**, 297–301.

MacLeod, A.K., Buckner, R.L., Miezin, F.M., Petersen, S.E. & Raichle, M.E. (1998). Right anterior prefrontal cortex activation during semantic monitoring and working memory. *Neuroimage*, **7**, 41–8.

Markowitsch, H.J. (1992). *Intellectual Functions and the Brain. An Historical Perspective.* Toronto: Hogrefe and Huber.

Markowitsch, H.J. (1995). Cerebral bases of consciousness: a historical view. *Neuropsychologia*, **33**, 1181–92.

Markowitsch, H.J. (1996). Organic and psychogenic retrograde amnesia: two sides of the same coin? *Neurocase*, **2**, 357–71.

Markowitsch, H.J. (1999a). Koma und Hirntod: Funktionelle Anatomie von Bewußtsein und Bewußtseinsstörungen [Coma and brain death: functional anatomy of consciousness and its disturbances]. In *Neurologie in Praxis und Klinik*, vol. 1, ed. H.C. Hopf, G. Deuschl, H.C. Diener & H. Reichmann, pp. 60–6. Stuttgart: Thieme.

Markowitsch, H.J. (1999b). Functional neuroimaging correlates of functional amnesia. *Memory*, **7**, 561–83.

Markowitsch, H.J. (1999c). Neuroimaging and mechanisms of brain function in psychiatric disorders. *Current Opinion in Psychiatry*, **12**, 331–7.

Markowitsch, H.J. (2000). Memory and amnesia. In *Principles of Cognitive and Behavioral Neurology*, ed. M.-M. Mesulam, pp. 257–93. New York: Oxford University Press.

Markowitsch, H.J., Calabrese, P., Haupts, M. et al. (1993a). Searching for the anatomical basis of retrograde amnesia. *Journal of Clinical and Experimental Neuropsychology*, **15**, 947–67.

Markowitsch, H.J., von Cramon, D.Y. & Schuri, U. (1993b). Mnestic performance profile of a bilateral diencephalic infarct patient with preserved intelligence and severe amnesic disturbances. *Journal of Clinical and Experimental Neuropsychology*, **15**, 627–52.

Markowitsch, H.J., Calabrese, P., Fink, G.R. et al. (1997a). Impaired episodic memory retrieval in a case of probable psychogenic amnesia. *Psychiatry Research: Neuroimaging Section*, **74**, 119–26.

Markowitsch, H.J., Fink, G.R., Thöne, A.I.M., Kessler, J. & Heiss, W.-D. (1997b). Persistent psychogenic amnesia with a PET-proven organic basis. *Cognitive Neuropsychiatry,* **2**, 135–58.

Markowitsch, H.J., Thiel, A., Kessler, J., von Stockhausen, H.-M. & Heiss, W.-D. (1997c). Ecphorizing semi-conscious episodic information via the right temporopolar cortex – a PET study. *Neurocase,* **3**, 445–9.

Markowitsch, H.J., Kessler, J., Van der Ven, C., Weber-Luxenburger, G. & Heiss, W.-D. (1998). Psychic trauma causing grossly reduced brain metabolism and cognitive deterioration. *Neuropsychologia,* **36**, 77–82.

Markowitsch, H.J., Kessler, J., Russ, M.O. et al. (1999). Mnestic block syndrome. *Cortex,* **35**, 219–30.

Markowitsch, H.J., Kessler, J., Schramm, U. & Frölich, L. (2000a). Severe degenerative cortical and cerebellar atrophy and progressive dementia in a young adult. *Neurocase,* **6**, 357–64.

Markowitsch, H.J., Kessler, J., Weber-Luxenburger, G., Van der Ven, C. & Heiss, W.-D. (2000b). Neuroimaging and behavioral correlates of recovery from 'mnestic block syndrome' and other cognitive deteriorations. *Neuropsychiatry, Neuropsychology, and Behavioral Neurology,* **13**, 60–6.

Markowitsch, H.J., Thiel, A., Reinkemeier, M. et al. (2000c). Right amygdalar and temporofrontal activation during autobiographic, but not during fictitious memory retrieval. *Behavioural Neurology,* **12**, 181–90.

McGuire, P.K., Silbersweig, D.A., Wright, I. et al. (1996). The neural correlates of inner speech and auditory verbal imagery in schizophrenia: relationship to auditory verbal hallucinations. *British Journal of Psychiatry,* **169**, 148–59.

Mesulam, M.-M. (2000). Behavioral neuroanatomy: large-scale networks, association cortex, frontal syndromes, the limbic system, and hemispheric specializations. In *Principles of Behavioral and Cognitive Neurology*, 2nd edn, ed. M.-M. Mesulam, pp. 1–120. New York: Oxford University Press.

Moscovitch, M. (2000). Theories of memory and consciousness. In *The Oxford Handbook of Memory*, ed. E. Tulving & F.I.M. Craik, pp. 609–26. New York: Oxford University Press.

Perner, J. & Ruffman, T. (1995). Episodic memory and autonoetic consciousness: developmental evidence and a theory of childhood amnesia. *Journal of Experimental Child Psychology,* **59**, 516–48.

Perry, E., Walker, M., Grace, J. & Perry, R. (1999). Acetylcholine in mind: a neurotransmitter correlate of consciousness? *Trends in Neurosciences,* **22**, 273–80.

Raichle, M.E. (2000). The neural correlates of consciousness: an analysis of cognitive skill learning. In *The New Cognitive Neurosciences*, 2nd edn, ed. M.S. Gazzaniga, pp. 1305–18. Cambridge, MA: MIT Press.

Romijn, H. (1997). About the origin of consciousness. A new, multidisciplinary perspective on the relationship between brain and mind. *Proceedings van de Koninklijke Nederlandse Akademie van Wetenschappen,* **100**, 181–267.

Rossi, A., Arduini, L., Prosperini, P. et al. (2000). Awareness of illness and outcome in schizophrenia. *European Archives of Psychiatry and Clinical Neurosciences,* **250**, 73–5.

Rueckert, L. & Grafman, J. (1996). Sustained attention deficits in patients with right frontal lesions. *Neuropsychologia,* **34**, 953–63.

Rugg, M.D., Fletcher, P.C., Chua, P.M.-L. & Dolan, R.J. (1999). The role of the prefrontal cortex in recognition memory and memory for source: an fMRI study. *NeuroImage,* **10**, 520–9.

Schacter, D.L. (1996). Illusory memories: a cognitive neuroscience analysis. *Proceedings of the National Academy of Sciences of the USA*, **93**, 13527–33.

Schacter, D.L., Curran, T., Galluccio, L., Milberg, W.P. & Bates, J.F. (1996). False recognition and the right frontal lobe: a case study. *Neuropsychologia*, **34**, 793–808.

Schacter, D.L., Koutstaal, W. & Norman, K.A. (1997). False memories and aging. *Trends in Cognitive Sciences*, **1**, 229–36.

Shammi, P. & Stuss, D.T. (1999). Humor appreciation: a role of the right frontal lobe. *Brain*, **122**, 657–66.

Sheldrake, R. (1988). *The Presence of the Past*. New York: Times Books.

Silbersweig, D.A., Stern, E., Frith, E. et al. (1995). A funtional neuroanatomy of hallucinations in schizophrenia. *Nature*, **378**, 176–9.

Smythies, J. (1999). Consciousness: some basic issues – a neurophilosophical perspective. *Consciousness and Cognition*, **8**, 164–72.

Spittler, J.F. (1992). Der Bewußtseinsbegriff aus neuropsychiatrischer und in interdisziplinärer Sicht [The term consciousness from neuropsychiatric and interdisciplinary views]. *Fortschritte der Neurologie und Psychiatrie*, **60**, 54–65.

Stuss, D.T. & Alexander, M.P. (2000). Affectively burnt in: a proposed role of the right frontal lobe. In *Memory, Consciousness, and the Brain*, ed. E. Tulving, pp. 215–27. Philadelphia, PA: Psychology Press.

Tononi, G. & Edelman, G.M. (1998). Consciousness and complexity. *Science*, **282**, 1846–51.

Tulving, E. (1993). Self-knowledge of an amnesic individual is represented abstractly. In *The Mental Representation of Trait and Autobiographical Knowledge about the Self. Advances in Social Cognition*, vol. V, ed. T.K. Srull & R.S. Wyer Jr, pp. 147–56. Hillsdale, NJ: Lawrence Erlbaum.

Tulving, E. & Markowitsch, H.J. (1998). Episodic and declarative memory: role of the hippocampus. *Hippocampus*, **8**, 198–204.

Tulving, E., Kapur, S., Craik, F.I.M., Moscovitch, M. & Houle, S. (1994). Hemispheric encoding/retrieval asymmetry in episodic memory: positron emission tomography findings. *Proceedings of the National Academy of Sciences of the USA*, **91**, 2016–20.

Vargha-Khadem, F., Gadian, D.G., Watkins, K.E. et al. (1997). Differential effects of early hippocampal pathology on episodic and semantic memory. *Science*, **277**, 376–80.

Wheeler, M.A. (2000). Episodic memory and autonoetic awareness. In *The Oxford Handbook of Memory*, ed. E. Tulving & F.I.M. Craik, pp. 597–608. New York: Oxford University Press.

Wheeler, M.A., Stuss, D.T. & Tulving, E. (1997). Towards a theory of episodic memory. The frontal lobes and autonoetic consciousness. *Psychological Bulletin*, **121**, 331–54.

Wilkes, K.V. (1988). ___, yìshì, duh, um, and consciousness. In *Consciousness in Contemporary Science*, ed. A.J. Marcel & E. Bisiach, pp. 16–41. New York: Oxford University Press.

Woolf, N.J. (1997). A possible role for cholinergic neurons of the basal forebrain and pontomesencephalon in consciousness. *Consciousness and Cognition*, **6**, 574–96.

Woolf, N.J. (1999). Cholinergic correlates of consciousness: from mind to molecules. *Trends in Neurosciences*, **22**, 540–1.

Young, G.B. & Pigott, S.E. (1999). Neurobiological basis of consciousness. *Archives of Neurology*, **56**, 153–7.

10

The neural nature of the core SELF: implications for understanding schizophrenia

Jaak Panksepp

Department of Psychology, Bowling Green State University, Bowling Green, OH, USA

Abstract

Schizophrenia is largely an organic disease that impacts many brain systems, especially those mediating cognition–emotion interactions. The present analysis is premised on the existence of a variety of basic emotional operating systems of the brain – birthrights that allow all newborn mammals to begin navigating the complexities of the world and to learn about the values and reward-related contingencies of the environment. Some of the basic emotional systems have now been provisionally characterized, and they help coordinate behavioural, physiological and psychological aspects of emotionality, including the valenced affective feeling states that provide internally experienced values for the guidance of behaviour. Converging lines of evidence suggest that emotional feelings emerge from the interaction of these systems with longitudinally organized brain process for self-representation that is concentrated in the medial strata of the brain. These include anterior cingulate, insular and frontal cortices, which are richly connected to various medial diencephalic and mesencephalic structures, especially the periaqueductal grey (PAG). This basic neural substrate for self-representation appears to be grounded in stable motor coordinates that generate emotion-specific *intentions in action*, yielding a variety of feeling states that help construct mood-congruent cognitive structures. These systems generate a sense of causality from correlated environmental events and hence promote the emergence of both adaptive and delusional cognitive states. Certain symptoms of schizophrenia may reflect the uncoupling of the higher cognitive and the lower affective processes, disrupting normal modes of emotion regulation and reality testing.

Introduction

Writing a short chapter on the neuropsychology of schizophrenia and the self is like navigating a vast ocean in a rowboat. The probability of being swamped is much greater than a successful passage. Initially, I was disposed to decline the editors' offer to participate in this journey, but ultimately I was tempted to navigate in this realm where metaphor may still provide a better tool for describing the relevant psychic spaces than more prosaic scientific approaches.

Although we now know a great deal about the many brain deficits that characterize schizophrenia (Sedvall & Terenius, 2000), we hardly comprehend how these
changes relate to the various psychic tendencies of schizophrenic minds. Although
brain-imaging technologies are beginning to localize some of the interrelations of
brain–mind activities (Toga & Mazziotta, 2000), including those that accompany
schizophrenia (see chapters 19 and 20 in this volume), the resolution of such techniques is not sufficient to offer insights into the underlying neuropsychological
details. Indeed, all modern brain-imaging pursuits are immediately confronted by
a conundrum: correlational analyses do not reveal causal relationships.

The difficulties entailed in doing causal studies in human beings as well as the
heterogeneity of those states of mind we label selves and schizophrenia confound
our desire to be definitive. A deep understanding of such processes must ultimately
emerge from our ability to fathom how the intrinsic psychobiological functions
of mammalian brains were designed in the crucible of evolution (Stevens & Price,
1996; Cartwright, 2000). Hence, a critical question is: Can we effectively use other
animals for such studies? I believe we can, and my perspective has been moulded
by such enquiries.

Without proper functional conceptualization of normal brain–mind organization, we will never be able to fathom the nature of its disorders. However, there
is no simple way to jump from a knowledge of molecules and neural circuits
in animals to the nature of their functions and disorders in humans. All neural
links to psychological issues must be inferential. Still, an attempt to conceptualize subtle neuropsychological functions, such as self-representation and the basic
emotional and cognitive abilities, is essential for understanding the mental imbalances that characterize schizophrenia. To make progress, we must find a rig-
orous scientific way to link brain dynamics and basic internal feeling processes,
and recently several new strategies for understanding the neurology of human
and animal emotions have been outlined (Panksepp, 1998a; Damasio, 1999; Rolls,
1999).

Neurochemistry provides an especially robust entry point into these issues. The
functions of neurochemical systems across all mammals remain remarkably well
conserved. Since schizophrenic symptoms prominently reflect interactive imbalances of dopaminergic, glutamatergic and GABAergic systems, which probably
perform homologous functions in the brains of all mammals, we may be able to
use animal models to fathom how imbalances in these systems create aberrant
mentations in humans (Panksepp, 1998a; Lipska & Weinberger, 2000).

Of course, all animal models have major problems. Not only is it risky to infer
mental processes simply from the study of behavioural responses, but some of the
key symptoms of schizophrenia (e.g. thought disorders) may be impossible to model
in creatures of modest cortical endowment. Indeed, certain investigators believe

schizophrenia may reflect brain dynamics uniquely related to human linguistic abilities (Crow, 2000). If that is correct, the useful information to be derived from animal work may be minimal. However, because of the deep functional homologies within the affected neurochemical systems and since the aetiology of schizophrenia is surely multiply determined, progress will be swiftest if all productive views are harmoniously integrated.

The present contribution proceeds from the assumption that data from preclinical and clinical studies be blended through creative inference to generate new ways of illuminating the basic nature of schizophrenic disorders. I believe that linking fundamental emotional and self-concepts to specific brain processes, especially when viewed in hierarchical neuroevolutionary terms where new levels of control open up new psychic possibilities, is a productive way to proceed. Indeed, I suspect those foundational systems were essential for consciousness to have emerged in neural evolution.

Neuroscepticism and the neural foundations of emotions

The manner in which a *sense of self* is created within the brain should be one of the foremost problems of neuroscience. This has not been the case for one simple reason: such hypothetical entities are remarkably difficult to study at the neuronal level. However, there are abundant reasons to believe such broad functional entities do exist and that they are fundamentally linked to our basic emotional and motivational capacities which derive a great deal of their affective impact from interacting with basic motor-integrative tendencies (i.e. instinctual emotional responses) that neurosymbolically reflect the organism as an active agent within the brain (Panksepp, 1998a, b). Such neural processes are bound to be represented widely in the brain, but the inevitable complexities have discouraged scientists from explicitly considering such matters until recently (Panksepp, 1998a; Damasio, 1999; Bekoff, 2000; Hauser, 2000).

By tradition, neuroscientists have felt more comfortable in analysing the input–output relations of the nervous systems than the intrinsic psychic structures and the underlying neurodynamics that exist in the *great intermediate net*. However, if that vast neuronal territory between inputs and outputs does contain intrinsic functional entities, created by evolutionary selection rather than simply through the unique experiences of each individual, then we must come to terms with the necessity of a neuroevolutionary approach to clarifying many of the remaining mysteries of the human brain/mind (Panksepp & Panksepp, 2000).

Despite the spectacular recent advances in brain imaging, we are still remote from visualizing the real-time neurodynamics of the vast ensembles of neurons that create the affective textures of human experience. None the less, relevant emotional territories have been glimpsed (Lane et al., 1997; Damasio et al., 2000) and they are remarkably similar to those mapped in animal studies (Panksepp, 1982, 1998a). Hence, we can be certain that there are a variety of evolutionarily derived and epigenetically refined emotional networks that constitute the fundamental substrates of mammalian minds. All mammalian brains have systems for SEEKING, RAGE, FEAR, LUST, CARE, PANIC and PLAY (Panksepp, 1998a, 2000a, e). Capitalizations are used to indicate that specific brain systems are the referents and to minimize part–whole confusions. These systems for distinct emotional–instinctual action tendencies probably generate self-referential affective frameworks for an organism's intrinsic sense of meaning or value. There are now excellent reasons to believe such embodied neuropsychic coherences are produced at comparatively low levels of the neuroaxis, and it has been proposed that an epicentre for self-representation resides in the periaqueductal/periventricular core of the brainstem (Panksepp, 1998a, b). However, this substrate for raw affective consciousness has extensive interrelations with higher brain functions (Damasio, 1999). Indeed, cognitions and emotions interact in specific areas of the brain (Borod, 2000), and a study of those dynamic interfaces may hold the key to understanding schizophrenic mentation (Tononi & Edelman, 1998, 2000).

On the primal nature of the SELF

At present, neural discussions of *the self* remain largely speculative patchworks based on data harvested for other reasons. The impoverished neurological–albeit rich conceptual–state of the field is captured in the recent compendium *Models of the Self* (Gallagher & Shear, 1999). Of the 27 contributions, a single contribution was unabashedly neurological (Panksepp, 1998b). I proposed that the foundation for *the self* is concentrated in centromedial mesencephalic tissues where all basic emotional circuits converge to generate instinctual survival-promoting behaviours and gut-level affective experiences which may constitute the primordial form of consciousness in mind/brain evolution. For semantic convenience, this neural system was designated as the SELF (simple ego-type life form) – a basic neuropsychic homunculus, grounded in action urges, from which a variety of core emotional *states of being* could emerge. This coherent brain function is extended in higher reaches of the brain through individual experiences, partly by the ability of the core SELF to modulate adjacent ascending reticulothalamic arousal systems (Newman, 1997), thereby providing mood-congruent control of higher sensory–perceptual processes. All my subsequent remarks are couched in the recognition that this is an ultracomplex integrative process that remains in desperate need of detailed empirical analysis.

The fundamental circuitry of the SELF appears quite similar (i.e. homologous) in all mammals, but its developmental ramifications within higher regions of the brain can take many species-typical trajectories. For instance, at the lower levels of integration in the midbrain and closely related limbic structures, the system presumably provides an unreflective, existential feeling of *I-ness* which organisms implicitly experience as a variety of basic psychomotor *states of being* (providing, perhaps, in Freudian terms, a variety of *id* structures for each animal). Within the higher sensory cortices (e.g. parietal, occipital and temporal), the developmental interactions of the SELF-system with various perceptual processes may generate a *me-ness* where one can actively contemplate one's state of being, which in highly cerebrated species leads to reflective self-recognition (providing *ego* structures for organisms). Within the higher executive motor regions of the brain such as the frontal lobes, the outgrowths of these processes may generate feelings of *mineness*, whereby one actively *possesses* perceptions of the world and egocentrically identifies one's place in the world and its cultural dynamics (ultimately providing *superego* functions for the human brain/mind).

Of course, these systems interpenetrate in dynamic gradients, which make all of our conceptual simplifications provisional ways to consider the underlying complexities. Although these hierarchical levels of self-representation are integrated in the healthy brain, presumably their interrelations become unravelled, to various degrees, in schizophrenia. This fraying could occur at multiple levels. If so, schizophrenia is surely a class of disorders in which some of the major types of psychic organization no longer operate harmoniously.

In terms of antecedent views of the primal self, one well-developed proposal put forward by Strehler (1991) sought to localize the epicentre of self-representation within the superior colliculus (SC) of the midbrain. In line with traditional thinking, Strehler's proposal is very much focused on sensory/perceptual processes of the brain.

My view (Panksepp, 1998a, b) is superficially similar to Strehler's, in that it recognizes the essential role of converging exteroceptive processes upon primitive multimodal brain areas such as the colliculi, but, along with related recent works (Watt, 2000), it advances that view in two distinct ways:

1. It emphasizes that self-representation must be closely linked to primal emotional value-generating mechanisms such as those that are concentrated within the underlying PAG.
2. It highlights the likelihood that self-representation has to be built upon stable motor coordinates, such as the somatic motor map nestled between the visceral integrations of the PAG ventrally and the somatosensory fields of the SC dorsally.

This primitive but coherent map of the body, receiving both exteroceptive and interoceptive guidance, has the necessary characteristics that a fundamental self-system should contain. The mental life of infants is presumed to be intimately and inextricably linked to this substrate for organismic coherence. Without this circuitry, no infant would survive, nor do adults (Bailey & Davis, 1942, 1943). In other words, babies and perhaps *lower* organisms in whom these systems are very active (Chugani, 1996) may primarily utilize these old parts for elaborating conscious awareness (Sewards & Sewards, 2000). Of course, this is only the *seed* of the extended adult self that projects to the highest reaches of the frontal lobes. In other words, the system grows and elaborates hierarchically in the brain as a function of the emerging developmental landscapes of individual lives.

Damasio's (1999) recent perspective on consciousness is also based on a core self constructed upon basic homeostatic systems of the brainstem. There seems to be one major difference between my view and that advanced by Damasio. His is premised very much on sensory processes, while I would advocate that motor coordinates exist at the very foundation of the SELF process. I believe a motor perspective helps save the present construct from the classic sensory-centric paradox of the infinite regress of observers (Panksepp, 2000c). The role of internal motor coordinates in the construction of consciousness has been surprisingly undervalued, but I cannot envision the evolution of consciousness without a stable integrated capacity for various instinctual action tendencies anchoring the emergence of higher brain/mind functions.

Perhaps the most striking point of agreement among all of the above proposals, and where they depart from most other formulations, is that they seek the foundational nature of the self at a rather low level of the neuroaxis. The above views are preconditioned by the widespread recognition that adjacent brainstem systems, classically conceptualized as the reticular-activating system, are essential for maintaining forebrain arousal (for a modernized overview, see Newman, 1997). However, it is now clear that there are intrinsic emotional functions, long neglected in consciousness studies, concentrated within nearby PAG zones which may help govern the emotion-specific quality of forebrain arousal, yielding internal affective feelings of evolutionary qualia (i.e. equalia) within the brain. Many of these feelings are not strictly linked to external events, but to internal interpretations of events and other internal neural activities.

Indeed, it is possible that this neural foundation for affective consciousness is necessary for the rest of the brain to create exteroceptive qualia: the extended SELF may constitute a global multimodal neurodynamic that allows sensory inputs to be resolved into an image of the world as the organism experiences it. Early studies highlighted how essential this tissue is for the conscious mental life of cats and monkeys (Bailey & Davis, 1942, 1943), and it is not much different for humans (Schiff & Plum, 1999, 2000).

I think the widespread failure to consider the role of such intrinsic motor-integrative systems in the creation of consciousness may be based on the faulty preconception that motor systems are psychologically passive output devices as opposed to complex systems with experienced feelings of their own that provide a unique substrate for the construction of consciousness. The felt urge to behave in various ways, albeit subtle in comparison to the perceptual impact of the exteroceptive senses, is here postulated to be a critical aspect of all other forms of consciousness.

Many are bound to find such a 'motor' view of primary-process consciousness baffling and counterintuitive, but close your eyes and imagine what it might be like within the mind's eye if that ever-present but psychologically subtle process that 'wants to do things' were to disappear. Would all of consciousness follow? I suspect it might. What if this entity were only partly disengaged from the sensory–perceptual world or destabilized? Would we have variants of the kinds of psychological chaos we call schizophrenia?

By considering such a view, we can solve many philosophical conundrums, including: (1) the infinite regress of recursive observers in the brain/mind; (2) the neurobiological nature of emotional experience; and (3) the existence of a basic *human/animal nature* that helps guide many developmental learning mechanisms. In such a scenario, the integrated bodily dynamics of emotions (e.g. the forcefulness of anger, the trembling of fear, the eager forward-directedness of seeking and the languishing despair of social loss), so evident in spontaneous human and animal body language, reflects the biologically dictated core values – the evolutionarily provided affects and motivations – of each organism.

In historical terms, such intrinsic processes of the brain/mind have been called *instincts*, and they have been viewed simply as complex motor capacities of the organism that are mere output functions and hence free of *mind stuff*. However, there are reasons to believe that the essential neuronal organizing principles that govern so-called instinctual actions add a critical dimension to mental existence. They appear to create a neurodynamic state of here-and-now affective consciousness, the experience of being an active organism in the world, that is not dependent on higher cognitive processes but which is highly interactive with them (Panksepp, 2000b, c, d).

The reason such a view has not been more attractive has curious historical threads, embedded in a widely accepted dualism – that mind and brain can be independently conceptualized – which still permeates our western intellectual tradition. In a nutshell, many assume that *I think and perceive, therefore I am* is the main path to understanding human nature and consciousness as opposed to giving equal attention to the notion that *I act and feel, therefore I am*. The perception-centric view of consciousness has led most to focus their efforts at high cortical levels with a benign neglect of subcortical issues. The implicit assumption has been that the primitive mesencephalic and diencephalic systems are merely permissive, providing simple *switches* for consciousness to be turned on upstairs in the brain.

The relevant human neurological evidence for the essential role of subcortical functions has been compelling for quite a while (Damasio, 1999; Mesulam, 2000;

Schiff & Plum, 2000). The animal data have also been remarkably concordant with the essential role of emotional processes and a primitive form of self-representation in guiding the emergence of consciousness (Panksepp, 1998b). Indeed, I have suggested three major criteria for identifying brain areas critical for constructing the emotional SELF, and they all affirm that a primordial epicentre for affect is probably situated in dorsal midbrain tissues that include the PAG:

1. Electrical stimulation there, at the lowest thresholds to be found anywhere in the brain, can produce the largest number of distinct emotional behavioural changes in animals and emotional subjective changes in humans.

2. The smallest amount of damage at this brain location can compromise the ability of the animal to exhibit a coherent emotional presence in the world.

3. This part of the brain has among the highest densities of visceral and somatic inputs from a diversity of brain areas, and an equally impressive set of outputs to both higher and lower regions of the brain (for the relevant literature, see Holstege et al., 1996).

This whole integrated system is here considered as the neural substrate of the SELF. Unfortunately, a depth of psychological conceptualization and corresponding empirical analyses of these primitive functions has barely been initiated. Since such primitive instinct-generating systems have been marginalized in our understanding of self-representation and consciousness, let me expand a bit on this issue before proceeding to some clinical implications.

The essential motor underpinnings of consciousness

The prevailing approach in consciousness studies is to comprehend how the rich sensorial/perceptual experience of conscious awareness is created. Indeed, it is now quite clear that even internally generated sensory images are tightly coupled to brain systems that generate exteroceptive perceptions (Nyberg et al., 2000; Wheeler et al., 2000). Important as those lines of enquiry are for understanding the *tools of consciousness* (Crick & Koch, 2000), the sensory-centric approach cannot yield a satisfactory understanding of primary process consciousness – that active feeling of a state of being that persists even when we shut our sensory portals (Panksepp, 2000f). There is much to commend the view that central motor representations provide an essential evolutionary grounding for the emergence of primary-process consciousness.

The primordial *I*–the SELF – that all of us experience seems to be a unified process that is critically dependent on our intrinsic capacity to exhibit spontaneous *intentions in action*. There is considerable evidence that our actions continually guide and focus our attentional and perceptual resources, for one end – the generation of effective behaviour to help us survive. In the evolution of consciousness, integrated action tendencies, perhaps still reflected in our emotional urges, came before any thought could be generated about how to act. Perceptions only allow appropriate guidance for those action processes, and there is no reason to believe that the posterior sensory cortices disconnected from the rest of the brain could elaborate any level of consciousness on their own. Accordingly, it may be impossible to fathom how the richness of sensorial experience is created without first considering the primacy of ancient psychomotor processes in creating a stable foundation for human and animal *minds.*

Since many people in neuroscience have trouble with the concept of mind, let me share one compelling perspective: minds came into existence when the evolved complexities of the nervous system allowed organisms *to know* more than is contained within their reflexive responses to the world (Godfrey-Smith, 1996). In my estimation, much of the knowledge is based upon the intrinsic systems of the brain that generate affect. In other words, the existence of mind can be inferred whenever a substantial amount of the variability in the behaviour of organisms can only be understood with reference to the brain's intrinsic representational abilities. For instance, the ability to experience raw affect may be an essential antecedent to foresight, planning, and thereby wilful intentionality. This allows brains to seek meaning intrinsically by dynamically *grasping* or comprehending the world in psychically energized, anticipatory ways (Freeman, 1999; Ikemoto & Panksepp, 1999). In short, mind reflects the intrinsic ways, often internally experienced, that brains reach out into the world in their attempts to make sense of internal imbalances and environmental circumstances that can help alleviate those imbalances.

In this view, intrinsic psychomotor tendencies can be considered the bedrock for the generation of this reaching-out process – the primordial neural substrates of the SELF – which is essential for integrating intrinsic fitness-related information to be derived from the external world. Thus, when we begin to view the ancient substrates of the mammalian brain in terms of endogenous systems that spontaneously guide behaviour, as opposed to simply ones that are constructed by reinforcement processes and other environmental constraints, we have a realistic way to conceptualize not only the nature of affect but the intrinsic, evolutionarily provided functional structure of the mind (Panksepp & Panksepp, 2000). This image of the fundamental neural systems for the generation of primary-process consciousness and intentionality (Panksepp, 2000a) may have some novel implications for our understanding of schizophrenia as well as some perplexing scientific curiosities.

Resolving the Libet paradox

Let me briefly consider one of the greatest paradoxes of consciousness studies from the above perspective. Twenty years ago Benjamin Libet demonstrated that, when humans generate voluntary movements, electroencephalographic changes are evident *before* the visually indexed awareness that one had intended to move (for recent summary, see Libet, 1999). In short, the brain initiates action before perceptual systems know about an individual's intentions. Accordingly, Libet suggested that the function of consciousness is not to initiate actions but only to edit behaviours that have been initiated unconsciously.

Libet's work was an enormous challenge to conventional thinking about the extent of our *free will*. However, by respecting the possibility that consciously experienced intentions may be more tightly linked to intrinsic brain motor processes than to sensory ones, the above paradox loses its impact: for instance, central psychomotor urges are the conscious substrates of willed action, and this type of arousal may be essential for the sensory–perceptual apparatus to harvest related information. Thus, willed actions and their correlated brain changes may occur *before* one can appreciate seeing the time at which one performs an action. In other words, perceptual consciousness may typically tend to follow the wilful responses that represent a more primary form of consciousness. If so, sensory consciousness may be fundamentally grounded upon some type of internal action capacities.

Although perceptions are the most evident aspects of our ongoing stream of conscious awareness, even modest contemplation of the inner life highlights that the internal generation of actions is essential for our perceptual systems to operate optimally. Although it is subjectively hard to dissociate sensory perception from internal motor processes, it seems likely from straightforward evolutionary perspectives that the capacity to perceive is closely linked to the capacity to act. Indeed, even cursory introspection suggests that action tendencies have a subtle feeling tone all their own. This view is also suggested by single-unit studies of primitive perceptual processes, where a stable motor apparatus determines how the perceptual surfaces of the brain operate (Sparks, 1988). In sum, the position advanced here is that the instinctual–emotional action systems of the mammalian brain constitute neuronal centres of gravity that provide an organic infrastructure and coherence for the rest of the neuropsychic apparatus. Such basic control processes may be absolutely essential for all other forms of consciousness. Of course, with higher cerebral evolution, the resonances of such systems became widely represented in the brain, both genetically and developmentally.

Neural hierarchies in the SELF-structures

The foundational structures of the core SELF, as represented in the centromedial structures of the brainstem, are closely linked to the more rostral brain structures that have been implicated in schizophrenic disorders. These include the dorsomedial thalamus (~30% neuronal loss in schizophrenia), nucleus accumbens (~50%

neuronal loss), anterior cingulate (selective loss of GABAergic interneurons) and the frontal lobes (diminished arousability, with no consistent neuronal loss). In other words, careful analyses of neural differences have implicated all of these structures in schizophrenic disorders (Thune & Pakkenberg, 2000), so let us inquire how these higher brain changes are related to the primordial SELF.

Anatomically, there are extensive neuronal interactions among these brain zones. For instance, there is a massive descending input from medial frontal areas to the PAG (Shipley et al., 1996). The nucleus accumbens receives descending inputs from the frontal cortex, and sends efferents to both the medial thalamus and the PAG (for summary, see Figure 1 in Ikemoto & Panksepp, 1999). The anterior cingulate is closely linked to medial thalamic, hypothalamic and PAG systems (Butler & Hodos, 1996). In short, these areas constitute an integrated system, where the lower components mediate basic emotional/affective action tendencies while the higher areas provide various regulatory controls better conceptualized in traditional cognitive terms. The higher parts of the SELF system in medial frontal and cingulate areas presumably provide affective interfaces to higher cognitive processes that would be operating without the guidance of feelings otherwise. If schizophrenia is fundamentally some kind of a neuronal disconnection syndrome, especially of small inhibitory–regulatory components such as GABAergic cells (Benes, 2000), which help mediate between higher and lower brain functions, then we can begin to understand why cognitive and affective activities may no longer be synchronized.

One way of viewing such circuits in action is that various higher cognitive components normally regulate more primitive emotional tendencies. This regulation may be substantially effected via glutamatergic influences on GABAergic interneurons, yielding a multitude of neural interfaces between cognitive activities and more primitive self-centred emotional urges. An individual suffering from schizophrenia may experience an inner world that is no longer clearly related to external events. As a result, external events may seem more novel, and thereby take on a stronger self-referential salience for which new meanings need to be constructed. This may lead to various schizophrenic symptoms such as paranoid delusions, the reduced ability to experience positive emotional states linked to incoming perceptions, and hence the dissolution of social relations and attachments.

The failure of the cognitive apparatus to connect with the primordial SELF may also help explain why schizophrenic speech is full of loose abstractions. In other words, instead of the individual SELF being woven into the fabric of external events, those events become dissociated from one's egocentric emotional concerns. Thus, the individual's psychic life may become more intimately intermeshed with the basic SELF processes, many of which, when not regulated by social systems, leave a negative feeling tone. In this regression, one is bound to experience emotions more intensely, perhaps in aversive and frightening ways that are disconnected from world events. Concurrently, one might anticipate that the regulation of cognitive spaces by the core SELF could become less effective, allowing the whole perceptual system to run free, yielding a characteristic hallucinatory overlay to everyday sensory experience.

Although there is insufficient space to get into detailed arguments, this may help explain why schizophrenia has been more closely linked to the frontal cortical motor executive processes than to the more posterior sensory processes (Andreasen et al., 1986; Benes et al., 1991) as well as to ascending dopamine systems which control frontal lobe functions (Grace, 2000). These are interface zones between primitive affective–instinctual and higher cognitive–experiential processes. The damage that has been observed in related dorsomedial thalamic and basal ganglia structures such as the amygdala which control emotional output systems of the brain (Bogerts et al., 1985; Rossi et al., 1994; Thune & Pakkenberg, 2000) are also consistent with the idea that the interface between emotional and cognitive processes has been disrupted in schizophrenia.

Toward animal models of schizophrenia

Imbalances in dopamine, GABA and glutamate systems figure most prominently in neurochemical theories of schizophrenia, albeit in ways that are not yet free of empirical contradictions (Sedvall & Terenius, 2000). This is not the place to detail the evidence, but to note that dopamine arousal promotes a coherent psychobiological message: seek resources vigorously (Ikemoto & Panksepp, 1999). Obviously, successful seeking behaviour can only be achieved effectively by interactions with cognitive, sensory/perceptual structures, at the heart of which are neocortical circuits critically dependent on glutamate and GABA.

Indeed, the mesolimbic dopamine system has now been conceptualized as part of a general-purpose appetitive motivation-*seeking* system of the brain that helps coordinate the construction of meaningful appetitive views of the world (Panksepp, 1998a; Ikemoto & Panksepp, 1999). It is positioned between bodily need states and environmental events so as to create and promote goal-directed activities, partially by establishing appetitive expectancies about events and objects. When this system is aroused, animal brains are especially likely to generate associations between world events and appetitive eagerness. In essence, this can be seen as facilitating the creation of unrealistic confirmation biases – beliefs that certain events are caused by certain other correlated events – which may be a key feature of schizophrenic delusions. In other words, excessively aroused brain dopamine which controls the gating of certain forms of information in the brain (Grace, 2000), may be an ideal neurochemical condition for solidifying internal convictions concerning the causal relationships among events (including internal psychological events), most of which are delusional (i.e. based merely on correlations). Precisely how this occurs can be studied in some detail in animal models (Ikemoto & Panksepp, 1999).

The GABA deficiency of schizophrenia may be most clearly highlighted by the deficiency in the automatic establishment of preparatory inhibitory sets in the schizophrenic brain. One of the clearest is the tendency of organisms to reduce their reflexive startle when attentional systems are aroused. This process is captured in the model of *prepulse inhibition* – namely the presentation of a mild sound just before the presentation of a startlingly loud stimulus (Swerdlow, 1996). This deficiency is also evident in schizophrenics, and to some extent, it reflects the diminution of GABA-mediated inhibition over emotional responses.

If one of the key deficits in schizophrenia is the diminution of GABAergic inhibition (Benes, 2000), perhaps created at some point in development by glutamatergic overactivity and eventual neurotoxicity, this may disconnect higher-brain regulatory and lower-brain emotional structures. To create an animal model of such a condition, we have injected rat pups during early development with the glutamate-like neurotoxin kainic acid (Gordon et al., 1998). The resulting brain injury (Olney & Farber, 1995), includes diffuse damage to many limbic structures, including pockets of damage in medial frontal areas, medial thalamic nuclei as well as extensive damage to reticular nuclei of the thalamus, yielding a characteristic syndrome of striking and lifelong temperamental change: such animals are generally hyperresponsive to handling (always squealing when handled) and they become socially incompetent (incapable of sustaining normal social interchange, as in social play). Although it would be premature to conclude that this is an animal model of schizophrenia, it allows us to study the specific symptoms of glutamate-induced neurotoxicities in the emergence of psychotic symptoms. From these data, we would suggest that one additional reasonable area to seek neuronal damage in the schizophrenic brain may be the inhibitory GABAergic neurons of the nucleus reticularis of the thalamus.

Future prospects

The view advanced here is that an understanding of how the brain mediates consciousness and the resulting disorders of consciousness cannot make much progress unless we vigorously confront the fundamental neural nature of affective processes and SELF-representation within the brain. Perhaps a clear conceptualization of such fundamental issues, which can only really be approached mechanistically through animal brain research, may have wider clinical implications for understanding schizophrenia and other psychiatric disorders than is commonly recognized (Panksepp, 1998a). Of course the complexity of the neural systems that have already been found to be disrupted in schizophrenia are so vast (Sevall & Terenius, 2000) that no simple conceptual scheme is likely to provide a satisfactory organizing principle for all findings.

In any event, the present view does suggest some critical observations that need to be made. Chronic schizophrenics seem to exhibit deficits in experiencing and expressing affect. To my knowledge, no one has yet characterized neuronal densities and patterns in more caudal midline regions such as the periventricular and PAG areas where primordial SELF structures are postulated to be situated. The neglect of such brain areas may simply have arisen because they are generally deemed irrelevant for the expression of schizophrenic symptoms. However, the same bias existed for Alzheimer's disease, but recent work has found dramatic neuropathologies within the PAG among Alzheimer's patients (Parvizi et al., 2000). Were it to turn out that there are no major disruptions in such periventricular systems in schizophrenia, then we might have to conclude that schizophrenic individuals have no fundamental deficits in elaborating primary-process emotionality. Then we might be more confident that their core deficits are restricted more to disconnections between the lower primary-process and higher cognitive mechanisms of the forebrain.

Finally, it may be worth noting that the old idea that schizophrenia may resemble the dream state, although largely abandoned in the modern era (Douglass, 1996), could have a new lease of life. It has been found that during rapid-eye-movement sleep, when much of the sleeping brain seems to wake up, certain frontal lobe areas tend to remain asleep (Marquet et al., 1996). Are these the same brain areas that are dysfunctional in the schizophrenic brain? If such frontal areas are relatively *offline* in certain schizophrenic syndromes, we may again need to consider that neural commonalities may exist in these bizarre forms of mentation which reflect the uncoupling of higher and lower brain functions. Just as dreaming is characterized by a regression toward primary-process mentation, schizophrenia may largely be a syndrome in which higher executive and lower emotional brain functions are uncoupled, leading to an incoherent sense of self and a disruption in the felt 'ownership' of qualia.

REFERENCES

Andreasen, N., Nasrallah, H., Dunn, V. et al. (1986). Structural abnormalities in the frontal system in schizophrenia. *Archives of General Psychiatry*, **43**, 136–44.

Bailey, P. & Davis, E.W. (1942). Effects of lesions of the periaqueductal gray matter in the cat. *Proceedings of the Society for Experimental Biology and Medicine*, **351**, 305–6.

Bailey, P. & Davis, E.W. (1943). Effects of lesions of the periaqueductal gray matter on the *Macaca mulatta*. *Journal of Neuropathology and Experimental Neurology*, **3**, 69–72.

Bekoff, M. (ed.) (2000). *The Smile of a Dolphin*. New York: Discovery Books.

Benes, F.M. (2000). Emerging principles of altered neuronal circuitry in schizophrenia. *Brain Research Reviews*, **31**, 252–69.

Benes, F.M., McSparren, J., Bird, E.D., SanGiovanni, J.P. & Vincent, S.L. (1991). Deficits in small interneurons in prefrontal and cingulate cortices of schizophrenic and schizoaffective patients. *Archives of General Psychiatry*, **48**, 996–1001.

Bogerts, B., Meertz, E. & Schonfeldt-Bausch, R. (1985). Basal ganglia and limbic system pathology in schizophrenia. *Archives of General Psychiatry*, **42**, 784–91.

Borod, J.C. (2000). *The Neuropsychology of Emotion*. New York: Oxford University Press.

Butler, A.B. & Hodos, W. (1996). *Comparative Vertebrate Neuroanatomy: Evolution and Adaptation* New York: Wiley-Liss.

Cartwright, J. (2000). *Evolution and Human Behavior*. Cambridge, MA: MIT Press.

Chugani, H.T. (1996). Neuroimaging of developmental nonlinearity and developmental pathologies. In *Developmental Neuroimaging: Mapping the Development of Brain and Behavior*, ed. R.W. Thatcher, G. Reid Lyon, J. Rumsey & N. Krasnegor, pp. 187–95. San Diego: Academic Press.

Crick, F. & Koch, C. (2000). The unconscious homunculus. *Neuro-Psychoanalysis*, **2**, 3–10.

Crow, T.J. (2000). Schizophrenia as the price that *Homo sapiens* pays for language: a resolution of the central paradox in the origin of the species. *Brain Research Reviews*, **31**, 118–29.

Damasio, A.R. (1999). *The Feeling of What Happens: Body and Emotion in the Making of Consciousness*. New York: Harcourt Brace.

Damasio, A.R., Grabowski, T.J., Bechara, A. et al. (2000). Subcortical and cortical brain activity during the feeling of self-generated emotions. *Nature Neuroscience*, **3**, 1049–56.

Douglass, A.B. (1996). Sleep abnormalities in major psychiatric illnesses: polysomnographic and clinical features. In *Advances in Biological Psychiatry*, vol. 2, ed. J. Panksepp, pp. 153–77. Greenwich, CT: JAI Press.

Freeman, W.J. (1999). *How the Brain Makes up Its Mind*. London: Blackwell.

Gallagher, S. & Shear, J. (eds) (1999). *Models of the Self*, Thorverton, UK: Imprint Academic.

Godfrey-Smith, P. (1996). *Complexity and the Function of Mind in Nature*. New York: Cambridge University Press.

Gordon, N., Panksepp, J., Secor, A. et al. (1998). Peripherally administered kainic acid induced brain damage effects on social and non-social behaviors. *Society for Neuroscience Abstracts*, **24**, 691.

Grace, A.A. (2000). Gating of information flow within the limbic system and the pathophysiology of schizophrenia. *Brain Research Reviews*, **31**, 330–41.

Hauser, M.D. (2000). *Wild Minds: What Animals Really Think*. New York: Henry Holt.

Holstege, G., Bandler, R. & Saper, C.B. (eds) (1996) *The Emotional Motor System. Progress in Brain Research*, vol. 107. Amsterdam: Elsevier.

Ikemoto, S. & Panksepp, J. (1999). The role of nucleus accumbens dopamine in motivated behavior: a unifying interpretation with special reference to reward-seeking. *Brain Research Reviews*, **31**, 6–41.

Lane, R.D., Reiman, E.M., Bradley, M.M. et al. (1997). Neuroanatomical correlates of pleasant and unpleasant emotion. *Neuropsychologia*, **15**, 1437–44.

Libet, B. (1999). Do we have free will? *Journal of Consciousness Studies*, **6**, 47–57.

Lipska, B.K. & Weinberger, D.R. (2000). To model a psychiatric disorder in animals: schizophrenia as a reality test. *Neuropsychopharmacology*, **23**, 223–39.

Maquet, P., Peters, J.-M., Aerts, J. et al. (1996). Functional neuroanatomy of human rapid-eye-movement sleep and dreaming. *Nature*, **383**, 163–6.

Mesulam, M.-M. (ed.) (2000). *Principles of Behavior and Cognitive Neurology*, 2nd edn. New York: Oxford University Press.

Newman, J. (1997). Putting the puzzle together: towards a general theory of the neural correlates of consciousness, *Journal of Consciousness Studies*, **4**, 47–66, 101–21.

Nyberg, L., Habib, R., McIntosh, A.R. & Tulving, E. (2000). Reactivation of encoding-related brain activity during memory retrieval. *Proceedings of the National Academy of Sciences of the USA*, **97**, 1120–24.

Olney, J.W. & Farber, N.B. (1995). NMDA antagonists as neurotherapeutic drugs, psychotogens, neurotoxins, and research tools for studying schizophrenia. *Neuropsychopharmacology*, **13**, 335–45.

Panksepp, J. (1982). Toward a general psychobiological theory of emotions. *Behavioral and Brain Sciences*, **5**, 407–67.

Panksepp, J. (1998a). *Affective Neuroscience: The Foundations of Human and Animal Emotion*. New York: Oxford University Press.

Panksepp, J. (1998b). The periconscious substrates of consciousness: affective states and the evolutionary origins of the self. *Journal of Consciousness Studies*, **5**, 566–82.

Panksepp, J. (2000a). Emotions as natural kinds within the mammalian brain. In: *The Handbook of Emotions*, 2nd edn, ed. M. Lewis and J. Haviland, pp. 137–56. New York: Guilford.

Panksepp, J. (2000b). The neurodynamics of emotions: an evolutionary-neurodevelopmental view. In *Emotion, Self-Organization, and Development*, ed. M.D. Lewis & I. Granic, pp. 236–64. New York: Cambridge University Press.

Panksepp, J. (2000c). Affective consciousness and the instinctual motor system: The neural sources of sadness and joy. In *The Caldron of Consciousness: Motivation, Affect and Self-Organization. Advances in Consciousness Research*, ed. R. Ellis & N. Newton, pp. 27–54. Amsterdam: John Benjamins.

Panksepp, J.(2000d). The neuro-evolutionary cusp between emotions and cognitions: implications for understand consciousness and the emergence of a unified mind science. *Consciousness and Emotion*, **1**, 17–56.

Panksepp, J. (2000e). Emotional circuits of the mammalian brain: implications for biological psychiatry. In *Biological Psychiatry*, ed. E.E. Bittar, pp. 27–58. Greenwich, CT: JAI Press.

Panksepp, J. (2000f). The cradle of consciousness: a periconscious emotional homunclus? *Neuro-Psychoanalysis*, **2**, 24–32.

Panksepp, J. & Panksepp, J.B. (2000). The seven sins of evolutionary psychology. *Evolution and Cognition*, **6**, 108–31.

Parvizi, J., Van Hoesen, G.W. & Damasio, A. (2000). Selective pathological changes of the periaqueductal gray in Alzheimer's disease. *Annals of Neurology*, **48**, 344–53.

Rolls, E.T. (1999). *The Brain and Emotion*. Oxford, UK: Oxford University Press.

Rossi, A., Stratta, P., Mancini, F. et al. (1994). Magnetic resonance imaging findings of amygdala-anterior hippocampus shrinkage in male patients with schizophrenia. *Psychiatry Research*, **52**, 43–53.

Schiff, N. & Plum, F. (1999). The neurology of impaired consciousness: global disorders and implied models. Target article for *Association for the Scientific Study of Consciousness Electronic Seminar*. http://athena.english.vt.edu/cgi.bin/netforum/nic/a/1

Schiff, N.D. & Plum, F. (2000). The role of arousal and 'gating' systems in the neurology of impaired consciousness. *Journal of Clinical Neuropsychology*, **17**, 438–452.

Sedvall, G. & Terenius, L. (eds) (2000). Schizophrenia: pathophysiological mechanisms. *Brain Research Reviews*, **31**, 106–404.

Sewards, T.V. & Sewards, M.A. (2000). Visual awareness due to neuronal activities in subcortical structures: a proposal. *Consciousness and Cognition*, **9**, 86–116.

Stevens, A. & Price, J. (1996). *Evolutionary Psychology: A New Beginning*. London: Routledge.

Strehler, B.L. (1991). Where is the self? A neuroanatomical theory of consciousness. *Synapse*, **7**, 44–91.

Swerdlow, N.R. (1996). Cortico-striate substrates of cognitive, motor, and sensory gating: speculation and implications for psychological function and dysfunction. In *Advances in Biological Psychiatry*, vol. 2, ed. J. Panksepp, pp. 179–207. Greenwich, CT: JAI Press.

Thune, J.J. & Pakkenberg, B. (2000). Stereological studies of the schizophrenic brain. *Brain Research Reviews*, **31**, 200–4.

Toga, A.W. & Mazziotta, J.C. (eds.) (2000) *Brain Mapping: The Systems*. San Diego, CA: Academic Press.

Tononi, G. & Edelman, G.M. (1998). Consciousness and complexity. *Science*, **282**, 1846–51.

Tononi, G. & Edelman, G.M. (2000). Schizophrenia and the mechanisms of conscious integration. *Brain Research Reviews*, **31**, 391–400.

Watt, D.G. (2000). The centrencephalon and thalamocortical integration: neglected contributions of periaqueductal gray. *Consciousness and Emotion*, **1**: 91–114.

Wheeler, M.E., Petersen, S.E. & Buckner, R.L. (2000). Memory's echo: vivid remembering reactivates sensory-specific cortex. *Proceedings of the National Academy of Sciences of the USA*, **97**, 11125–9.

Part III

Disturbances of the self: the case of schizophrenia

i Phenomenology

11

Self and schizophrenia: a phenomenological perspective

Josef Parnas

Department of Psychiatry, Hvidovre Hospital and Danish National Research Foundation: Center for Subjectivity Research, University of Copenhagen, Denmark

The greatest hazard of all, losing one's self, can occur very quietly in the world, as if it was nothing at all. No other loss can occur so quietly; any other loss – an arm, a leg, five dollars, a wife etc. – is sure to be noticed (Søren Kirkegaard).

Abstract

The purpose of this chapter is to present in clinical detail phenomenology of the disorders of self-experience that are observable in the schizophrenia spectrum conditions. Schizophrenia was considered by the founders of its concept as an instance of a severe affliction of the self, and psychiatric literature, especially of the phenomenological tradition, contains descriptions and analyses of the self-disorders. Recent empirical, phenomenologically informed research conducted in Denmark, Germany and Norway has provided empirical data demonstrating that not-yet-psychotic anomalies of self-experience occur frequently in the beginning stages of schizophrenia and in the schizotypal conditions. The most fundamental level of selfhood that appears to be affected in early schizophrenia is the automatic, preflective articulation of the first-person perspective. It is suggested that these subtle phenotypes may be of potential value as target phenomena for pathogenetic research (especially for research in the neurodevelopmental antecedents) and also of crucial importance for early differential diagnosis.

Introduction

Typically, psychiatric, cognitive and philosophical studies of anomalous experience and belief in schizophrenia focus on the well-crystallized psychotic stages, dominated by the so-called Schneiderian first-rank symptoms (Frith, 1992; Campbell, 1999). This unilateral emphasis on the symptoms of the advanced illness risks overlooking informative, though less spectacular, antecedents of such symptoms and syndromes (Parnas & Bovet, 1995; Parnas et al., 1996). Subtle experiential antecedents may indeed set important constraints on theoretical considerations, construction of pathogenetic models and ensuing empirical hypotheses. This issue becomes quite critical if one assumes that the *early* ontogenetical features, rather than the symptoms of the advanced illness, mirror the disorders indicative of the pathogenetic illness core. In all likelihood, advanced illness stages reflect accumulated sediments of long-standing interactions between the primary causal factors, variety of stress impacts, secondary illness adversities (e.g. isolation), treatment effects, and attempts to cope and adapt. Potential effects of the primary pathogenetic factors may simply fade out in the phenotypic noise of the advanced disease (Parnas, 1999a, 2000).

In line with this general epistemological concern, this contribution will focus on the clinical manifestations of self-disorders that may be detectable in the prodromal and premorbid phases of schizophrenia (*preonset* or *prepsychotic* phases). In addition to its potential theoretical value, such a task is also of obvious pragmatic significance given the recent emphasis on the prognostic importance of early diagnostic detection and therapeutic intervention in schizophrenia (McGlashan & Johannessen, 1996; Parnas, 1999a). Behaviourally defined prodromal features of schizophrenia are for this purpose prohibitively common in the general population (Mc Gorry et al., 1995) and 'behavioural deviations alone, without exploring subjective experience, lack the specificity necessary to predict future schizophrenia' (Weiser et al., 2001; p. 962). For this reason, nearly all early therapeutic programmes target *already psychotic* cases, albeit in their early stages (Larsen et al., 2001).

However, addressing self-disorders quickly runs into significant obstacles and ambiguities. The term *depersonalization* was coined in 1899 (Cattell & Cattell, 1974). The term is retained in the contemporary psychiatric vocabulary, but with confused usage (Spitzer, 1988; Cutting, 1997). Current diagnostic systems (*Diagnostic and Statistical Manual of Mental Disorders* (DSM-IV: American Psychiatric Association, 1994) and *International Classification of Diseases* (ICD-10: World Health Organization, 1992)) contain this category as a *separate disorder*, but there is no agreement whether it is empirically justified. The notion of self is removed from the psychiatric terminology of DSM-IV and ICD-10. It is rarely used in the psychiatric literature, and if it is, then it is used either in a colloquial or a psychoanalytic sense. Empirical psychology and cognitive science usually understand the self as a theoretical *construct*, an approach that is of limited clinical–descriptive utility, because it is strongly saturated by specific metaphysical (representational–computational) views on the nature of mind (Parnas & Bovet, 1995). Yet, in spite of these difficulties, a search for a faithful *description of experience* must be considered a necessary first step towards a possibility of its scientific reduction (Parnas & Zahavi, 2002). This prerequisite, articulated in psychopathology by Karl Jaspers in 1913, has more recently been expressed by Thomas Nagel (1974, p. 437) in relation to consciousness research: 'a necessary requirement for any coherent reductionism is that the entity to be reduced is properly understood'.

In order to meet these descriptive needs, a phenomenological approach is adopted here (see chapter 3, this volume): the self has an experiential mental reality, primarily as a *first-person givenness of experience* (Zahavi & Parnas, 1998; Zahavi, 1999; Parnas & Zahavi, 2002). This basic and foundational form of selfhood is an *implicit, prereflective egocentricity*, automatically saturating the very manifestation of experience. Thus the basic self equals a dimension of 'myness' of experience, a dimension that is not purely spiritual or cognitive but embodied, rooted in the basic affective tonalities (Depraz, 2001) and intimately linked to the object-directedness of consciousness (see below). At a more explicit and complex level, self-awareness is a reflective consciousness of an *I* as the invariant and persisting subject pole of experience and action (Reflective I-consciousness is phenomenologically derivative and dependent on the more elementary sense of ipseity. Phenomena such as feelings of agency, coherence, unity, temporal identity and demarcation presuppose ipseity in order to be articulated. For example, if a memory of a past event is to contribute to my sense of temporal identity, a claim widely held in cognitive science, it can only do this job in so far as the past event is being remembered *as haven taken place in my field of awareness*, as something which was originally experienced from my first-person perspective.). Finally, one can speak of self-image or social self, the self-referential structures endowed with *personal* particularities of style, habit and history.

The morbid self-experience in early schizophrenia reflects the *primary alterations* of the very basic, prepersonal or prereflective sense of self (*ipseity*; Latin: *ipse* = self, itself). These may be, and usually are, followed by the changes in the reflective *I* awareness and in the social self, thus resulting in the profound disturbances of identity, clinically manifest on all three levels of selfhood.

Morbid self-experience is defined in this contribution as an experience in which one's first-person experiential perspective or one's status as a subject of experience and action is somehow distorted. Consequently only the experiences whose subject-aspects are somehow at stake will be addressed here – an approach which *does not exhaust* the range of anomalous experiences in the preonset phases of schizophrenia.

It is important to reemphasize that morbid self-experiences described in this chapter are of *not-yet psychotic intensity*, since our focus is on the premorbid (preonset) phases of schizophrenia. In other words, we are not dealing here with delusional elaborations, hallucinatory phenomena or experiences of external influence thematized by delusional explanatory efforts. The patient is able to keep a distance from his or her altered experience, a distance frequently expressed in conditional *as-if* statements, e.g. 'it feels *as if* my body does not belong to me'. (For a comprehensive description of the *as-if* experiential mode [*als-ob Erlebnismodus*], see Klosterkötter (1988). This mode occurs in connection with many morbid experiences in schizophrenia.) Moreover, such abnormalities of self-experience are, in general, *only* observable in the early illness stages. Apart from a continuous presence in a minority of patients, they become incorporated and transformed in the emerging psychotic symptomatology (Parnas, 2000).

Self and schizophrenia: early descriptive approaches

A variety of self-disorders in schizophrenia have always been recognized, at least implicitly, as the essential components of its clinical picture. An absent reference to a self is frequently merely terminological, because the relevant phenomena are addressed in other terms and/or in another theoretical framework.

Self-disorders were described in detail at the turn of the nineteenth and twentieth century. French psychiatrists published numerous case histories of patients who would today be diagnosed as suffering from schizophrenic and schizotypal disorders, characterized by profoundly altered self-experience (Janet, 1903; Hesnard, 1909; de Clérambault, 1942). Eugene Bleuler (1911, 1979) considered *basic disorder* of personality (the expression 'basic disorder of personality', also used in ICD-8 and 9, refers to universal impersonal aspects of a person, i.e. the fundamental structure of the self, and not to individuated, unique personality features), including various alterations of behaviour and the schizophrenic *dementia* as the so-called *complex fundamental* (diagnostic) features of schizophrenia, stating that the illness invariably involves affection (splitting) of the self: '*Ganz intakt ist dennoch das Ich nirgends*' ('The I is, however, never completely intact': Bleuler, 1911, p. 58). Schizophrenic autism, another *fundamental* symptom, may likewise be viewed as inclusive of self-disorders (Bleuler, 1972; Parnas & Bovet, 1991). Kraepelin (1896, 1913) claimed that a *disunity of consciousness* ('orchestra without a conductor') is the core feature of the illness. The disunity was closely linked to 'a peculiar destruction of the psychic personality's inner integrity, whereby emotion and volition in particular are impaired' (1913, p. 668, my translation).

A contemporary of Bleuler and Kraepelin, Joseph Berze (1914) was the first explicitly to propose that a *basic alteration of self-consciousness* was a primary disorder of schizophrenia (what he called a 'primary insufficiency') and he provided rich clinical material to illustrate this hypothesis. Berze described the *primary insufficiency* as a peculiar change, a diminished luminosity and affectability of self-awareness. Jaspers (1923) suggested the following experiential modes in which a *self is aware of itself*: (1) *activity*, comprising awareness of one's existence and action; (2) *unity*; (3) temporal–diachronic *identity*; and (4) me/not me *demarcation*. The sense of self, says Jaspers, may be affected in any of these modes. The vignettes that Jaspers provided are often suggestive of schizophrenia, but he stopped short of pursuing potential theoretical significance of self-disorders. Kurt Schneider (1959) addressed self-disorders in his description of passivity phenomena, allegedly reflective of a loss of *ego-boundaries*. Scharfetter (1980, 1981) modified Jaspers' domains of self-experience to comprise, in increasing order of complexity, vitality, activity, continuity, demarcation and identity. He considered many delusional phenomena as being compensatory reactions to self-disorders. Most of his clinical examples of altered self-experience in schizophrenia are, however, of a clearly psychotic intensity.

Detailed descriptions of self-disturbances, usually associated with the explorations of the sense and the nature of self, are to be found in the phenomenologically oriented work (Minkowski, 1927, 1997; Blankenburg, 1969, 1971, 1986; Tatossian, 1979; Bin Kimura, 1997). The main implication from this line of work is that self-disorders represent the *core feature* of schizophrenia, conferring on it a unique gestalt and reflecting its pathogenetic nucleus:

> The madness . . . does not originate in the disorders of judgement, perception or will, but in the derangement of the innermost structure of the self (Minkowski, 1997, p. 114; my translation).

Recent studies

There is little empirical research that offers *prospective* data on subjective aspects of self-experience in schizophrenia. One follow-back study using objective data did, however, reveal that fluidity of self-demarcation, lack of a coherent narrative–historical self-identity and other self-disturbances were prominent features of the preschizophrenic states at school age (Hartmann et al., 1984). None of the prospective high-risk projects or birth cohort studies collected data pertaining to the anomalies of self-experience.

An important contribution in this field is the work of Gerd Huber and his colleagues in Germany (which may be seen as a continuation of the research done by Berze, 1914): in a series of retrospective and, more recently, prospective studies, they identified subtle affective, cognitive, perceptual, motor and corporeal disturbances, designated as *basic symptoms*, some of which are specific to schizophrenia and frequently precede its onset (Huber et al., 1979; Huber, 1983; Klosterkötter, 1988; Klosterkötter et al., 1997, 2001). Several of these disturbances reflect self-disorders (e.g. varieties of depersonalization, disturbances of the stream of consciousness, distorted bodily experiences) and are thoroughly described in the Bonn Scale for the Assessment of Basic Symptoms (BSABS: Gross et al., 1987), translated into Danish and routinely used in our own studies.

In a Norwegian study using naturalistically oriented indepth interviews with 20 first-onset schizophrenic patients (Møller & Husby, 2000), three domains of the prodromal subjective change were revealed: *all* patients had profound and alarming changes of self-experience; nearly all patients complained of ineffability of self-alteration; and the great majority reported preoccupations with metaphysical, supernatural or philosophical issues.

Our own pilot retrospective study of schizophrenic prodromes in 19 first-onset patients admitted to the Copenhagen University Department of Psychiatry at

Hvidovre Hospital (Parnas et al., 1998) indicated a nearly identical profile of results. More recently, we completed systematic and detailed data collection, including items pertaining to self-disorders and basic symptoms (BSABS), on 155 first-admission cases diagnosed according to the ICD-10 research criteria: 57 suffered from a schizophrenia spectrum psychosis, 43 from schizotypal disorder and the remaining 55 patients suffered from other, nonschizophrenia spectrum disorders (The Copenhagen Prodromal Study: Handest, 2003). In a separate project, the occurrence of the BSABS-defined self-disorders on the lifetime basis was compared between 21 ICD-10 patients with residual schizophrenia and 23 remitted bipolar patients (Parnas et al., 2003). Analysis of these data indicates that self-disorders are highly specific for the schizophrenia spectrum conditions (note that self-disorders are *not* a part of the ICD-10 diagnostic criteria of schizophrenia), mark the picture of the preschizophrenic prodromes and frequently occur in hospitalized schizotypal conditions. Self-disorders correlate positively with the duration of the preonset social dysfunction and aggregate significantly in patients having a *positive* family history of schizophrenia. Self-disorders correlate both with the *negative* and *positive* symptom-scales of the positive and negative syndrome scale for schizophrenia (PANSS: Kay et al., 1987).

The clinical descriptions of self-disorders, which appear below, are drawn from several sources: our own empirical research and clinical experience and reports from the literature. The vignettes and quotes from the patients stem from our own studies unless otherwise indicated.

Presentation of complaints upon the initial medical contact

The vast majority of first-admitted schizophrenia spectrum patients in our series had been seen and treated *prior* to their first hospitalization by practising psychologists or psychiatrists, usually with a diagnosis of depression and an attempt at treatment with selective serotonin reuptake inhibitor antidepressant drugs (only 35% of schizophrenic and 6% of schizotypal patients had never been exposed to such a contact). One reason for this lack of correct early diagnosis is linked to the cryptic ways in which patients verbalize their complaints. Early misdiagnosis may also be attributed to a widespread ignorance of the nonpsychotic subjective experience in schizophrenia. They present nonspecific complaints such as depression, fatigue or anxiety. Blankenburg (1971) speaks here of 'specific nonspecificity': a trivial (nonspecific) complaint of fatigue turns out, on closer evaluation, to be caused by a pervasive inability to grasp the everyday significance of the world and a correlated paralysing perplexity (a condition highly suggestive of schizophrenia, hence *specificity*). Self-disorders reveal themselves only after some attempt to penetrate beyond the surface level of such complaints. As already observed by Berze (1914), only a clinician who is familiar with the scope of manifestations of self-disorders can perform such a penetration. The difficulty patients have in describing their experiences is multidetermined. The linguistic resources for characterizing dimensions of subjectivity, especially of the nonpropositional type, are not readily available. This is doubly true of the prereflective experiences that have taken on an unusual and unfamiliar quality, and which, as is more specifically the case with self-disorders, affect the very conditions of experience and its reportability. Adding to these difficulties is the fragility of the forms of consciousness in question, with their unstable wavering of implicit/prereflective into explicit/reflective modalities.

A case example of anomalous self-experiences in schizophrenia

The following vignette from the Copenhagen series of first-admission cases is a paradigmatic example of early schizophrenic experiences. I will return to selected aspects of this vignette in the descriptions of specific aspects of preschizophrenic self-experience.

Case 1

Robert, a 21-year-old unskilled worker, complained that for more than a year he had been feeling painfully cut-off from the world and had a feeling of some sort of indescribable inner change, prohibiting him from normal life. He had lost his initiative and energy, and had a tendency to an inverse sleep pattern. He was troubled by a strange, pervasive and very distressing feeling of not being really *present*, or fully alive, of not participating in interactions with his surroundings. He was never entirely *involved in the world*, in the sense of engaged absorption in daily activities and daily life. This experience of disengagement, isolation or ineffable distance from the world was accompanied by a tendency to observe or monitor his inner life. He summarized his affliction in one exclamation: 'my first personal life is lost and replaced by a third-person perspective' (He was not at all philosophically read.) In order to exemplify this statement more concretely, he said that, for instance, listening to music on his stereo would give him an impression that the musical tune somehow lacked its natural fullness; 'as if something was wrong with the sound itself', and he tried to regulate the sound parameters on his stereo equipment, to no avail, and only to realize finally that he was somehow 'internally watching' his own receptivity to music, his own mind receiving or registering musical tunes. So to speak, he witnessed his own sensory processes rather than living them. It applied to most of his experiences that, instead of living them, he experienced his own experiencing.

He reflected on self-evident daily matters and had difficulties 'in letting things and matters pass by' and linked it to a long-lasting attitude of 'adopting multiple perspectives', a tendency to regard any matter from all possible points of view. When younger he considered this ability as a gift, a source of creativity, despite the fundamental indecisiveness it caused. Now it had become more like an affliction, associated with a feeling of floating around, social withdrawal and abstention from action. Periodically he experienced his own movements as reflected upon and deautomatized. His thinking processes could acquire an acoustic quality, becoming a loud monologue confined to his skull. He considered all these experiences to be morbid, or at least, unusual and certainly very distressing, preventing him from having a normal life. However, he also claimed that, perhaps due to such experiences, he was sometimes brought for fleeting moments face-to-face with other, nonphysical and normally hidden dimensions of reality (Parnas, 2000, pp. 124–125).

Phenomenological description of self-disorders

The classification which follows below reflects phenomenological aspects of morbid self-experience as defined above – aspects that are *intimately interrelated*, but distinguished here for the sake of clarity of clinical exposition.

Presence and its alterations

The phenomenological concept of *presence* refers to a prereflective first-person perspective of experience (*ipseity*), intimately linked to a sense of immersion in the surrounding world: 'Subject and object are two abstract moments of a unique structure which is presence' (Merleau-Ponty, 1945, p. 430). We are normally self-aware through our absorption in the world of objects. We reside actively among things and other people and in this absorption our self-awareness operates at a prereflective or tacit level. We may distinguish here two aspects: a prereflective self-awareness or ipseity and a correlative, unreflective dwelling in the world. These experiential *moments* (i.e. nonindependent parts) deserve a more detailed exposition, because disturbances of presence seem to be the earliest type of prodromal experience in schizophrenia (Parnas et al., 1998; Møller & Husby, 2000). Most likely these disturbances constitute a foundation of the experientially more articulated or explicit anomalies of selfhood described in the following sections.

Ipseity may be described as a certain unreflected presence to oneself, certain *luminosity* or welling-up of self-awareness (Henry, 1963). (The term 'luminosity' indicates a fundamental mode of self-awareness, equal to the very being or emergence of consciousness. It is different from the concept of 'clarity' (disturbed in delirious conditions); luminosity is a condition of the latter. It denotes a certain welling-up of (self)-awareness, its *phenomenality* (Henry, 1963).) We may speak of ipseity or a prereflective self-awareness whenever we are *directly*, noninferentially or nonreflectively conscious of our own ongoing thoughts, perceptions, feelings or pains; these always appear in a first-person mode of presentation that immediately tags them as our own, i.e. it entails an automatic self-reference. First-person givenness is not just a varnish that the experience could lack without ceasing to be an experience. It is precisely its first-person givenness that makes the experience *subjective*. To be aware of one*self* is not to apprehend a self *apart* from experience, but to be acquainted with an experience in its first-person mode of presentation, that is, from within. The subject of experience is a *feature or function of its presentation*.

Unreflected immersion in the world is considered by phenomenology as a mode of intentionality, i.e. a mode of consciousness' object-directedness. Phenomenology distinguishes between a thematic, explicit or objectifying intentionality (e.g. when I am aware of *this chair* to the left from me), and a nonreflective, tacit sensibility, constituting our primary *presence to the world*. This prereflective *operative intentionality* (Merleau-Ponty, 1945) is functional without being engaged in any *explicit* epistemic acquisition. It procures a background texture or organization to the field of experience. It is upon such texture that explicit intentionality configures its perceptual (e.g. seeing *this particular chair*) or judgemental disclosures. It is in the prereflective mode that habits or dispositions become acquired. Operative intentionality may therefore be considered as a condition of our nonreflective, automatic attunement to the world, i.e. *common sense* (Parnas & Bovet, 1991).

The most prominent feature of altered presence in the preonset stages of schizophrenia is disturbed ipseity, a disturbance in which the sense of self no longer saturates the experience. For instance, the sense of *myness* of experience may become subtly affected: one of our patients reported that his feeling of his experience *as his own experience* only 'appeared a split-second delayed'.

The patient in Case 1 complains of unstable fullness or reality of his self-awareness. He feels that a profound change is afflicting him, yet he cannot pinpoint *what exactly* is changing because it is not a *something* that can easily be expressed in propositional terms. What has become problematic is the pregiven, pervasive and normally unnoticed medium of being. The patient appears to be saying that he feels bereft of the foundation of his existence. The phrasings of such complaints may range from a trivial 'I don't feel myself' or 'I am not myself' to 'I am losing contact with myself', 'I am turning inhuman' or 'I am becoming perverse, a monster' (Møller & Husby, 2000). The patient senses an inner void, a lack of an indefinable *inner nucleus*, which is normally constitutive of his field of awareness and *crucial to its very subsistence*. Some of these complaints point to alterations of self-consciousness, as if the *luminosity* of consciousness was somehow disturbed or diminished (the term 'luminosity' refers to the very manifestation or phenomenality of self-awareness; Henry, 1963). The patient does not feel *fully awake or conscious*: 'I have no consciousness'; 'My consciousness is not as whole as it should be'; 'I am simply unconscious'; 'I am half-awake'; 'I have no self-consciousness'; 'My I-feeling is diminished'; 'My I is disappearing for me'; 'My feeling of consciousness is fragmented'; 'It is a continuous universal blocking' (Berze, 1914; pp. 126–9).

The intentional aspect of altered presence is usually described as lack of immersion in the world, a lack of presence or a sense of imposed detachment from the world. It may also manifest itself as a *phenomenological distance* within perception and action. In a normal perceptual experience, the object perceived is given directly, in the flesh, so to say, but now it appears somehow filtered and deprived of fullness. Perception is not lived but is more like a mechanical, receptive, sensory process, unaccompanied by its affective feeling-tone (Case 1).

We should note here that psychiatrists sometimes describe such patients as *anhedonic* (deficient in feeling pleasure), but anhedonia is only one particular aspect of this diminishment of basic tonality, luminosity or reactivity–*affectabilility* of self-awareness (A similar description is found in Berze (1914).), accompanied by a sense of inexplicable inner fissure or void. The subjective effort required to grasp the meaning of these experiential changes may dominate the clinical picture that becomes thematized through hypochondriacal preoccupations.

In Robert's case, the incertitude, a sort of polyvalence (rather than ambivalence) is linked to a more global fragmentation of meaning, a loss of *natural evidence*, which is the hallmark of schizophrenic autism and perplexity (Parnas & Bovet, 1991). Robert resembles Anne, a patient described by Blankenburg (1969), whose main and monotonous complaint was her inability to grasp the world's natural significance and appeal. Nothing was self-evident and Anne had distressing difficulty in the automatic understanding of people and situations: 'it is not the question of knowledge; it is *prior to* knowledge . . . ; it is so small, so trivial; every child has it!' This experience of meaning fragmentation is linked to a lack of *perspectival abridgement*, a lack of a *dominant point of view*, blocking out potential rival perspectives and necessary for fluid attunement to the world (Sass, 1992). Such abridgement can only be realized in the experiential medium of reliable selfhood. As Robert's case illustrates, fragmentation of meaning may be associated with hyperreflexive forms of awareness, discernible in the emotional life, perception, cognition and action (see below).

Sense of corporeality and its alterations

Consciousness has always an experiential bodily background (embodiment, incarnation). (For a phenomenological discussion of the concepts *body image/body schema* in relation to the neurocognitive models of schizophrenia, see Gallagher (2000).) The body has an ambiguous experiential status, wavering between two opposite experiential modes: at the one pole as a *lived*, spiritualized, subjective body (*Leib*), identical or superposable with the subject (as when *we are* our body in a graceful movement) and, at the other extreme, as a physically spatial, thing-like objective body, as when we visually inspect our hands (*Körper*) (Husserl, 1972). Incessant gradations, oscillation and interplay between these bodily modes of being self-aware constitute a smooth and hardly noticed foundation of all experiencing (Depraz, 2001). The corporeal aspect of self-awareness is considered a necessary condition for the constitution of the sense of the mind-independent, perceptual world of objects – a position shared by phenomenology (Merleau-Ponty, 1945) and contemporary analytic philosophy (Evans, 1994; Cassam, 1997).

In incipient schizophrenia there is a variety of dissociations of the bodily experiential modes, with a striking tendency to experience one's body *predominantly as an object*: there is an increasing experiential distance between subjectivity and corporeality. The following vignette illustrates many experiential aspects of such a fissure or disjunction.

Case 2

'I am no longer myself…I feel strange, I am no longer in my body, it is someone else; I sense my body but it is far away, some other place. Here are my legs, my hands, I can also feel my head, but cannot find it again. I hear my voice when I speak, but the voice seems to originate from some other place'. He has difficulty in localizing his own person: 'Am I here or there? Am I here or behind?' When he does something, he has a feeling of observing his actions as a witness, without being actively involved: 'One might think that my person is no longer here…I walk like a machine; it seems to me that it is not me who is walking, talking, or writing with this pencil. When I am walking, I look at my legs which are moving forward; I fear to fall by not moving them correctly'. When he watches himself in a mirror, he is afraid of staying there or is not sure on which side of the mirror he actually is….

The patient's reason is intact; *he knows very well* that he is himself (Hesnard, 1909, p. 138, my translation; the last sentence of Hesnard presumably indicates that the patient is not psychotic, i.e. his experiences happen in the *as-if* mode).

The most frequent early change is a sense of being detached, disconnected from one's body, which feels somehow alien or not *fitting* the subject. For examples, a patient may say that he feels 'as if his body was too small to be inhabited', or as somehow indefinably uncomfortable to live with.

A clearer distortion of experience consists of the loss of bodily coherence: bodily parts are felt as if they were disconnected or isolated from each other. This feeling may take on an alarming intensity, where psychocorporeal unity disintegrates and there is a sense of fragmentation accompanied by a (pre)psychotic panic of literal dissolution ('going to pieces').

Yet another, experientially more articulated disturbance consists of a *feeling* of morphological change: the body or its parts *feel* heavier/lighter/smaller/larger/longer/shorter, a feeling which may be accompanied by optical illusions involving an actual visual experience of bodily change. The best known example of this is the *mirror phenomenon* (*signe du miroir* (Abely, 1930), *Spiegelphänomen*) where the patient inspects his or her face in the mirror because of feelings of self-alteration: the eyes may look dead and empty, the face may seem deformed. A subtler variety of this phenomenon consists of avoiding one's mirror image because it is perceived as somehow threatening or provoking (Case 2), having difficulty in recognizing oneself in photographs or becoming amazed by one's look in photographs.

Disturbance of subjectivity may manifest itself in motor performance. Motor or verbal acts may occur without or despite the patient's will and interfere with his or her actions or speech but are *not* (yet) regarded as being made by external forces.

Case 3
A former paramedic reported that many years prior to the onset of his illness he occasionally experienced (for example, when driving in an ambulance and to the driver's surprise) that he could involuntarily utter a few words, totally unconnected with his occurrent thoughts. He then immediately continued to speak in a relevant way or made some clichéd remarks in order to cover up this embarrassing episode.

Motor block (complete blockage of intended actions) occurs as a sudden and brief sense of paralysis when the patient is unable to move or speak. Another, frequent phenomenon is *deautomatization of motor action*, in which habitual performance (such as dressing, walking, teeth-brushing) suddenly requires conscious attention and a sense of mental and physical effort (see also Case 2).

Case 4
A female library assistant reported that prior to the onset of her illness she was alarmed by a frequently recurring experience that replacing the returned books from a trailer on the library shelves suddenly required attention: she had to think *how* she was to lift her arm, grasp a book with her hand and turn herself to the shelf.

Mimetic experiences occur rarely, and are sometimes accompanied by a feeling of centrality (see Solipsism, below): the patient, while in motion, experiences similar movements of inanimate objects or of people. He may feel, in the *as-if* mode, that he is somehow forced to imitate others or that others imitate him.

Case 5
Luc, 17 years old, reports: 'I made the same gestures as others, but *ahead of* them'. Then he corrects himself: '*following* them', but this does not seem satisfactory either. He hesitates between these two versions, and ends up choosing the one in which he *precedes* the others (Grivois, 1995, p. 107, translation and italics mine).

Stream of consciousness and its alterations

The stream of consciousness (also designated as a *stream of thoughts*) is a sense of *consciousness as a temporal flow* (James, 1890; Bergson, 1927; Husserl, 1966) oscillating between explicit, introspectable *static* moments of explicit cognitive–emotional activity and vaguely articulated tendencies of transition into new and different mental contents (fringes of consciousness: James, 1890). Even though the transitions and shifts may be quite abrupt or saccadic (especially for thoughts), self-awareness is fundamentally uninterrupted, as the *same temporal flow*. In a given temporal moment of the stream, its constituent contents (e.g. thoughts, images and sensations) form an experiential whole (Dainton, 2000). The self permeates the mental contents as its first-person perspective: *There is no distance between my thoughts and myself.* Apart from certain reflective acts, my thinking is at the 'zero point of orientation' which is my embodied subjectivity (Husserl, 1972, paragraph 43). Consciousness is essentially nonspatial in the sense of physical space, although certain *perceptual* contents are experienced with spatial dimensions. Consciousness is never experienced as a *thing* with a specific location or with spatial coordinates; its introspective contents are transparent or immediately given in a nonspatial way (i.e. the contents are not like physical objects lending themselves to a description in spatial terms).

A fundamental change of the stream of consciousness in the early phases of schizophrenia consists of an emerging experiential gap between the self and its contents (in a similar way as described above for the changed sense of corporeality). Mental contents become quasiautonomous, bereft of their natural dimension of *myness*. Thoughts may appear as if from nowhere, are felt as egoless, decentred from the self, and may sometimes evoke unusual and pregnant significance (Conrad, 1958). They interfere with the ongoing stream of thoughts (*thought interference*), and may be described by the patient in specific designations such as 'automatic', 'acute' thoughts or 'thought-tics'. Patients still self-ascribe their thoughts as their own, their content is often neutral and there is no internal resistance or mental struggle (as in the case of obsessions).

Robert (Case 1) reports increasing objectification of the introspective experience. Inner speech becomes transformed from a *medium of thinking* into an object-like entity with quasiperceptual characteristics (*Gedankenlautwerden*). Other patients may exhibit a subtler *spatialization* of inner experience. They describe their thoughts or feelings in physical terms, as if possessing an object-like quality ('my thoughts are dense and encapsulated') or locate them spatially ('my thoughts feel mainly in the right side of the brain'; 'it feels *as if* my thoughts were slightly behind my skull').

It also seems that shrinking of *myness* makes the experience stripped of its lived context, inviting an introspective, hyperreflexive awareness (Case 1) (Sass, 1992, 2000).

Case 6

If a thought passed quickly through his brain without him being fully aware of it, he was forced to direct back his attention and scrutinize his mind in order to know exactly what he had been thinking. In one word he is preoccupied by the continuity of his thinking. He fears that he may stop thinking for a while, that there might have been 'a time when my imagination had been arrested'...He wakes up one night and asks himself: 'Am I thinking? Since there is nothing which can prove that I am thinking, I cannot know whether I exist'. In this manner he annihilated the famous aphorism of Descartes...(quoted in Hesnard, 1909, p. 179, my translation).

Hyperreflexivity may have a compensatory nature, making up for enduring perplexity and 'loss of natural evidence' (Blankenburg, 1971) (Case 7), or it may operate as a more autonomous affliction (Case 8). The thinking process loses its sense of subjective mastery and is experienced as increasingly alienated.

Case 7

A 34-year-old university graduate reported that for many years trivial matters frequently came to occupy his mind. For example, while reading a novel written in the first person, and encountering a sentence like 'she said that he must return tomorrow' he immediately started to reflect on the reasons for using the personal pronouns, and finally to conclude that 'it has something to do with communication'. He then turned his attention to the word 'communication' and continued to think on the necessity to communicate etc. He could also reflect upon the fact that the air distributed itself in the rooms of his apartment. He called this type of thinking 'chopping up a sentence, taking a word out of its flow'.

Case 8

'I bypass a window display of a shop in which there are exposed bicycles and bicycle parts; [in a wheel] all the metal spokes cross each other in mutually sharp angles before they reach the axle...the axle turns around with the spokes. No, it is not the axle that rotates; it is the bar, a piece of steel. The axle does not exist; it is just a mathematical line, perpendicular to the plane of the wheel that is determined by the spokes, by 40 straight lines. But this is not necessary either: only two lines are needed to determine a flat surface. And the circumference? $2\pi r$ is the expression for the length of the felloe, or more precisely, for the theoretical circumference, outlined by this inexact circle (i.e. the felloe). Are we able to conceive an ideal line by paying attention to the lines in nature? Is Spencer's claim that mathematics originates from experience and induction correct?...These associations...would not seem to me as sick if I were able to master them, like someone who calmly reflects on the matters that he is working with, contemplating some professional problems. But when I am thinking in this way, without being able to stop it...I have no mastery over the course of these ideas...it seems to me *as if it is not me* who generates them...' (Hesnard 1909, p. 146, my translation and italics).

This state of mind may intensify into a *thought pressure* (*Gedankenjagen*), where the patient is overwhelmed by a myriad of unconnected thoughts going in different directions; loss of meaning or lack of an organizing theme is a cardinal feature of this symptom, in addition to the fact that the contents may appear affectively neutral (as opposed to depressive ruminations). Patients may use spatial metaphors to describe their experience ('my thoughts feel like a swarm of bees pressing from the inside of my skull'). One patient reported a feeling *as-if* his consciousness consisted of multiple emanating sources, disconnected from each other and each 'pulsating' at its own pace. A seemingly opposite experience is of a *thought block*, where thoughts abruptly disappear from the stream or more gradually fade away. A variant of this phenomenon is a sudden and total *discontinuity of self-awareness*: a patient may report that for some seconds she loses awareness of her activity, e.g. she does not know how and why she got from her living room to the kitchen or she finds herself somewhere in the city without knowing how she got there (see also Case 6). Less characteristic phenomena comprise difficulties in initiating and carrying through the thinking process: the patient may complain of a diminished ability to generate thoughts or of a general slowness of cognition and inability to reach the desired goal (*disturbances in thought intentionality and goal-directedness*). Communication of meaning to other people may also be distorted (*disturbed self-expression*). Patients have an experience of a disaccord between the cognitive-emotional state and its outward expression. They perceive their own behaviour, gestures, facial expression or language as somehow disfigured and out of control – a condition usually associated with hyperreflexive forms of self-awareness.

Hyperreflexivity and diminished *myness* are often associated with a peculiar *splitting or doubling of the self* (*Ich-Spaltung*) into an *observing* and *observed* ego, neither of which assures ipseity function (see Case 1). Such experience becomes especially prominent immediately before the onset of a frank psychotic episode. It may be felt as a form of inner struggle or an oscillation between the good and the evil parts or between different selves (which themselves may be described in spatialized terms). This is, at least initially, felt and communicated on the *as-if* metaphorical level. Normal processes of reflection and imagination also involve an ego-split, but they possess a natural flexibility and happen in a unified field of experience in which the sense of *myness* or self-presence never questions itself.

Self-demarcation and its alterations

Inability to discriminate self from nonself in schizophrenia was coined as *transitivism* by Bleuler (1911). This phenomenon attracted attention from numerous authors in connection with psychotic symptoms such as delusions of external influence, mind reading, thought broadcasting, certain hallucinations and of psychotic *projection* in psychoanalytic terms (loss of ego-boundaries: see Fenichel, 1945) and in the more recent neurocognitive investigations (Frith, 1992). Typically, in the neurocognitive literature the sense of mental self-possession is regarded as being generated by inferential self-monitoring mental processes. From a phenomenological perspective, the *me/not-me* demarcation (deficient in transitivistic experience) is automatically constituted in every experience; such border is just an *aspect* of nonreflexive self-awareness. Inferential reflection seems to arise only post hoc, as a consequence of a deficient sense of *myness*:

Case 9

A young schizotypal patient frequently contemplated his 'ego-boundary'. He thought about 'this fluid transition between me and the world': 'it must consist of a mixture of air molecules, sweat droplets and tiny fragments of skin debris'.

In the prodromal phases of schizophrenia and in the schizotypal conditions, one may observe subtle transitivistic phenomena which are purely experiential, i.e. unaccompanied by delusional elaborations (i.e. a *loss of reality testing*). The following case is paradigmatic of such experiences:

Case 10

A young man was frequently confused in a conversation, being unable to distinguish between himself and his interlocutor. He tended to lose the sense of whose thoughts originated in whom, and felt 'as if' his interlocutor somehow 'invaded him', an experience that shattered his identity and was intensely anxiety-provoking. When walking on the street, he scrupulously avoided glancing at his mirror image in the windowpanes of the shops, because he felt uncertain on which side *he actually was*. He used to wear a wide and tight belt in order to feel 'more whole and demarcated'. He was very attracted by the philosophy of Maurice Merleau-Ponty, whom he considered as the only philosopher who had truly grasped the fundamental subject–object reversibility (see also Case 2).

Transitivistic tendency may also manifest itself in less characteristic complaints of *increased impressionability*: certain events, previously unassociated with emotional reactions, are now overwhelming and lead to affective arousal (e.g. tension, nervousness, sleep disturbance, obsessive-like ruminations). The patient feels as if 'having a thinner skin', 'no barriers or filters'. Increased impressionability may concern everyday events, behaviours, comments of others or misfortune/unhappiness of others (e.g. TV news, newspaper reports, etc.). *Heightened perception*, a feeling of being overwhelmed by light, sounds, colours, object movements, may be construed in a similar way.

Solipsism

Møller & Husby note in their study (confirming a common clinical experience) that many preschizophrenic patients become preoccupied with philosophical, supernatural and metaphysical themes. It seems as if for many patients a fundamental transformation of their world view is taking place: 'Had to define and analyse everything I was thinking about; needed new concepts for the world and human existence; absorbed by new ideas or interests, gradually taking over my way of life and thinking' (Møller & Husby, 2000). This search for a *transcendent meaning* (i.e. metaphysical quest) is of course not restricted to schizophrenia but is a distinctive and pervasive characteristic of all human thought. It is fuelled by a paradox or a discordance intrinsic to *human self-relation* – what Dieter Henrich, a contemporary German philosopher, designates as the *basic relation* (Henrich, 1997). On the one hand, we experience ourselves as spiritual, unique and autonomous free beings; on the other hand, we are also self-aware as finite, causally determined entities, belonging to the world order of natural objects:

The origins of transcending thinking arise out of the following states of affairs . . . : the unintelligible self-relation due to which self-consciousness exists; the . . . opposition of reality and self-consciousness . . . and the unintelligibility of finite individuality in the world order. Taken together, they constitute what can be experienced as the *darkness that inheres in the basic relation.* That darkness calls for a [metaphysical] thinking in which these states of affairs can be comprehended . . . with a clarity that is not available in the basic relation itself (Henrich, 1997; p. 126; my italics).

Anomalies of experience so far described, involving subjectivization of the world, disembodiment and instability of the self, shatter the experiential equilibrium normally characteristic of the *basic relation* and intensify the metaphysical quest, thereby leading to the existential reorientations described by Møller and Husby. The patient experiences phenomena which are beyond common sensical, naturalistic folk metaphysics: *reality* is increasingly mind-dependent, *other minds* are enigmatic projective constructions, causality seems nonphysical, the I–world polarity or subject–object articulation is blurred and self-awareness endures a transformation in which the constitutive and therefore normally tacit mental processes become available for an introspective gaze (Parnas, 1999b). The term 'solipsism', denoting here a paradoxical mixture of increasing subjectivization of the world and of self-dissolution, adequately captures such a position (Sass, 1994), a position motivated by a profoundly altered self-experience and cognitively elaborated into a nexus of interests and beliefs pointing to a new existential orientation.

Case 11
A young patient reported that he had, in brief moments, a feeling that only the objects in his current field of vision were real, *as if* the rest of the world, including most familiar places and persons, did not really exist. Probed about suicidal intentions, he replied: 'No, I could never kill myself. *I can't imagine the world not being represented* [by me]'.

It is the solipsistic sentiment that inspires the patient to suspect an existence of a hidden ontological domain, only accessible to him or her. Feelings of *centrality* may be quite prominent in such conditions:

Case 12
A former physician, when working in the emergency room of a small provincial hospital, experienced, during fleeting moments, a feeling that he was the only true doctor in the entire world and that the fate of humanity was in his hands. He immediately suppressed this feeling as entirely nonsensical.

Case 13
When I hear a dog barking or a cat screaming far away, I instantly get a feeling that they bark and scream *at me.* When I listen to the radio, I get this thought that one is trying to let me understand something. I *know* that it is pure rubbish (Gross et al., 1984, p. 78, my translation and italics).

Solipsism may be a source of a quite specific type of subtle grandiosity observable in the schizophrenia spectrum conditions: the patient may regard other people as pitiable, ontologically ignorant morons, solely chasing the material aspects of life. In the more chronic stages of the disease, the entire ontological–epistemological framework of experience, normally revolving around *naïve realism* (in the western world) is dramatically transformed (Bovet & Parnas, 1993), leading to *beliefs*, which, on the face of their implausible or impossible content, are classified as so-called bizarre delusions (American Psychiatric Association, 1994). Yet, what is being perceived as bizarre in this kind of delusion is not only the content as such, but also an *altered way of the patient's experiencing*, transparent through this content (Bovet & Parnas, 1993). The *metaphysical taint* indicates something of the nature of the experienced self-relation; that is to say, it points to a disturbance of the 'self as a founding instance' (Blankenburg, 1988).

Self-experience and negative symptoms

Important clinical features of the prodromal stages of schizophrenia comprise anergia, avolition and asociality (Parnas, 1999a). However, such symptoms cannot be reduced to simple mechanical shortages of energy and initiative, as is portrayed in standard texts on schizophrenia and described as the so-called deficit or *negative* symptoms (Parnas & Bovet, 1994; Sass, 2000). First of all, such symptoms are *not only* deficits or shortages; their *negativity* or deficiary nature is often a consequence of inadequate and uninformed psychiatric interview. As noted above, negative symptoms in the Copenhagen Prodromal Study correlate positively with the quite *positive* anomalies of self-experience. In many cases, isolation, asociality and poverty of speech are simply varieties of avoidant coping behaviour (see Mundt, 1985, for a multifactorial approach). *Negative* symptoms such as anergia and avolition may also follow from a more fundamental but also more complex dissolution of the structure of experience, linked to the anomalies of self-awareness. To be moved and inspired to action, in other words to be *affected* by an object (heteroaffection), presupposes self-affectability or self-affection (Henry, 1963). Prior to a volitional *I-can* sense of agency, there is a more elemental and prereflective experience of self-affection, in which I am the one who is both the affected as well as the affecting: *I have a capacity that I have not created.* The *I-can* structure of agency arises from this self-affection as its emergent moment. This moment is the *constitutive core* around which the complex whole of willed action crystallizes itself by clustering, in a smooth, self-organizing way, affectivity–affection, desire–motive, cognition and perceptual–motor response. Successful realization or completion of acting requires a steady embeddedness in the tacit medium of *myness*/ipseity. A failing phenomenal *myness* contributes to the distortions of flow of affective and conative processes and results in *varieties of disjunction* in this domain. Action may be inhibited, inconsequential, intersubjectively inappropriate (described as 'autistic activity' by Minkowski, 1927) or having a paradoxical, internally contradictory or ambiguous structure. It is usually no longer spontaneous because it is *not lived*, and this may apply both to automatic unreflective action as well as to action organized by a focal, thematic core. Moreover, hyperreflexive ruminations, another aspect of anomalous self-experience, may further impede the emergence of a dominant theme, necessary to initiate and sustain action.

Transition to psychosis

In the psychotic phases, self-disorders become thematized in the emergence of delusions, hallucinations and passivity phenomena (see chapter 12 in this volume). The patient loses his or her sense of autonomy and feels 'at the mercy' of the world (*Beeinflussungsstimmung*). Pervasive sentiment of centrality and self-reference (to the point of literal resonance between inner experience and external world events) precedes the emergence of psychotic phenomena (*Anastrophé*, Conrad, 1958). Many of these psychotic symptoms involve fundamental alterations of the sense of possession and control of one's own thoughts, action, sensations, emotions and bodily experience (Scharfetter, 1980). Such self-disorders (either explicitly recognized as such, or implicit in the nature of a psychotic symptom) seem to arise upon the background of a more primary transformation of *myness*, described above (Parnas, 2000). The following reconstruction of the progression of symptoms illustrates the transition from a prodromal phase into frank psychosis.

Case 14

Peter's history of illness: January 1985: 'strange change is affecting him, diminished self-presence, feels 'self-disgust', has 'lost contact to himself'. August 1985: increasingly preoccupied by existential themes and Indian philosophy, 'perhaps meditation could help'. Increasingly isolated. January 1987: feels fundamentally transformed, 'something in me has become inhuman', 'no contact to his body', 'feels empty', has to 'find a new path in his life'. January 1988: is of the opinion that Indians are superior compared to other human races; they perhaps have a mission to save our planet. September 1992: preoccupied by recurring thoughts about extraterrestrials. January 1993: is convinced that Indians are reincarnated extraterrestrials. April 1994: feels that he is being brought here each day from another planet in order to assist Indians in their salvatory mission. Delusions of external influence and auditory hallucinations. June 1994: first admission to a psychiatric ward, 24 years old (Møller, 2001; expanded after personal communication).

We notice that the initial and ineffable self-transformation is becoming progressively articulated and thematized: there is a new interest in existentialism and Buddhist philosophy reflective of the emergence of charismatic and eschatological mental contents. These initial disturbances evolve through *odd or overvalued* ideas and culminate in the emergence of *bizarre delusions* and auditory hallucinations.

Implications

A revival of the clinical interest in the anomalies of subjective experience seems necessary today for any further progress in the pathogenetic research and for a more accurate early detection of the schizophrenia spectrum conditions.

Contrary to the classical view, schizophrenia is portrayed here as a disorder of consciousness, yet of a *different kind* than pathologies observed in organic delirious conditions. These essential phenomenological features are already present in the very initial stages of the illness. Psychotic developments appear to take place as progressive organizations of novel coherence patterns with various degrees of stability and temporal constancy (Bovet & Parnas, 1993; Parnas & Bovet, 1995; Parnas, 1999a, 2000). An emphasis on the pathogenetic import of self-disorders gives the perspective on schizophrenia another turf: the schizophrenia spectrum disorders need no longer be defined as contingent agglomerations of essentially disconnected symptoms, held together by a convention. Rather, these disorders may constitute a unitary group, qualitatively distinct from affective and organic conditions, and organized around fundamental anomalies of the self (Parnas, 1999b). Such unitary view is, of course, not new. It was behind countless attempts to extract a specific, unifying gestalt from the polymorphic picture of schizophrenia (Wyrsch, 1946), although, as aptly observed by Bleuler, this gestalt is quite elusive: 'the disease is characterized by a peculiar transformation of feeling, thinking and perceiving, found *nowhere* else in this particular fashion' (Bleuler, 1911).

Pathogenetic research, if guided by phenomenological considerations, should focus on the early illness stages and even on its earlier, infantile antecedents. Data are rapidly accumulating which demonstrate that preschizophrenic phenotypic abnormalities are traceable to the neonatal period and to early childhood (Murray & Lewis, 1987; Asarnow et al., 1995; Waddington et al., 1995; Parnas, 1999a; Parnas & Carter, 2002). We have proposed elsewhere that disruptions in the ontogenesis of corticocortical connectivity may represent a crucial aetiological element in the origins of schizophrenia (Parnas et al., 1996). Development of the elemental self–object relation is on the biological level most likely heavily dependent on a progressive sophistication of intra- and intermodal sensory and sensorimotor integrations. An intact and very precise intracortical and corticocortical connectivity is a necessary condition for such developments. Therefore, developmental trajectories in infants and children at high risk for schizophrenia should be studied in detail, in conjunction with research on the normal formation of self and self–world relation. An interdisciplinary approach, with a specific focus on the infantile selfhood

(Stern, 1985; Neisser, 1995; Rochat, 2001), might be a suitable framework for such a research programme.

REFERENCES

Abely, P. (1930). De signe du miroir dans les psychoses et plus spécialement dans la démence précoce. *Annales Médico-psychologiques*, **88**, 28–36.

American Psychiatric Association. (1994). *Diagnostic and Statistical Manual of Mental Disorders* (DSM-IV), 4th edn. Washington: American Psychiatric Association.

Asarnow, R.F., Caplan, R. & Asarnow, J.R. (1995). Neurobehavioral studies of schizophrenic children: a developmental perspective on schizophrenic disorders. In *Search for the Causes of Schizophrenia*, vol. III, ed. H. Häfner & W.F. Gattaz, pp. 87–113. Berlin: Springer.

Bergson, H. (1927). *Essai sur les Données Immédiates de la Conscience*. Paris: PUF.

Berze, J. (1914). *Die primäre Insuffizienz der psychischen Aktivität. Ihr Wesen, ihre Erscheinungen und ihre Bedeutung als Grundstörungen der Dementia Praecox und der hypophrenen Überhaupt*. Leipzig: Franz Deuticke.

Bin Kimura, B. (1997). Cogito et le je. *L'Évolution Psychiatrique*, **62**, 335–48.

Blankenburg, W. (1969). Ansätze zu einer Psychopathologie des 'common sense'. *Confinia Psychiatrica*, **12**, 144–63.

Blankenburg, W. (1971). *Der Verlust der natürlichen Selbstverständlichkeit. Ein Beitrag zur Psychopathologie symptomarmer Schizophrenien*. Stuttgart: Enke.

Blankenburg, W. (1986). Autismus. In *Lexicon der Psychiatrie. Gesammelte Abhandlungen der gebräuchlisten psychiatrischen Begriffe*, 2nd edn, ed. C. Müller, pp. 83–9. Berlin: Springer.

Blankenburg, W. (1988). Zur Psychopathologie des Ich-Erlebens Schizophrener. In *Psychopathology and Philosophy*, ed. M. Spitzer, F.A. Uehlein & G. Oepen, pp. 184–97. Berlin: Springer.

Bleuler, E. (1911). Dementia Praecox oder Gruppe der Schizophrenien. In *Handbuch der Psychiatrie*, ed. G. Aschaffenburg. Leipzig: Franz Deuticke.

Bleuler, M. (1972). Klinik der schizophrenen Geistesstörungen. In *Psychiatrie der Gegenwart. Klinische Psychiatrie I*, ed. K.P. Kisker, J.-E. Meyer, M. Müller & E. Strömgren, pp. 7–82. Berlin: Springer Verlag.

Bleuler, E. (1979). *Lehrbuch der Psychiatrie*, vol. 14. Berlin: Springer Verlag.

Bovet, P. & Parnas, J. (1993). Schizophrenic delusions: a phenomenological approach. *Schizophrenia Bulletin*, **19**, 579–97.

Campbell, J. (1999). Schizophrenia, the space of reasons and thinking as a motor process. *The Monist*, **82**, 609–25.

Cassam, Q. (1997). *Self and World*. Oxford: Oxford University Press.

Cattell, J.P. & Cattell, J.S. (1974). Depersonalization: psychological and social perspectives. In *American Handbook of Psychiatry*, 2nd ed, vol. III. *Adult Clinical Psychiatry*, ed. S. Arieti & E.B. Brody, pp. 766–99. New York: Basic Books.

Conrad, K. (1958). *Die beginnende Schizophrenie. Versuch einer Gestaltanalyse des Wahns*. Stuttgart: Thieme Verlag.

Cutting, J. (1997). *Principles of Psychopathology. Two Worlds – Two Minds – Two Hemispheres.* Oxford: Oxford University Press.

Dainton, B. (2000). *Stream of Consciousness. Unity and Continuity in Conscious Experience.* London: Routledge.

Ďe Clérambault, G. (1942). *Oeuvre Psychiatrique*, ed. J. Fretet. Paris: PUF.

Depraz, N. (2001). *Lucidité du Corps. De l'Empirisme Transcendental en Phénoménologie.* Dodrecht: Kluwer Academic.

Evans, G. (1994). Self-identification. In *Self-Knowledge*, ed. Q. Cassam, pp. 184–209. Oxford: Oxford University Press.

Fenichel, O. (1945). *The Psychoanalytic Theory of Neurosis.* New York: Norton.

Frith, C.D. (1992). *The Cognitive Neuropsychology of Schizophrenia.* Erlbaum: Hove.

Gallagher, S. (2000). Self-reference and schizophrenia: a cognitive model of immunity to error through misidentification. In *Exploring the Self. Philosophical and Psychopathological Perspectives on Self-Experience*, ed. D. Zahavi, pp. 203–42. Philadelphia: John Benjamins.

Grivois, L. (1995). *Le Fou et le Mouvement du Monde.* Paris: Éditions Grasset et Fasquelle.

Gross, G., Huber, G., Klosterkötter, J. & Linz, M. (1987). *Bonner Skala für die Beurteilung von Basissymptomen.* Translated by P. Handest & M. Handest; ed. J. Parnas & P. Handest (1995). Copenhagen: Synthélabo Scandinavia.

Handest, P. (2003). *The Prodromes of Schizophrenia.* Doctoral thesis. Copenhagen: University of Copenhagen.

Hartmann, E., Milofsky, E., Vaillant, G. et al. (1984). Vulnerability to schizophrenia. Prediction of adult schizophrenia using childhood information. *Archives of General Psychiatry*, **41**, 1050–6.

Henrich, D. (1997). Self-consciousness and speculative thinking. In *Figuring the Self: Subject, Absolute, and Others in Classical German Philosophy*, ed. D.E. Klemm & G. Zöller, pp. 99–133. Albany: State University of New York Press.

Henry, M. (1963). *L'Essence de la Manifestation.* Paris: PUF.

Hesnard, A.-L.M. (1909). *Les Troubles de la Personalité dans les États d'Asthénie Psychique. Étude de Psychologie Clinique.* Thèse de médecine. Bordeaux: Université de Bordeaux.

Huber, G. (1983). Das Konzept substratnaher Basissymptome und seine Bedeutung für Theorie und Therapie schizophrener Erkrankungen. *Nervenarzt*, **54**, 23–32.

Huber, G., Gross, G. & Schüttler, R. (1979). *Schizophrenie. Eine Verlaufs- und sozialpsychiatrische Langzeitstudie.* Springer: Berlin.

Husserl, E. (1966). *Zur Phänomenologie des inneren Zeitbewusstseins.* The Hague: Martinus Nijhoff.

Husserl, E. (1972). *Ideas Pertaining to a Pure Phenomenology and to a Phenomenological Philosophy*, vol. 2. Translated by R. Rojcewicz & A. Schuwer. Dodrecht: Kluwer Academic.

James, W. (1890). *The Principles of Psychology.* London: Macmillan.

Janet, P. (1903). *Les Obsessions et la Psychasthénie.* Paris: Alcan.

Jaspers, K. (1923). *Allgemeine Psychopathologie*, 3rd edn. Berlin: Springer.

Kay, S., Fishbein, A. & Opier, L. (1987). The positive and negative syndrome scale (PANSS) for schizophrenia. *Schizophrenia Bulletin*, **13**, 261–75.

Kirkegaard, S. (1980). *The Sickness Unto Death. Kirkegaard's Writings*, vol. 19, ed. and translated by H.V. Hong & E.H. Hong, pp. 32–3. Princeton, NJ: Princeton University Press.

Klosterkötter, J. (1988). *Basissymptome und Endphänomene der Schizophrenie. Eine empirische Untersuchung der psychopathologischen Übergangsreihen zwischen defizitären und produktiven Schizophreniesymptomen.* Berlin: Springer.

Klosterkötter, J., Schultze-Lutter, F., Gross, G., Huber, G. & Steinmeyer, E.M. (1997). Early self-experienced neuropsychological deficits and subsequent schizophrenic diseases: an 8-year average follow-up prospective study. *Acta Psychiatrica Scandinavica*, **95**, 396–404.

Klosterkötter, J., Hellmich, M., Steinmeyer, E.M. & Schultze-Lutter, F. (2001). Diagnosing schizophrenia in the initial prodromal phase. *Archives of General Psychiatry*, **58**, 158–64.

Kraepelin, E. (1896). *Psychiatrie*, 4th edn. Leipzig: J.A. Barth.

Kraepelin, E. (1913). *Psychiatrie*, vol. 3. *Klinische Psychiatrie.* Leipzig: J.A. Barth.

Larsen, T.K., Friis, S., Haahr, U. et al. (2001). Early detection and intervention in first-episode schizophrenia: a critical review. *Acta Psychiatrica Scandinavica*, **103**, 323–34.

McGlashan, T.H. & Johannessen, J.O. (1996). Early detection and intervention with schizophrenia: rationale. *Schizophrenia Bulletin*, **22**, 201–22.

Mc Gorry, P.D., Mc Farlane, C., Patton, G.C. et al. (1995). The prevalence of prodromal features of schizophrenia in adolescence: a preliminary study. *Acta Psychiatrica Scandinavica*, **92**, 241–9.

Merleau-Ponty, M. (1945). *Phénoménologie de la Perception.* Paris: Gallimard. Translated by C. Smith. *Phenomenology of Perception* (1962). London: Routledge & Kegan Paul.

Minkowski, E. (1927). *La Schizophrènie. Psychopathologie des Schizoïdes et des Schizophrènes.* Paris: Payot.

Minkowski, E. (1997). Du symptome au trouble gènèrateur. (Originally published in *Archives Suisses de Neurologie et de Psychiatrie*, 1928; 22.) In *Au-delà du Rationalisme Morbide.* Paris: Éditions l'Harmattan.

Møller, P. (2001). Duration of untreated psychosis: are we ignoring the mode of initial development? *Psychopathology*, **34**, 8–14.

Møller, P. & Husby, R. (2000). The initial prodrome in schizophrenia: searching for naturalistic core dimensions of experience and behavior. *Schizophrenia Bulletin*, **26**, 217–32.

Mundt, C. (1985). *Das Apathiesyndrom der Schizophrenen. Eine psychopathologische und computertomographische Untersuchung.* Berlin: Springer Verlag.

Murray, R.M. & Lewis, S.W. (1987). Is schizophrenia a neurodevelopmental disorder? *British Medical Journal*, **295**, 681–2.

Nagel, T. (1974). 'What is it like to be a bat?' *Philosophical Review*, **83**, 435–50.

Neisser, U. (1995). Criteria for an ecological self. In *The Self in Infancy: Theory and Research*, ed. P. Rochat, pp. 17–34. Amsterdam: Elsevier.

Parnas, J. (1999a). From predisposition to psychosis: progression of symptoms in schizophrenia. *Acta Psychiatrica Scandinavica*, **99**(suppl. 395), 20–9.

Parnas, J. (1999b). On defining schizophrenia. In *Schizophrenia*, ed. M. Maj & N. Sartorius, pp. 43–5. *WPA Series: Evidence and Experience in Psychiatry*, vol. II. New York: John Wiley.

Parnas, J. (2000). The self and intentionality in the pre-psychotic stages of schizophrenia: a phenomenological study. In *Exploring the Self. Philosophical and Psychopathological Perspectives on Self-Experience*, ed. D. Zahavi, pp. 115–48. Philadelphia: John Benjamins.

Parnas, J. & Bovet, P. (1991). Autism in schizophrenia revisited. *Comprehensive Psychiatry*, **32**, 7–21.

Parnas, J. & Bovet, P. (1994). Negative/positive symptoms of schizophrenia: clinical and conceptual issues. *Nordic Journal of Psychiatry*, **48**(suppl. 31), 5–14.

Parnas, J. & Bovet, P. (1995). Research in psychopathology: epistemologic issues. *Comprehensive Psychiatry*, **36**, 167–81.

Parnas, J. & Carter, J.W. (2002). High-risk studies and developmental hypothesis. In *Risk and Protective Factors in Schizophrenia: Towards a Conceptual Disease Model*, ed. H. Häfner. Darmstadt: Steinkopff Verlag, pp. 71–82.

Parnas, J. & Zahavi, D. (2002). The role of phenomenology in psychiatric classification and diagnosis. In *Psychiatric Diagnosis and Classification*, ed. M. Maj, W. Gaebel, J.J. Lopez- Ibor & N. Sartorius, pp. 137–62. New York: John Wiley.

Parnas, J., Bovet, P. & Innocenti, G. (1996). Schizophrenic trait features, binding and cortico-cortical connectivity: a neurodevelopmental pathogenetic hypothesis. *Neurology, Psychiatry and Brain Research*, **4**, 185–96.

Parnas, J., Jansson, L., Sass, L.A. & Handest, P. (1998). Self-experience in the prodromal phases of schizophrenia. *Neurology, Psychiatry, and Brain Research*, **6**, 97–106.

Parnas, J., Handest, P., Jansson, L. & Saebye, D. (2003). Anomalies of subjective experience in schizophrenia and psychotic bipolar illness. *Acta Psychiatrica Scandinavica*, **107**, 1–8.

Rochat, P. (2001). *The Infant's World*. Cambridge, MA: Harvard University Press.

Sass, L.A. (1992). *Madness and Modernism. Insanity in the Light of Modern Art, Literature, and Thought*. New York: Basic Books.

Sass, L.A. (1994). *The Paradoxes of Delusion. Wittgenstein, Schreber, and the Schizophrenic Mind*. Ithaca: Cornell University Press.

Sass, L.A. (2000). Schizophrenia, self-experience, and the so-called 'negative symptoms'. In *Exploring the Self. Philosophical and Psychopathological Perspectives on Self-Experience*, ed. D. Zahavi, pp. 149–84. Philadelphia: John Benjamins.

Scharfetter, C. (1980). *General Psychopathology. An Introduction*. Translated by H. Marshall. Cambridge: Cambridge University Press.

Scharfetter, C. (1981). Ego-psychopathology: the concept and its empirical evaluation. *Psychological Medicine*, **11**, 273–80.

Schneider, K. (1959). *Clinical Psychopathology*. Translated by M.W. Hamilton. New York: Grune and Stratton.

Spitzer, M. (1988). Ichstörungen: in search of a theory. In *Psychopathology and Philosophy*, ed. M. Spitzer, F.A. Uehlein & G. Oepen, pp. 167–83. Berlin: Springer.

Stern, D.N. (1985). *The Interpersonal World of the Infant. A View from Psychoanalysis and Developmental Psychology*. New York: Basic Books.

Tatossian, A. (1979). *Phénoménologie des Psychoses*. Paris: Masson.

Waddington, J.L., O'Callaghan, E., Youssef, H.A. et al. (1995). The neurodevelopmental basis to schizophrenia: beyond a hypothesis? In *Schizophrenia: An Integrated View*, ed. R. Fog, J. Gerlach & R. Hemmingsen, pp. 43–53. Copenhagen: Munskgaard.

Weiser, M., Reichenberg, A., Rabinowitz, J. et al. (2001). Association between nonpsychotic psychiatric diagnoses in adolescent males and subsequent onset of schizophrenia. *Archives of General Psychiatry*, **58**, 959–64.

World Health Organization (1992). *International Classification of Diseases*, 10th edn. Geneva: World Health Organization.

Wyrsch, J. (1946). Ueber die Intuition bei der Erkennung des Schizophrenen. *Schweizerische Medizinische Wochenschrift*, **46**, 1173–6.

Zahavi, D. (1999). *Self-Awareness and Alterity. A Phenomenological Investigation*. Evanston: Northwestern University Press.

Zahavi, D. & Parnas, J. (1998). Phenomenal consciousness and self-awareness: a phenomenological critique of representational theory. *Journal of Consciousness Studies*, **5**, 687–705.

12

Self-disturbance in schizophrenia: hyperreflexivity and diminished self-affection

Louis A. Sass

Rutgers University, Piscataway, NJ, USA

Abstract

The present chapter offers a unifying but nonreductive interpretation of schizophrenia, one that attempts to show how the diverse signs and symptoms of this illness may all be rooted in certain fundamental alterations in the acts of consciousness that constitute both self and world. Schizophrenia, I argue, can best be understood as a two-faceted disturbance of self-experience. Phenomena that would normally be inhabited – and in this sense experienced as part of the self – come instead to be taken as objects of focal or objectifying awareness (*hyperreflexivity*). Intimately connected with this development is a profound weakening of the sense of existing as a subject of awareness, as a presence for oneself and before the world (diminished self-affection). Both facets imply a key disturbance of *ipseity*, i.e. of the basic sense of existing as a vital and self-coinciding subject of experience or first-person perspective on the world. (*Ipse* is Latin for self or itself.)

To explain the nature of this self-disturbance, I borrow the philosopher Merleau-Ponty's concept of the *intentional arc* along with Michael Polanyi's notion of an experiential continuum stretching between the object of awareness and what has a more *tacit* form of existence. I also distinguish between *compensatory, consequential* and more *basic* forms of hyperreflexivity. I consider the *positive, negative* and *disorganized* syndromes or types of schizophrenic symptom; and attempt, in each case, to illuminate the role of shared disturbances of consciousness and the sense of self.

Introduction

Ever since Kraepelin brought patients with hebephrenic, catatonic and paranoid symptoms together under a new disease concept – dementia praecox – there has been controversy about the unity of the entity he created. In his influential revisioning, Eugen Bleuler proposed four 'fundamental' symptoms, each supposedly typical of schizophrenia (perhaps pathognomonic), and present in all cases of the disease. Only one, however – the famous *association disturbance* – was consistently given a primary pathogenetic role; and all four symptoms proved to be elastic concepts that were difficult to operationalize or to define with adequate specificity (Hoenig, 1983).

Bleuler's (1950) equivocating title, *Dementia Praecox, or the Group of Schizophrenias*, conveys uncertainty about the unity of the entity he renamed. Even more keenly aware of the difficulty of specifying the essence of schizophrenic illness was the third great figure of twentieth-century psychiatry, Karl Jaspers (1963), who believed that the only unifying psychological factor would turn out to be the sheer fact of strangeness itself:

> search has been made for *a central factor*...Theoretically we talk of incoherence, dissociation, fragmenting of consciousness, intrapsychic ataxia, weakness of apperception, insufficiency of psychic activity and disturbance of association, etc. We call the behavior crazy or silly but all these words simply imply in the end that there is a common element of 'the ununderstandable' (p. 581).

The contemporary status of the concept and diagnosis of schizophrenia is not very different from what it was early in the last century. The aetiology remains largely unknown and the nosology persistently in dispute (McKenna, 1994, chapters 4 and 5). While some experts argue that schizophrenia will inevitably break down into a small group of distinct conditions, others defend the notion of schizophrenia as '*essentially* one entity, one clearly definable mental disorder that must be studied in unity along the whole continuum of its manifestations' (Gottesman, 1991, p. 20; Maj, 1998; Andreasen, 1999).

One of the most vigorous trends is that of contemporary cognitive neuropsychology and neuropsychiatry. Here the diverse psychopathology of schizophrenia is typically divided into distinct symptoms or symptom groups, which are then examined independently in an attempt to identify distinct underlying cognitive and neurobiological processes associated with the group in question (Persons, 1986; Costello, 1992; Cahill & Frith, 1996a, p. 373; Cahill & Frith, 1996b, p. 282, p. 373; Spitzer, 1997; see also Mojtabai & Rieder, 1998). Researchers who follow this strategy are not necessarily committed to denying that schizophrenia is a legitimate disease entity; but they generally accept the apparent, radical differentness of the various syndromes, both as these appear to the average observer and as they are conceptualized by conventional psychopathological understanding. The emphasis they place on the distinctness of the syndromes and the pursuit of 'independent disease processes underlying schizophrenia' (Johnstone & Frith, 1996, p. 670) can make it difficult to see what the individual symptoms and purported causal mechanisms might have in common, or even how they could be part of a single psychological condition. (Cahill & Frith (1996a) acknowledge, e.g., that their model implies that 'persons experiencing "negative" symptoms could not also experience "positive" symptoms' (p. 392).)

The original reasons for retaining a unified concept of schizophrenia remain valid; they are, if anything, reinforced by recent family-incidence research showing that schizophrenia subtypes do not 'breed true', and by long-term symptomatic studies that document the overlapping and interpenetration of syndromes, especially the fact that patients often shift over time from one syndrome to another (Fenton & McGlashan, 1991). This evidence for the unity of schizophrenia as a diagnostic entity raises the question of a unity of underlying psychological processes. In this chapter, I offer a unifying but nonreductive interpretation of schizophrenia, one that acknowledges the diversity of its features while also showing how these may all be rooted in certain fundamental and distinctive alterations in the acts of consciousness that constitute both self and world.

Schizophrenia, I shall argue, can best be understood as a self- or ipseity-disorder (*ipse* is Latin for self or itself; see Ricoeur, 1992) in which phenomena that would normally be inhabited, and in this sense experienced as part of the self, come instead to be taken as objects of focal or objectifying awareness (hyperreflexivity; Sass, 1992). Intimately connected with – indeed, implicit in – this development is a profound weakening of the sense of existing as a subject of awareness, as a presence for oneself and before the world (diminished self-affection; Parnas & Sass, 2001). 'I am somehow strange to myself. I am not myself', said one patient with schizophrenia. 'I was simply there, only in that place, but without being present' (Blankenburg, 1991, pp. 94, 77). Both these complementary alterations affect the most fundamental aspect of selfhood or self-experience, which is the basic sense of ipseity, i.e. the sense of existing as a vital centre or source that anchors, possesses and often controls its own experiences and actions. William James (1981) called this the 'central nucleus of the self' (p. 286). It involves a kind of experiential self-coinciding, a coherent subjectivity that involves the sense of existing as a vital conscious presence or first-person perspective whose experiences are unified and owned rather than merely 'fly[ing] about loose' (p. 330). Gallagher (2000) describes this as the 'prereflective point of origin for action, experience and thought' (p. 15). Damasio (1999) speaks of the 'sense of self in the act of knowing': 'Besides [the sensory] images there is also this other presence that signifies you, as observer of the things imaged, owner of the things imaged, potential actor on the things imaged ... There is a presence of you in a particular relationship with some object ... The presence is quiet and subtle ...' (p. 10).

My approach is phenomenological (in the continental sense of the term; Bernet et al., 1993; Tatossian, 1997) and, as such, largely descriptive or interpretative rather than explanatory in nature. I attempt to describe and to evoke what it may be like to suffer these experiences, and also to bring out key affinities, on the subjective plane, between what can appear to be divergent or even antithetical signs and symptoms. My main goal is not to hypothesize causal chains that might lead from one symptom to another but rather, to recast our understanding of the various symptoms so that we can discern common features pervading them all. Such an approach should be helpful to those who wish to empathize with the patient, to communicate understanding and to grasp the subjective impact of therapeutic interventions. But it may also contribute something to the contemporary project of pathogenetic explanation (Sass & Parnas, in press). Phenomenology offers, at the very least, a description of experiential dimensions that must be included in any account that aspires to integrate subjective, cognitive and neurobiological aspects (Gallagher, 1997; Petitot et al., 1999). I recognize the valuable contributions of the symptom or syndrome-oriented research programme (Cahill & Frith, 1996a; Gray et al., 1991; Goldman-Rakic, 1994). I suggest, however, that these approaches will remain radically incomplete so long as they fail to recognize and to account for aspects of the illness that may have a more fundamental and encompassing status. Current cognitive neuropsychiatric accounts may well identify specific cognitive or neurobiological factors that underlie particular syndromes. But these factors could also reflect, at least in part, the more general conditions (viz. the alterations of the intentional arc), to be described later in this chapter. (Consider the flattening of associational hierarchies and various disturbances suggesting problems with working memory (which are associated with *disorganization* symptoms; Goldman-Rakic, 1994; Spitzer, 1997). These may be, at least in part, consequences of the attitude of indifference characteristic of lowered self-affection or of the erosion of focus inherent in hyperreflexivity. One might argue as well that a neurophysiological and neurocognitive factor like decline of efferent feedback (often associated with *positive* symptoms; Frith & Done, 1989) may partly result from the detached attitude toward one's own actions and thoughts that is characteristic of hyperreflexivity.)

The hypothesis offered here is preliminary, with much that needs to be clarified and worked out in more detail. I hope, nevertheless, that it will help to organize our comprehension of the full range of schizophrenic symptoms as well as to orient future research (Sass & Parnas, 2001).

In order to survey the wide range of schizophrenic symptoms, I shall adopt the most widely accepted current subtyping of symptoms and syndromes: the tripartite distinction between so-called positive, negative and disorganized symptoms. Whereas positive symptoms, mainly hallucinations and delusions, are said to involve the *presence* of experiences that would normally be *absent*, the negative symptoms – including poverty of speech, affective flattening and apparent apathy – are defined by an apparent *diminution* of what would normally be *present* (Marneros et al., 1991). These two categories are often supplemented by a third group of *disorganization* symptoms, mainly aspects of formal thought disorder (Liddle, 1987; Liddle et al., 1994). These latter are generally conceptualized in quantitative terms: as a diminishment of the degree of structure or organization inherent in an individual's thought and language.

The empirical evidence for the distinctness of the positive and negative syndromes is far from definitive and has been hotly debated (McGlashan & Fenton, 1992; Häfner et al., 1998). However, the distinction itself clearly has great intuitive appeal in anglophone psychiatry. The very notion of positive-versus-negative, or more-versus-less, suggests the possibility of a straightforward, noninterpretative assessment of signs and symptoms – an assessment not of *what* one may be observing but merely of whether, or to what extent, something is present; this seems to hold out the promise of both quantification and high reliability. Also important is the way the positive–negative distinction resonates with the widespread mechanistic and often reductionistic assumption that the key schizophrenic symptoms are manifestations or consequences of a defective cognitive mechanism or 'broken brain' (Andreasen, 1984), and largely involve a decline of the higher or more quintessentially human faculties of the mind. (For more extensive discussion of negative symptoms, see Sass, 2000.)

As I shall argue below, close phenomenological analysis suggests that the characteristically schizophrenic abnormalities of experience do indeed share certain underlying features, but that these features are not consistent with traditional mechanistic and reductionistic assumptions. Indeed, the abnormalities seem to defy any simple quantitative description, and force us to seek a richer and more qualitative set of concepts. Before turning our attention to schizophrenia, it is necessary to lay some groundwork necessary for conceptualizing relevant aspects of consciousness and the self.

Hyperreflexivity and diminished self-affection

Below I shall argue that, despite the variety of its manifestations, schizophrenia nearly always involves two mutually interdependent mutations of the act of consciousness – what can be termed *hyperreflexivity* and diminished *self-affection*. The term 'reflexive' refers to situations or processes whereby some being, especially an agent or self, takes itself or some aspect of itself as its own object of awareness. The exaggerated way in which this occurs in schizophrenia can be described as a hyperreflexive tendency (Sass, 1992). *Self-affection* (or *autoaffection*) refers to the basic and implicit sense of existing as a vital centre of consciousness or source of luminosity that is characteristic of what is sometimes called the *prereflective cogito* (Grene, 1968). Hyperreflexivity and diminished self-affection are the two aspects of the self- or ipseity-disturbance that are at the heart of schizophrenia.

The sense of vital self-affection may verge on ineffability or may seem a mere tautology. It is nevertheless something quite real, having very real consequences.

What the philosopher Michel Henry (1973) has called the 'self-feeling of self', 'being-affected by self', is a kind of unmediated feeling, sense of aliveness or tonality that provides the foundation or ontological condition for both 'the Being and the possibility of the Self' and our encountering of the external world (pp. 465, 479, 481; Zahavi, 1999). We encounter a solid object as the terminus of actual, potential and infinitely repeatable movements of our arm and hand; our knowing of that solid object is therefore grounded in a more primordial awareness of our own actions. In this sense, self-awareness or autoaffection is a logically prior, necessary and foundational condition for intentional directedness toward the world. It should be noted that the awareness of one's arm movement is normally an implicit or non-objectifying type of self-awareness. To have focal or objectifying awareness of one's arm (a form of hyperreflexivity) would disrupt the experience of both self and world.

The writer Antonin Artaud (1976), who suffered from schizophrenia and will serve as a key example below, spoke of self-feeling as the 'essential illumination' and the 'very substance of what is called the soul' (p. 169; 1965, p. 20). Michel Henry (1973) describes consciousness as like a flame that, in illuminating objects, illuminates itself as well. Similarly, Artaud speaks of a 'phosphorescent point' that illuminates itself at the same time as it illuminates and organizes the objects of one's awareness, and that seems to be bound up with the tacit sense of self-coinciding and vital self-presence: 'What is difficult is to find one's place and to reestablish communication with one's self', Artaud writes. 'Everything depends on a certain flocculation [coming together] of things, on the clustering of all these mental gems around a point which has yet to be found...a phosphorescent point at which all reality is recovered' (p. 82). Without this basic sense of self-affection, and the ipseity it grounds, Artaud experiences what he calls 'a kind of constant leakage of the normal level of reality' (p. 82); there can emerge no charged purpose or idea, no 'criterion' (p. 169) that can compel the attention or around which the mind can organize itself.

Although hyperreflexivity or diminished self-affection may be more prominent or obvious in a given patient at a given moment, these two facets of the self- or ipseity-disturbance are equally important, playing an equally primordial pathogenetic role. Indeed, their relationship is of the most intimate kind, involving something more like mutual phenomenological implication than causal interaction; they are, in a sense, different aspects of the very same phenomenon, but described from two different standpoints. The hyperreflexive aspect is emphasized in this chapter, but this is not meant to imply any causal or conceptual priority; I shall conclude with examples that illustrate their essential interdependence.

To understand the essential complementarity of hyperreflexivity and diminished self-affection, it is useful to recall the phenomenological philosopher Maurice

Merleau-Ponty's concept of the *intentional arc* – a term he uses to refer to the fundamental dynamic structuring of our field of awareness and lived world, and which he describes as a 'mobile vector, active in all directions... through which we can orient ourselves towards anything *outside and inside us*' and which 'endows experience with its degree of vitality and fruitfulness' (1945, pp. 158, 184; 1962, pp. 135–136, 157, translation altered). (As used here, the term 'intentional' refers to the object-directed nature of awareness rather than to the issue of volition or choice; Bernet et al., 1993, pp. 88–101.) The nature of the intentional arc or vector of awareness is clarified by Michael Polanyi's (1964, 1967; Grene, 1968) notion of a continuum that stretches between the objectified or focally known *object* of awareness and that which exists more in the *tacit dimension*, that is, which is known in a more subsidiary, proximal, implicit or tacit manner. Tacit knowledge can be profoundly unconscious, but it may also involve a peripheral kind of awareness (Polanyi, 1968, p. 420); it includes our awareness of the perceptual background or worldly context of awareness as well as the structures and processes of the embodied, knowing self.

One might exemplify these two ways of knowing – focal versus tacit – by distinguishing the body *image* from what might be called the bodily or corporeal *subject*. Whereas the first refers to an objectified or objectifiable representation *of* one's own body, the second refers to the body as a sensori-motor agent and witness that not only encounters, but in some sense constitutes the world of our awareness as well as our most basic sense of self (Gallagher & Meltzoff, 1996; Dillon, 1997, pp. 121–123; Merleau-Ponty, 1962, pp. 99–104). The human being is, of course, a *bodily* subject; and a person's self-feeling or ipseity is based, at least in part, on awareness of proprioceptive and kinesthetic sensations. Normally, however, these sensations are not in the objectifying focus of attention; nor do they have their significance 'in themselves,' but rather as the subjective correlates of other- or object-directed forms of intentionality. As the perceptual psychologist J.J. Gibson (1979) noted, perceptual awareness of the external world always includes a preconceptual awareness of one's relationship *to* the world. 'To perceive the world is to coperceive oneself', wrote J.J. Gibson (quoted in E.J. Gibson, 1993, p. 25).

Thus we see something as located near or far *from us*, and we see the world primarily in terms of *affordances*, for instance, whether an object allows for (affords) walking on or jumping over. The prereflective *intentionality* of the bodily or corporeal subject could be said to encompass all the implicitly felt and tacitly constitutive, subjective correlates of these Gibsonian affordances.

Normal self-affection involves an amalgam of appetite, vital energy and point of orientation: it is what motivates human actions and organizes our experiential world in accordance with needs and wishes, thereby giving objects their significance for us as obstacles, tools, objects of desire, and the like. Although clearly associated with a sense of energy and vitality, self-affection cannot be reduced to this factor alone. It is something more basic: a matter of 'mattering' – of constituting a lived point of orientation and the correlated pattern of significances that make for a coherent and meaningful world.

We see, then, that object-directedness and subjective self-affection are inseparable and interdependent aspects of the intentional arc, which can be understood as a vector having dimensional gradations from one end to the other. In the proximal end of the intentional arc, the infrastructure is tacit or implicit; this is the realm of prereflective, nonfocal self-awareness, which normally occurs in conjunction with a focal or explicit positing of an object of awareness. Tacitness is crucial; it is, in a sense, the very medium of autoaffection – of the prereflective ipseity or self-awareness that is, in turn, the *medium* through which all intentional activity is realized. Any disturbance of this tacit-focal structure, or of the ipseity it implies, is likely to have subtle but broadly reverberating effects; such disturbances must necessarily upset the balance and shake the foundations of both self and world.

The intentional arc or vector is a very general feature of consciousness that, at the most fundamental level, always involves a relatively passive, automatic or unreflective dimension of operation – what Merleau-Ponty (1962), following Husserl, called 'operative intentionality' (*fungierende Intentionalität*). But it can also be imbued, at higher levels, with a sense of activity and volition – with the 'reflective intentionality' that is characteristic of our explicit judgements and of 'those occasions when we voluntarily take up a position' (p. xviii). The determination of which elements of awareness will be focal and which tacit will be affected by factors that are partially volitional, such as focal attention. The actual structuring of the vector of awareness occurs automatically, however, as part of the *fundamental receptivity* of the automatic or *passive syntheses* that structure the basic act of consciousness and constitute the most fundamental relationship of self to world (Blankenburg, 1991, pp. 93, 130, 132).

As we shall see, hyperreflexive qualities can be manifest on a number of distinct levels or in a variety of different ways – involving different degrees of sophistication and intellectual self-consciousness and not necessarily implying a significant amount of volition, intellectual activity or reflective self-control. I shall distinguish between *operative* and *reflective* forms of hyperreflexive intentionality. I shall also distinguish according to whether the reflexivity is *compensatory*, *consequential* or *basal* in nature – that is, whether it occurs in some kind of defensive compensation *for* or as a consequence *of* some more basic defect or abnormality, or else as a facet of the basic defect itself. (The reflective–operative distinction is meant to refer primarily to the *nature* of the phenomenon in question; the basal–consequential–compensatory distinction pertains to its *causal status*. Whereas compensatory hyperreflexivity tends to be of the reflective sort, basal hyperreflexivity tends to be of the operative kind. Consequential hyperreflexivity seems equally likely to be reflective or operative; in this chapter, I emphasize the reflective forms.)

The portrayal of schizophrenia offered here is congruent with the notion that the underlying, unifying feature across all the schizophrenic syndromes is a defective *preconceptual attunement* between the individual and the world (the original meaning of 'autism'; Parnas & Bovet, 1991). I go beyond this traditional view by offering a more specific account of the disturbances in the constitution of both self and world (of the intentional arc) that underlie this defective attunement. This defective attunement accounts, in large measure, for the *praecox feeling* that schizophrenia so often evokes in the interviewer: that sense of encountering someone who can seem 'totally strange, puzzling, inconceivable, uncanny', and from whom one may feel separated by 'a gulf which defies description' (Jaspers, 1963, p. 447; Bleuler, 1978, p. 15; Rümke, 1990). As we shall see, however, the alienation felt by the interviewer may not indicate a simple failure to comprehend the patient or resonate with her affective life; it may actually mirror forms of *self*-alienation that the patient herself experiences from within.

Positive symptoms

The most prominent *positive* symptoms are the well-known *first-rank symptoms* of schizophrenia (Mellor, 1970). Most of these symptoms are actually *defined* by diminished self-affection, i.e. by loss of the sense of inhabiting one's own actions, thoughts, feelings, impulses, bodily sensations or perceptions, often to the point of feeling that these are possessed or controlled by some alien being or force. As the following quotation suggests, the alteration in question seems to involve something more basic than a belief, some actual diminishment of the sensations of ownership and agency that are normally intrinsic to action itself: 'When I reach my hand for a comb it is my hand and arm which move, and my fingers pick up the pen, but I don't control them . . . I sit there watching them move, and they are quite independent, what they do is nothing to do with me' (p. 18).

Jaspers (1963) considered these symptoms to be quintessential examples of schizophrenic incomprehensibility, recalcitrant to any kind of empathy or psychological explanation. By contrast, many psychoanalysts have interpreted these symptoms as manifestations of regression to early-infantile states of consciousness that precede differentiation of self from other. The most influential recent attempts at an explanation are the intriguing neurocognitive hypotheses of Frith (1987). He has postulated a neurophysiologically based decline in the feedback (*efference copy*) that indexes the willed or intentional nature of human action or, in a more recent formulation, a failure in the mechanism that derives predicted consequences of an action from a cognitive model of an intended sequence of motor commands (Frith et al., 2000). Frith has sometimes interpreted this disturbance as a consequence of a more general incapacity for *metarepresentation*, i.e. of the general ability of patients 'to reflect (consciously) upon their own mental activity' (Frith, 1992; Mlakar et al., 1994, p. 557), or to 'represent [one's] own states, including [one's] intentions' (p. 154).

The account I offer contrasts with each of these approaches. I will argue that these manifestations of external influence and diminished self-possession are in fact open to a kind of psychological comprehension, but that, far from involving regression to infantile adualism or an absence of self-conscious awareness, the diminished self-affection is actually associated with forms of *exaggerated* self-consciousness that are rooted in disturbed ipseity and hyperreflexive distortion of the normal structure of the intentional arc.

To understand how exaggerated self-consciousness could be associated with diminished self-affection and disturbed ipseity, recall Polanyi's discussion of the tacit dimension – the realm of sensations, stimuli or other components of experience that are known implicitly and that serve as the *proximal* term in the *from–to* structure inherent in the intentional arc. On Polanyi's account, the most basic sense of self does not require a separate channel of self-monitoring or a second, self-directed act of reflection or representation (as various theorists would claim, e.g. Frith, 1992, p. 116; Armstrong, 1993; Rosenthal, 1997). Tacitness itself is the medium or index of selfhood or normal self-affection: for, what we tacitly know, we inhabit or indwell. Processes of self-monitoring or self-reflection are likely to have the effect of alienating or dividing the self; for what is explicitly known cannot, by virtue of that fact, be fully inhabited as part of the intimate, and always only implicit, sense of an inner or core self.

Perhaps the clearest instance of indwelling is the relationship a person has with her own body in the course of normal, world-directed activity. 'It is the subsidiary sensing of our body that makes us feel that it is *our* body', Polanyi (1968) explains. 'The subsidiary sensing is *the meaning our body normally has for us*' (p. 405). But indwelling is not restricted to the body alone. By using a cane in the service of skilfully exploring the world: 'we incorporate [the cane] in our body ... so that we come to dwell in it' (p. 16; also Polanyi, 1964, pp. 55–59). In this way, 'we may be said to interiorize these things or to pour ourselves into them' (1968, p. 405). To focus explicit or focal attention on what had been tacitly experienced is, however, to objectify or alienate that phenomenon, to cause it to be experienced as existing at a remove (what is *focal* is also *distal* in Polanyi's terminology). What happens in schizophrenia, I suggest, is that this kind of attending continues until otherwise inalienable aspects of the self come to seem separate or detached. One's arms or legs, one's face, the feelings in the mouth or throat, the orbital housing of the eyes, even one's speaking, thinking or feeling can come to seem objectified, alien and apart, perhaps even like the possessions of some foreign being.

The symptomatic progression that often occurs – from mild to more extreme self-alienation – is clearly documented in the important German research on the basic symptoms (Koehler & Sauer, 1984), which will be discussed in the following section. The process may begin with a basal and operative hyperreflexivity, that is, with some disruptive breakdown of the normal, automatic structuring of the intentional arc that is experienced as a mostly *passive* process. (At the proximal end of the intentional arc, the same phenomenon will be experienced as a loss of self-affection.) But the process may be exacerbated and sustained by more reflective forms of hyperreflexivity that develop in consequence or by way of compensation. It is known, in fact, that patients with schizophrenia do not habituate readily, or use memory-based schemas to disattend to irrelevant information or familiar stimuli (Gray et al., 1991; van den Bosch, 1994; Hemsley, 1998). Since the latter category includes kinaesthetic sensations and other self-directed experiences, this cognitive abnormality might provide the source of the hyperreflexive sensations that soon come to attract more volitional forms of attention. (See also Hemsley (1998) for an analysis of first-rank symptoms that is compatible with the view presented here.) It seems, however, that this initially automatic process of progressive estrangement may often be potentiated and exaggerated by adopting a passive, observational stance; also relevant is the fact that many schizophrenics are able, at times, to minimize such symptoms by throwing themselves into some kind of habitual and unthinking activity (Breier & Strauss, 1983).

This progression is well illustrated in a classic article from 1919, Victor Tausk's 'On the origin of the 'influencing machine' in schizophrenia'. Tausk describes Natalija, a young woman with schizophrenia who felt a subtle sense of alienation from her own body, saliva and name, and who eventually came to experience her own actions, sensations and perceptions as but mechanical reflections – epiphenomena – of what she imagined was actually happening to a distant machine that resembled her own body. This distant yet intimate influencing machine had certain characteristics (e.g. the absence of a visible head, velvet on the torso) that suggest that it should be seen as a projected image not of the literal, physical body, but of Natalija's lived body – a lived body that had, in a sense, been turned inside out, reified and extruded in a process whereby normally tacit phenomena come into explicit focal awareness (Sass, 1992, p. 227).

This analysis also helps clarify some additional first-rank symptoms of schizophrenia: namely, thought echo and thought broadcasting, as well as running

commentary and voices arguing (the latter involving hallucinatory or quasihallu-
cinatory voices that describe the patient's ongoing actions or thoughts or discuss
the patient in the third person).

Over the last century, various authors have suggested that auditory hallucinations
of verbal material actually involve unrecognized perceptions of one's own 'inner
speech' (Johnson, 1978; Hoffman, 1986; Cahill & Frith, 1996a, p. 381). Others have
noted the occurrence of certain altered states of self-awareness that tend to precede
these auditory verbal hallucinations (e.g. Ey, 1973; Tissot, 1984; Naudin et al., 2000).
What happens is that the patient experiences his own subjectivity as becoming in
a certain way *ready* for something strange to happen. His stream of consciousness
feels somehow disembodied, at a distance, and he himself has a sense of emptiness.
Thinking and inner speech no longer exist at what Husserl (1989, section 41) called
the 'zero point of orientation'; they are no longer inhabited as the very medium of
selfhood, but have become more like introspected objects, with increasingly reified,
spatialized and externalized qualities.

Mutations of this kind may initially impose themselves on the patient; they tend
however to attract further attention, thereby initiating processes of scrutiny and
self-exacerbating alienation (*consequential* hyperreflexivity) that have a more active or *reflective* quality (which is not to say, however, that they are *fully* conscious
or volitional). Such mutations may also become the object of defensive or *compensatory* forms of hyperreflexivity, as when patients attempt to reassert control or to
reestablish a sense of self by means of introspective scrutiny or pseudo-obsessive
intellectual ruminations. But there is reason to believe that these more active or
reflective forms of hyperreflexivity, whether compensatory or consequential, may
well have largely counterproductive effects, serving as the source of further alienation, diminished self-affection and disturbed perceptual meaning. Introspectionist studies with normal individuals show that a kind of hyperreflection – in this
case produced in a purely volitional manner – can in fact bring on some alterations of the sense of both self and world that are strikingly reminiscent of what
occurs in schizophrenia (Hunt, 1985, 1995; Sass, 1994, p. 90). And, we might
now add, these further alterations could also inspire further forms of a hyperreflexivity that can take on a life of its own. All this suggests the possibility of a
veritable cascade of hyperreflexivity – of the basal, consequential and compensatory sort, and involving hyperreflexivity of the operative as well as more reflective
kinds.

A schizophrenic patient named Jonathan Lang (1938) offers an excellent autobiographical account of this process, a veritable centrifuging of the self in which
mental contents seem to migrate ever outward and away, leading to a loss of the normal sense of self-coinciding or self-affection. The process appears to involve focal

awareness of the sort of phenomena that are normally tacit yet come to be noticed by subjects in introspectionist experiments. Thus Lang describes his 'thoughts-out-loud' as being associated with 'a minimal tonus of vocal muscles and a sensation of proprioceptive pressure', and states: 'In so far as there is any hallucinatory factor in the experience, the sensation of proprioceptive pressure probably provides it' (Lang, 1938, p. 1091).

It is worth noting that the sentences or phrases that are 'heard' in thought-echo or thought-broadcasting experiences often have the grammatical peculiarities characteristic of normal inner speech, which usually serves as the tacit medium of thinking itself. These peculiarities include omission of explicit causal and logical connections, a tendency to presuppose rather than assert and absence of explicit markers of identity of speaker, listener, time or place (Vygotsky, 1962; Sokolov, 1972; Sass, 1992, p. 194). The specific content of the audioverbal hallucinations is also relevant. Among the most characteristic auditory hallucinations in schizophrenia are a voice describing the patient's ongoing behaviour or experience, and two or more voices discussing the patient in the third person. Whereas thought echo and thought broadcasting appear to involve an externalization of a more *basic* level of thinking, these characteristic auditory hallucinations (running commentary, voice arguing) are emblematic of the self-consciousness that *generates* this self-alienation. It is remarkable that not only the more *basic* level of thinking, but also self-consciousness itself (manifest in voices discussing and voices commenting on the patient) can come to be projected outward, as if it too were located in some alien being.

To account for the apparent failure to recognize the source of one's auditory hallucinations, Frith (1987) postulates a deficit in the *self-monitoring system*, which he considers a module or 'sub-component of the willed action system' (Cahill & Frith, 1996a, pp. 378, 392). Alterations of self-monitoring obviously do occur. But, as mentioned above, the auditory–verbal hallucinations typical of schizophrenia involve not diminished but exaggerated self-consciousness, that is, a sense of alienation from and a bringing-to-explicit-awareness of the processes of consciousness itself. Such an interpretation tends to undermine the conceptual basis of the very distinction between so-called *positive* and *negative* symptoms: in a sense, these positive symptoms do not involve the addition of anything new but only an *awareness* of what is always present (e.g. of inner speech, the perfectly *normal* medium of much of our thinking) in the context of diminished self-presence. But, of course, this very awareness itself constitutes a radical mutation, a key transformation of the modality (the degree of implicitness) in which the now-emergent phenomenon occurs. We might say, in fact, that thought echo and thought broadcasting (like Natalija's influencing machine) represent the perfectly *normal* phenomena of ordinary human experience but lived in the perfectly *abnormal* condition of hyperreflexive awareness and diminished self-affection.

These experiential transformations occurring in schizophrenia will certainly be accompanied by changes on the neural plane. To some extent, in fact, they may be fairly direct manifestations on the phenomenal level of progressive organic changes that occur in the brain and nervous system. But the preceding analysis suggests that these phenomenal changes are not likely to be *mere* epiphenomena. What elicits the ever-more intense forms of reflective concentration is not, after all, neural events *per se* but, rather, certain kinds of *experiences*; certain irreducible features of subjective life are what provide both the motivation and the field of possibility for the progressive developments. In this sense, the experiential phenomenology of abnormal experiences does not merely *constrain* explanations on the cognitive or neurobiological levels; it seems likely to play an important causal role in contributing to the progressive experiential transformations of a developing schizophrenic illness (McClamrock, 1995; Sass & Barnes, in press).

Negative symptoms

The concept of *negative* symptomatology is often said to be perfectly atheoretical, a purely behavioural description of an observable absence or diminishment of normal activity or expression: namely, poverty of speech, affective flattening, avolition, apathy, anhedonia and a general inattentiveness to the social or practical world. Actually, however, this overt behavioural lack has often been taken to indicate an underlying diminishment of an 'inferred function one normally expects to be present' (Sommers, 1985), that is, a paucity of psychological activity or subjective life, and in particular of the higher mental processes involving self-awareness, reasoning, abstraction, volition and complex emotional response. For example, *Diagnostic and Statistical Manual of Mental Disorders* (DSM-IV: American Psychiatric Association, 1994) refers to an apparent 'diminution of thoughts' and to 'diminution or absence of affect' (pp. 276–277), while Frith (1987; Cahill & Frith, 1996a, p. 376) postulates 'a specific deficit concerning the production of "internally generated" or "willed" action', a 'failure in a particular branch of the willed action system' such that goals simply 'fail to generate' willed intentions. Such views have significant affinities with the original conceptualization of negative symptoms that was offered by Hughlings Jackson and his followers at the end of the nineteenth century (Berrios, 1985). On this view, deficit is the essential feature of serious mental illness: 'The affection of function is always in the direction of loss, of deficit, or diminution . . . degradation of action to a lower plane' (quoted in Clark, 1981, p. 284).

Until recently, anglophone psychiatry had paid little attention to the subjective experiences associated with the so-called 'negative syndrome' (Selten et al., 1998). The failure of some patients to report subjective experiences consistent with their negative-symptom presentation has sometimes been dismissed as a manifestation of the lack of insight characteristic of schizophrenia. Recent research suggests, however, that the underlying experiences are not, in fact, direct analogues of what is observed at the behavioural level (van den Bosch et al., 1993; Selten et al., 2000). Patients who, from the observer's standpoint, demonstrate absence of thoughts, lack of motivation or energy, anhedonia, asociality or inability to feel intimacy and closeness do not seem to have the subjective experience one might expect (Selten, 1995, p. 212; Selten et al., 1998). Negative-symptom patients sometimes do have an inner sense of lacking thoughts, but just as often they deny such experiences (Selten, 1995, pp. 135, 138, 139), and they may even report a speeding-up or proliferation of thought processes (see below).

Earlier reports had already indicated that patients displaying catatonic withdrawal are often acutely conscious of surrounding events, and that asocial behaviour is often accompanied by an underlying yet fearful yearning for contact (Arieti, 1978; McGlashan, 1982). Recently it has been shown that patients who display flat affect report an intense emotional reactivity that contradicts their lack of overt affective expression (Bouricius, 1989; Hurlbut, 1990, p. 254; Berenbaum & Oltmanns, 1992; Kring et al., 1993), a claim nicely corroborated by electrodermal measurements showing equal or even higher reactivity than for normal subjects (Kring & Neale, 1996). So far, however, there has been very little attempt, at least in the English-language literature, to offer a detailed or theoretically informed understanding of the experiences in question.

The richest account of the subjective side of the negative or seemingly deficit syndrome is provided in a classic of German phenomenological psychiatry, Wolfgang Blankenburg's *The Loss of Natural Self-Evidence: A Contribution to the Study of Symptom-Poor Schizophrenics* (1991, French translation; German original, 1971; also 1969). In Blankenburg's view, the central defect or abnormality in schizophrenia is best described as a loss of the usual common-sense orientation to reality, of the unquestioned sense of obviousness and of the unproblematic background quality that normally enables a person to take for granted so many aspects of the social and practical world. Blankenburg's approach is consistent with empirical studies showing that, although schizophrenics often do well on intellectual tasks requiring abstract or logical thought, they have particular difficulties in attempting to solve more practical or common-sensical problems, perhaps especially when these relate to the social world (Cutting & Murphy, 1988, 1990.) Although 'loss of natural self-evidence' is characteristic of all schizophrenic patients, according to Blankenburg, it is easier to recognize in negative-symptom patients. As we shall see, it goes a long way toward explaining the social withdrawal as well as the slowing and inactivity characteristic of such patients.

At first, loss of natural self-evidence might seem a fairly straightforward negative symptom – a privation of something normally present, namely, common sense. Blankenburg, however, puts considerable emphasis on heightened or unusual forms of awareness that tend to accompany the loss of natural self-evidence in many negative-symptom patients. As he points out (p. 12), patients with schizophrenia often experience states of hyperreflexive consciousness in which they are explicitly aware of aspects or processes of action and experience that, for the normal person, would be simply presupposed and unnoticed. His central case example, Anne, speaks of being 'hooked to' or 'hung up on' (pp. 79–80) obvious or self-evident problems and questions that healthy people simply take for granted. 'It is impossible for me to stop myself from thinking', she said (pp. 82, 91). Anne's constant need to think was accompanied by a constant inability to understand or to act in spontaneous or practical ways (pp. 11, 72). Results from an ongoing study in Copenhagen demonstrate a high correlation between negative-symptom presentation and 'perplexity', a variable involving several *positive* aberrations including ambivalence, hyperreflectivity, disturbed perception of the meaning of things, aroused state of perceptual awareness, and deautomatization (Handest, 2002).

Blankenburg's portrayal is consistent with the view that the schizophrenic 'attentional disturbance' involves 'excessive *self*-awareness', including abnormal awareness of the '*cognitive* unconscious' (Frith, 1979). Research shows that persons with schizophrenia do often rely on analytic, sequential, conscious and quasivoluntary cognitive procedures in circumstances that normally call forth more automatic or spontaneous forms of holistic and parallel processing (Cutting, 1985, pp. 294–300, 305; Sass, 1992, pp. 390–396). 'I have to do everything step by step, nothing is automatic now. Everything has to be considered', reported one patient with schizophrenia (McGhie & Chapman, 1961, p. 108). '[I am] not sure of my own movements any more', said another such patient:

It's not so much thinking out what to do, it's the doing of it that sticks me . . . I take more time to do things because I am always conscious of what I am doing. If I could just stop noticing what I am doing, I would get things done a lot faster (p. 107).

The relationship between this hyperreflexivity and loss of self-evidence is likely to be complex. The analytic, self-conscious focus may well occur in compensation for failures of schema-controlled, automatic processing that have a more basal and operative status; but such focusing may also precipitate failures of such processing. It seems likely, in any case, to contribute to the sense of overload, effortfulness and perplexity (*Ratlosigkeit*) that is characteristic of schizophrenia. (*Ratlosigkeit* refer to a self-aware, anguishing and (to the patient) perfectly inexplicable sense of being unable to maintain a consistent grasp on reality or to cope with normal situational demands, usually accompanied by withdrawal into the self: Storring, 1987.) It would also tend to block the spontaneity necessary both for graceful movement and for the exercise of subtle intuitive discernment, thus helping to account for the awkwardness as well as the loss of a certain *esprit de finesse* that is common in persons with schizophrenia (Blankenburg, 1991, pp. 94, 128); see also Kim et al., 1994, p. 432, regarding a correlation, between loss of smoothness of action and disturbed sense of self.)

To understand this characteristic schizophrenic perplexity, it is not sufficient to recognize that the patient's consciousness may be in a state of cognitive overload (the usual emphasis of interpretations of schizophrenia as a disorder of the attentional filter; Cutting, 1985, chapter 8). Even more important is a radical *qualitative* shift: when the tacit dimension becomes explicit, it can no longer perform the grounding, orienting, in effect *constituting* function that only what remains in the background can play. Anne herself speaks of the 'way', 'manner of thinking' or 'framework' that each person needs in order to know how to conduct him- or herself. Normally this develops over time and largely unnoticed, like one's character itself, she says. But whereas others have a *natural* relationship to this framework, she says that she herself feels at an enormous distance from any such thing: 'In my case, everything is just an *object* of thought' (Blankenburg, 1991, p. 127).

It is important to consider the complementary but nomothetic and longitudinal work on basic symptoms done by a group of German researchers who, over 40 years or more, have been gathering first-person data and carefully mapping subjective experiences in the prodromal, active and residual states of schizophrenia (Klosterkötter, 1992). Whereas Blankenburg draws our attention to abstract preoccupations that can give schizophrenic thought and speech a quasiphilosophical or hyperabstract quality, e.g. conventions of social interaction, framework assumptions, and the like, the basic-symptom research documents how the larger unities of experience and action, with their 'hierarchies of habituation' (Armbruster & Klosterkoetter, 1986, p. 1148) can break down due to preoccupation with the sensations or other experiential particulars that constitute what Klosterkötter et al. (1997) term the forms of 'basal irritation'.

The basic symptoms are believed to represent the subjective dimension of seeming deficiency states that are presumably 'substrate-close' (Gross, 1986, p. 1142) since they occur in virtually identical form both before and after the development of productive, positive symptoms. This is in contrast to the negative symptoms, which have often been altered by 'processes of working out and transformation' (Armbruster & Klosterkoetter, 1986, p. 1150) and can reflect defensive withdrawal, demoralization and reactive apathy (Huber, 1986, p. 1137).

The basic-symptom research clearly demonstrates that even the most clearly *negative* symptoms, such as apathy or avolition, are accompanied by a panoply of *positive* experiential disturbances in the domains of cognition, perception, bodily experience, action and emotion.

One cluster of early-stage basic symptoms are the cenaesthesias: sensations of movement or pressure inside the body or on its surfaces; electric or migrating sensations; awareness of kinaesthetic or thermic sensations; and sensations of diminution, enlargement or emptiness, or of numbness or stiffness of the body or its parts. Generally unpleasant, and frequently accompanied by feelings of decline of vital energy, these experiences are combined with a loss of automatic skills and with interference with the smooth flow of motor activity. They appear to involve hyperreflexive awareness of bodily sensations that would not normally be attended to in any direct or sustained fashion, and that can no longer serve as a medium of self-affection. Basic symptoms do not normally occur in healthy persons or in neurotic or character disorders (Huber, 1986, p. 1137). They are, however, remarkably similar to the experiences reported by normal subjects who adopt a detached, introspective stance toward their own experiences (see Angyal, 1936; Hunt, 1985, p. 248; 1995, p. 201; Sass, 1994, pp. 90–97, 159–161).

It is not surprising that good first-person descriptions of schizophrenic negative symptoms are extremely rare: everyday language is badly suited to describing such unusual and inner experiences, and the states themselves tend to undermine the capacity for sustained or coherent thought or discourse (see below). We are therefore especially fortunate to have the writings of Antonin Artaud, a writer and general man-of-the-theatre who has recently been described as almost the only person with schizophrenia who has managed to describe his negative symptoms in real detail (Sass, 1996; Selten et al., 1998, p. 79). In a work called *The Umbilicus of Limbo*, Artaud conveys his sense of vertigo and bewilderment, and the consequent withdrawal that occurs when bodily appendages and movements come to seem distant, devitalized, dislocated and strange:

Unconscious incoherence of steps, of gestures, of movements. Will power constantly inhibited in even the simplest gestures, renunciation of simple gestures, . . . state of painful numbness, sort of localized numbness on skin surface . . . but felt like the radical suppression of a limb, transmitting to the brain no more than images of bloody old cottons pulled out in the shape of arms and legs, images of distant and dislocated members. Sort of inward breakdown of entire nervous system.

A shifting vertigo, a sort of oblique bewilderment which accompanies every effort (Artaud, 1965, pp. 28–29; 1976, p. 65; translations combined).

In another passage he describes: 'The limbo of a nightmare of bone and muscles . . . Larval images that are pushed as if by a finger and have no relation to any material thing' (p. 44).

Artaud also describes experiences akin to both the *direct* and the *indirect* or secondary types of *dynamic deficiency* discussed in the basic-symptom research. He senses a basic and painful lack of vital energy and directedness that prevents actions from having a natural or spontaneous sort of coherence and flow: 'a staggering and central fatigue, a kind of gasping fatigue. Movements must be recomposed, a sort of deathlike fatigue'. But this brings on a secondary sort of fatigue (what Blankenburg, 1991, pp. 132–133, 153, 155–156, calls 'schizophrenic asthenia'), for it forces Artaud to expend effort in order to achieve forms of bodily and cognitive integration that would normally occur in an effortlessly automatic fashion. Artaud describes:

a fatigue of cosmic Creation, the sense of having to carry one's body around . . . state of painful numbness, sort of localized numbness on skin surface which does not hinder a single motion but alters nevertheless that internal feeling in your limbs so that the mere act of standing vertical is achieved only at the price of a victorious struggle (1965, pp. 28–29; 1976, pp. 64–65; translations combined).

Here we see, on a brute, bodily level, the kinds of experiences that can underlie Blankenburg's 'loss of natural self-evidence' and that can lead to motoric slowing or even complete withdrawal from action. Artaud appears to be describing processes whereby phenomena that would normally recede as part of a sensed but unnoticed background or medium of consciousness – the planes and protrusions of one's body and limbs, physical sensations of movement, tension or release – move out of the tacit dimension and emerge into hyperreflexive awareness. It is easy to see how such basic experiences of self-alienation, rooted in hyperreflexive disruptions of the intentional arc, might be conducive to the forms of inactivity and social withdrawal, the detachment from emotion and desire and the sense of effortfulness and associated fatigue that characterize the negative-symptom syndrome.

Disorganization symptoms

The disorganization syndrome comprises a variety of abnormalities in the organization of thought, speech and attention, including tangentiality and derailment, incoherence and pressure of speech, poverty of content of speech and diminished self-affection. Each of these signs suggests abnormalities of cognitive focus that can be seen as consistent with the above discussion of hyperreflexivity and ipseity disturbance. There seems to be a loss of the ability to be focused on or committed to a particular topic or goal, along with a concomitant awareness, distracting and disruptive, of issues, dimensions and processes that would usually be presupposed. There is indeed disorganization, but of a kind that can be described in fairly precise, qualitative terms, and that can be distinguished from those more characteristic of other psychopathological groups. I shall first stress the role of hyperreflexivity, then turn to diminished self-affection.

The specifically schizophrenic *attentional disturbance* appears to involve a heightened awareness of what has been called the 'cognitive unconscious', that is, of features of cognitive processing that are normally presupposed (Frith, 1979). This distinguishes it from the attentional abnormalities characteristic of the manic, depressed or organic patient. Schizophrenic *language disturbances* are distinct from the aphasias, for they particularly affect what linguists call the pragmatic dimension of speech (Schwartz, 1982; Sass, 1992, chapter 6), especially the subtle and shifting relationships between what can be asserted and what would normally be presupposed – that is to say, between what emerges as the shared focus at a given moment of a conversation and what would normally serve as the tacit and taken-for-granted background.

What of the types of *formal thought disorder* that are particularly common in schizophrenic and schizotypal individuals? Research shows that, whereas manic thought disorder is 'extravagantly combinatory, usually with humor, flippancy, and playfulness', schizophrenic thinking appears 'disorganized, confused, and ideationally fluid', with 'interpenetrations of one idea by another [and] unstable verbal referents'; schizophrenic thinking often conveys 'an impression of inner turmoil and bewilderment, and may cause confusion in the listener as well' (Solovay et al., 1987, pp. 13, 20). Unlike manic patients, who often fail to stay focused on particular *objects* of awareness, persons with schizophrenia demonstrate a more fundamental failure to stay anchored within a single frame of reference, perspective or orientation (Angyal, 1964; Holzman et al., 1986; Sass, 1992, chapter 4). Often there is a shift among conceptual levels, including hyperabstract as well as hyperconcrete or hyperliteral perspectives, both of which may represent emerging awareness of normally presupposed components of thought and experience (Sass, 1992, chapter 5). This suggests not acceleration or easing of inhibitions, as in mania, but a more basic disruption of fundamental processes of consciousness (viz. of the intentional arc) whereby the objects of awareness are normally constituted and fixed.

Still another disorganization symptom is *poverty of content of speech*. While this listener-defined category almost certainly comprises heterogeneous phenomena, many instances seem to represent the confusing impact on the listener of this framework drift, or else the hyperabstract, and therefore hard-to-follow, nature of certain hyperreflexive concerns. Poverty of speech, it should be noted, is often described as 'vague' or 'hyperabstract', or as sounding like 'empty philosophizing' (Andreasen, 1979, p. 1318), 'fruitless intellectualizing' or 'pseudo-abstract reasoning' (Ostwald & Zavarin, 1980, p. 75).

Most attempts to explain these disorganization symptoms have assumed they are rooted in purely cognitive and often rather modular dysfunctions, such as particular kinds of associational disturbance, failure of attention or working memory or an incapacity for the planning or monitoring of discourse or thought (Hoffman et al., 1982; Goldman-Rakic, 1994; Spitzer, 1997). I agree that such functions are disrupted. But it is important to note that, as indicated above, the disruptions in question are especially likely to involve hyperreflexive distortion of the normal intentional arc, and are closely bound up with basic mutations of vital self-affection. (Research on the basic symptoms shows that a decline in dynamic aspects is to be found among the earliest symptoms, e.g. disturbances of concentration, of immediate recall and of thought initiative or 'thought energy', as well as a retardation and impediment of thought processes (Klosterkötter et al., 1997).)

In the absence of vital self-affection and the lines of orientation it establishes, the structured nature of the worlds of both thought and perception will be altered or even dissolved. The world will be stripped of all the affordances and vectors of concern by which the fabric of normal, common-sense reality is knitted together into an organized and meaningful whole.

One (so-called) disorganization symptom not yet mentioned is *incongruous affect* – a condition in which the quality or kind of emotion expressed seems inappropriate to the context or eliciting event. Many theorists, including Darwin and William James, have argued that affective experiences are rooted in experiences of bodily states – in what Damasio (1994) has described as 'representations' or 'images of the body' that have come to be associated as 'somatic markers' with particular contexts or stimulus situations. But it seems likely that, at least under normal conditions, emotional experience involves not representations of the objectified body *image* so much as implicitly felt experiences involving the body *subject*: somatic markers, patterns or tension states are normally experienced not as focal objects but as the tacitly inhabited medium of an attitude – such as fear, desire or disgust – that is directed toward some object in the world.

When normally tacit experiences come to be the objects of a more focal and objectifying awareness (as in Artaud's description above of experiencing his arms and legs as 'images of distant and dislocated members'), then the emotion-related sensory configurations are no longer serving as an attitude and impetus *toward* the world; they would instead be experienced at a subjective distance, almost as objects in themselves, while others might simply fail to coalesce at all. This would lead to a sense of awkwardness, artificiality and distance, both in the patient's affective experience as well as in what is visible to others. It would also undermine the very sentiment of being, the sense of existing as a subject with attitudes, intentions and an impetus toward action, thereby 'weakening...those emotional activities which permanently form the mainsprings of volition' (Kraepelin, 1913, quoted in Frith, 1987, p. 646).

We see, then, that despite striking differences between the positive, negative and disorganization syndromes, the symptoms in each group also seem to have fundamental affinities: a disturbance of the intentional arc involving both hyperreflexivity and diminished self-affection. It is possible that these pervasive abnormalities could represent some kind of final common pathway deriving from several wholly distinct abnormal neurocognitive mechanisms. It seems more probable, however, that the shared abnormalities indicate a more fundamental disturbance, a disturbance that is likely to play some kind of generative role in the pathogenesis of each of the syndromes.

This is not the place for an extended discussion of possible neurobiological or neurocognitive factors. I will simply note that the phenomenological analysis offered above suggests that the most fundamental neurocognitive factors seem likely to involve relatively low-level processes implicated in the basic constitution of the act of awareness (that is, aspects of operative intentionality). Contemporary hypotheses that seem consistent with the conceptualization offered here include theories about the role of the comparator system in organizing focal attention (Hemsley, 1987; Gray et al., 1991) as well as theories that postulate a deficit or malfunction of the more spontaneous, context-oriented mental processes, perhaps accompanied by dysfunctional hypertrophy of the more volitional, conscious or analytic modes of awareness (Cutting, 1990). Although the higher-level processes emphasized in some theories, such as the Supervisory Attentional System or the capacity for normal forms of metarepresentation (Frith, 1992, p. 117; Cahill & Frith, 1996a, p. 378), can certainly be affected, these seem likely to play a less primordial pathogenetic role.

Artaud: interdependence of the syndromes

Given the experiential focus of this chapter, it is fitting to conclude with some autobiographical reflections in which Artaud rehearses all the main themes of the chapter. In a letter written in 1932, Artaud offers what can be read as a spontaneous critique of the conceptual foundations of the positive–negative–disorganization distinction, one that illustrates the interdependence of these three aspects while also showing the complementarity of hyperreflexivity and diminished self-affection.

In his letter, Artaud (1976) describes a 'sense of monstrous, horrible fatigue' and 'total exhaustion', feelings of emptiness (what he calls 'lack of nervous density'), and especially an 'inability to form or develop thoughts'. 'It is', he writes, 'as if each time my thought tries to manifest itself it contracts, and it is this contraction that shuts off my thought from within, makes it rigid as in a spasm' (p. 293). At first, Artaud's fatigue and thought contraction might appear to be straightforward negative symptoms – deficits of both energy and ideation. Yet in the very next sentence, Artaud informs us that his experiences of mental stammering and thought blocking actually result from a *surfeit* of mental content: 'the thought, the expression stops because the flow is too violent, because the brain wants to say too many things which it thinks of all at once, ten thoughts instead of one rush toward the exit ...'.

Then, a few lines later, Artaud reverses himself again, now saying that, at a more profound level, his mind really is too empty: 'But if one really analyzes a state of this kind it is not by being too full that consciousness errs at these moments but by being too empty, for this prolific and above all unstable and shifting juxtaposition is an illusion' (p. 293). As it turns out, the violent flow and consequent disorganization that he describes is really a kind of hyperreflexive cascade – a collapse of metalevels, of hyperabstract metaperspectives whose proliferation suggests a loss of perspectival abridgement and natural self-evidence and a tendency to experience his own mind almost as if it were being seen from the perspective of an outside observer: 'the brain sees the whole thought at once with all its circumstances, and it also sees all the points of view it could take and all the forms with which it could invest them, a vast juxtaposition of concepts' (p. 293). Artaud describes himself as 'losing contact *with*' but, at the same time, becoming focally aware *of* 'all those first assumptions which are at the foundation of thought' (p. 290). What is most characteristic of 'this slackening, this confusion, this fragility', he writes, 'is a kind of disappearance or disintegration or collapse of first assumptions which even causes me to wonder why, for example, red (the color) is considered red and affects me as red, why a judgment affects me as a judgment and not as a pain, why I feel a pain, and why this particular pain, which I feel without understanding it' (p. 294).

Here we seem to have a hyperreflexive proliferation of viewpoints, a slippage among possible perspectives as well as among perspectives *on* perspectives that erodes any capacity for conceptual or perceptual focusing. But this is the counterpart of an *absence* of something equally basic – a disturbance of self-affection involving decline of the vital reactivity and spontaneous directedness that gives orientation and a kind of organization to one's thinking. As Artaud explains with his characteristic precision:

in every [normal] state of consciousness there is always a dominant theme, and if the mind has not 'automatically' decided on a dominant theme it is through weakness and because at that moment nothing dominated, nothing presented itself with enough force or continuity in the field of consciousness to be recorded. The truth is, therefore, that [in my case] rather than an overflow or an excess there was a deficiency; in the absence of some precise thought that was able to develop, there was slackening, confusion, fragility (p. 293).

What Artaud describes as his 'incorrigible inability to concentrate upon an object' does not appear to be a purely cognitive disorder. It is bound up with disturbances in the basic sense of selfhood – with what Artaud calls 'the very substance of what is called the soul and that is the emanation of our nervous force which coagulates around objects' (1965, p. 20). As we have seen, hyperreflexivity and diminished self-affection are two facets of a fundamental experiential transformation that erodes the capacity for perceptual focus or conceptual grip. Together they provide what Artaud calls 'the destructive element which de-mineralizes the mind and deprives it of its first assumptions', thereby making 'the ground under my thought crumble' (pp. 94, 290).

Acknowledgement

This article is indebted to collaborative work carried out with Josef Parnas.

REFERENCES

American Psychiatric Association. (1994). *Diagnostic and Statistical Manual of Mental Disorders* (DSM-IV). Washington, DC: American Psychiatric Press.

Andreasen, N. (1979). Thought, language, and communication disorders: I. *Archives of General Psychiatry*, **36**, 1315–21.

Andreasen, N. (1984). *The Broken Brain: The Biological Revolution in Psychiatry*. New York: Harper and Row.

Andreasen, N. (1999). A unitary model of schizophrenia: Bleuler's 'fragmented phrene' as schizencephaly. *Archives of General Psychiatry*, **56**, 781–7.

Angyal, A. (1936). The experience of the body-self in schizophrenia. *Archives of Neurology and Psychiatry*, **35**, 1029–53.

Angyal, A. (1964). Disturbances of thinking in schizophrenia. In *Language and Thought in Schizophrenia*, ed. J.S. Kasanin, pp. 115–23. New York: Norton.

Arieti, S. (1978). Volition and value: a study based on catatonic schizophrenia. In *On Schizophrenia, Phobias, Depression, Psychotherapy, and the Farther Shores of Psychiatry*, ed. S. Arieti, pp. 109–20. New York: Brunner/Mazel.

Armbruster, B. & Klosterkoetter, J. (1986). Basic versus negative symptoms. In *Biological Psychiatry 1985*, ed. C. Shagass, R.C. Josiassen, W.H. Bridger et al. pp. 1148–50. New York: Elsevier.

Armstrong, D.M. (1993). *A Materialist Theory of the Mind*. London: Routledge.

Artaud, A. (1965). *Antonin Artaud Anthology*, ed. J. Hirschman. San Francisco, CA: City Lights Books.

Artaud, A. (1976). *Antonin Artaud: Selected Writings*, ed. S. Sontag, translated by H. Weaver. New York: Farrar, Straus, & Giroux.

Berenbaum, H. & Oltmanns, T.F. (1992). Emotional experience and expression in schizophrenia and depression. *Journal of Abnormal Psychology*, **101**, 37–44.

Bernet, R., Kern, I. & Marbach, E. (1993). *An Introduction to Husserlian Phenomenology.* Evanston, IL: Northwestern University Press.

Berrios, G.E. (1985). Positive and negative symptoms and Jackson. *Archives of General Psychiatry,* **42**, 95–7.

Blankenburg, W. (1969). Ansätze zu einer Pschopathologie des 'common sense'. *Confinia Psychiatrica,* **12**, 144–63. [First steps toward a psychopathology of 'common sense', English translation in *Philosophy, Psychiatry, Psychology,* **8**, 303–15 (2001).]

Blankenburg, W. (1991). *La Perte de l'Evidence Naturelle: Une Contribution a la Psychopathologie des Schizophrenies Pauci-Symptomatiques.* Translated by J.-M. Azorin & Y. Totoyan. Paris: Presses Universitaires de France. Originally published in 1971: *Der Verlust der Naturlichen Selbstverstandlichkeit: Ein Beitrag zur Psychopathologie Symptomarmer Schizophrenien.* Stuttgart: Ferdinand Enke Verlag.

Bleuler, E. (1950). *Dementia Praecox, or The Group of Schizophrenias.* Translated by J. Zinkin. New York: International Universities Press.

Bleuler, M. (1978). *The Schizophrenic Disorders.* Translated by S.M. Clemens. New Haven, CT: Yale University Press.

Bouricius, J.K. (1989). Negative symptoms and emotions in schizophrenia. *Schizophrenia Bulletin,* **15**, 201–7.

Breier, A. & Strauss, J.S. (1983). Self-control in psychotic disorders. *Archives of General Psychiatry,* **40**, 1141–5.

Cahill, C. & Frith, C. D. (1996a). A cognitive basis for the signs and symptoms of schizophrenia. In *Schizophrenia: A Neuropsychological Perspective,* ed. C. Pantelis, H.E. Nelson & T.R.E. Barnes, pp. 373–95. New York: John Wiley.

Cahill, C. & Frith, C.D. (1996b). False perceptions or false beliefs? Hallucinations and delusions in schizophrenia. In *Method in Madness: Case Studies in Cognitive Neuropsychiatry,* ed. P.W. Halligan & J.C. Marshall, pp. 267–91. Howe, East Sussex, UK: Erlbaum.

Clark, M.J. (1981). The rejection of psychological approaches to mental disorder in late nineteenth-century British psychiatry. In *Madhouses, Mad-Doctors, and Madmen: The Social History of Psychiatry in the Victorian Era,* ed. A. Scull, pp. 271–312. Philadelphia: University of Pennsylvania Press.

Costello, C.G. (1992). Research on symptoms versus research on syndromes: arguments in favour of allocating more research time to the study of symptoms. *British Journal of Psychiatry,* **160**, 304–8.

Cutting, J. (1985). *The Psychology of Schizophrenia.* Edinburgh: Churchill Livingstone.

Cutting, J. (1990). *The Right Cerebral Hemisphere and Psychiatric Disorders.* Oxford: Oxford University Press.

Cutting, J. & Murphy, D. (1988). Schizophrenic thought disorder: a psychological and organic interpretation. *British Journal of Psychiatry,* **152**, 310–19.

Cutting, J. & Murphy, D. (1990). Impaired ability of schizophrenics, relative to manics or depressives, to appreciate social knowledge about their culture. *British Journal of Psychiatry,* **157**, 355–8.

Damasio, A.R. (1994). *Descartes' Error: Emotion, Reason, and the Human Brain.* New York: Avon Books.

Damasio, A.R. (1999). *The Feeling of What Happens: Body and Emotion in the Making of Consciousness*. New York: Harcourt Brace.

Dillon, M. (1997). *Merleau-Ponty's Ontology*, 2nd edn. Evanston, IL: Northwestern University Press.

Ey, H. (1973). *Traité des Hallucinations*. Paris: Masson.

Fenton, W.S. & McGlashan, T. (1991). Natural history of schizophrenia subtypes: II. Positive and negative symptoms and long-term course. *Archives of General Psychiatry*, **48**, 978–86.

Frith, C.D. (1979). Consciousness, information processing, and schizophrenia. *British Journal of Psychiatry*, **134**, 225–35.

Frith, C.D. (1987). The positive and negative symptoms of schizophrenia reflect impairments in perception and initiation of action. *Psychological Medicine*, **17**, 631–48.

Frith, C. (1992). *The Cognitive Neuropsychology of Schizophrenia*. Hove, UK: Lawrence Erlbaum.

Frith, C.D. & Done, D.J. (1989). Experiences of alien control in schizophrenia reflect a disorder in central monitoring of action. *Psychological Medicine*, **19**, 359–63.

Frith, C.D., Blakemore, S.-J. & Wolpert, D. M. (2000). Explaining the symptoms of schizophrenia: abnormalities in the awareness of action. *Brain Research Reviews*, **31**, 357–63.

Gallagher, S. (1997). Mutual enlightenment: recent phenomenology in cognitive science. *Journal of Consciousness Studies*, **4**, 195–214.

Gallagher, S. (2000). Philosophical concepts of the self: implications for cognitive science. *Trends in Cognitive Science*, **4**, 1–35.

Gallagher, S. & Meltzoff, A. (1996). The earliest sense of self and others: Merleau-Ponty and recent developmental studies. *Philosophical Psychology*, **9**, 211–33.

Gibson, J.J. (1979). *The Ecological Approach to Visual Perception*. Boston: Houghton Mifflin.

Gibson, E.J. (1993). Ontogenesis of the perceived self. In *The Perceived Self*, ed. U. Neisser, pp. 25–42. Cambridge, UK: Cambridge University Press.

Goldman-Rakic, P. (1994). Working memory dysfunction in schizophrenia. *Journal of Neuropsychiatry and Clinical Neurosciences*, **6**, 348–57.

Gottesman, I. (1991). *Schizophrenia Genesis: The Origins of Madness*. New York: W.H. Freeman.

Gray, J.A., Feldon, J., Rawlins, J.N., Hemsley, D.R. & Smith, A.D. (1991). The neuropsychology of schizophrenia. *Behavioral and Brain Sciences*, **14**, 1–20.

Grene, M. (1968). Tacit knowing and the pre-reflective cogito. In *Intellect and Hope: Essays in the Thought of Michael Polanyi*, ed. T.A. Langford & W.H. Poteat, pp. 19–57. Durham, NC: Duke University Press.

Gross, G. (1986). The Bonn scale for the assessment of basic symptoms. In *Biological Psychiatry 1985*, ed. C. Shagass, R.C. Josiassen, W.H. Bridger et al. pp. 1142–4. New York: Elsevier.

Hafner, H., Maurer, K., Loeffler, W. et al. (1998). The ABC schizophrenia study: a preliminary overview of the results. *Social Psychiatry and Psychiatric Epidemiology*, **33**, 380–6.

Handest, P. (2002). *The Prodromes of schizophrenia*. Doctoral dissertation. In Danish with English summary. Copenhagen: medical faculty, University of Copenhagen.

Hemsley, D.R. (1987). An experimental psychological model for schizophrenia. In *Search for the Causes of Schizophrenia*, vol. 1, ed. H. Hafner, W.F. Gattaz, & W. Janzarik, pp. 179–88. New York: Springer.

Hemsley, D.R. (1998). The disruption of the 'sense of self' in schizophrenia: potential links with disturbances of information processing. *British Journal of Medical Psychology*, **71**, 115–24.

Henry, M. (1973). *The Essence of Manifestation*. Translated by G. Etzkorn. The Hague: Martinus Nijhoff. Original in 1963: *L'Essence de la Manifestation*. Paris: PUF.

Hoenig, J. (1983). The concept of schizophrenia: Kraepelin–Bleuler–Schneider. *British Journal of Psychiatry*, **142**, 547–56.

Hoffman, R. (1986). Verbal hallucinations and language production processes in schizophrenia. *Behavioral and Brain Sciences*, **9**, 503–48.

Hoffman, R., Kirstein, L., Stopek, S. & Cichetti, D. (1982). Apprehending schizophrenic discourse: a structural analysis of the listener's task. *Brain and Language*, **15**, 207–33.

Holzman, P.S., Shenton, M.E. & Solovay, M.R. (1986). Quality of thought disorder in differential diagnosis. *Schizophrenia Bulletin*, **12**, 360–72.

Huber, G. (1986). Negative or basic symptoms in schizophrenia and affective illness. In *Biological Psychiatry 1985*, ed. C. Shagass, R.C. Josiassen, W.H. Bridger et al., pp. 1136–41. New York: Elsevier.

Hunt, H.T. (1985). Cognition and states of consciousness. *Perceptual and Motor Skills*, **60**, 239–82.

Hunt, H.T. (1995). *On the Nature of Consciousness*. New Haven, CT: Yale University Press.

Hurlbut, R.T. (1990). *Sampling Normal and Schizophrenic Inner Experience*. New York: Plenum.

Husserl, E. (1989). *Ideas Pertaining to a Pure Phenomenology and to a Phenomenological Philosophy*, vol. 2. Translated by R. Rojcewicz & A. Schuwer. Dordrecht: Kluwer.

James, W. (1981). *The Principles of Psychology*. Cambridge, MA: Harvard University Press.

Jaspers, K. (1963). *General Psychopathology*. Translated by J. Hoenig & M.W. Hamilton. Chicago: University of Chicago Press.

Johnson, R. (1978). *The Anatomy of Hallucinations*. Chicago: Nelson Hall.

Johnstone, E.C. & Frith, C.D. (1996). Validation of three dimensions of schizophrenic symptoms in a large unselected sample of patients. *Psychological Medicine*, **26**, 669–79.

Kim, Y., Takemoto, K., Mayahara, K., Sumida, K. & Shiba, S. (1994). An analysis of the subjective experience of schizophrenia. *Comprehensive Psychiatry*, **35**, 430–6.

Klosterkötter, J. (1992). The meaning of basic symptoms for the development of schizophrenic psychoses. *Neurology, Psychiatry, and Brain Research*, **1**, 30–41.

Klosterkötter, J., Gross, G., Huber, G. et al. (1997). Evaluation of the 'Bonn Scale for the Assessment of Basic Symptoms' (BSABS) as an instrument for the assessment of schizophrenia proneness. *Neurology, Psychiatry, and Brain Research*, **5**, 137–50.

Koehler, K. & Sauer, H. (1984). Huber's basic symptoms: another approach to negative psychopathology in schizophrenia. *Comprehensive Psychiatry*, **25**, 174–82.

Kring, A.M. & Neale, J. (1996). Do schizophrenic patients show a disjunctive relationship among expressive, experiential, and psychophysiological components of emotion? *Journal of Abnormal Psychology*, **105**, 249–57.

Kring, A.M., Kerr, S.L., Smith, D.A. et al. (1993). Flat affect in schizophrenia does not reflect diminished subjective experience of emotion. *Journal of Abnormal Psychology*, **102**, 507–17.

Lang, J. (1938). The other side of hallucinations. *American Journal of Psychiatry*, **94**, 1089–97.

Liddle, P.F. (1987). The symptoms of chronic schizophrenia: a re-examination of the positive–negative dichotomy. *British Journal of Psychiatry*, **151**, 145–51.

Liddle, P.F., Carpenter, W.T. & Crow, T. (1994). Syndromes of schizophrenia: classic literature. *British Journal of Psychiatry*, **165**, 721–7.

Maj, M. (1998). Critique of the DSM-IV operational diagnostic criteria for schizophrenia. *British Journal of Psychiatry*, **172**, 458–60.

Marneros, A., Andreasen, N.C. & Tsuang, M.T. (eds) (1991). *Negative versus Positive Schizophrenia*. Berlin: Springer-Verlag.

McClamrock, R. (1995). *Existential Cognition: Computational Minds in the World*. Chicago: University of Chicago Press.

McGhie, A. & Chapman, J. (1961). Disorders of attention and perception in early schizophrenia. *British Journal of Medical Psychology*, **34**, 103–15.

McGlashan, T.H. (1982). Aphanasis: the phenomenon of pseudo-depression in schizophrenia. *Schizophrenia Bulletin*, **8**, 118–34.

McGlashan, T.H. & Fenton, W.S. (1992). The positive–negative distinction in schizophrenia: review of natural history indicators. *Archives of General Psychiatry*, **49**, 63–72.

McKenna, P.J. (1994). *Schizophrenia and Related Syndromes*. Oxford, UK: Oxford University Press.

Mellor, C.S. (1970). First rank symptoms of schizophrenia. *British Journal of Psychiatry*, **117**, 15–23.

Merleau-Ponty, M. (1945). *Phenomenologie de la Perception*. Paris: Gallimard.

Merleau-Ponty, M. (1962). *The Phenomenology of Perception*. Translated by C. Smith. New York: Routledge and Kegan Paul.

Mlakar, J., Jensterle, J. & Frith, C.D. (1994). Central monitoring deficiency and schizophrenic symptoms. *Psychological Medicine*, **24**, 557–64.

Mojtabai, R. & Rieder, R.O. (1998). Limitations of the symptom-oriented approach to psychiatric research. *British Journal of Psychiatry*, **173**, 198–202.

Naudin, J., Banovic, I., Schwartz, M.A. et al. (2000). Définir l'hallucination acoustico-verbale comme trouble de la conscience de soi. *Evolution Psychiatrique*, **65**, 311–24.

Ostwald, P. & Zavarin, V. (1980). Studies of language and schizophrenia in the USSR. In *Applied Psycholinguistics and Mental Health*, ed. R.W. Rieber, pp. 69–92. New York: Plenum.

Parnas, J. & Bovet, P. (1991). Autism in schizophrenia revisited. *Comprehensive Psychiatry*, **32**, 7–21.

Parnas, J. & Sass, L. (2001). Self, solipsism, and schizophrenic delusions. *Philosophy, Psychiatry, Psychology*, **8**, 101–20.

Persons, J. (1986). The advantages of studying psychological phenomena rather than psychiatric diagnoses. *American Psychologist*, **41**, 1252–60.

Petitot, J., Varela, F.J., Pachoud, B. & Roy, J.-M. (eds) (1999). *Naturalizing Phenomenology: Issues in Contemporary Phenomenology and Cognitive Science*. Stanford, CA: Stanford University Press.

Polanyi, M. (1964). *Personal Knowledge*. New York: Harper Torchbooks.

Polanyi, M. (1967). *The Tacit Dimension*. Garden City, NY: Anchor Books.

Polanyi, M. (1968). Sense-giving and sense-reading. In *Intellect and Hope: Essays in the Thought of Michael Polanyi*, ed. T.A. Langford & W.H. Poteat, pp. 402–31. Durham, NC: Duke University Press.

Ricoeur, P. (1992). *Oneself as Another*, translated by K. Blamey. Chicago: University of Chicago Press.

Rosenthal, D.M. (1997). A theory of consciousness. In *The Nature of Consciousness*, ed. N. Block, O. Flanagan & G. Guzeldere, pp. 729–53. Cambridge, MA: MIT Press.

Rumke, H.C. (1990 [1941]). The nuclear symptom of schizophrenia and the praecox feeling. *History of Psychiatry*, **1**, 331–41.

Sass, L. (1992). *Madness and Modernism: Insanity in the Light of Modern Art, Literature, and Thought.* New York: Basic Books (Harvard University Press peperback, 1994).

Sass, L. (1994). *The Paradoxes of Delusion: Wittgenstein, Schreber, and the Schizophrenic Mind.* Ithaca, NY: Cornell University Press.

Sass, L. (1996). 'The catastrophes of heaven': modernism, primitivism, and the madness of Antonin Artaud. *Modernism/Modernity*, **3**, 73–92.

Sass, L. (2000). Schizophrenia, self-experience, and the so-called 'negative symptoms.' In *Exploring the Self: Philosophical and Psychopathological Perspectives on Self-experience*, ed. D. Zahavi, pp. 149–82. Amsterdam: John Benjamins.

Sass, L. & Parnas, J. (2001). Phenomenology of self disturbances in schizophrenia: some research findings and directions. *Philosophy, Psychiatry, Psychology*, **8**, 347–56.

Sass, L. & Parnas, J. (in press). Explaining schizophrenia: the relevance of phenomenology. In *The Philosophical Understanding of Schizophrenia*, ed. M.C. Chung, K.W.M. Fulford & G. Graham. Oxford: Oxford University Press.

Schwartz, S. (1982). Is there a schizophrenic language? *Behavioral and Brain Sciences*, **5**, 579–88.

Selten, J.P. (1995). *The Subjective Experience of Negative Symptoms.* Doctoral dissertation. Rijksuniversiteit Groningen, The Netherlands.

Selten, J.-P., van den Bosch, R.J. & Sijben, A.E.S. (1998). The subjective experience of negative symptoms. In *Insight and Psychosis*, ed. X.F. Amador & A.S. David, pp. 78–90. New York: Oxford University Press.

Selten, J.-P., Wiersma, D. & van den Bosch, R.J. (2000). Discrepancy between subjective and objective ratings for negative symptoms. *Journal of Psychiatric Research*, **34**, 11–13.

Sokolov, A.N. (1972). *Inner Speech and Thought.* New York: Plenum.

Solovay, M.R., Shenton, M.E. & Holzman, P.S. (1987). Comparative studies of thought disorder: mania and schizophrenia. *Archives of General Psychiatry*, **44**, 13–20.

Sommers, A.A. (1985). Negative symptoms: conceptual and methodological problems. *Schizophrenia Bulletin*, **11**, 364–79.

Spitzer, M. (1997). A cognitive neuroscience view of schizophrenic thought disorder. *Schizophrenia Bulletin*, **23**, 29–50.

Stanghellini, G. & Monti, M.R. (1993). Influencing and being influenced: the other side of 'bizarre delusions.' *Psychopathology*, **26**, 165–9.

Storring, G. (1987). Perplexity. In *The Clinical Roots of the Schizophrenia Concept*, ed. J. Cutting & M. Shepherd, pp. 79–82. Cambridge, UK: Cambridge University Press.

Tatossian, A. (1997). *La Phenomenologie des psychoses.* Paris: L'Art du Comprendre.

Tausk, V. (1933 [1919]). On the origin of the 'influencing machine' in schizophrenia. *Psychoanalytic Quarterly*, **2**, 519–56.

Tissot, T. (1984). *Fonction Symbolique et Psychopathologie.* Paris: Masson.

van den Bosch, R. (1994). Context and cognition in schizophrenia. In *Advances in the Neurobiology of Schizophrenia*, ed. J.A. den Boer, H.G.M. Westenberg & H.M. van Praag. pp. 343–66. Chichester, UK: Wiley. Available at http://www.psy.med.rug.nl/0014.

van den Bosch, R.J., Rombouts, R.P. & van Asma, M.J.O. (1993). Subjective cognitive dysfunction in schizophrenic and depressed patients. *Comprehensive Psychiatry*, **34**, 130–6.

Vygotsky, L. (1962). *Thought and Language*. Translated by E. Hanfmann & G. Vakar. Cambridge, MA: MIT Press.

Zahavi, D. (1999). Michel Henry and the phenomenology of the invisible. *Continental Philosophy Review*, **32**, 223–40.

13

The self-experience of schizophrenics

Christian Scharfetter

Psychiatric University Hospital, Zurich, Switzerland

Abstract

A severe disorder of the self-experience is conceived as the common experiential denominator of the heterogeneous group of schizophrenic psychoses. The ego-pathology focuses on this ego-disorder in its five basic dimensions (vitality, activity, consistency/coherence, demarcation, and identity).

A population of 664 probands (552 schizophrenics, 25 borderline personality disorder, 87 depressive disorder, *Diagnostic and Statistical Manual of Mental Disorders* (DSM-III-R) American Psychiatric Association, 1987) was systematically studied using the Ego Pathology Inventory (53 items). The most important evaluation was the confirmatory factor analysis.

The self-experience of schizophrenics concerns the uncertainties, deficits or even annihilation of the five basic dimensions. Confirmatory factor analysis allows comparison between theoretical and empirical item allocation and shows a high congruence (kappa 0.95). Analysis of variance between the three diagnostic groups on the level of items as well as scales shows differences in the respective proband groups. External measurements serve as arguments for the validity of the model.

The concept of five basic dimensions of self-experience can be shown as a reliable, valid and viable approach to study empirically the disordered ego/self of schizophrenics and other diagnostic groups. Concerning therapeutic consequences, some hints for a need-adapted treatment are given with the aim of reconstructing the disordered self-experience, even in body awareness.

A detailed presentation of the psychopathology research reported in this article is published in Scharfetter (1996). The first article was published in English in 1981.

The aim of psychopathology

Psychopathology's task is not only to list and operationalize symptoms and signs and to incorporate them as pathognomonic signs in a categorical nosological system. Psychopathology serves more than 'psychiatric symptom hunting' (Ornstein, 1976) to establish a diagnosis, or eventually to identify target symptoms for psychopharmacological treatment.

Psychopathology not only has to identify symptoms and signs in an interpersonal context, but to read them, to interpret them as an indicator of the patient's therapeutic needs and accessibility. Thus, psychopathology serves to clarify the fundaments for the construction of a need-adapted treatment plan with pharmaco-, psycho- and sociotherapeutic strategies.

Psychopathological symptoms indicate:
1. which functions, certainties, capacities the patient has lost
2. what he/she mostly is in need of (what should be reestablished, regained, reconstructed)
3. which autotherapeutic strategies are to be found in a patient and with what effect
4. what kind of treatment offer a patient can accept, to which he/she is accessible.

Focusing the self-experience of schizophrenics

The common experiential denominator, i.e. the awareness of oneself (I myself), of the heterogeneous group of schizophrenic disorders is severe disorganization of the ego as the personified centre of wakeful self-consciousness: This disordered self-experience of schizophrenics can be learnt from their self-accounts as well as by a functional interpretation of their behaviour. The psychiatrists of the nineteenth century already knew such accounts of some of their patients (Some nineteenth-century authors are quoted in Scharfetter, 1996, pp. 64–67, and in German in Scharfetter, 1995, pp. 21–28.)

The following verbal quotations of patients' self-accounts (collected by the author) illustrate the disordered self-experience in the respective dimensions:
1. *Ego vitality*: 'I feel myself a corpse, dead.' 'I have to breathe forcefully to regain the certainty that I am still alive.'
2. *Ego activity*: 'I feel directed by alien forces.' 'I have to open and close my fingers to reassure myself that I am still able to move on my own intention.'
3. *Ego consistency and coherence*: 'I am in a process of dissolution; feelings and thoughts are split apart.'
4. *Ego demarcation*: 'I am not aware of my boundaries and feel myself unsheltered.'
5. *Ego identity*: 'I do not know who I am.' 'My gestalt, physiognomy and identity are changed.'

Thus, patients' spontaneous communication of their self-experience and their own interpretation of their behaviour as an attempt at self-rescue lead us to the core of the self-experience of humans with a schizophrenic syndrome, whether the nosological category of schizophrenic disorder (according to DSM-IV: American Psychiatric Association, 1994) or a schizophrenia-like syndrome of shorter duration with or without a triggering life event or induction by psychedelic drugs.

What Kraepelin and Bleuler saw as the common characteristic of schizophrenics is the 'peculiar destruction of the inner coherence of the personality' (Kraepelin, 1913), the 'disorder of personality by splitting, dissociation' (Bleuler, 1911). Both authors did not give a detailed description and did not comment on their concept of 'personality' (which could be understood as character).

Long before the somewhat crude nosological construction of dementia praecox by Kraepelin and the naming as schizophrenia of this group of disorders by Bleuler, psychiatrists had reported in their texts unsystematic observations of the disordered self-experience. Some of them had already seen the struggle for self-rescue and described autotherapeutic efforts. Ideler (1835) wrote: 'We see in the psychosis the serious effort of the consciousness to reestablish and maintain its reorganization'.

The empirical ego as the centre of self-awareness

Leaving aside various philosophical, psychological and metapsychological concepts of self and ego, we have to restrict ourselves to the self-experience, the instance Kant called the *empirical ego*. This empirical ego means the human experience of being present as a living, self-governing, delimited and self-identical person with a certain consistency and a coherent self-organization. In order to prepare a systematization as the basis for empirical studies, the following terminology was introduced (Scharfetter, 1981, 1995, 1996).

Ego vitality

Ego vitality can be defined as being present as a living being: the awareness and certainty (1) of being alive, experiencing oneself as a living being and (2) existing actually present in a given situation.

Self-accounts illustrating disorder of ego vitality

I am not alive anymore

I do not exist at all

That is the core question: do I really exist?

Am I still alive?

I am afraid that I will lose all life

My ego does not exist any longer

My watch is broken, stands still

I do not feel/sense myself as living

I am dying, my heart stopped beating

I have to breathe forcedly and repeatedly to reassure myself that I am alive

I have to see my blood, to inflict pain on myself, so that I know I am still alive

I am rotting

I am destroyed – the world is destroyed

I am totally dried up, tomorrow everything is dead

My face, my cheeks are of plastic, not living

Ego activity

Ego activity involves functioning as a self-directing unity, governing the integration of afferent (e.g. perceptive), cognitive (e.g. thinking), cognitive–affective (relation of thoughts and emotions/affects) and efferent (e.g. speaking, movements, reactions and actions) functions.

Self-accounts illustrating disorder of ego activity

I am directed by strange powers

My thoughts are manipulated from outside myself

I have to open and close my fists to reassure myself that I am able to move on my own

I am not able to control and direct my thoughts and activities

I feel paralysed

I do not have any power

I felt as if tied

I feel mechanized

I am directed by hypnosis, by magic influences

The devil possessed me, inducing my activities

It is not me who shouts – that is done by influences on my nerves

One can be severely handicapped by insertion into the brain

I do not have arms

My thoughts are made, induced, inserted, directed, taken off, broken

I am no longer governor of myself

Ego consistency and coherence

Ego consistency and coherence can be defined as being mentally and bodily a united consistent (concerning quality) and coherent being.

Self-accounts illustrating disorders of ego consistency and coherence

I feel split apart

I am an amorphous mass, dropping down from the couch

I am decaying

My thoughts and feelings are disintegrated

My brain is perforated

Bones and teeth are broken

I feel myself dissolving

I feel myself cut into pieces

I do not feel myself as a unity

My genitals are ripped open

My body is halved

I am four people

I am split into pieces

I am unable to bring together thoughts and feelings

My soul was taken away and distributed

My skeleton is broken

In my right shoulder and chest is my father, on the left side my mother

Ego demarcation

Ego demarcation involves being distinct from other things and beings, aware of the boundary between ego/self and nonego.

Self-accounts illustrating disorders of ego demarcation

I do not know my boundaries

I am unable to differentiate between inside and outside myself

I feel unsheltered

Parts of my body are outside myself

My brain is outside myself

I feel unprotected

Everything is intruding into me, penetrates me

What others think is transferred into me

What I suffer all others have to bear

I cannot keep my thoughts to myself, everybody can know them

I feel unsheltered and open to every external influence

Ego identity

Ego identity involves certainty of one's own personal self-sameness concerning morphology, physiognomy, gender, genealogical origin, social function and biographical (lifetime) continuity.

Self-accounts illustrating disorders of ego identity

I am me, myself

I am a human being like you

My flesh is not of human type

I do not know who I am

Leave me my shape and figure belonging to me

I do not want another body

I am male and female at the same time

On the right side I am my father, on the left my mother – and on the nose there is the skin of a cow

I have to control my face in the mirror, I am afraid it is changing

Now I am certain again who I am

The voices say 'you are not Josef' [his correct name]

I was not sure whether I was still Ueli

I have another nose

I am an animal, a monster

Blood – only half of it is my own

This exposition of five basic dimensions of the empirical ego helps to organize the main topics of the patient's self-experience. This step prepares the systematic study of ego-pathology in schizophrenics.

The construct of ego-pathology of schizophrenics

From this organization of the patient's self-accounts follows the following schedule of the pathology of the five basic ego dimensions (Box 13.1).

Box 13.1 The pathology of the five basic ego dimensions

Ego vitality
- Experience of (or fear of) one's own death, of dying, the fading away of liveliness, of nonexistence of self
- Experience of (or fear of imminent) ruin of the world, of humanity, of the universe
- Overcompensation can be seen in delusions of being a healer, a world renewer

Ego activity
- Lack of or deficit in one's own ability/potency/power for self-determined acting, thinking, feeling, perceiving
- Control by outside powers, manipulation by others
- Thoughts, feelings, perceptions made by others, inserted, taken away, stopped
- Feeling of being weak or paralysed or possessed by strange powers
- Awareness and certainty of intentionally directing one's own thinking, speech, action mean autonomy in self-government
- Disorders of ego activity correspond to the well-known symptom of being influenced, directed by alien forces
- Overcompensation is the megalomaniac self-inflation of omnipotence

Ego consistency and coherence
- Destruction of the consistency and coherence of one's self, the body, soul, the world, the universe as a unitary being, dissolution, splitting, multiplication
- Disruption of the connection of thinking and feeling, of will, impulse and fulfilment of action

Ego consistency has a broader connotation than coherence. It means the *quality* of self-experience as structured and organized (against chaotic disorganization, dissociation, disintegration) into a coherent living being:
- in coenaesthetic self-sense (body experience)
- in a harmonious fitting together of experienced mental content and corresponding feeling
- in experiencing a coherent process of reasoning
- in experiencing a coherent, structured, organized external and internal world

Megalomaniac overcompensation in multiplicatory delusions is rare.

Ego demarcation
- Uncertainty, weakness or lack of the differentiation between ego and nonego spheres
- Deficit of a private sheltered realm of body experience, thinking, feeling
- Disturbance of the discrimination of inner and outer, of personal and external fields

Ego demarcation not only allows us to be sure of our own private realm of experiencing mental events but also, at the same time, to communicate by the passage through the transparent boundary outwards (centrifugally) and inwards (centripetally).

Ego demarcation may be seen as a basic prerequisite as well as a result of a defined, i.e. delimited, ego identity.

> **Ego identity**
> • Loss of, changes of, or doubts concerning one's own identity in respect of (human) gestalt (morphology), physiognomy, gender, genealogical origin and biography
> Ego identity means a prereflexively 'naturally' given certainty of one's own definite selfhood despite changes in life course, in various situations. As self-definition, or development of a self-concept, it includes a definition of one's own limits or boundaries.

The schizophrenic symptoms evolving from the disordered self-experience

The clinical elaboration of this ego-pathology concept (see Scharfetter, 1996) can be only presented here in a short sketch. Most of the psychopathological symptoms of schizophrenics described in textbooks can be understood as reactions to the acuteness and severity with which the ego-disorder manifests itself in a vulnerable individual.

The acute and severe experience of a loss of or disordered self-experience does not allow autotherapeutic, self-rescue strategies or defensive, adaptive, coping efforts. Thus, the reactions of the organism are rather uniform and do not vary greatly according to the individual hit by the experience. Therefore, the reactions can be seen as phylo- or ontogenetically 'primitive': stupor or agitation, movement disorders.

But if the respective ego-disorder develops gradually, is not too severe and thus is not too overwhelming, the individual experiencing the disorder has a much greater variability of reactions to the experience: he can defend himself, by avoiding the situation, withdrawing, adapting by emotional reactions, using private cognitive–affective constructs (delusion, paranoid) taking elements of personal biographical as well as cultural material for the content and elaboration of his private explanatory mythologems (which we call delusion).

Reactions to the threat of ego disintegration
Motor behaviour

Stupor and mutism	Flight
Flexibilitas cerea	Self-mutilation
Automatism	Parakinesia
Stereotypia	Echopraxia, echolalia
Agitation, aggression, fight	

Affective behaviour

Anxiety, panic, bewilderment	Delusional mood
Shy, suspicious, distrustful	Aggressive, dysphoric affect

Unstable, ambivalent, 'undecided'

Parathymia (reflecting ambivalence, splitting, inconsistency of affect and content of mind or interpreted as an attempt to overcome overwhelming anxiety)

Maniform self-elevation (interpreted as overcompensation)

Cognitive behaviour

Thinking disturbances (reflection of overwhelming anxiety and bewilderment, splitting – sign of an attempt to flee or defend against threat and danger – sign of reaching new framework and fence for ego)

Suspicious, distrustful interpretations

Detection of 'new' meanings

Delusional interpretation

(autistic–derealisitic self- and world concept)

Naming and thematization (mainly *negative* delusions)

Creation of private symbols, signs, language creation of new self-concept, role, identity creation of a new world, realm, science, religion

Activity determined by delusional belief

Interactive behaviour

Shy, suspicious, dysphoric behaviour

Withdrawal, isolation, shelter

Mannerism (odd, stylized, artificial, nonspontaneous behaviour)

New approach to society in new role (as healer, prophet, messiah)

Avoidance of communication by:
• miming
• gesture
• language
  • mutism
  • schizophasia
  • kryptolalia, kryptographia

Cognitive–affective overcompensation

Megalomanic self-surmount

Delusions of omniscience, omnipotence (healing, creating a new religion, founding a new world, even a new cosmos)

Maniform self-elevation

Empirical studies

After the construction of the theoretical model of a general factor ego/self-disorder, subdivided into five subfactors in the schizophrenic syndrome, the next step in the preparation of the empirical studies was construction of the Ego Pathology Inventory (EPI).

The ego pathology inventory

In a series of steps, an interview schedule was developed to evaluate in a systematic way the presence of the five ego disorders, constituting together the superordinated or general factor *ego-pathology*. The present (fifth) version of the interview schedule contains 53 items, covering nine sections: the five basic ego dimensions (1–23), items of overcompensation (24–29), body experience (30–39), thought disorders (40–46) and items of increased control (47–53). The inverview schedule is presented in the appendix to this chapter.

Inquiry into the ego-pathology of self-experience takes place within a free clinical interview which can be flexibly adapted to the topics introduced by patients. The various sections of the interview schedule can be investigated according to the themes the patient mentions spontaneously or, if he/she does not do so, they may be covered in a structured form of questioning. The interview lasts about 1 h. The enquiry covers the whole life experience (it questions: did you ever experience . . . ?). Thus, there is no time window (but it could be used).

The item rating is trichotomous: never experienced (0); fear of or uncertainty about the respective experience (1); frequently positive and/or intensely experienced (2). The rating was done by colleagues after special training in investigating and assessing ego-pathology items.

Study population

Probands of the study were recruited from inpatients of Swiss mental hospitals. The diagnoses were evaluated in DSM-IIIR categories (American Psychiatric Association, 1987). All diagnoses were evaluated from the information of personal interview, case history and Present State Examination Scale (Wing et al., 1974).

The study population included a total of 664 probands: 552 with a diagnosis of schizophrenia, 25 borderline personality disorder and 87 with depressive disorder. The 87 probands with depressive disorder were heterogeneous: there were 43 major depressive disorder, 19 depressive episodes of bipolar affective disorder and 25 dysthymic disorder.

Results

Reliability studies concerned the diagnosis (kappa 0.92), interrater reliability (kappa 0.9) and retest reliability (kappa 0.65).

The most important step was to test the empirical distribution of ego-pathology items with the theoretical data matrix. This was done by confirmatory factor analysis.

Confirmatory factor analysis

The empirical data matrix which contains the ego-pathology ratings of the 552 schizophrenic subjects is compared with the theoretical matrix in which the items

Table 13.1 Confirmatory factor analysis

The items congruently indicating disorders of ego *identity* are:

1. I didn't know who I was	5. My ancestry changed
2. I often had to look in the mirror	27. I thought I had children
3. I had to say repeatedly 'I am who I am'	30. My body or parts of it changed
4. My sex changed	

The items congruently indicating disorders of ego *demarcation* are:

6. I felt vulnerable, without protection	37. I had to rub my skin
7. I had to withdraw from other people	40. Others could read my thoughts
8. I melted together with other people	42. I coded my words or thoughts
9. I felt I was someone or something else	43. My thoughts spread out
35. I had to hurt myself	

The items congruently indicating disorders of ego *consistency* are:

10. My whole self was split into pieces	31. Parts of my body didn't match any more
11. I felt the world exploding	32. My body was torn to pieces or dissolving
12. My feelings and thoughts didn't match	33. Parts of my body lay outside me
13. I was torn between good and evil	44. My thoughts were split up
14. I heard voices within me or outside me	

The items congruently characterizing disorders of ego *activity* are:

15. I felt hampered	41. I could read others' thoughts
16. I felt persecuted/spied upon	45. Strange thoughts were put into my head
17. I felt controlled by others	46. My thoughts were cut short
18. I was possessed/conquered	48. I particularly controlled my movements
24. I could control people or nature	49. I repeated my own movements or words
25. I could cure other people	51. I froze with fear
26. I could see in distant times or places	

The items congruently characterizing disorders of ego *vitality* are:

19. I felt myself dying	34. My body or parts of it changed
20. I felt myself dead (like a mummy)	36. I had to see my blood
21. I felt the world coming to an end	38. My sexuality changed
22. My soul was stolen	39. I had to breathe heavily
23. I felt that others tried to annihilate me	52. I panicked (catatonic excitation)

were allocated to the five dimensions. This procedure of confirmatory factor analysis revealed a nearly 100% correspondence between the theoretical model and the empirical data. The exact percentage of congruence is 96, kappa being 0.95.

The optimal congruence in the allocation of items in the theoretical and the empirical matrix was an important factor (Table 13.2).

Table 13.2 Confirmatory factor analysis

Empirical matrix	Theoretical matrix					
	Identity	Demarcation	Consistency	Activity	Vitality	Uncertain
Identity	1, 2, 3, 4, 5, 27, 30		29	50		28
Demarcation		6, 7, 8, 9, 35, 37, 40, 42, 43				47, 53
Consistency			10, 11, 12, 13, 14, 31, 32, 33, 44			
Activity	(26)			15, 16, 17, 18, 24, 25, (26), 41, 45, 46, 48, 49, 51		
Vitality					19, 20, 21, 22, 23, 34, 36, 38, 39, 52	

Validity

The validity of the ego-pathology concept can be argued for by the following considerations.

Face validity

Every psychiatrist who listens thoroughly to what his or her patients say about their self-experience, and who observes their behaviour and the extent to which that behaviour is motivated by their self-experience knows these central topics which are systematically presented in ego-pathology. And long before the concept of schizophrenia was established by Kraepelin and Bleuler, psychiatrists described such 'disorders of the ego' (see the references in Scharfetter 1995, 1996).

Content validity

Content validity means that the components of the instrument fit to the features we want to achieve. Generally, content validity is ascribed to an instrument by experts in the respective field. The 'experts' in ego-pathology are primarily the patients themselves as 'purveyors' of that self-experience which we want to explore. The pool of items contained in the instrument was collected directly from the reports and self-accounts of patients. The historical forerunners of systematically elaborated

ego-pathology cover principally the same main topics of their patient's self-experience (i.e. disorders of ego vitality, activity, consistency, demarcation, identity). The
high frequency of positive answers in the EPI may serve as a further argument that
schizophrenic patients really accept the content of the items as covering important
aspects of their self-experience. This was also expressed spontaneously by many
probands: they felt that the questions asked showed that they were being understood.

Thus, in so far as content validity of ego-pathology is concerned, it seems justified
to assume that the EPI really records the patient's ego/self-experience with sufficient accuracy.

Criterion validity

Criterion validity is the correlation of the instrument's measure with other measures
of the subject studied. These other measures have to be directly or at least indirectly
related to the same subject and they should likewise be valid in performing their own
task. The subcategories of criterion validity are concurrent and predictive validity.
External validation criteria by other instruments, measuring independently the
same topic, do not exist. Thus we are not able to determine a validity coefficient
(Pearson) determining the correlation of two scales.

Concurrent validity

Concurrent validity means, according to Messick (1980), diagnostic utility. The
EPI instrument allows us to separate diagnostic categories significantly, especially
schizophrenic from nonschizophrenic probands. In this ability to discriminate between diagnoses the EPI is associated with (1) traditional psychopathology as the
basis for diagnosis and (2) other diagnostically differing instruments, e.g. ego assessment. Thus ego-pathology is useful in differential diagnosis, in spite of the fact that it
was not conceived as a diagnostic instrument, but as an instrument for systematic exploration of the ego/self-experience of a certain diagnostic group (schizophrenics).

Predictive validity

The other subcategory of criterion validity, predictive validity, can only be applied
to ego-pathology in a follow-up, which we did in a small catamnestic study covering
2 years. A relatively stable ego-pathology was shown.

Construct validity

Construct validity concerns the model construct, not only the instrument used to
test it. Clinical observation of patients' behaviour and their statements about their
ego/self-experience and the relationship between behaviour and experience (the
latter motivating the former) led to the hypothetical construct of ego-pathology.
This construct serves to explain relationships between various types of behaviours

and self-experiences. The EPI is the only instrument developed for systematic study of disorders of ego-consciousness in schizophrenics. At the present stage of evaluation of the ego-pathology construct, we have only a few confirmative arguments for construct validity.

Construct validation by extreme groups in ego-pathology research can be seen when we compare schizophrenics with depressives. The EPI can clearly separate a diagnostic group with high scores in ego-pathology (schizophrenics) from the group of depressives with (virtually) no positive answers to the EPI items.

Convergent validity

So far as convergent validity of the construct of ego-pathology is concerned, the relevant arguments lie in the positive correlation of the severity indices (scores) in ego-pathology with the ones of 'basic disorders', especially 'loss of automatism' (Pearson correlation 0.7, $P = 0.50$) and of the ego-assessment scale of Bellak (1976) (Spearman correlation 0.7–0.8, $P = 0.0001$), as well as in the positive correlation with traditional psychopathology (Pearson correlation 0.35, $P = 0.09$). The correlation with some subscales of the positive and negative syndrome scales (PANSS) (Scharfetter, 1996, pp. 151–155) and with certain speech and voice characteristics can serve as a further argument in that direction.

Discriminant validity

Concerning discriminant validity, we can show that ego-pathology does not correlate with theoretically unrelated variables (e.g. sex, education, diagnostic subtype of schizophrenia, duration or course of illness).

Treatment of schizophrenics: reconstruction, resynthesis

As mentioned before, psychopathology should serve to establish a treatment plan adapted to patients' needs and accessibility. The ego-pathology concept helps us to understand better the therapeutic needs of the patient: what is it that should be reconstructed? What should be helped by what means in regaining a resynthesis of the self (ego-consolidation therapy by informed empathy)? I mention here only some very elementary principles of the treatment programme.

Principles of treatment programme

1. Overcoming of dualistic mind–body splitting: the body has to be included in therapeutic reconstruction, especially in severe acute ego disintegration.
2. The schizophrenic experience, developed in interpersonal and social context, means isolation and alienation. Treatment happens in mutual relations, carefully

tuned concerning stimulation, closeness and distance and clear concrete ways of communication.

3. The schizophrenic breakdown results from an impairing process of self-development, i.e. personification in family and extrafamilial society. Treatment has to include family and life-mates and to consider the socioeconomic life situation.

4. Individual psychotherapy: overcoming isolation, offering and serving the therapist as an alternative ego or temporary substitute for identification, reality testing, insight (psychodynamic–genetic and meaning of symptoms), strengthening healthy functions.

5. Psychopharmacological treatment.

6. Cognitive–behaviour therapy of symptoms for strengthening reality testing, observer ego, self-monitoring and control.

7. The basic attitude of the therapist: nonegoistic presence, therapeutic love, sensitivity, sense of reality.

Body-including treatment can be seen as contributing to the reconstruction of: (1) the disordered body-ego (*Leibbewußtsein*); (2) the interpersonal relation; and (3) the commonly shared reality.

Some suggestions for including the patient's body in the resynthetic therapeutic work are given here because this therapeutic tool is still not sufficiently known and valued (Box 13.2).

Box 13.2 Body-including treatment as suggested by ego psychopathology

Vitality	Breathing
	Pulsation of blood in fingers, face, abdominal aorta
	Centre the body in abdominal–pelvic region
	Sensory awareness (Gindler, Selver) in gripping, keeping (patient him- or herself)
Activity	Intentional movements (fingers), reassuring self-directedness, self-determination
Consistence	Focusing on centre of the body
	Breathing, becoming aware of continuous flow throughout the whole body
	Closing the arms around the own trunk
	Hedgehog or turtle position
Demarcation	To mark one's own territory (mat, circle made by chalk, ring)
	Patient determines distance and closeness him- or herself (instrumental, verbal)
Identity	Focusing on face and palms (together) (feeling the warmth, pulsation, calming)
	Mirror

Concluding remarks

The self-experience of schizophrenics, conceived as the common experiential denominator with regard to aetiology, pathogenesis, course and outcome of a heterogeneous group of mental disorders, can be determined empirically with sufficient reliability. The concept of ego-pathology can be seen as a valid and viable instrument for studying the self-experience of schizophrenics, for guiding our treatment strategies as well as stimulating further studies.

I conclude with a few remarks on further research in this field. The instrument serves to study ego-pathology in an intercultural comparative perspective. Child psychiatrists may be interested in the question of the ontogenesis of the empirical ego and its pathology in certain stages of development. Studies in the long-term course of ego-pathology would show the correlation of ego disorder, course and outcome, e.g. the *negative schizophrenia* seen as a result of 'burned-out ego' in energetic exhaustion, resignation and demoralization or in a climate of understimulation. Studies in psychedelic states of mind, with so-called experimental psychosis, combined with modern techniques of measuring brain metabolism and topographic physiology, are already going on (Vollenweider, 1998).

APPENDIX   THE EGO PATHOLOGY INVENTORY

The research instrument Ego Pathology Inventory (EPI) is available in six languages: English, German, French, Italian, Spanish and Polish.

Identity
1. I was no longer sure that I was still the same person or I had the feeling I was someone different.
2. I checked my appearance in the mirror more often than I used to.
3. I repeatedly said to myself: I am me, or I am a human being.
4. My gender had changed. I felt I was a man (a woman).
5. I thought I had a different family, a different life history, compared to what I used to believe.

Demarcation
6. I felt I was defenceless, at the mercy of influences beyond my control. I could not defend myself and I was not aware of my own boundaries any more.
7. I had to withdraw physically or mentally from other people in order to protect myself. I did not allow anybody to come too close to me any more. I shut myself off from others.

8. I became one with other creatures or objects. I lost the sense of my own boundaries.
9. When I had an experience I often did not know if it was mine or the experience of someone else.

Consistency/coherence
10. I felt an internal split (splits) or felt that I was being torn apart, fragmented as a person or I felt that I was dissolving or falling to pieces.
11. I had the feeling that the whole world was exploding and falling to pieces.
12. My feelings did not match with my thoughts, experiences or actions. My experience of life was paradoxical and mixed up.
13. I felt torn between two powers/opposites (good/bad). Opposing feelings or incompatible emotions tore me apart.
14. I heard internal voices or external voices even though nobody was there.

Activity
15. Some mysterious or awesome force hindered my movements, my actions and speech. My activity was obstructed, I felt slowed down or paralysed.
16. I felt spied upon, persecuted, watched and followed. I was no longer free in my actions and decisions.
17. I could no longer do what I intended to do, my movements and actions were directed and controlled. I felt like a tool, a puppet.
18. I felt overwhelmed, possessed by alien forces, powers or people.

Vitality
19. I felt that my life was disintegrating, that I was dying.
20. I felt lifeless, dead as a mummy.
21. I felt that the world was about to end and all living beings would die.
22. My soul, my inner liveliness was taken from me, was annihilated or killed.
23. Some people or alien forces tried or planned to destroy and kill me.

Overcompensation
24. I had tremendous power and influence and was able to direct and control people, natural forces or world affairs.
25. I was able to heal sick people by spiritual means.
26. I had visions. I was able to see things which happened far away and at other times.
27. I had one or several children.
28. I gave birth to living beings (without requiring sexual relations).
29. I felt doubled or multiplied. I consisted of many living beings or these beings lived inside of me.

Body

30. The appearance, the shape of my body had partially or totally changed.
31. My limbs did not fit together in the usual way. Their connection was loosened, everything was disarranged or out of place. I felt disoriented in my body.
32. My body or parts of it were torn to pieces, dissolved or fell apart.
33. Parts of my body separated themselves from the whole so that I experienced them outside of me.
34. My whole body or parts of it were dead or dying (possibly already decaying).
35. I had to hurt myself deliberately in order to cause pain.
36. I had to hurt myself in order to see my own blood.
37. I did not feel my skin any more, so I had to rub or pinch or punch it.
38. My sexual behaviour changed.
39. I had to breathe fast, or my breathing was reduced or stopped completely.

Thought process

40. Other people were able to read my thoughts.
41. I was able to read other people's thoughts.
42. I coded my language or my thoughts so that only I understood and nobody else could understand them.
43. My own thoughts left my head, they spread out everywhere. I could not keep them within me or for myself. They slipped away and everybody knew them.
44. My thoughts were torn apart. I had a tremendous confusion in my head.
45. Alien thoughts were given to me (through telepathy or hypnosis). My thoughts and feelings came from outside of me.
46. My thoughts were disrupted from the outside. My chain of thought was interrupted or some thoughts were taken away from me.

Psychomotoric behaviour

47. Everything that happened around me seemed dangerous, menacing, strange. I felt alarmed and watched everything attentively and anxiously.
48. I had to pay close attention to my movements. I had to control them strictly.
49. I repeated my own movements or words several times.
50. I automatically imitated other people's movements or words, like an echo.
51. I froze stiff with fear and remained motionless for a long period of time.
52. I was seized by a wild and uncontrollable panic. I was overwhelmed with fear.
53. I assaulted people or banged into objects out of pure desperation.

REFERENCES

American Psychiatric Association. (1987). *Diagnostic and Statistical Manual of Mental Disorders*, 3rd edn revised. Washington, DC: American Psychiatric Association.

American Psychiatric Association. (1994). *Diagnostic and Statistical Manual of Mental Disorders*, 4th edn. Washington, DC: American Psychiatric Association.

Bellak, L. (1976). *The Broad Scope of Ego Function Assessment*. New York: Wiley.

Bleuler, E. (1911). Dementia Praecox oder die Gruppe der Schizophrenien. In *Handbuch der Psychiatrie*, ed. G. Aschaffenburg, pp. 6, 296–8. Leipzig: Deuticke.

Ideler, D.W. (1835/38). *Grundriss der Seelenheilkunde*, vols I, II. Berlin: Enslin.

Kraepelin, E. (1913). *Psychiatrie*, vol. III, 8th edn. Leipzig: Barth.

Messick, S. (1980). Test validity and the ethics of assessment. *American Psychologist*, **35**, 1012–27.

Ornstein, R. (1976). *The Mind Field*. New York: Viking Press.

Scharfetter, C. (1981). Ego psychopathology: the concept and its empirical evaluation. *Psychological Medicine*, **11**, 273–80.

Scharfetter, C. (1995). *Schizophrene Menschen*, 4th edn. Weinheim: Psychologie Verlagsunion.

Scharfetter C. (1996). *The Self-experience of Schizophrenics. Empirical Studies of the Ego/Self in Schizophrenia, Borderline Disorders and Depression*, 2nd edn. Zürich: University of Zürich.

Vollenweider, F.X. (1998). Recent advances and concepts in the search for biological correlates of hallucinogen-induced altered states of consciousness. *Heffter Review of Psychedelic Research*, **1**, 21–32.

Wing, J.K., Coper, J.E. & Sartorius, N. (1974). *The Measurement and Classification of Psychiatric Symptoms*. Cambridge: Cambridge University Press.

ii Social psychology

14

The paranoid self

Richard Bentall

Department of Psychology, University of Manchester, Manchester, UK

Abstract

The idea that delusions often reflect an abnormal attitude towards the self has a long history. Consistent with this idea, the most common delusional themes – persecution and grandiosity – seem to reflect individuals' preoccupations about their position in the social universe. Psycho-analysts have interpreted persecutory delusions as the consequence of defensive strategies that serve the function of protecting the individual from negative perceptions of the self, and the well-replicated finding of an abnormal stye of explaining negative events in paranoid patients seems consistent with this idea. However, attempts to test the hypothesis of a paranoid defence by measuring self-esteem in deluded patients has led to inconsistent and even contradictory results.

These findings may reflect false assumptions about the unity and stability of self-representations. The self consists of a cluster of fluidly related constructs, for example the self as it actually is, the ideal self and the self as it ought to be. Furthermore, evaluations of the self can change dramatically from day to day, and some people consistently make less stable self-evaluations than others. These observations point to the need for a dynamic account of the relationship between self-representations, other cognitive structures and environmental influences.

In this chapter a model is presented of the dynamic interactions between causal explanations (attributions) and self-representations. It will be shown that this kind of model can accommodate the apparently inconsistent findings obtained when self-esteem has been measured in paranoid patients, and leads to novel predictions that can be experimentally tested.

It is striking that the delusional beliefs observed in psychiatric practice nearly always concern the self and the individual's position within the social universe. When specific delusional themes are analysed, the most common type is paranoid or persecutory, in which the self is seen as the object of the malign intentions of other people, resulting in threats of violence or humiliation. For example, of 55 British psychiatric patients surveyed by Garety et al. (1988), the largest group of 19 suffered from persecutory delusions. Seventeen had delusional beliefs about the self that were unrealistically negative and 14 had delusional beliefs about the self that were unrealistically positive. In contrast, delusions classified as negative or positive beliefs about the world were very few in number (3 patients and 1 patient respectively). Similarly, when Jorgensen & Jensen (1994) surveyed the delusional beliefs of psychotic patients admitted for the first time to psychiatric wards in Denmark, they found that 37 out of 88 deluded patients had persecutory beliefs. This observation of a high prevalence of persecutory ideation in psychotic patients seems to have some cross-cultural validity; studies comparing the delusional beliefs of patients in Europe, the Indian subcontinent and the Far East have also reported very high rates of persecutory delusions in nearly all samples (Ndetei & Vadher, 1984; Stompe et al., 1999).

Attempts to explain delusions have been hampered by the erroneous assumption, attributable to Jaspers (1913/1963) amongst others, that delusional beliefs are qualitatively different from the kinds of beliefs and attitudes expressed by ordinary people. According to Jaspers, the abnormal beliefs of psychiatric patients are held with extraordinary conviction, tend to be impervious to experience or counterarguments and often have bizarre or impossible content. However, Jaspers concluded that true delusions, as opposed to delusion-like ideas, are *ununderstandable* in the technical sense that they are not amenable to empathy, and therefore cannot be understood in terms of the patient's personality or experiences (Sims, 1995). According to Jaspers, delusions and other psychotic experiences must therefore be explained in terms of some underlying disease processes. This general viewpoint has been echoed in Berrios' (1991) more recent assertion that delusions are 'Empty speech acts, whose informational content refers to neither world or self. They are not the symbolic expression of anything'.

In contrast to these opinions, empirical research has consistently pointed to a continuum between delusions and normal beliefs. Strauss (1969) first reported that he could discern beliefs reported by his patients that seemed to fall between the extremes of the mundane and the delusional, and argued that they could be classified along four dimensions of conviction, cultural congruence, preoccupation and implausibility. Subsequent studies have confirmed that a dimensional model of delusions best fits the phenomenological data, although additional dimensions, for example, bizarreness and distress, have been suggested (Kendler et al., 1983; Garety & Hemsley, 1987). It has also become apparent that, although many delusional beliefs persist for years (Harrow et al., 1988, 1995), patients' delusional conviction can vary in the short term, so that beliefs that are held to be undoubtedly true on one day may be held to be only possibly true on the next (Brett-Jones et al., 1987).

This evidence against a categorical distinction between delusions and normal beliefs has been supplemented by recent studies which have shown that quasidelusional ideas are surprisingly common in normal population samples. For example, when van Os et al. (2000) gave psychiatric interviews to a large general-population sample in the Netherlands, they found that 3.3% were found to have 'true' delusions and 8.7% had delusions that were not clinically relevant (that is, which were not associated with distress and therefore did not require treatment). Poulton et al. (2000) found comparable results in a long-term follow-up study of New Zealand residents born between 1 April 1972 and 31 March 1973, of whom 20.1% were recorded as having delusions by early adulthood, and 12.6% were judged to be paranoid.

This high rate of delusional ideation in ordinary people, together with the apparent difficulty in drawing a clear dividing line between delusions and everyday beliefs and attitudes, suggests that we should look to normal psychological processes to explain even the most bizarre beliefs of psychiatric patients. The most commonly observed contents of such beliefs further suggests that the processes involved in *self-representation* are likely to play a central role in delusions. Recent studies of persecutory delusions, which are the specific focus of this chapter, bear out these intuitions.

Paranoia as a defence

The idea that paranoid ideation reflects some kind of abnormal attitude towards the self has a long history. The early psychoanalysts argued that persecutory delusions protect the self against desires and impulses that would be unacceptable to the self and hence traumatic. For example, Freud (1911/1950) concluded his celebrated analysis of the autobiography of the psychotic judge Daniel Schreber (1903/1955) by arguing that his paranoid delusions were the consequence of repressed homosexual desires towards his father, which had been displaced on to his physician Dr Fleishig. According to Freud, awareness of these unacceptable impulses was warded off in further series of defensive manoeuvres, which culminated in Schreber's conviction that he was the victim of a supernatural conspiracy to turn him into a woman.

More recent accounts inspired by psychoanalysis have continued to assume that paranoia has a defensive function, but have attributed less complex underlying psychopathologies to the paranoid patient. The work of Kenneth Colby (Colby et al., 1971, 1979; Colby, 1977) is a case in point. Colby argued that paranoid patients ward off feared humiliation by attributing the cause of their misfortunes to the deliberate actions of others, and was able to create a primitive computer program that simulated the cognitive processes involved. The implication of this account was that paranoid patients suffer from fragile self-esteem. However, neither Colby nor any other researchers of the period were able to devise methods of measuring the hypothesized cognitive processes in patients.

Since that time, there has been considerable progress in understanding the psychological processes involved in knowledge of the self and in attributing intentions to others. The application of these new ideas to the study of paranoid patients has facilitated the development of a model of the psychological processes involved in persecutory delusions that in many ways reflects Colby's earlier ideas.

The attributional style and paranoia

Attribution theory is the area of psychology that is concerned with the way in which people generate causal explanations (or 'attributions', that is, statements that either include or imply the word 'because') for events. Ordinary people make attributions very frequently, usually at the rate of one for every few hundred words of speech (Zullow et al., 1988). Initial attempts to link this process to psychopathology focused on depression. Abramson et al. (1978) argued that people who are vulnerable to depression have a depressogenic attributional style, which involves attributing negative events to causes that are internal (that is, some characteristic of the individual rather than of the environment), global (that are likely to affect all areas of life) and stable (that are unchangeable). According to this model, depression occurs when real-life negative events are experienced as uncontrollable but are at the same time explained in this pessimistic way. An example would be a person who attributes failing to pass an exam to 'stupidity', a cause that implicates the self, which has pessimistic implications for other life domains such as employment and relationships, and which the individual can do little to change. Although this model has undergone a series of revisions since it was first proposed (Abramson et al., 1989), it has survived the test of time remarkably well. A metaanalysis of no less than 106 studies published by Sweeny et al. (1986) found strong evidence of the predicted relationship between a pessimistic attributional style and depression, and subsequent research has generally replicated this finding (Robins & Hayes, 1995). More recently, the Temple-Wisconsin Cognitive Vulnerability to Depression project (Alloy et al., 1999) demonstrated that apparently healthy students who had a pessimistic attributional style and dysfunctional attitudes towards self-evaluation were at much higher risk of depression over the following 2 years (17% for major depression as defined by DSM-IV criteria (American Psychiatric Association, 1994) and 39% for minor depressive symptoms) in comparison with students who did not have these characteristics (1% and 6% respectively).

Although many paranoid beliefs appear to reflect patients' attempts to account for their experiences, attribution theory was first applied to this phenomenon some time after attributional research on depression had become well established. However, earlier work on the related construct of locus of control – the tendency, conceived as a personality trait, to attribute life experiences in general to the self or to external causes – provided some hints that abnormal attributions may play an important role in paranoid beliefs. Using Levenson's (1974) multidimensional locus of control scale, which measures an individual's general tendency to attribute life experiences to the self (internal locus), the actions of powerful others or to chance, Rosenbaum & Hadari (1985) found that paranoid patients in comparison with controls showed an excessive tendency to attribute their experiences to powerful others. This finding was later replicated by Kaney & Bentall (1989) and Lasar (1997).

Attributional research differs from research on locus of control in assuming that individuals make different kinds of explanations for different kinds of events, and that explanations can be classified along more than one dimension. Kaney & Bentall (1989) included the first attempt at study of attributional style in paranoid patients, using Peterson et al.'s (1982) attributional-style questionnaire, which has been widely used in depression research, and which requires respondents to state the likely causes of a series of hypothetical positive ('you obtain a pay rise') and negative ('you go on a date and it turns out badly') events. After generating each causal statement, participants are then asked to self-rate their explanations along three bipolar scales: internality (anchor points: the cause was 'totally due to other people and circumstances' versus 'totally due to me'), globalness (anchor points: the cause 'influences just this particular area' versus 'influences all areas of life') and stability (anchor points: the cause 'will never be present' versus 'will always be present'). Paranoid patients, like depressed patients, made excessively global and stable attributions for negative events. However, unlike depressed patients, they made excessively external attributions for negative events and excessively internal attributions for positive events. This finding has been quite well replicated. For example, Candido & Romney (1990) compared the attributional styles of paranoid patients, depressed-paranoid patients and depressed patients, finding that their paranoid patients made excessively external attributions for negative events, that their depressed patients made excessively internal attributions for negative events and that the internality scores for negative events of the depressed-paranoid patients fell midway between these two extremes. Fear et al. (1996) demonstrated the paranoid attributional style in patients diagnosed as suffering from delusional disorder and, in a later study, showed that this style was only evident in patients whose delusions were of a persecutory or grandiose nature, and not in patients with other kinds of delusions (Sharp et al., 1997). Lee & Won (1998) replicated our observation of a paranoid attributional style in paranoid patients from South Korea, whereas Kristev et al. (1999) partially replicated this finding in a study of Australian patients recovering from their first episode of psychosis, in which those with paranoid delusions were compared with those without.

There are several important qualifications to these findings. The first concerns the poor psychometric properties of attributional measures such as the attributional state questionnaire (Reivich, 1995), and the difficulty that people experience when trying to make internality judgements (White, 1991). Kinderman & Bentall

(1996a) argued that these limitations reflected the method of classifying attributions developed by Peterson, Seligman and their colleagues, which failed to distinguish between two types of external attributions that have different implications for mental health: external-situational attributions (in which events are attributed to circumstances) and external-personal attributions (in which events are attributed to the intentions and actions of other people). According to this view, whereas external-personal attributions for negative events lead individuals to suspect the intentions of other people, external-situational attributions are psychologically benign, requiring individuals to blame their misfortunes neither on themselves nor on the malevolence of others. Kinderman & Bentall found that this typology was more reliable than the traditional typology of attributional loci (see also Day & Maltby, 2000) and, in a further study (Kinderman & Bentall, 1997), that paranoid patients made excessively external-personal attributions for negative events, and few external-situational attributions for any kind of events. More recently, Craig et al. (in submission) devised a more ecologically valid method of assessing attributional style in which attributions were coded from patients' verbal responses to hypothetical scenarios and similarly found an excess of external-personal attributions for negative events in paranoid patients. These findings are clearly consistent with the earlier work assessing paranoid attributions from the locus of control perspective (Rosenbaum & Hadari, 1985; Kaney & Bentall, 1989; Lasar, 1997). One possible interpretation of this finding is that paranoid patients feel compelled to avoid internal attributions and, for want of some kind of inability to generate external-situational events, are left only with the option of generating external-personal attributions.

Are paranoid attributions self-protective?

In healthy people, the tendency to attribute positive events more internally than negative events, known as the *self-serving bias*, tends to become more evident in conditions in which the self is under some kind of threat (Campbell, 1990). This observation suggests that people deploy attributions partly as a way of regulating their feelings about themselves. A natural extension of this idea is the hypothesis that the abnormal self-serving bias observed in paranoid participants reflects patients' need to protect their fragile self-esteem, perhaps because they harbour more implicit or underlying beliefs about the self which are very negative. This hypothesis amounts to an elaboration of the earlier theory of paranoia suggested by Kenneth Colby (Colby et al., 1971, 1979; Colby, 1977).

Some commentators have objected to the idea that paranoid attributions are self-protective in this way. Freeman et al. (1998), for example, in a study of patients participating in a trial of cognitive–behaviour therapy for psychosis, found that many patients with paranoia had low self-esteem, although they did not have control data and instead reported a comparison with published norms. In fact, the available data on the relationship between paranoia and self-esteem are contradictory. Havner & Izard (1962) found that paranoid patients, in comparison with other schizophrenia patients, reported high consistency between their beliefs about themselves and their ideals. Candido & Romney (1990), in their comparison of paranoid patients, depressed patients and patients who were both paranoid and depressed, reported high self-esteem in the paranoid patients, low self-esteem in the depressed patients and intermediate scores in patients with both sets of symptoms, although like Freeman et al. (1998), they did not report data from normal controls. Lyon et al. (1994) reported that paranoid patients scored as high as matched normal controls on Rosenberg's (1965) self-esteem scale, whereas Bowins & Shugar (1998) reported low self-esteem in deluded patients compared to controls but did not specifically assess the self-esteem of paranoid patients.

In contrast, the evidence that paranoid patients harbour implicit negative beliefs about the self is fairly consistent. For example, whether or not they are currently depressed, paranoid patients score highly on the Dysfunctional Attitude Scale (Bentall & Kaney, 1996; Fear et al., 1996), a questionnaire measure of overly perfectionist standards of self-evaluation on which depressed patients typically score highly. As perfectionist standards of these sort render individuals vulnerable to negative self-evaluation, they can be thought of as an indirect indication of negative beliefs about the self.

Perhaps more persuasive evidence of underlying self-esteem difficulties in paranoid patients has emerged from studies employing the emotional Stroop task, in which individuals are required to name the print colours (but not the words themselves) of words written in different coloured inks. Typically, people are slower at colour-naming words that are emotionally salient than words that are emotionally neutral so that, for example, depressed people are slow at colour-naming depression-related words (Williams & Broadbent, 1986) and anorexic patients are slow at colour-naming food words (Channon et al., 1988). Although the mechanisms underlying this effect are not completely understood, the slowed colour-naming of emotionally salient words is thought to reflect response competition between the tendency to say the word itself and the requirement to state the colour. Not surprisingly, paranoid patients are slow to colour-name threat-related words (Bentall & Kaney, 1989; Fear et al., 1996).

In an interesting variation of the Stroop procedure, Kinderman (1994) asked paranoid patients first to state whether various positive and negative self-esteem words were self-descriptive, before asking them to perform the colour-naming task with those words. He found that paranoid patients, like normal controls but in contrast to depressed patients, tended to endorse as self-descriptive a large number of positive self-esteem words. They also endorsed more negative self-esteem words than the normal controls, but not as many as the depressed patients. However, during the colour-naming phase of the experiment they showed marked slowing for both the positive words and especially negative words. These findings were essentially replicated by Lee (2000) in South Korea. Kinderman argued that the endorsement data indicated an attempt to maintain a positive view of the self; the Stroop data indicated that the paranoid patients found the positive and especially the negative self-esteem words emotionally challenging.

When findings are as inconsistent as those obtained using simple self-esteem measures, it is reasonable to suppose that researchers have been asking the wrong question, or at least approaching the right question in the wrong way. In this case, a major stumbling block seems to be the assumption that beliefs about the self can be captured by a simple unidimensional scale. Kinderman's (1994) findings indicate that different ways of measuring attitudes towards the self may yield dramatically different results. Even the concept of self-esteem, which might be thought of as the simplest way in which individuals can describe themselves, has been criticized by Robson (1989) on the grounds that 'it is an idea rather than an entity', so that 'the term signifies different things to different people'. Robson's own self-esteem scale, developed from this fairly sceptical position and employed in Freeman et al.'s study, samples as wide a range of self-esteem-related constructs as possible, including the belief that other people have negative beliefs about the self ('Most people would take advantage of me if they could'; 'I often worry about what other people are thinking of me'); it is hardly surprising therefore that paranoid patients score low on this scale. Other self-esteem questionnaires, for example Rosenberg's scale, which measures perceived self-worth, are likely to yield different results.

Even more problematic is the assumption that self-esteem is a stable trait. After all, the idea that paranoid attributions are defensive is a dynamic hypothesis, which is presumably best tested by examining how attributions affect beliefs about the self over time, rather than the average value of the same beliefs in a large number of people. Kernis (1993) has shown that, when individuals are asked to rate their self-esteem on a regular basis using a specially adapted form of the Rosenberg scale, great variations in the stability of their scores can be observed. People with highly unstable self-esteem tend to have lower average scores than people with stable self-esteem, but high average scoring but highly unstable individuals can be found. Interestingly, Greenier et al. (1995) reported that individuals with unstable self-esteem tend to make more extreme attributions for everyday positive and negative events than people with stable self-esteem. These findings point to a much more dynamic relationship between judgements about the self and symptoms than assumed by most psychopathology researchers. It is as if some people are locked in a constant struggle to maintain their self-esteem, which they sometimes win and sometimes lose.

This dynamic struggle is also reflected in evidence on the nature of attributional style which, despite researchers' best attempts to treat it as a stable trait, appears to fluctuate, at least in the short term. For example, although Alloy et al. (1999) found that a pessimistic attributional style predicted future depression in euthymic students, other researchers conducting longitudinal investigations have found that attributions for negative events are markedly more internal during the depressed state (Segal & Ingram, 1994; Robins & Hayes, 1995). In a study of attributions coded from the speech of a patient undergoing psychological treatement for depression, Peterson et al. (1983) found that marked changes in the patient's attributions could be detected, so that pessimistic attributions preceded dysphoric mood. Finally, in a series of experiments, Forgas et al. (1990) reported that healthy participants exposed to contrived failure experiences showed changes in their attributional style, which became more pessimistic. Overall, these findings point to a complex relationship between attributions and beliefs about the self that evolves over time in a nonlinear way. If we are to understand paranoia we will therefore require a much more sophisticated understanding of this relationship. We will begin by considering the processes involved in representing the self to the self.

What is the self?

To many hard-nosed biological scientists, the self might seem an almost meta-physcial concept. As Baumeister (1999) has commented:

> Providing a satisfactory definition of the self has proven fiendishly difficult. It is what you mean when you say 'I'. Most people use 'I' and 'self' many times each day, and so most people have a secure understanding of what the self is – but articulating that understanding is not easy.

It would therefore be wrong to regard the self as a 'thing', or to expect that it has some kind of easily definable ontological status. Rather, it is best regarded as a set of ideas, images or beliefs (or, to use a generic term, mental representations) of who we are. Some of these representations are implicit and therefore easy to articulate, whereas others are more implicit and take the form of vague assump-tions or 'schemas'. Like all mental representations, the self is therefore fluid and has boundaries that overlap with other related concepts. When we think about our-selves, we can generate verbal descriptions of our attributes, talents and deficiencies; remember defining moments in our lives; consider how we match or fail to match our moral, social and material aspirations; contemplate the quality of our relation-ships; compare ourselves to other people; and imagine how those other people see us. Although each of these activities invokes the self, none encompasses it entirely. To use a metaphor suggested by the philosopher Dan Dennett (1991), the self is like the narrative centre of gravity of the individual, which cannot be separated from the rest, but around which the stories we tell ourselves about ourselves are constructed.

It is possible to examine the process of self-representation from developmental, cultural and neurobiological perspectives. Some developmentalists have sought origins of the self in the protoconversational exchanges between the infant and caregiver, during which the infant first demonstrates an ability to distinguish between self and other (Trevarthen, 1993). After the child has acquired language she is able to internalize increasingly elaborate descriptions of the self, based on accumulated memories, her interpretation of her experiences and also what she has been told about herself by significant others. By adulthood, we have acquired a reservoir of knowledge about the self that allow us to define our identity ('I am a slightly overweight family man with a good sense of humour'), our membership of groups of like-minded people ('I belong to the tribe of clinical psychologists'), claim our rights ('I want my colleagues to take notice of my ideas about the self'), plan our future achievements ('I have the skills and motivation to carry out more research') and acknowledge our limitations ('...but not to climb Mount Everest').

Because the self develops in the context of social relationships, people growing up in different cultures learn to think about themselves in different ways. For this reason, historical and geographical differences in self-representation can be documented (Baumeister, 1987). For example, during the Middle Ages, most people saw life on earth as a prelude to heavenly bliss, and the self was mainly construed in terms of visible manifestations and actions. In modern individualist societies, on the other hand, there is a preoccupation with self-actualization, accompanied by the widespread belief that the self is difficult to know except perhaps in the context of special techniques such as psychoanalysis. In contrast to this way of thinking about the self, however, in collectivist societies such as Japan people usually define themselves in terms of their harmonious relationships with other people (Markus & Kitayama, 1991).

Like other conceptual structures, the self does not have clear boundaries that allow it to be unambiguously distinguished from other kinds of mental representations. It would therefore be foolish to expect it to be located in a specific neuroanatomical structure. Equally foolish would be the contrary assumption that the self is somehow separate from the physical body in the manner imagined by Descartes; clearly something 'brainy' is happening when we think about ourselves. The role of different brain regions in this process is beyond the scope of this discussion; here I merely note that specific neuroactivations have been detected in functional imaging experiments in which participants have been asked to make judgements that are relevant to the self (Kircher et al., 2000a, 2000b).

The process of self-representation

In the light of the self's fluid nature and indistinct boundaries, it is doubtful whether it would ever be possible to provide an exhaustive description of an individual's self-representations. None the less, the kinds of crude questionnaire measures developed by psychologists have enabled helpful distinctions to be made between important ways in which we think about the self.

We have already seen that beliefs about the self may vary from one point in time to another (Kernis, 1993). Indeed, a moment's reflection will reveal that we spend much of the time thinking about things other than ourselves, and that how we feel about ourselves changes in response to our ongoing experiences. Markus & Wurf (1987) have suggested the term *the working self* to describe our online representations of the self, the collection of thoughts and beliefs about ourselves that we are currently aware of and that help to determine our immediate goals. The specific model of the self that we currently hold in mind has been described by Higgins (1987) as the *actual self*, but both Higgins and Markus have pointed out that other domains of self-representation are usually also available within the working self. These include, for example, the self that I would like to be (or *ideal self*), the self that I ought to be (or *ought self*) and the self that I imagine I might become in the future (or *possible self*, cf. Markus & Nurius, 1986). A further complication noted by Higgins is that we can imagine the self from different *perspectives*. Not only do I have beliefs about the sort of person I am, would like to be and ought to be, but I can also imagine how my mother (or any other significant person) thinks about me, would like me to be and thinks that I ought to be.

Higgins refers to the ideal self and the ought self as *self-guides*, because they appear to have motivational properties. He argues that discrepancies between the actual self and self-guides are associated with distinct emotional states, so that actual–ideal discrepancies are associated with depressed mood whereas actual–ought discrepancies are associated with feelings of anxiety and agitation. A substantial body of empirical research has supported these predictions. For example, when asked to write descriptions of different domains of the self, depressed students and psychiatric patients with a diagnosis of unipolar depression report a large number of actual–ideal discrepancies (Strauman & Higgins, 1988; Strauman, 1989; Scott & O'Hara, 1993). Socially anxious students and patients, on the other hand, report substantial discrepancies between the actual self and the ought self. Not surprisingly, given the strong correlation between depression and anxiety symptoms observed in both healthy and clinical samples (Goldberg & Huxley, 1992), most researchers have reported a strong correlation between the two types of discrepancy, leading some to question whether they are qualitatively distinct (Boldero & Francis, 1999).

That these emotional effects are determined by online self-representations is shown by studies demonstrating that feelings of dysphoria can be provoked by making ordinary people think about their self-discrepancies. Not only does this lead to negative mood, but it also leads to changes in speech rate (speech becomes momentarily more sluggish as individuals contemplate actual–ideal discrepancies), a detectable electrodermal response indicative of emotional arousal (Strauman & Higgins, 1987) and a temporary reduction in immune system functioning (Strauman et al., 1993).

The relationship between self-discrepancies and delusional ideation has been explored by Kinderman & Bentall (1996b), in a study in which paranoid, depressed and normal participants were asked to generate descriptions of their selves and their ideals, and were also asked to say how their parents would describe them. (We first asked the participants to say how their friends would describe them, but this approach floundered because the paranoid patients appeared to have very few friends.) As expected, the normal controls reported high consistency between their selves, their ideals and the believed views of their parents, all of which were very positive. Also, as expected, the depressed patients reported considerable discrepancies between their selves and their ideals, and also some degree of discrepancy between their selves and the believed views of their parents. (On further analysis, it was found that this often reflected the participants' expectations that their parents would describe them in unrealistically positive ways.) The paranoid participants reported considerable consistency between their selves and their ideals, but attributed very hostile views about themselves to their parents. We interpreted this finding as evidence that they had maintained a positive view of the self by attributing negative experiences to the actions of their parents (and, presumably, other people), with the consequence that they assumed their parents disliked them.

The model of the working self that I have just outlined, in which different self-representations come to the fore, and perhaps become discrepant with each other under different circumstances, is clearly a step towards the more dynamic account that a theory of paranoia seems to require. However, it is worth noting that, behind the contents of the working self, there must be a more enduring reservoir of *stored knowledge about the self*, consisting of semantic representations, memories of relevant life experiences and implicit standards of self-evaluation (or self-schemas) as envisaged in Beck's (1976) theory of depression. Indeed, it seems reasonable to assume that the contents of the working self reflects the extent to which current circumstances bring forth (or 'prime', in the language of cognitive psychology) these different kinds of self knowledge.

The attribution–self-representation cycle

We are now in a better position to understand the relationship between attributions and self-representations, and the role that both of these processes play in psychopathology (both depression and paranoia). To achieve this understanding it will be necessary to solve two problems: firstly, to understand how attributions are generated and secondly, to understand how attributions affect the kinds of

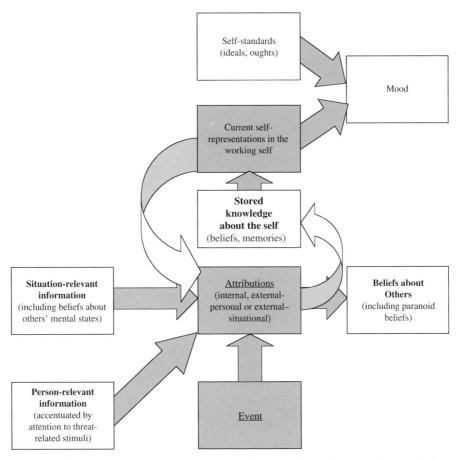

Figure 14.1   The attribution–self-representation cycle. Reproduced from Bentall & Kaney, in submission.

representations in the working self. When these two problems are considered, it becomes apparent that attributions and self-representations are linked together in a cyclical process, in which attributions influence self-representations, which in turn influence future attributions (Figure 14.1). This cycle, driven partly in response to environmental events, is responsible for the dynamic changes in attributions and self-representations that I have already described. It is presumably endless (at least until death), so to ask which is primary – attributions or self-representations – misses the point.

How the working self influences attributions

Strangely, most researchers working on attributional models of psychopathology have ignored the first of these problems. Because attributional *style* has been as-sumed to be a stable trait, the mechanisms involved in generating attributional *responses* have been almost entirely neglected. We can begin considering this problem by acknowledging that most attribution-eliciting events include some kinds of attributional cues. For example, the exam script returned with the comment, 'You have not studied the material sufficiently to write an adequate essay' clearly includes an attributional signpost, as does a violent attack from a stranger.

In the 1960s, Kelley (1967) argued that information about the consistency (has it happened before?) and distinctiveness (does it only happen in particular circumstances?) of events, together with consensus information (does the event affect only me or everyone else?) may be particularly important in influencing attributional responses. For example, an apparently random assault experienced by a civilian during warfare may be attributed to causes external to himself because he knows that attacks have been ongoing for some time (high consistency), occur only when enemy troops are present (high distinctiveness) and are experienced by many other civilians (high consensus). However, even such well-signposted events allow some freedom in the kind of attribution generated. For example, consider the following attempt by a concentration camp survivor to explain the death of his older brother in the closing days of the Second World War:

My brother died in my arms from dysentery. He faded away to nothing. A man who was a giant died a skeleton. I held him in my arms when he died. There was just nothing I could do. When I think about it, I sometimes blame myself. He did so much to keep me alive. I feel that had he saved some of that energy for himself he would have had a better chance to survive (Gilbert, 1996, p. 236).

In this case, an internal attribution is made despite apparently overwhelming evidence that the cause should be allocated elsewhere, presumably because the speaker's judgement is also influenced by relevant beliefs about himself (that he was insufficiently strong). In this way, beliefs about the self form an additional source of information when individuals attempt to determine the causal locus of an event. To take a more trivial example than that given above, if an individual already believes himself to be stupid, his failure to pass an exam will almost certainly be attributed internally, because there is an available self-representation that 'fits' the event. Hence, people who score low on global self-esteem measures typically make internal attributions for negative events (Flett et al., 1995) whereas those with high self-esteem tend to make internal attributions for successful outcomes (Ickes & Layden, 1978).

There is evidence that the process of integrating this information from the world and the working self to generate an attribution typically requires more than one step. Gilbert et al. (1988) observed that normal people, when explaining the actions of others, tend to make dispositional or personal attributions when handicapped by a cognitive load (being required to perform a competing task) but more situational attributions under less demanding conditions. The implication of this finding is that the actions of others are first attributed to some enduring trait, before being later adjusted to take into account situational data if the necessary cognitive resources are available. Adding this insight to what we already know about the influence of the working self on attributions, the final explanation generated to account for a social encounter might be thought of as the answer to two sequentially posed questions: 'Is it me?' (if the answer is 'yes' the attribution will be internal) and 'Is it the situation?' (if the answer is 'No', or if this question does not get asked, the nature of the social encounter will be attributed to some kind of enduring trait in the other person).

How attributions influence the working self

We have already seen that negative mood tends to be elicited when individuals experience discrepancies between their current beliefs about themselves and their ideals (Higgins, 1987). It seems reasonable to assume that attributions therefore influence mood by changing beliefs about the self. Consistent with this hypothesis, studies using path analysis indicate that the relationship between a pessimistic attributional style and depression is entirely mediated by low self-esteem (Tennen et al., 1987; Romney, 1994). If you discover that you are not really the sort of person you would like to be, you will inevitably feel bad about yourself.

The impact of attributions on self-representations becomes more apparent when we consider each of the three attributional loci described in Kinderman & Bentall's (1996a, 1997) typology. Internal attributions for negative events presumably prime stored knowledge about the self, making representations of the actual self more negative. The external-personal attributions for negative events made by paranoid patients, on the other hand, presumably allow the individual to maintain a positive view of the self, but at the terrible expense of attributing malicious intentions to others. In this way paranoid beliefs are formed. (Kinderman & Bentall's self-discrepancy data obtained from paranoid patients, described earlier, are obviously consistent with this account.) External-situational attributions, on the other hand, appear to be psychologically benign. They do not lead to negative views about the self or to the attribution of malicious intentions to others. Hence, they are the essence of good excuse-making (as in, 'I'm sorry I'm late but the traffic was dreadful').

Biases in the cycle

Although attributions and self-representations are free to change over time according to the account of their relationship that I have just given, we have already seen that different groups of individuals have a tendency to make some types of attributions more than others. Ordinary people typically show a self-serving bias, attributing positive events more to the self than negative events (Campbell & Sedikides, 1999), depressed patients lack this bias or may even have a tendency to make internal attributions more for negative events than for positive events (Abramson et al., 1978) and, in paranoid patients, the self-serving bias appears to be exaggerated (Kaney & Bentall, 1989). There therefore appear to be different biases in the cycle in these different groups.

We can begin to understand the implications of these biases by considering the function of the self-serving bias in ordinary people. If the bias is absent in an individual who has even modestly negative beliefs about the self, there is clearly a possibility that a negative event will elicit an internal attribution. In this eventuality, stored negative information about the self is likely to be primed, increasing the negative content of the working self. This in turn will increase the probability of an internal attribution being elicited for a negative event during some future iteration of the cycle. It is not difficult to see that, under some circumstances, this process will lead to a negative spiral, in which there is a progressive loss of self-esteem and in which the individual's apparent attributional style becomes ever more pessimistic. These consequences are, of course, characteristics that are regularly observed in depressed people. Indeed, on this account, depression is the end stage of many iterations of the cycle in individuals who are not protected by a self-serving bias sufficiently robust to counter whatever slings and arrows of outrageous fortune they happen to be exposed to.

The idea that the self-serving bias in ordinary people is self-protective gives us some insight into its function in paranoid patients. The data on the self-representations of these patients reviewed earlier are clearly consistent with the hypothesis that they are motivated by a need to maintain positive beliefs about the self, even in the face of adversity. Recall that, on indirect measures of self-representation, paranoid patients fairly consistently show evidence of negative beliefs about the self (Kinderman, 1994; Bentall & Kaney, 1996; Fear et al., 1996; Lee, 2000) but that, on simple self-esteem measures, no consistent pattern is observed (Candido & Romney, 1990; Freeman et al., 1998). The motivation to avoid internal attributions for negative events presumably springs from the underlying negative view of the self. The inconsistent observations on simple self-esteem measures, on the other hand, presumably reflect the extent to which the struggle to maintain positive beliefs about the self is successful in different patients under different circumstances.

The impact of life events

According to the account of the attribution–self-representation cycle given above, different kinds of life events are likely to elicit different types of attributions. This is because, as we have seen, different types of life events contain attributional cues that, all other things being equal (which, of course, they are often not), will tend to point to particular types of attributions (internal, external-personal or external-situational) and so start the cycle moving in one direction or another. These effects are likely to be particularly profound when the attributional cues are consistent with existing biases so that the life events, so to speak, push at an open door. Not surprisingly, therefore, events that are readily interpreted as involving personal failure are particularly troublesome to people who are vulnerable to depression (Brown & Moran, 1998).

On this account, cues that shift attention to the actions of other people should facilitate external-personal attributions and hence paranoid ideation. This phenomenon has been demonstrated in normal individuals by Bodner & Mikulincer (1998), in a series of studies in which participants were asked to explain their performance following a contrived failure experience. When their attention was focused on the experimenter (for example, by having a video camera obviously pointing at the experimenter and a monitor showing the experimenter's image in clear view) the participants were especially likely to make paranoid attributions. However, when the participants' attention was focused on themselves (for example, because the camera was pointing at them) they tended to make more internal attributions.

Not surprisingly, it is events that implicate the actions of other people that seem to be most clearly associated with the onset of paranoid ideation. Harris (1987) argued that these can be characterized as intrusive. They might include threats from landlords, police enquiries, burglaries and unwanted sexual propositions, but all involve someone imposing demands or experiences on the patient. Harris (1987) found a 20-fold difference in the number of these events in a comparison of schizophrenic patients who were about to relapse and ordinary people, a finding which was largely replicated in the World Health Organization study of the Determinants of Outcome of Severe Mental Disorders (Day et al., 1987) and in a recent study of late-onset paraphrenia (Fuchs, 1999).

Testing and developing the model

In this chapter I have outlined a theory that attempts to account for the relationship between the self and the attributions that we generate for significant life events. The focus of the account has been persecutory delusions, which are seen as one output of this process. By making a series of external-personal attributions for negative life experiences, the individual develops the belief that others have negative attitudes towards the self, and in this way a paranoid world-view is established.

However, we have also seen that research findings on the role of cognitive processes in depression can also be accommodated within this model. Indeed, the findings support the view that these conditions are under the control of the same cognitive mechanisms and suggests reasons why they often occur together. (A para-noid person who develops substantial discrepancies between beliefs about the self and ideals, despite a robust self-serving bias, should become depressed according to the model.)

A further advantage of this model over previous attempts to account for paranoia and depression is that it begins to account for changes in psychopathology over time. The attribution–self-representation cycle clearly constitutes a nonlinear system. In ordinary people the self-serving bias ensures that the system maintains a degree of stability, even in adversity. However, in psychiatric patients we must expect symptoms to fluctuate regularly and unpredictably as individuals pass through iterations of the cycle and are buffeted by daily events. This kind of instability is often observed in clinical practice, and is equally often dismissed as 'noise' or a nuisance by researchers in psychopathology. In future studies it will be useful to find ways of tracking and analysing these kinds of fluctuations, in the hope of achieving a better understanding of the long-term course of patients' symptoms.

The fact that it is difficult or even impossible to make precise predictions about the self-esteem scores of paranoid patients may be troublesome to some readers, perhaps raising the spectre of untestability that has dogged psychoanalytic theories of psychopathology (Eysenck, 1985). However, this property of the theory does not preclude the possibility that it might be subjected to other kinds of experimental tests. In fact, three sets of predictions derived from the model have already been subjected to empirical investigation.

The first concerns the time required to generate an internal attribution. If these kinds of explanations for events are made partly by accessing relevant self-representations, it follows that ordinary people with mostly positive beliefs about the self should more rapidly generate internal attributions for positive events than for negative events. People with more negative beliefs about the self, on the other hand, should be just as quick to generate internal attributions for both types of events or (if their beliefs about themselves are overwhelmingly negative) quicker to generate internal attributions for negative events. Bentall et al. (1999) asked nor-mal, depressed and paranoid individuals to read attributional scenarios out aloud before generating verbal attributions, and timed the period between completion of the reading of each scenario and the beginning of each attributional response. As expected, internal attributions were quicker for positive than for negative events in the ordinary people. This bias was absent in both the depressed and paranoid patients.

The second set of predictions concerns the dynamic influences of self-representations on attributions and vice versa. In an attempt to observe these di-rectly, Kinderman & Bentall (2000) conducted two experiments in which normal participants were asked to describe themselves, their ideals and the believed views of others about the self both before and after generating a series of attributions for hypothetical negative events. As expected, those who showed most actual–ideal discrepancies at the outset were most likely to make internal attributions for the negative events. However, when this effect was controlled for it was found that the different kinds of attributions had different impacts on the participants' self-representations. As expected, internal attributions for negative events tended to lead to an increase in actual–ideal discrepancies. Also as expected, individuals who made predominantly external-situational attributions tended to preserve a positive view of themselves, and also continued to believe that others had positive beliefs about them. External-personal attributions of the kind made by paranoid patients, on the other hand, tended to leave the actual self unaffected, but led to increased discrepancies between the participants' beliefs about themselves and the apparent beliefs of others about the self, which were more negative by the end of the experiments.

A final set of predictions concerned the lability of attributional responses. According to the theory of the attribution–self-representation cycle, attributional responses for negative events should become more internal following experiences that prompt negative beliefs about the self. Forgas et al. (1990) had previously demonstrated this effect in ordinary people. In a recent study, Bentall & Kaney (submitted) measured attributional style for negative events in ordinary, depressed and paranoid people before and after exposing them to a contrived failure experience in the form of insoluble anagrams. Before this experience, the attributional differences between the groups were consistent with previous studies: the paranoid patients made predominantly external attributions, the depressed patients made predominantly internal attributions and the attributions of the ordinary people fell between these two extremes. Following the insoluble anagrams task, however, both the paranoid and depressed patients made far more internal attributions than before. In contrast to the findings of Forgas et al. (1990), however, our normal group showed very little shift in their attributions, perhaps because the insoluble anagram task was too mild to prime negative self-representations in this group.

Perhaps the most important scientific question that remains to be addressed concerns the developmental origins of the attributional biases and dysfunctional self-representations observed in paranoid patients. Although it has become somewhat unfashionable to implicate dysfunctional family relationships in psychotic symptoms, studies of depressed patients clearly indicate that the development of the cognitive processes I have described in this chapter is influenced by relationships with significant others. Thus, a depressogenic cognitive style is predicted by emotional abuse (Alloy et al., 1999), a cold and unaccepting maternal parenting style (Garber & Flynn, 2001; Hammen, 1991) and inappropriate feedback given by parents to children following negative experiences (Alloy et al., 2001). Although virtually no longitudinal data exist on future paranoid patients, there is a considerable amount of 'smoking gun' evidence that suggests that family factors and the early environment may be appropriate targets for future investigation. For example, studies of people at high risk of psychotic disorders indicate that suspiciousness (Cannon et al., 2001) and an external locus of control (Frenkel et al., 1995) are predictors of future positive symptoms, suggesting that abnormal functioning of the attribution–self-representation cycle may considerably predate the onset of florid symptoms. Moreover, clinical studies (Dozier et al., 1991; Dozier & Lee, 1995) and population surveys (Mickelson et al., 1997; Cooper et al., 1998) both indicate that paranoid ideation in patients and in normal individuals is associated with an insecure, and especially an avoidant attachment style.

Of course, even if future research should establish beyond a doubt that early relationships play a causal role in the development of paranoid ideation, this would not preclude the possibility that biological and neurocognitive factors also make a contribution. Although beyond the scope of this chapter, there is ample evidence that such factors may be important in the development of psychosis. It may eventually be possible to specify in some detail how biological factors impact on the cycle itself, or underlie its components. Indeed, work on establishing the functional neuroanatomy of these components has already begun (Blackwood et al., 2000).

REFERENCES

Abramson, L.Y., Seligman, M.E.P. & Teasdale, J.D. (1978). Learned helplessness in humans: critique and reformulation. *Journal of Abnormal Psychology*, **78**, 40–74.

Abramson, L.Y., Metalsky, G.I. & Alloy, L.B. (1989). Hopelessness depression: a theory-based subtype of depression. *Psychological Review*, **96**, 358–72.

Alloy, L.B., Abramson, L.Y., Whitehouse, W.G. et al. (1999). Depressogenic cognitive styles: predictive validity, information processing and personality characteristics, and developmental origins. *Behaviour Research and Therapy*, **37**, 503–31.

Alloy, L.B., Abramson, L.Y., Tashman, N.A. et al. (2001). Developmental origins of cognitive vulnerability to depression: parenting, cognitive and inferential feedback styles of the parents of individuals at high and low cognitive risk for depression. *Cognitive Therapy and Research*, **25**, 397–423.

American Psychiatric Association (1994). *Diagnostic and Statistical Manual of Mental Disorders*, 4th edn. Washington, DC: American Psychiatric Association.

Baumeister, R.F. (1987). How the self became a problem: a psychological review of historical research. *Journal of Personality and Social Psychology*, **52**, 163–76.

Baumeister, R.F. (1999). The nature and structure of the self: an overview. In *The Self in Social Psychology*, ed. F. Baumeister, pp. 1–20. Philadelphia, PA: Psychology Press.

Beck, A.T. (1976). *Cognitive Therapy and the Emotional Disorders.* New York: International Universities Press.

Bentall, R.P. & Kaney, S. (1989). Content-specific information processing and persecutory delusions: an investigation using the emotional Stroop test. *British Journal of Medical Psychology,* **62**, 355–64.

Bentall, R.P. & Kaney, S. (submitted). Attributional lability in depression and paranoia: psychopathology and the attribution–self-representation cycle.

Bentall, R.P. & Kaney, S. (1996). Abnormalities of self-representation and persecutory delusions. *Psychological Medicine,* **26**, 1231–7.

Bentall, R.P., Kinderman, P. & Bowen-Jones, K. (1999). Response latencies for the causal attributions of depressed, paranoid and normal individuals: availability of self-representations. *Cognitive Neuropsychiatry,* **4**, 107–18.

Berrios, G. (1991). Delusions as 'wrong beliefs': a conceptual history. *British Journal of Psychiatry,* **159** (suppl. 14), 6–13.

Blackwood, N., Howard, R.J., ffytche, D.H. et al. (2000). Imaging attentional and attributional biases: an fMRI approach to paranoid delusions. *Psychological Medicine,* **30**, 873–83.

Bodner, E. & Mikulincer, M. (1998). Learned helplessness and the occurrence of depressive-like and paranoid-like responses: the role of attentional focus. *Journal of Personality and Social Psychology,* **74**, 1010–23.

Boldero, J. & Francis, J. (1999). Ideals, oughts, and self-regulation: are there qualitatively distinct self-guides? *Asian Journal of Social Psychology,* **2**, 343–55.

Bowins, B. & Shugar, G. (1998). Delusions and self-esteem. *Canadian Journal of Psychiatry,* **43**, 154–8.

Brett-Jones, J., Garety, P. & Hemsley, D. (1987). Measuring delusional experiences: a method and its application. *British Journal of Clinical Psychology,* **26**, 257–65.

Brown, G.W. & Moran, P. (1998). Emotion and the etiology of depressive disorders. In *Emotions in Psychopathology: Theory and Research,* ed. W.F. Flack & J.D. Laird, pp. 171–84. New York: Oxford University Press.

Campbell, J.D. (1990). Self-esteem and the clarity of the self-concept. *Journal of Personality and Social Psychology,* **59**, 538–49.

Campbell, W.K. & Sedikides, C. (1999). Self-threat magnifies the self-serving bias: a meta-analytic integration. *Review of General Psychology,* **3**, 23–43.

Candido, C.L. & Romney, D.M. (1990). Attributional style in paranoid vs depressed patients. *British Journal of Medical Psychology,* **63**, 355–63.

Cannon, M., Walsh, E., Hollis, C. et al. (2001). Predictors of later schizophrenia and affective psychosis among attendees at a child psychiatry department. *British Journal of Psychiatry,* **178**, 420–6.

Channon, S., Hemsley, D.R. & de Silva, P. (1988). Selective processing of food words in anorexia nervosa. *British Journal of Clinical Psychology,* **27**, 259–60.

Colby, K.M. (1977). Appraisal of four psychological theories of paranoid phenomena. *Journal of Abnormal Psychology,* **86**, 54–9.

Colby, K., Weber, S. & Hilf, F.D. (1971). Artificial paranoia. *Artificial Intelligence,* **2**, 1–25.

Colby, K.M., Faught, W.S. & Parkinson, R.C. (1979). Cognitive therapy of paranoid conditions: heuristic suggestions based on a computer simulation. *Cognitive Therapy and Research*, **3**, 55–60.

Cooper, M.L., Shaver, P.R. & Collins, N.L. (1998). Attachment style, emotion regulation, and adjustment in adolescence. *Journal of Personality and Social Psychology*, **74**, 1380–97.

Craig, J., Hatton, C. & Bentall, R. P. (submitted). Theory of mind and attributions in persecutory delusions and Asperger's syndrome.

Day, L. & Maltby, J. (2000). Can Kinderman and Bentall's suggestion for a personal and situational attributions questionnaire be used to examine all aspects of attributional style? *Personality and Individual Differences*, **29**, 1047–55.

Day, R., Neilsen, J.A., Korten, A. et al. (1987). Stressful life events preceding the onset of acute schizophrenia: a cross-national study from the World Health Organization. *Culture, Medicine and Psychiatry*, **11**, 123–206.

Dennett, D.C. (1991). *Consciousness Explained*. London: Allen Lane.

Dozier, M. & Lee, S.W. (1995). Discrepancies between self and other-report of psychiatric symptomatology: effects of dismissing attachment strategies. *Development and Psychopathology*, **7**, 217–26.

Dozier, M., Stevenson, A.L., Lee, S.W. & Velligan, D.I. (1991). Attachment organization and familiar overinvolvement for adults with serious psychopathological disorders. *Development and Psychopathology*, **3**, 475–89.

Eysenck, H.J. (1985). *The Decline and Fall of the Freudian empire*. Harmondsworth: Penguin.

Fear, C.F., Sharp, H. & Healy, D. (1996). Cognitive processes in delusional disorder. *British Journal of Psychiatry*, **168**, 61–7.

Flett, G.L., Pliner, P. & Blankstein, K.R. (1995). Preattributional dimensions in self-esteem and depressive symptomatology. *Journal of Social Behavior and Personality*, **10**, 101–22.

Forgas, J.P., Bower, G.H. & Moylan, S.J. (1990). Praise or blame? Affective influences on attributions for achievement. *Journal of Personality and Social Psychology*, **59**, 809–19.

Freeman, D., Garety, P., Fowler, D. et al. (1998). The London–East Anglia randomized controlled trial of cognitive-behaviour therapy for psychosis IV: self-esteem and persecutory delusions. *British Journal of Clinical Psychology*, **37**, 415–30.

Frenkel, E., Kugelmass, S., Nathan, M. & Ingraham, L.J. (1995). Locus of control and mental health in adolescence and adulthood. *Schizophrenia Bulletin*, **21**, 219–26.

Freud, S. (1911/50). *Psychoanalytic Notes upon an Autobiographical Account of a Case of Paranoia (Dementia Paranoides), Collected Papers*, vol. III, pp. 387–466). London: Hogarth Press.

Fuchs, T. (1999). Life events in late paraphrenia and depression. *Psychopathology*, **32**, 60–9.

Garber, J. & Flynn, C. (2001). Predictors of depressive cognitions in young adolescents. *Cognitive Therapy and Research*, **25**, 353–76.

Garety, P.A. & Hemsley, D.R. (1987). The characteristics of delusional experience. *European Archives of Psychiatry and Neurological Sciences*, **236**, 294–8.

Garety, P.A., Everitt, B.S. & Hemsley, D.R. (1988). The characteristics of delusions: a cluster analysis of deluded subjects. *European Archives of Psychiatry and Neurological Sciences*, **237**, 112–14.

Gilbert, M. (1996). *The Boys: Triumph over Adversity*. London: Weidenfeld and Nicolson.

Gilbert, D.T., Pelham, B.W. & Krull, D.S. (1988). On cognitive busyness: when person perceivers meet persons perceived. *Journal of Personality and Social Psychology*, **54**, 733–40.

Goldberg, D. & Huxley, P. (1992). *Common Mental Disorders: A Bio-social Model*. London: Routledge.

Greenier, K.D., Kernis, M.H. & Waschull, S.B. (1995). Not all high (or low) self-esteem people are the same: theory and research on stability of self-esteem. In *Efficacy, Agency, and Self-esteem*, ed. M.H. Kernis, pp. 51–71. New York: Plenum.

Hammen, C. (1991). *Depression Runs in Families: The Social Context of Risk and Resilience in Children of Depressed Mothers*. London: Springer-Verlag.

Harris, T. (1987). Recent developments in the study of life events in relation to psychiatric and physical disorders. In *Psychiatric Epidemiology: Progress and Prospects*, ed. B. Cooper, pp. 81–102. London: Croom Helm.

Harrow, M., Rattenbury, F. & Stoll, F. (1988). Schizophrenic delusions: an analysis of their persistence, of related premorbid ideas and three major dimensions. In *Delusional Beliefs*, ed. T.F. Oltmanns & B.A. Maher, pp. 184–211. New York: John Wiley.

Harrow, M., MacDonald, A.W., Sands, J.R. & Silverstein, M.L. (1995). Vulnerability to delusions over time in schizophrenia and affective disorders. *Schizophrenia Bulletin*, **21**, 95–109.

Havner, P.H. & Izard, C.E. (1962). Unrealistic self-enhancement in paranoid schizophrenics. *Journal of Consulting Psychology*, **26**, 65–8.

Higgins, E.T. (1987). Self-discrepancy: a theory relating self and affect. *Psychological Review*, **94**, 319–40.

Ickes, W. & Layden, M.A. (1978). Attributional styles. In *New Directions in Attribution Research*, vol. 2, ed. J.H. Harvey, W. Ickes & R.F. Kidd, pp. 119–92. Hillsdale, NJ: Lawrence Erlbaum.

Jaspers, K. (1913/63). *General Psychopathology*. Translated by J. Hoenig & M.W. Hamilton. Manchester: Manchester University Press.

Jorgensen, P. & Jensen, J. (1994). Delusional beliefs in first admitters. *Psychopathology*, **27**, 100–12.

Kaney, S. & Bentall, R.P. (1989). Persecutory delusions and attributional style. *British Journal of Medical Psychology*, **62**, 191–8.

Kelley, H.H. (1967). Attribution theory in social psychology. In *Nebraska Symposium on Motivation*, vol. 15, ed. D. Levine, pp. 192–240. Lincoln: University of Nebraska Press.

Kendler, K.S., Glazer, W. & Morgenstern, H. (1983). Dimensions of delusional experience. *American Journal of Psychiatry*, **140**, 466–9.

Kernis, M.H. (1993). The role of stability and level of self-esteem in psychological functioning. In *Self-esteem: The Puzzle of Low Self-regard*, ed. R.F. Baumeister, pp. 167–82. New York: Plenum.

Kinderman, P. (1994). Attentional bias, persecutory delusions and the self concept. *British Journal of Medical Psychology*, **67**, 53–66.

Kinderman, P. & Bentall, R.P. (1996a). The development of a novel measure of causal attributions: the Internal Personal and Situational Attributions Questionnaire. *Personality and Individual Differences*, **20**, 261–4.

Kinderman, P. & Bentall, R.P. (1996b). Self-discrepancies and persecutory delusions: evidence for a defensive model of paranoid ideation. *Journal of Abnormal Psychology*, **105**, 106–14.

Kinderman, P. & Bentall, R.P. (1997). Causal attributions in paranoia: internal, personal and situational attributions for negative events. *Journal of Abnormal Psychology*, **106**, 341–5.

Kinderman, P. & Bentall, R.P. (2000). Self-discrepancies and causal attributions: studies of hypothesized relationships. *British Journal of Clinical Psychology*, **39**, 255–73.

Kircher, T.T.J., Senior, C., Phillips, M. et al. (2000a). Towards a functional neuroanatomy of self-processing effects of faces and words. *Cognition and Brain Research*, **10**, 133–44.

Kircher, T.T.J., Senior, C., Phillips, M. et al. (2000b). Recognising one's own face. *Cognition*, **78** B1–15.

Kristev, H., Jackson, H. & Maude, D. (1999). An investigation of attributional style in first-episode psychosis. *British Journal of Clinical Psychology*, **88**, 181–94.

Lasar, M. (1997). Cognitive evaluation of action in chronic schizophrenia: locus of control beliefs in an inpatient group. *Psychologische Bietraege*, **39**, 297–311.

Lee, H.J. (2000). Attentional bias, memory bias and the self-concept in paranoia. *Psychological Science*, **9**, 77–99.

Lee, H.J. & Won, H.T. (1998). The self-concepts, the other-concepts, and attributional style in paranoia and depression. *Korean Journal of Clinical Psychology*, **17**, 105–25.

Levenson, H. (1974). Activism and powerful others: distinctions within the concept of internal–external control. *Journal of Personality Assessment*, **38**, 377–83.

Lyon, H.M., Kaney, S. & Bentall, R.P. (1994). The defensive function of persecutory delusions: evidence from attribution tasks. *British Journal of Psychiatry*, **164**, 637–46.

Markus, H. & Kitayama, S. (1991). Culture and the self: implications for cognition, emotion, and motivation. *Psychological Review*, **98**, 224–53.

Markus, H. & Nurius, P. (1986). Possible selves. *American Psychologist*, **41**, 954–69.

Markus, H. & Wurf, E. (1987). The dynamic self-concept: a social psychological perspective. *Annual Review of Psychology*, **38**, 299–337.

Mickelson, K.D., Kessler, R.C. & Shaver, P.R. (1997). Adult attachment in a nationally representative sample. *Journal of Personality and Social Psychology*, **73**, 1092–106.

Ndetei, D.M. & Vadher, A. (1984). Frequency and clinical significance of delusions across cultures. *Acta Psychiatrica Scandinavica*, **70**, 73–6.

Peterson, C., Luborsky, L. & Seligman, M.E.P. (1983). Attributions and depressive mood shifts: a case study using the symptom-context method. *Journal of Abnormal Psychology*, **92**, 93–103.

Peterson, C., Semmel, A., Von Baeyer, C. et al. (1982). The Attributional Style Questionnaire. *Cognitive Therapy and Research*, **3**, 287–300.

Poulton, R., Caspi, A., Moffitt, T.E. et al. (2000). Children's self-reported psychotic symptoms and adult schizophreniform disorder: a 15-year longitudinal study. *Archives of General Psychiatry*, **57**, 1053–8.

Reivich, K. (1995). The measurement of explanatory style. In *Explanatory Style*, ed. G.M. Buchanan & M.E.P. Seligman, pp. 21–48. Hillsdale, NJ: Lawrence Erlbaum.

Robins, C.J. & Hayes, A.H. (1995). The role of causal attributions in the prediction of depression. In *Explanatory Style*, ed. G.M. Buchanan & M.E.P. Seligman, pp. 71–98. Hillsdale, NJ: Lawrence Erlbaum.

Robson, P. (1989). Development of a new self-report measure of self-esteem. *Psychological Medicine*, **19**, 513–18.

Romney, D.M. (1994). Cross-validating a causal model relating attributional style, self-esteem, and depression: an heuristic study. *Psychological Reports*, **74**, 203–7.

Rosenbaum, M. & Hadari, D. (1985). Personal efficacy, external locus of control, and perceived contingency of parental reinforcement among depressed, paranoid and normal subjects. *Journal of Abnormal Psychology*, **49**, 539–47.

Rosenberg, M. (1965). *Society and the Adolescent Self-image*. Princeton, NJ: Princeton University Press.

Schreber, D. (1903/55). *Memoirs of my Nervous Illness*. Translated by I. Macalpine & R.A. Hunter. London: Dawsons.

Scott, L. & O'Hara, M.W. (1993). Self-discrepancies in clinically anxious and depressed university students. *Journal of Abnormal Psychology*, **102**, 282–7.

Segal, Z.V. & Ingram, R.E. (1994). Mood priming and construct activation in tests of cognitive vulnerability to unipolar depression. *Clinical Psychology Review*, **14**, 663–95.

Sharp, H.M., Fear, C.F. & Healy, D. (1997). Attributional style and delusions: an investigation based on delusional content. *European Psychiatry*, **12**, 1–7.

Sims, A. (1995). *Symptoms in the Mind*, 2nd edn. London: W.B. Saunders.

Stompe, T., Friedman, A., Ortwein, G. et al. (1999). Comparisons of delusions among schizophrenics in Austria and Pakistan. *Psychopathology*, **32**, 225–34.

Strauman, T.J. (1989). Self-discrepancies in clinical depression and social phobia: cognitive structures that underlie emotional disorders? *Journal of Abnormal Psychology*, **98**, 14–22.

Strauman, T.J. & Higgins, E.T. (1987). Automatic activation of self-discrepancies and emotional syndromes: when cognitive structures influence affect. *Journal of Abnormal Psychology*, **98**, 14–22.

Strauman, T.J. & Higgins, E.T. (1988). Self-discrepancies as predictors of vulnerability to distinct syndromes of chronic emotional distress. *Journal of Personality*, **56**, 685–707.

Strauman, T.J., Lemieux, A.M. & Coe, C.L. (1993). Self-discrepancy and natural killer cell activity: immunological consequences of negative self-evaluation. *Journal of Personality and Social Psychology*, **64**, 1042–52.

Strauss, J.S. (1969). Hallucinations and delusions as points on continua function: rating scale evidence. *Archives of General Psychiatry*, **21**, 581–6.

Sweeny, P., Anderson, K. & Bailey, S. (1986). Attributional style and depression: a meta-analytic review. *Journal of Personality and Social Psychology*, **50**, 774–91.

Tennen, H., Herzenberger, S. & Nelson, H.F. (1987). Depressive attributional style: the role of self-esteem. *Journal of Personality*, **55**, 631–60.

Trevarthen, C. (1993). The self born in intersubjectivity: the psychology of an infant communicating. In *The Perceived Self: Ecological and Interpersonal Sources of Self-knowledge*, ed. U. Neisser, pp. 121–73. Cambridge: Cambridge University Press.

van Os, J., Hanssen, M., Bijl, R.V. & Ravelli, A. (2000). Strauss (1969) revisited: a psychosis continuum in the normal population? *Schizophrenia Research*, **45**, 11–20.

White, P.A. (1991). Ambiguity in the internal/external distinction in causal attibution. *Journal of Experimental Social Psychology*, **27**, 259–70.

Williams, J.M.G. & Broadbent, K. (1986). Distraction by emotional stimuli: use of a Stroop task with suicide attempters. *British Journal of Clinical Psychology*, **25**, 101–10.

Zullow, H.M., Oettingen, G., Peterson, C. & Seligman, M.E.P. (1988). Pessimistic explanatory style in the historical record: CAVEing LBJ, Presidential candidates, and East versus West Berlin. *American Psychologist*, **43**, 673–82.

15

Schizophrenia and the narrative self

James Phillips

Yale School of Medicine, New Haven, CT, USA

Abstract

In this study of schizophrenia and narrative identity, the author begins with a description of narrative identity and a discussion of the debate over narrative identity: a debate that pits theorists arguing that narrative structures are embedded in lived life against those claiming that self-narratives are fictive structures that bear no relation to life as actually lived. The author defends a centrist position that finds narrative identity in part emerging from the life of the individual and in part constructed by the individual. Against the background of this discussion he then presents the histories of three schizophrenic patients. The first is an example of a highly fragmented self-narrative. The second is a delusional self-narrative. Finally, the third history is that of a woman struggling over whether to think of herself in terms of a schizophrenic 'illness' narrative.

Introduction

In addressing the narrative self in schizophrenia, I will begin with the broader topic of the self as such. Contemporary discussions of the self divide into positions that view the self as an essence or substance and those that view it as a construct. The notion of self as essence or substance implies that there is something like a human nature that dictates the course of self-development through the life span. Philosophically, Aristotle is the central figure at the origin of this point of view; he argued that man has a 'form' which he realizes over the course of a life. Although Aristotle's views on substance and the teleology of human life have long since been rejected in the modern era, he has many heirs in contemporary times, including neuroscientific models that locate the origins of selfhood in the complex neural structures of the brain and point to a neurobiologically based self-development, as well as biological models of schizophrenia that posit a normal course of self-development and understand schizophrenia in terms of a deviation from that course. In the area of psychology, we have a major example of the essentialist self in psychoanalytic developmental theory, that traces a predictable development of the self or person over time and interprets psychopathology in terms of deviations from the developmental norm and treatment in terms of a return to the norm. David Winnicott readily comes to mind as a theoretician and practitioner whose views about psychopathology and treatment (including the psychotic disorders and their treatment) are in this tradition. He describes psychopathology in terms of a defensive false self-structure that has been erected to protect a hidden, true self, and the path to health as facilitating the patient's recovery of his or her true self. Writing about psychotic conditions, he says:

> Here could be brought in the concept of the true and the false self. It is essential to include this concept in the attempt to understand the deceptive clinical picture presented in most cases of schizophrenic-type illness. What is presented is a false self, adapted to the expectations of various layers of the individual's environment. In effect the compliant or false self is a pathological version of that which is called in health the polite, socially adapted aspect of the healthy personality . . . A mental breakdown is often a 'healthy' sign in that it implies a capacity of the individual to use an environment that has become available in order to re-establish an existence on a basis that feels real (Winnicott, 1965, p. 225).

With respect to the notion of the self as a construct, there has been a tendency in much twentieth-century philosophy to reject the notion of a substantial self, or anything like it. Sartre and Heidegger come to mind as philosophers who reject the notion that there is anything like a human nature or natural self-development, or like a natural Aristotelian form whose task it is for the individual to realize. If Aristotle stands at the origins of the substantial self, we may assign an analogous role to Nietzsche for the constructed self. Following this latter view of the self, pathology and treatment will focus, not on the failure to achieve a natural process, as with the Aristotelian self, but rather on the failure to construct a self.

The focus of this chapter is the narrative self, and more specifically the narrative self in schizophrenia. I begin the discussion with questions about the nature of narrative and the narrative self. What is the narrative self, and where does it fit in the above debate? Is the narrative self an unfolding natural product, grounded in a common human nature, or is it a construct? Not surprisingly, the debate just described over the nature of the self is repeated in discussions of narrative theory and narrative identity. In these discussions, as will be seen below, the debate is reframed in terms of narrative reference.

The narrative self

The self of narrative identity is the 'I' that tells stories about itself, exists in those stories and conceives its identity in the terms of those stories. In Peter Brooks' words:

Our lives are ceaselessly intertwined with narrative, with the stories that we tell and hear told, those we dream or imagine or would like to tell, all of which are reworked in that story of our own lives that we narrate to ourselves in an episodic, sometimes semi-conscious, but virtually uninterrupted monologue. We live immersed in narrative, recounting and reassessing the meaning of our past actions, anticipating the outcome of our future projects, situating ourselves at the intersection of several stories not yet completed (Brooks, 1984, p. 3).

As suggested in the introduction, questions of narrative and narrative identity are not as simple as might be implied in the Brooks quotation. A major debate has emerged in recent decades concerning the exact nature of narrative – whether, to put the matter simply, narrative belongs only to fiction or also to life. The very idea of a narrative identity or narrative self hangs on the outcome of that debate. Does an actual, lived life have a narrative structure, as suggested by Peter Brooks, or are self-narratives merely fictions that bear no real reference to our lives? In the terminology of the introduction, this question could be reframed by saying that, while self-narratives are always in some fashion constructed by the individual, the question remains whether that construction emerges from, and reflects, the life of the individual, or whether the constructed self-narrative is a pure fiction that does *not* emerge from the individual life. If the self-narrative emerges *from* the individual life, it is then both construct and essence. If, however, the self-narrative bears no real reference to the individual life, it is then pure construct. In this section I will review the debate over narrative and argue for a centrist position that will be most helpful in understanding the course of the narrative self in schizophrenia.

The debate over the relation of narrative to the real world has been carried out on several fronts – or fields of specialization – history, literary theory and philosophy. In the field of history the debate was engaged in the 1960s with the publication of works by W.B. Gallie (1964), Morton White (1965) and Arthur Danto (1965), all of whom emphasized the importance of narrative in the historian's work and thus defended the narrativist traditions of nineteenth-century historiography. In contrast, other traditions of historiography rather dramatically dismissed the narrative dimension of historical work. Carl Hempel (1962) had already presented a positivist view of historical knowledge that required causal laws and was dismissive of narrative history-telling. And on a larger scale, the Annales group in France (Braudel, 1980) has been highly critical of narrative history, dismissing it as superficial in comparison with the study of long-term impersonal trends in demography, economics, etc.

An ambiguous position is held by those theoreticians who have defended the role of narrative in history but in turn argue for its fictive nature. Louis Mink (1970) may be cited here, but the most influential writer is Hayden White (1973, 1978, 1987), who has written extensively on the question of narrative and history. While defending and analysing the variety of narrative styles that are an inevitable component of history writing, White arrives at a thoroughly sceptical conclusion concerning the relation of narrative to historical reality.

> What I have sought to suggest is that this value attached to narrativity in the representation of real events arises out of a desire to have real events display the coherence, integrity, fullness, and closure of an image of life that is and can only be imaginary. The notion that sequences of real events possess the formal attributes of the stories we tell about imaginary events could only have its origin in wishes, day-dreams, reveries. Does the world really present itself to perception in the form of well-made stories, with central subjects, proper beginnings, middles, and ends, and a coherence that permits us to see 'the end' in every beginning? Or does it present itself more in the forms that the annals and chronicle suggest, either as mere sequence without beginning or end or as sequences of beginnings that only terminate and never conclude? And does the world, even the social world, ever really come to us as already narrativized, already speaking itself from beyond the horizon of our capacity to make scientific sense of it? (White, 1987, pp. 24–25)

While the relation of narrative to lived reality has been a matter of debate among historians, it is in the field of literary theory that the purely fictive nature of narrative has been most strongly promoted. In the Anglo-American world Frank Kermode has written forcefully of a longing for order that is found wanting in the world and fulfilled only in fiction. He questions in *The Genesis of Secrecy*, 'why do we labor to reduce fortuity first, before we decide that there is a way of looking which provides a place for it? I have still no satisfying answer; but it does appear that we are programmed to prefer fulfilment to disappointment, the closed to the open' (1979, p. 64). And he writes in *The Sense of an Ending* that 'in "making sense" of the world we still feel a need, harder than ever to satisfy because of an accumulated skepticism, to experience that concordance of beginning, middle, and end which is the essence of our explanatory fictions' (Kermode, 1966, p. 36).

It is however in contemporary French literary criticism that the breach between narrative and reality has been most stridently made. In both the structuralist (e.g. Levi-Strauss) and poststructuralist (e.g. Derrida, Foucault, Kristeva) waves of recent French criticism, the rupture of narrative from its referent can be found. Roland Barthes, who attacked the narrative connection both in history and literature, wrote typically with respect to the latter:

> Claims concerning the 'realism' of narrative are therefore to be discounted ... The function of narrative is not to 'represent,' it is to constitute a spectacle ... Narrative does not show, does not imitate ... 'What takes place' in a narrative is from the referential (reality) point of view literally *nothing*; 'what happens' is language alone, the adventure of language, the unceasing celebration of its coming (Barthes, 1977, p. 124).

It should be noted that this strongly sceptical vein in French narratological thinking derives rather directly from Nietzsche, the Nietzsche of *On the Advantage and*

Disadvantage of History for Life (1980), *On the Genealogy of Morals* (1969), and *The Gay Science* (1974) with its 'infinite interpretations' of the world. (In concluding this discussion of the opponents of narrative reference, I will take note of Daniel Dennett (1991), who enters the discussion from a completely different background, that of analytic philosophy and cognitive neuroscience. In arguing for a kind of self-narrative, a 'center of narrative gravity', that is a product of the brain's language-producing activity, Dennett joins forces with those historians and literary theorists who view the narrative self as a fiction of the living individual.)

In the face of all this doubt concerning the reality claims of narrative, it is of interest that the strongest defence of narrative's connection to the real world has come from three philosophers, Paul Ricoeur, David Carr and Alasdair MacIntyre. In the terminology of the introduction, these philosophers assume a centrist position. That is, while they do not argue for a literal Aristotelian substantial self, they insist that human life has a natural narrative structure. To that degree they are essentialists. On the other hand, they view the self-narrative not just as a given but as a task to be accomplished. In that sense they are also constructionists.

In his extensive three-volume treatise, *Time and Narrative* (1984, 1985, 1988), Paul Ricoeur elaborates a general thesis that narrative is the manner in which human time is articulated. He locates an ultimate narrative referentiality both in the abstractest specimens of history writing and in the most antinarrative examples of fiction. Ricoeur argues for an anchorage of narrative in lived reality by describing the ways in which the composition of plot is grounded in a 'preunderstanding' of the world of action, its symbolic structures and its temporal character. With respect to the first, the world of action, 'every narrative presupposes a familiarity with terms such as agent, goal, means, circumstance, help, hostility, cooperation, conflict, success, failure, etc., on the part of its narrator and any listener' (Ricoeur, 1984, p. 55). The point is that these terms are not the product of fictive invention but are lifted from the practical world. The second form of practical understanding that grounds narrative construction is the symbolic structures of the practical field. 'If, in fact, human action can be narrated, it is because it is always already articulated by signs, rules, and norms. It is always symbolically mediated' (ibid., p. 57). Ricoeur calls on the work of anthropologists such as Clifford Geertz (1973), who make use of *Verstehen* sociology, and of Cassirer's *The Philosophy of Symbolic Forms* (1957), to show that through symbolic structures human action is in fact prenarrated. 'In this way, symbolism confers an initial *readability* on action' (ibid., p. 58). Finally, turning to Heidegger's *Being and Time* (1962), Ricoeur describes the temporal structures that are part of practical understanding and that ground the temporal categories of formal narrative.

In his analysis of narrative Alasdair MacIntyre argues that human action is only comprehensible as intelligible action, and that this intelligibility means the embeddedness of action in a historical sequence. 'An action is a moment in a possible or actual history or in a number of such histories. The notion of a history is as fundamental a notion as the notion of an action' (MacIntyre, 1981, p. 214). He describes this interconnection of action, intelligibility and history further:

It is now becoming clear that we render the actions of others intelligible in this way because action itself has a basically historical character. It is because we all live out narratives in our lives and because we understand our own lives in terms of the narratives that we live out that the form of narrative is appropriate for understanding the actions of others. Stories are lived before they are told – except in the case of fiction (ibid., pp. 211–212).

Human activities are thus 'enacted narratives'. As such they share some of the formal properties of narrative. They have beginnings, middles and endings, as do literary works. They may be evaluated according to different genres – as, for instance, a particular sequence of events may be judged to be tragic or comic. And as in literary productions, '[actual conversations] embody reversals and recognitions; they move towards and away from climaxes. There may within a longer conversation be digressions and subplots, indeed digressions within digressions and subplots within subplots' (ibid., p. 211).

MacIntyre says further of lived narratives that they have both an unpredictable and a partially teleological character. The meaningfulness of a life is always in part a function of a projected future, but this future is marked by inevitable uncertainty. About the authorship of a lived narrative he says that one is never fully the author of the narrative that one lives out. 'We enter upon a stage which we did not design and we find ourselves part of an action that was not of our making. Each of us being a main character in his own drama plays subordinate parts in the dramas of others, and each drama constrains the others' (ibid., p. 213).

Finally, MacIntyre associates the notion of personal identity with that of narrative identity, insisting that the concept of personal identity has no meaning if it does not include the idea of narrative intelligibility. The unity of an individual life is the unity of a narrative enacted through the course of that life. He concludes that '[t]he unity of a human life is the unity of a narrative quest' (ibid., p. 219).

In his *Time, Narrative, and History* (1986) David Carr focuses on the narrative dimension of history. Modelling Husserl's effort to describe a prescientific 'lifeworld' that grounds the natural sciences, he attempts a similar task in the area of history.

What I am saying is that in a naive and prescientific way the historical past is *there* for all of us, that it *figures* in our ordinary view of things, whether we are historians or not. We have what the phenomenologists call a *non-thematic* or *pre-thematic awareness* of the historical past which functions as background for our present experience, or our experience of the present (Carr, 1986, p. 3).

Narrative is central to his study because it is our primary way of organizing our experience of time: 'understood in this sense it can elucidate our pre-theoretical past' (ibid., p. 5). In examining the pretheoretical foundations of temporality and history, Carr offers a more extensive description than either Ricoeur or MacIntyre of the narrative character of ordinary lived experience.

Following Husserl's studies of time-consciousness and expanding on them, Carr begins his analysis by demonstrating the temporally configured quality of the most basic (and brief) experiences, such as listening to a melodic line or initiating a tennis serve. He then moves on to more extended sequences to show that they also have a configured, and now fully narrative, structure. The most basic narrative configuration, which is present in life before – and whether – it is narrated in fiction, is that of the temporal whole: 'each constitutes a temporal closure, which can only be expressed by speaking of a beginning, a middle, and an end' (ibid., p. 47). He then elaborates on the ways in which this basic structure can be developed:

> Let us now take stock: though we have not yet departed from the sort of simple, short-term actions and experiences that have so far served as examples, we have found that the notion of 'temporal configuration' can be elaborated in a number of ways: first as closure or beginning, middle, and end, the most general designation of the phenomenon; then as departure and arrival, departure and return, means and end, suspension and resolution, problem and solution (ibid., p. 49).

To the objection that true narrative involves a separation of the roles of author, characters and audience, Carr responds that in the lived narrative of one's own life, one indeed assumes in some fashion all of these roles.

Carr then takes his analysis a step further by taking up, in a manner similar to MacIntyre, the theme of narrative identity. He argues that narrative structure is 'the organizing principle not only of experiences and actions but of the self who experiences and acts' (ibid., p. 73). Building on Dilthey's concept of the coherence (*Zusammenhang*) of life structures, and its further development by Heidegger in his *Being and Time*, he develops the notion of one's entire life as a narrative structure. He is however quick to add that a lived life never enjoys the orderliness of a constructed narrative. Echoing MacIntyre's felicitous idea of a 'narrative quest', he speaks of the life narrative as a task to be achieved rather than a finished project.

> at no level, and certainly not at the scale of the life-story itself, is the narrative coherence of events and actions simply a 'given' for us. Rather it is a constant task, sometimes a struggle, and when it succeeds it is an achievement. As a struggle it has an adversary, which is, described in the most general way, temporal disorder, confusion, incoherence, chaos. It is the chaos and dissolution represented, paradoxically, by the steady running-off of mere sequence. To experience, to act, to live in the most general sense, is to maintain and if necessary to restore the narrative coherence of time itself, to preserve it against this internal dissolution into its component parts (ibid., p. 96).

Finally, to the notions of narrative quest, task and challenge, as elaborated by MacIntyre and Carr, I will add another dimension of narrative identity described by Ricoeur in a book written after the series cited above. In *Oneself as Another* (Ricoeur, 1992) he introduces the notions of avowal and commitment. In projecting my life into the future, I am not only assuming the task and challenge of constructing a meaningful life, I am also assuming my commitments as part of that life.

In the analysis of 'normal' and schizophrenic self-narratives studied in this chapter, I will follow the guidelines provided by Ricoeur, MacIntyre and Carr. Their studies have the virtue of transcending the debate over narrative referentiality by arguing that while human life has a narrative structure, this structure, to use the terminology of the introduction, is *both* natural process *and* construct. Biological development, life cycle and culture provide narratives (and prenarratives, to employ Ricoeur's term) that in some manner structure an individual's life. But it remains the challenge of the individual to mould all of these givens into a more-or-less coherent, individual self-narrative. The use by the authors of terms like task, struggle and narrative quest points to the fact that the individual narrative is not simply a given structure that is laid out in advance but rather a product that is accomplished by the individual. The cultural narratives studied by Brunner (1990), for instance, represent possibilities to be realized, not formulas dictated for compliance.

A 'normal' self-narrative is one in which – to quote Peter Brooks again – '[w]e live immersed in narrative, recounting and reassessing the meaning of our past actions, anticipating the outcome of our future projects, situating ourselves at the intersection of several stories not yet completed' (Brooks, 1984, p. 3). As this quotation, and the above analyses by Ricoeur, MacIntyre and Carr suggest, narrative identity does not imply that the individual lives out one coherent life story, with beginning, middle and end. It means rather that we can only think about ourselves in a temporal, narrativized fashion, situated in a present that bears the past and projects itself imaginatively into the future. As Heidegger has emphasized (1962), we live very much in the future perfect, thinking about ourselves in the present from the point of view of a future time – I orient myself *now* from a perspective of looking back at myself from a projected future, *how I will have been*. And as Heidegger has also emphasized, one's past is always in some manner refashioned from the perspective of the present and future. At any given point in my life, my past represents the preparation for my current and future projects. As those projects change, so will my interpretation of my past.

The temporal sequences in which we live our lives form not one but many narratives, some large, some small, some embedded in other narratives. There will be many beginnings, middles and endings. For most individuals two of the larger narratives are those of career and personal life. The narrative of one's career, for instance, will be both planned and subject to unexpected contingencies and changes in focus. It will be composed of larger trajectories and many subplots. It will contain satisfactions and regrets over past accomplishments and failures, and hopes and anticipations of future accomplishments that will fulfil or redeem the past. All of this may also be said of that other larger narrative, that of one's personal life. It too will be filled with larger trajectories and smaller subplots. The raising of children is a subplot in a marriage. And the frequency of divorce attests to the way in which marriage narratives encounter breaks in the plot line that were not anticipated in the initial projections. The end of a relationship or marriage, or of a particular job, is both an ending of one episode and a beginning of another.

Still another dimension of life narratives is revealed by the psychoanalytic approach and what may be called the psychoanalytic or psychodynamic narrative (Phillips, 1999). What the psychoanalytic approach suggests is the possibility of an 'unconscious' narrative – that is, the possibility that there are themes being lived out of which the individual is unaware. To suggest a simple example, a man may be pursuing his career in a fully self-aware fashion and at the same time be engaging in an unconscious, competitive battle with his father. Thus there are not one but two self-narratives here, one conscious, the other unconscious. This man may not become aware of the second narrative unless it gets him into trouble and provides the occasion for therapeutic reflection. Then he might discover, for instance, that the aggressive behaviour toward his superiors that has caused trouble in his professional life has less to do with his superiors' treatment of him than with old, forgotten battles with his father. In this case, then, the original self-narrative – the way in which the man would have described his life – is modified with the interpellation of the second, psychoanalytically oriented narrative.

Finally, to these various narratives and subnarratives, conscious and not, that compose a life, we need to add that each life narrative has its final ending in death, an ending that is unique in that it is anticipated but not available for retrospective reflection.

The narrative self in schizophrenia

Narrative identity can take many turns – undergo many deformations – in schizophrenia. In the remainder of the chapter I will illustrate with case histories three such deformations. While the three styles of schizophrenic narrative described here are typical of this condition, I hasten to add that, firstly, they are not the only styles of schizophrenic self-narrative, and secondly, any case may mix the styles described. The first case, a man with long-standing chronic schizophrenia, is an example of a rather impoverished and fragmented self-narrative, a narrative that is limited by the cognitive and emotional deficits that are central to the chronic schizophrenic condition. This is an example of the way in which the schizophrenic process itself imposes cognitive limitations on the narrativizing activity. The second case, a man with rather flamboyant delusional experiences, represents a style of self-narrative in which the challenges of developing a self-narrative are resolved through the creation of a delusional narrative. The final case, a woman with schizoaffective disorder, demonstrates the style of attempting to deal with the schizophrenic condition through the use of a 'sick' narrative.

The first case is that of a man who is now 58 years old and whom I have had in treatment for the past 25 years. The patient, whom I will call Mr B, had an uneventful early life and suffered his first schizophrenic breakdown following his marriage and the birth of a first child in his early 20s. The next several years were marked by efforts to work, repeated psychotic breaks and hospitalizations, and attempts at outpatient treatment. Another child was born during these years. The acute psychotic episodes were described as episodes in which he would become acutely psychotic with vivid hallucinatory and delusional experiences, and would become violent, threatening his wife and throwing and breaking objects in the house. The most persistent and recurrent delusion was that he would be burned at the stake for his sins. Before going to the hospital he would generally spend time at his mother's house, as she had more capacity than his wife to calm him down.

Gradually Mr B assumed a disabled status and limited himself to doing minor household chores and a limited amount of child care. His wife, who was a trained secretary, returned to work as soon as the children were of school age. For most of the next two decades the family life of the B family was relatively calm. Mr B remained at home, Mrs B worked, and the children were raised and did well. The pattern changed about 3 years ago when, for reasons that have remained unclear, Mr B would decide abruptly to stop taking his medication for several days at a time. His behaviour and self-care would deteriorate dramatically, he would become vaguely psychotic, but he would not become violent as in his younger years. These episodes would produce a crisis in the home – the children were all out of the house by this point – and the patient would at times resume his medication and at other times have to be committed for a brief hospitalization. After this pattern repeated itself several times, the patient's wife instituted divorce proceedings during one of the hospitalizations. The patient returned to his parents' house, where he now lives. He still continues the pattern of not taking medication for days at a time – now exasperating his mother rather than his wife – but for the most part he has assumed a new role of offering considerable help to his ageing parents, his mother now rather frail and his father having suffered a stroke and being partially paralysed.

Mr B presents a self-narrative that is fragmentary, impoverished and clearly a product of his disordered thinking style. I should add that on the few occasions when I have asked him directly for his view of his self, he has responded by laughing and telling me not to ask stupid questions. In his own spontaneous, nonreflective manner, the ingredients he has tried to integrate into a self-narrative include the nature and origin of his condition, his inability to work, his strong but barely acknowledged feelings about not being the working man of the house, his marriage and children, and now his life out of the marriage, with his parents and his grandchildren. In the early years of treatment he would talk a lot about working and not working. He would refer to himself as mentally ill and unable to work, and he would intersperse comments about being burned at the stake – not, however, directly relating these to his failures as a bread-winner. He would talk about managing the family garden and cutting wood for the wood stove in winter, obviously taking some satisfaction in these accomplishments. He would often break into an ongoing conversation with statements about how it all started when . . . , and he would generally fill this in with some moment in his early marriage when his wife said something, which was supposedly the start of his mental illness. Over the years his comments about his wife became increasingly disparaging. He clearly felt himself to be in an emasculated position as the disabled mental patient with a wife who was both working and raising the two children. In recent years the major focus of our conversation has been his pattern of going off the medication and getting into trouble. He complains about the side-effects and insists that he does not really need the medication and is more himself without it. He doesn't seem to mind the life disruptions and hospitalizations and denies that there is any problem with going off the medication.

Mr B has always, from my point of view, been unable to present a coherent life narrative or sense of self. He does not articulate a life history that incorporates the schizophrenia in a way that can be adapted to and lived with. The dimension of constructed or fictive self is occasional, unpredictable, fragmented, at times delusional, and not very coherent. It contains the burning at the stake, the various moments at which the illness started, and the frequent, imagined accusations toward his wife. It does *not* involve the projection of an imagined future that connects with the present and past in a constructive and hopeful manner. The integration of future into his narrative has always been minimal. When he thinks about it, he imagines a future in which he will be living on the street, or more positively, in which he will simply be living comfortably in a hospital. His efforts to locate a self that is not that of the mentally ill man take the form of occasional pathetic denials of his illness and the insistence that he is more himself off the medication, whatever the devastations that occur in that state. In his best moments now, he seems pleased to be out of a marriage in which he felt inadequate, and back with his parents where he has found a helpful and productive family role. With his fragmented and impoverished self-narrative, Mr B presents a self that is barren and minimally unified.

The second case, Mr S, is a 35-year-old single man whose difficulties began at some point in the later years of high school with problems relating to other students.

He went away to college and again experienced a lot of difficulty both with his social life and his studies. In the course of the college years he affiliated himself with a religious cult that provided a lot of structure for him psychologically. Following college he returned to his parents' house and, following a temper outburst, accepted the recommendation of a family friend to seek psychiatric help for the first time. His initial presentation suggested a probable course of a developing thought disorder over the previous years. He described dramatic symptoms of thought insertion, ideas of reference and paranoid feelings about how he was treated by other people. He had no fixed delusions, although his religious system allowed for vivid identifications with historical figures of whom he was the reincarnation. He described a couple of visual and auditory hallucinatory experiences from the past year. Following the initial several months of outpatient psychotherapy Mr S made a serious suicide attempt and was psychiatrically hospitalized. He was then referred to another city for a several-year treatment that involved a long inpatient hospitalization and intensive outpatient psychotherapy. Eventually, he returned to his mother's house and resumed treatment with me. For the next several years, he worked in the accounting field, in which he had been trained, lived independently, remained actively involved in his religious group and remained in treatment. Despite the extended inpatient hospitalization and extended outpatient treatment with his hospital psychiatrist, as well as ample use of neuroleptic medication, and also despite the fact that he was able to work and go about his life, Mr S remained in some sense chronically psychotic. He believed that his entire mental life was controlled by other people. At times this would take the form of his guru putting good thoughts into his head; at other times it had the more paranoid quality of other individuals implanting destructive thoughts. He would regularly misinterpret the actions and motivations of others, assuming that events or actions were intended for him that bore no relation to him. An active topic of therapy sessions was the question of coincidence, whether things could just happen by coincidence and did not necessarily have to have a relation to him.

Mr S had a good memory and a very clear sense of his past and future. He frequently talked about events from his past, and he regularly considered what the future had in store for him. Unlike Mr B, his thought pattern was internally clear, and his self-narrative was fully smooth and coherent. On the other hand, the self-narrative was marked by all the idiosyncratic and flamboyant aspects of this man's view of himself. Since he saw himself as the vehicle of forces greater than himself, the narrative was always presented in the passive voice. In the patient's narrative, he was the reincarnation of an assortment of past historical figures – important figures, it should be noted – and his current life was thus the continuation of those previous lives. In this particular life and incarnation, he was destined to live out his existence as he was doing at this moment but was destined for greater religious achievements in the coming years. He would often express some uncertainty about the future, raising the question about whether he had read the signs correctly. If he made a prediction that did not come to pass, he interpreted that as his having misread the inspiration rather than his being wrong about the phenomenon of inspiration.

From the perspective of the theme of this chapter, this patient presents an excess of the constructed and the fictive in his self-narrative. The balance of construct and reference in his narrative tilts a long way in the direction of construct. His sense of the past and future are quite strong, but they are so delusionally coloured that they present a parody of the Heideggerian self (*Desein*) projecting itself into the future out of its past. The delusional embellishments with which he adorns his narrative bear little reference to his life, but they do manage, most of the time, to maintain a cheerful, optimistic mood. In the variations on self-narrative in schizophrenia, he represents the delusional resolution to the schizophrenic problem. If the previous patient, Mr B, presents a *fragmented* schizophrenic narrative, this man presents a *delusional* schizophrenic narrative.

The third and final case is that of a woman, Mrs M, in her early 40s, who had her first psychotic experience when she was away at college. A several-month period of deteriorating academic functioning and social withdrawal led finally to a florid psychosis with an abundance of bizarre and religious delusions. After a failed brief hospitalization, she was hospitalized at the age of 20 in a long-term hospital for over a year. The next several years were marked by efforts to live independently and to work and support herself. There were several psychotic decompensations with brief hospitalizations during these years. During the past decade she has gradually done better, completing her education, working in accounting, getting married and having a child. She has not been hospitalized in several years. It is during this recent decade that she has been my patient.

In our sessions Mrs M has focused on a great variety of relevant topics, but a prevailing theme has been the illness itself. She has struggled unceasingly to find a way to think of herself as something other than 'mentally ill'. She has also acted this out in her use of psychotropic medication, going for periods with no medication, always trying to find the most minimal dose that maintains her stability. She has become an expert in the art of recognizing early signs of psychosis and adjusting her medication quickly upward, thus aborting further decompensation and the need for hospitalization. Although this use of the medication is an acquired skill of which the patient might be proud, it is also a strong reminder that she *does* need the medication and becomes sick when off it for any period of time. The medication, instead of being an automatic ritual that is barely focused on, remains an active object of attention and an active reminder of the painful reality of her mental illness.

The central issue in this woman's sense of self and self-narrative is the place of the illness in the narrative. The resolution we would probably all suggest – that of thinking of herself as *having* an illness but *being* more than the illness – is not easily available to her. When she thinks of herself as mentally ill, the illness becomes almost her total reality, and her story becomes simply that of the progression of a mental illness. In reaction to the 'mental illness' self-interpretation, she tries to develop self-narratives that diminish the mental illness – usually to the point of nonexistence. She has tried many of these, but has not been able to sustain any of them because of their blatant irreality. She has, for instance, tried to convince herself that the mental illness is merely some kind of an allergy. She has tried many variations on a theme in which the diagnosis is a kind of mistake – that, for instance, she was simply immature and away from home too soon, or that her self-assertion and reasonable disagreements have been misinterpreted as mental illness. Of course these self-interpretations always break down when the need for medication intrudes itself, and at that point she flips back into the illness narrative.

Mrs M's sense of her future alternates with the self-interpretation that is dominant at any moment. When she is feeling overwhelmed by the prospect of unremitting psychiatric illness, she is pessimistic and cannot see a future beyond that of the illness. When she is escaping into fantasies of not being ill, she can imagine a future, but it is one that is founded on the denial of illness.

In the context of our theme her self-narratives show an attempt to come to terms with her schizophrenic condition by developing a balanced 'illness narrative' (Kleinman, 1988), that is, a narrative that combines a realistic acknowledgement of her condition with an assurance that there is more to her than the schizophrenia. Her struggle – and frequent failure – to achieve this balance is a reminder of the fact that the illness narratives of the chronic psychiatric conditions tend to be totalizing in a way that physical illness narratives are not. In the case of the latter, even when the physical illness is a severe one, it remains easier for the patient to say, 'I am not my illness'. In contrast with the first two patients, Mrs M's narrative is neither fragmented nor delusional (except to the extent that the fantasies of not being psychiatrically ill assume delusional proportions). It is an effort to cope with her condition with the use of an illness narrative, and her difficulties with the narrative reflect the uniqueness of her psychiatric condition in developing such a narrative.

Conclusion

In concluding this chapter I will make note of the fact that this discussion of the narrative self in schizophrenia has not dealt at all with the current and recent findings regarding the biological basis of schizophrenia. This neglect does not reflect a disregard for the importance of such findings but rather an effort to approach schizophrenia from a perspective – that of self, identity and self-narratives – that is also important and that will eventually have to be correlated with the findings of the biological sciences.

I will close by pointing to one such current effort in the direction of that correlation. I am referring to Antonio Demasio's recent *The Feeling of What Happens* (1999). In his integrated view of consciousness, Demasio presents the 'autobiographical self' as a product of a higher form of consciousness – extended consciousness – that involves language and an awareness of one's past and future. Demasio's 'autobiographical self' is in fact quite close to what I am describing as the narrative self. In his investigation of the disruptions of the autobiographical self by various neurological conditions, he approaches the question of schizophrenia.

We can also find examples of impaired extended consciousness in a number of psychiatric conditions, although, given the complexity of these conditions, any interpretation in terms of this framework should be regarded as tentative... Some manifestations of schizophrenia, for instance, thought insertion and auditory hallucinations, may be interpreted in part as disorders of extended consciousness. In all likelihood, the patients so affected have anomalous autobiographical memories and deploy anomalous autobiographical selves. It should be noted, however, that during the appearance of such manifestations, the 'objects' of their perceptions may be in and of themselves anomalous, and that their proto-selves and core consciousness may be anomalous as well (Demasio, 1999, pp. 215–216).

Demasio of course offers nothing conclusive on this topic. His work is, however, of great interest in that it points to the challenge before us in understanding schizophrenia – that of integrating the kind of analysis attempted in this chapter with the ever-increasing findings from the biological sciences.

(A thorough review of neuroscientific findings concerning schizophrenia and narrative identity may be found in Shaun Gallagher's contribution to this volume (chapter 16). He identifies four capacities – temporal integration of information, minimal self-reference, encoding and retrieving episodic–autobiographical memories and engaging in reflective metacognition – that are both neurobiologically grounded and necessary for the development of self-narrative. Testing those capacities against the case histories detailed in this chapter points to the usefulness of the capacities approach and at the same time to the elusiveness of schizophrenics in conforming to research protocols. Mr B, the most chronic of the patients, with a full range of negative symptoms, readily demonstrates failures in all of the four capacities. Mr S, on the other hand, shows no impairment in either temporal integration of information or episodic–autobiographical memories. His pathology is in the areas of delusional thinking and significant disturbance of ego boundaries. His capacity for self-reference is thus significantly disturbed and, as suggested by Gallagher, his elaborate delusions also suggest an impairment of reflective metacognition. Finally,

Mrs M is striking in that, when taking her medication, she does not exhibit a clear impairment in any of the four capacities. Her conflict over her psychotic condition is certainly troubling for her, but the conflict is not in itself different from that of a nonpsychotic person struggling against the acceptance of a physical illness. What Mrs M reminds us of is the role of medication and negative symptoms in schizophrenic research. In the absence of chronic negative symptoms, she does not exhibit impairment in the capacities while on medication, although she would display dramatic impairment if psychotic. At the other end of the schizophrenic spectrum, Mr B, with a full gamut of negative symptoms, gives ample evidence of impairment in the capacities while fully medicated.)

REFERENCES

Barthes, R. (1977). *Image, Music, Text*. Translated by S. Heath. New York: Hill and Wang.

Braudel, F. (1980). *On History*. Translated by S. Matthews. Chicago: University of Chicago Press.

Brooks, P. (1984). *Reading for the Plot*. New York: Vintage Books.

Brunner, J. (1990). *Acts of Meaning*. Cambridge, MA: The Harvard University Press.

Carr, D. (1986). *Time, Narrative, and History*. Bloomington: University of Indiana Press.

Cassirer, E. (1957). *The Philosophy of Symbolic Forms*, vol. 3. *The Phenomenology of Knowledge*. Translated by R. Manheim. New Haven: Yale University Press.

Danto, A. (1965). *Analytic Philosophy of History*. Cambridge: Cambridge University Press.

Demasio, A. (1999). *The Feeling of What Happens: Body and Emotion in the Making of Consciousness*. New York: Harcourt Brace.

Dennett, D. (1991). *Consciousness Explained*. Boston: Little, Brown.

Gallie, W.B. (1964). *Philosophical and Historical Understanding*. London: Chatto and Windus.

Geertz, C. (1973). *The Interpretation of Cultures*. New York: Basic Books.

Heidegger, M. (1962). *Being and Time*. Translated by J. Macquarrie & E. Robinson. New York: Harper and Row.

Hempel, C.G. (1962). Explanation in science and history. In *Frontiers of Science and Philosophy*, ed. R. Colodny, pp. 7–34. Pittsburgh: Pittsburgh Press.

Kermode, F. (1966). *The Sense of an Ending*. London: Oxford University Press.

Kermode, F. (1979). *The Genesis of Secrecy*. Cambridge, MA: The Harvard University Press.

Kleinman, A. (1988). *The Illness Narratives: Suffering, Healing and the Human Condition*. New York: Basic Books.

MacIntyre, A. (1981). *After Virtue*. Notre Dame: University of Notre Dame Press.

Mink, L. (1970). History and fiction as modes of comprehension. *New Literary History*, **I**: 541–58.

Nietzsche, F. (1969). *On the Genealogy of Morals*. Translated by W. Kaufmann. New York: Vintage Books.

Nietzsche, F. (1974). *The Gay Science*. Translated by W. Kaufmann. New York: Vintage Books.

Nietzsche, F. (1980). *On the Advantage and Disadvantage of History for Life*. Translated by P. Preuss. Indianapolis: Hackett.

Phillips, J. (1999). The psychodynamic narrative. In *Healing Stories: Narrative in Psychiatry and Psychotherapy*, ed. G. Roberts & J. Holmes, pp. 27–48. Oxford: Oxford University Press.

Ricoeur, P. (1984). *Time and Narrative*, vol. I. Translated by K. McLaughlin & D. Pellauer. Chicago: University of Chicago Press.

Ricoeur, P. (1985). *Time and Narrative*, vol. II. Translated by K. McLaughlin & D. Pellauer. Chicago: University of Chicago Press.

Ricoeur, P. (1988). *Time and Narrative*, vol. III. Translated by K. McLaughlin & D. Pellauer. Chicago: University of Chicago Press.

Ricoeur, P. (1992). *Oneself as Another*. Translated by K. Blamey. Chicago: University of Chicago Press.

White, M. (1965). *Foundations of Historical Knowledge*. New York: Harper and Row.

White, H. (1973). *Metahistory, The Historical Imagination in Nineteenth Century Europe*. Baltimore: Johns Hopkins University Press.

White, H. (1978). *Tropics of Discourse*. Baltimore: Johns Hopkins University Press.

White, H. (1987). *The Content of the Form*. Baltimore: Johns Hopkins University Press.

Winnicott, D.W. (1965). *The Maturational Processes and the Facilitating Environment*. New York: International Universities Press.

16

Self-narrative in schizophrenia

Shaun Gallagher

Department of Philosophy and Cognitive Science, Canisius College, Buffalo, NY, USA

Abstract

Proper structures of self-narrative depend on at least four capacities in the narrator: (1) a capacity for temporal integration of information; (2) a capacity for minimal self-reference; (3) a capacity for encoding and retrieving autobiographical memories; (4) a capacity for engaging in reflective metacognition. This chapter explicates the cognitive, phenomenological, narratological and neurological details of these four capacities and their dysfunction in schizophrenia, as evidenced by schizophrenic self-narrative.

Introduction

The concept of the narrative self involves a diachronic and complex structure that depends on reflective experience and on factors that are conceptual, emotional and socially embedded. According to a narrative approach, persons constitute their own identity by formulating autobiographical narratives – life stories (Schechtman, 1996). In this chapter I want to explore issues pertaining to the generation and structure of the narrative self in schizophrenia. Normal generation of a narrative self depends on the proper functioning of a variety of cognitive capacities, including capacities for short-term temporal processing (working memory), self-awareness, episodic memory and reflective metacognition. Neuropsychological research suggests that in schizophrenia the mechanisms responsible for each of these elements are frequently disrupted. It should not be surprising that, as a result, schizophrenic narratives, and the self that is constituted through them, are problematic, both in structure and content. (Problems with narrative self-identity begin at the prodromal stage for preschizophrenic subjects at school age (Hartmann et al., 1984).)

Self-narrative

We think of ourselves as entities extended in time, and this is reflected in the way that we speak of ourselves. We have memories that extend to our past and we make plans that project into an uncertain future. As individual selves, we encompass a multiplicity of experiences that are linked in causal and intentional continuities. To some degree each of us has a sense of being a continuous and temporally extended self.

Some philosophers, however, think that the continuity of the self is illusory. Hume (1739: reprinted 1975), for example, famously suggested that the self consists of nothing but a bundle of momentary impressions that are strung together by memory or the imagination. On this view an extended self is simply a fiction. It may be a useful fiction because it lends to life a practical sense of continuity, or operates as a defence mechanism against a fundamental anxiety (Sartre, 1936). Narrative theories of self are more recent versions of the Humean view, informed now by social psychology (see, for example, Bruner and Kalmar, 1998). The invention of a self is not a private affair that happens in the confines of an individual mind. Rather, a self is constructed at the intersections of communicative and social practices. On some theories of the narrative self I am nothing other than the character that appears in the stories that I tell about myself and that others tell about me.

Dennett (1988, 1991) proposes a version of narrative theory consistent with recent developments in neuroscience. He finds in the brain something analogous to what Hume had found in the mind, a collection of distributed processes with no central theatre, no real, neurological centre of experience. (Hume had used the metaphor of the theatre, but immediately set it aside: 'The mind is a kind of theatre, where several perceptions successively make their appearance ... The comparison of the theatre must not mislead us. They are the successive perceptions only, that constitute the mind; nor have we the most distant notion of the place, where these scenes are represented' (p. 253). Dennett (1991) critiques the notion of a Cartesian theatre.) Thus, there is no real simplicity of experience at one time nor real identity across time that we could label the self. The physical brain is real, however, and it generates a minimal biological distinction between self and nonself – a distinction, however, that is not sufficient for the purpose of creating an identical self at the level of personal experience. Importantly, however, the brain is capable of generating virtual connections that traverse the human social environment. That is, the brain, operating in social settings produced by evolutionary fortuity, generates language. Language allows us to weave stories that trace our experiences in relatively coherent plots over extended time periods. In these stories we extend our biological identities through the use of words like 'I' and 'you'. A self emerges from such practices: what I call myself comes to be called my *self*.

On Dennett's account, biological organisms with brains like ours cannot prevent themselves from inventing selves. We are hardwired to become language users. Once caught in the web of language we begin spinning our own stories. But we are not totally in control of the product. As Dennett puts it, 'for the most part we don't spin them [the stories]; they spin us' (1991, p. 418). The self that is produced in this spinning, however, has no substantial reality. Rather, the narrative self is an empty abstraction. Dennett defines it as an abstract 'center of narrative gravity', and he likens the self to the theoretical construct of the centre of gravity found in any physical object. A narrative self is an abstract and movable point where various fictional or biographical stories about ourselves, told by ourselves or by others, intersect.

Philosophically there is some question as to whether an account of the narrative self is a sufficient account of the self more generally, that is, whether the whole story about the self is that it is *nothing more than* a story about the self. There is, nevertheless, a growing consensus that the concept of the narrative self captures something essential about human existence. Still, within the general consensus there are disagreements. In contrast to Dennett, for example, Ricoeur (1992) conceives of the narrative self, not as an abstract point at the intersection of various narratives, but as something richer and more concrete. He emphasizes the fact that one's own self-narrative is always entangled in the narratives of others, and that out of this entanglement comes a unified life narrative that helps to shape the individual's continuing behaviour.

Let me extend these remarks with two further observations. Firstly, although my own self-narrative is greatly influenced by what others say about me, and is more generally constrained by the kinds of things that can be said, and that are said about persons in my culture, my own self-narrative has, from a first-person perspective, a priority in shaping my self-identity. What others say can have an effect on my self-identity from a first-person perspective only in so far as it can be related, positively or negatively, with my own self-narrative. What someone else says about me *matters* only so far as it fits or fails to fit into my own self-narrative. This priority is important for the following discussion.

Secondly, in contrast to either a simple abstract point of intersecting narratives (Dennett), or a unified product of a consistent narrative (Ricoeur), it is also possible to conceive of the self as a complex narrative product that is not fully unified – a product of incomplete summation and selective subtraction, imperfect memories and multiple reiterations. The self so conceived can provide a good model to explain the various equivocations, contradictions and struggles that find expression within an individual's personal life. On a psychological level, a narrative model like this could account for conflict, moral indecision and self-deception, in a way that would be difficult to work out in terms of more traditional theories of self-identity.

A narrative model of the self may also lend itself to developing an account of certain pathological experiences. To pursue this idea we first need to identify those elements that seem essential to the normal formation of self-narratives. We will then ask which of these elements are problematic in cases of schizophrenic narrative.

There are at least four cognitive capacities that condition the formation of self-narratives:

1. a capacity for temporal integration of information;
2. a capacity for minimal self-reference;
3. a capacity for encoding and retrieving episodic–autobiographical memories;
4. a capacity for engaging in reflective metacognition.

If any one of these mechanisms fails we would expect that failure to be reflected in the subject's self-narrative. In schizophrenia the situation is far more complex. There is good evidence that in some instances more than one, and possibly all of these mechanisms fail. In the following sections we examine each of these capacities in turn, exploring questions that ultimately throw light on the nature of the self in schizophrenia.

Temporal integration

In general, narrative involves a twofold temporal structure. First, there is always a timeframe that is internal to the narrative itself, a serial order in which one event follows another. This internal timeframe allows for the composition of narrative structure. Although in some way each event in the narrative is something new and different ('discordance'), in another way each event is part of a series ('concordance'), determined by what came before and constraining what is to come (Ricoeur, 1992). Configurations of concordance and discordance make possible the basic structure of narrative, the plot.

In contrast to this internal time structure, a second, external temporality defines the narrator's temporal relation to the events of the narrative. Even if this relation is left unspecified ('Once upon a time...') it is usually open to a specification that these events happened in the past, or will happen in the future, relative to the narrator's present. Of course it is possible that if the events never happened and never will happen (as in the case of fictional events) we might think of them precisely as not having a specifiable place in time relative to the narrator. Since this cannot be the case with respect to self-narrative, however, this possibility need not concern us here. Even if the event in question never did happen (for example, an event falsely remembered) or never will happen (for example, a planned event that never comes to be actualized) in self-narrative it is still set in a temporal relation to the narrator.

The external timeframe is perspectival in a way that the internal timeframe is not. The external timeframe is defined relative to the narrator who defines the present. From the perspective of the narrator telling the story, the events of the story, which internally maintain their serial relations (x happens before y), may be more or less remotely past (or future). In self-narrative it is always the case that the narrator (oneself) is related to the events in the narrative in a perspectival way. The events recounted in the narrative are part of the narrator's immediate or remote past, or are projected to be part of the narrator's future, or are happening to the narrator in the present. Someone who is incapable of maintaining a normal perspectival frame of reference is unable to generate a self-narrative properly specified in its temporal framework.

There is a large body of evidence indicating that some schizophrenic subjects experience problems pertaining to temporal experience in ways that interfere with both internal and external temporal frameworks. Future time-perspective is curtailed in schizophrenia (Dilling & Rabin, 1967). Minkowski describes schizophrenia as involving 'acts without concern for tomorrow'. He quotes a patient: 'There is an absolute fixity around me. I have even less mobility for the future than I have for the present and the past. There is a kind of routine in me which does not allow me to envisage the future. The creative power in me is abolished. I see the future as a repetition of the past' (Minkowski, 1933, p. 277).

Schizophrenics also experience difficulties in indexing events in time, and these difficulties are positively correlated to symptoms of auditory hallucinations, feelings of being influenced and problems that involve distinguishing between self and nonself (Melges, 1982; Melges & Freeman, 1977). Some schizophrenic narratives are characterized by a derailing of thought; by constant tangents, the loss of goal, the loosening of associations or the compression of a temporally extended story to a single gesture (Cutting, 1998). Self-narratives of some schizophrenic patients reflect more general problems in the proper sequencing of events and self-placement in appropriate temporal frameworks. (The impoverished and fragmented self-narratives of James Phillips' patient, Mr B, reflect both problems with future perspective and sequencing (see chapter 15, this volume). Problems with proper sequencing of events can also be found in patients interviewed by Bernal (2001).) One patient reports:

> I felt as if I had been put back, as if something of the past had returned, so to speak, toward me ... so that not only time repeated itself again but all that had happened for me during that time as well ... In the middle of all this something happened which did not seem to belong there. Suddenly it was not only 11:00 again, but a time which has passed a long time before was there ... In the middle of time I was coming from the past toward myself ... Before there was a before and after. Yet it isn't there now ... [When someone visits and then leaves] it could very well have happened yesterday. I can no longer arrange it, in order to know where it belongs (cited by Minkowski, 1933, (reprinted 1970), pp. 284–286).

Schizophrenics have difficulty planning and initiating action (Levin, 1984), problems with temporal organization (DePue et al., 1975) and experienced continuity (Pöppel, 1994). Bovet & Parnas (1993, p. 584) describe these problems in general terms as an 'impairment of self-temporalization'.

Impairment of self-temporalization manifests itself not only across these internal and external frames, but also in short-term integration. Working memory involves the temporal integration of experience over very short periods of time. Studies of spatial (Keefe et al., 1997), temporal ordering (Dreher et al., 2001) and verbal (Wexler et al., 1998) tasks in schizophrenics show marked deficits of working memory (Goldman-Rakic, 1994; Park & Holzman, 1992; Gold et al., 1997; Carter et al., 1998; Cohen et al., 1999). Difficulties with the processing of working memory sometimes manifest themselves as 'formal thought disorders' – a breakdown of the temporal organization of reasoning and speech (Fuster, 1999), 'cognitive dysmetria' (Andreasen et al., 1998) and relatively slow speeds of cognitive processing (Fuster, 1997, 1999; Tauscher-Wisniewski, 1999). Problems that some schizophrenics have in keeping track of recent actions (Mlakar et al., 1994), and with respect to the sense of agency may involve their inability to anticipate or sequence in working memory their own actions (Gallagher, 2000b). They also perform poorly on delayed-response tasks (Strous et al., 1995; Fleming et al., 1997). (Disorganized cognition includes perspectival shifts that disrupt the subject's ability to block out alternative perspectives (Sass, 1992, p. 144), an ability that is necessary for unconfused action and clear communication.)

Singh and his colleagues have linked these temporalization problems with the same neurological dysfunctions involved in the schizophrenic's voluntary movement (Singh et al., 1992; also see Graybiel, 1997). Schizophrenics show a greater propensity to misattribute a perceived self-movement that is delayed from the actual movement, reflecting a difficulty in the perception of slight temporal differences (Daprati et al., 1997; Franck et al., 2001). They are unable to discriminate between different velocities of a moving vertical grating (Chen et al., 1999) or a moving dot (Schwartz et al., 1999). This suggests an inability to integrate efficiently temporal cues in their perception of movement. A failure of temporal integration may explain the schizophrenic's difficulty in generating spontaneous actions, as well as difficulties in performing self-directed search (Frith, 1992).

As a result of disturbances in temporal integration, the continuity (semantic binding) of experience often breaks down in schizophrenia (Pöppel & Schwender, 1993; Pöppel, 1994). Studies have found evidence for the failure of intermodal sensory integration in schizophrenic experience (Parnas et al., 1996; de Gelder et al., 1997, in press). It is not surprising, then, that problems with temporal integration and intermodal binding are reflected in the narratives of schizophrenics. One patient reports: 'sometimes everything is so fragmented, when it should be so unified. A bird in the garden chirps, for example. I heard the bird, and I know that he chirps; but that it is a bird and that he chirps, these two things are separated from each other' (cited by Minkowski, 1933, p. 285).

Neurologically, temporal integration and self-temporalization are linked to frontal brain structures (von Steinbüchel et al., 1996; Pöppel, 1997). The sequencing of events in proper order is disrupted after frontal lobe lesions, especially in damage to the left frontal lobe (Milner, 1974; Pöppel, 1978). Integration of experienced content in the time domain, the temporal integration of sensory information (intermodal binding) in behavioural and linguistic sequences and the proper functioning of working memory depend on brain activity in the prefrontal cortex (Fuster, 1997; Fuster et al., 2000). There is good evidence to suggest that schizophrenia involves just such prefrontal dysfunction. Schizophrenic patients, compared with controls, show significantly lower relative blood flow in prefrontal regions during working memory tasks (Rubin et al., 1994). There is evidence from positron emission tomography (PET) studies for reduced metabolic rate in bilateral prefrontal regions in schizophrenics during behavioural performance (Singh et al., 1992; Andreasen et al., 1996; Goldberg & Weinberger, 1996). Neuropsychological and neurophysiological studies show similarities of impairments in schizophrenic patients and in those with frontal lobe damage (Frith & Done 1988; Goldman-Rakic, 1995). Both categories of patients demonstrate impairments on a variety of cognitive and behavioural tests. It is well noted, however, that dysfunction in the prefrontal cortex necessarily implicates the basal ganglia, thalamus, brainstem, hippocampal formation and other neocortical areas since the prefrontal cortex interacts with a complex distributed network (Goldman-Rakic & Selemon, 1997).

Capabilities related to temporal integration and the linear ordering of events within a temporal framework are essential to the formation of the narrative perspective and to the sequential order that characterizes narrative. The proper functioning of working memory is also a necessary condition for capabilities that are directly relevant to the formation of self-narrative, namely, capabilities that involve minimal self-reference and episodic–autobiographical memory.

Minimal self-reference

To begin to form a self-narrative one must be able to refer to oneself by using the first-person pronoun. In turn, the development of the ability to use the first-person pronoun depends on a primitive sense of differentiation between self and nonself. Experiments on neonate imitation clearly show that the sense of this differentiation is present in the human infant from birth (Meltzoff & Moore, 1977; Gallagher & Meltzoff, 1996). This sense of differentiation is the basis for a minimal self – a self that is accessible to immediate and present self-consciousness. It is this minimal self which is extended and enhanced in the self-narrative. Without the basic sense of differentiation between self and nonself I would not be able to refer to myself with any specification, and self-narrative would have no starting point.

Certain forms of access that I have to my minimal self cannot be mistaken, and as a result certain uses of the first-person pronoun in self-reference are immune to error through misidentification (Shoemaker, 1968). For example, if I say 'I think it is going to rain today', I may be entirely wrong about the rain, but I cannot be wrong about the I. I cannot say 'I' and mean to identify someone else by that word. If I say 'I see that John is at his desk', I can be wrong about it being a desk; I can be wrong about it being John; and I can even be wrong about my cognitive act (it may be hallucination rather than visual perception). It would be nonsensical, however, to ask me 'Are you sure that *you* are the one who sees that John is at his desk?'

Importantly, even in cases where I do *objectively* misidentify myself (e.g. if I mistakenly claim that I am the one who hit the target, when in fact it is somebody else who hit the target), I am not mistaken in my *subjective* self-reference (Wittgenstein, 1958; Strawson, 1994). When I say 'I', I am referring to myself, even though I may be wrong about who hit the target. Indeed, I can objectively misidentify myself in this respect only because I have correctly self-referred. In such cases, it is precisely myself about whom I am wrong. The immunity principle holds for such cases of self-reference because they are cases in which there is no need for identification, and thus no chance of misidentification (Shoemaker, 1968). In other words, we are immune to error in this regard, not because we are so proficient, or so infallible at judging who we are, but because this kind of self-awareness doesn't involve a judgement at all. In this way I can never subjectively misidentify myself when I say 'I'. This makes the minimal self an extremely secure anchor for self-narratives.

The minimal self has a structure that can be articulated into several elements. There is good evidence from developmental and behavioural studies to suggest that the minimal self involves at least two distinguishable aspects: a differentiation between self and nonself, and a sense of one's own body that is based on proprioceptive–motor processes (Bermúdez, 1996, 1998; Gallagher, 1996). In the case of movement, the latter aspect may be specified further to include both a sense of ownership for movement (that is, a sense that I am moving) and a sense of agency (that is, a sense that I am the one causing the movement).

For the construction of self-narrative the sense of agency, and the ability to attribute action to oneself, are essential. Ricoeur (1992) makes it clear that in narrative a character is either (or alternatively) an agent or a sufferer. In self-narrative the construal of the character (the self) as agent or sufferer depends on the ability of the narrator to self-attribute action. This means that even if other aspects of the minimal self are intact, a lack of a sense of agency will be disruptive to self-narrative.

In certain symptoms of schizophrenia, such as thought insertion, delusions of control and auditory hallucinations, various aspects of self-awareness are disrupted. Specifically, it has been suggested that such schizophrenic experiences involve a lack of a sense of ownership and/or agency (Stephens & Graham, 1994; Georgieff & Jeannerod, 1999; Gallagher, 2000a, 2000b). Campbell (1999) goes so far as to suggest that these phenomena represent a failure of the immunity principle. That is, phenomena like thought insertion seem to involve errors of self-identification. The patient who suffers from thought insertion is not in error about the thought content, but is wrong about whose thought it is. For reasons outlined elsewhere, however, I have argued that certain aspects of minimal self-awareness and self-reference remain intact even in cases of thought insertion, delusions of control and auditory hallucinations (Gallagher, 2000b). Moreover, in these cases, the aspects that remain intact are sufficient to prevent a violation of the immunity principle. Patients who suffer from these symptoms wrongly attribute their experiences to someone else only with respect to agency (that is, they claim that someone else caused the action) but they correctly self-attribute these experiences in terms of ownership (that is, they acknowledge that they themselves are the ones who undergo the experience) and they correctly and with immunity use the first-person pronoun to formulate their complaints.

A patient may be seemingly lost in a confusion of self and other, but is none the less able to use the first-person pronoun properly and consistently. For example, a schizophrenic woman describes what she experiences when she is in a conversation: 'then I, through this combination of myself projecting into the other person, and the other person in itself, am monitored to react as expected ... and that happens so rapidly that I, even if I had wanted to, am unable to stop myself. And after that, I am left by myself and very lonely' (quoted in Sass, 1998, p. 334). One patient with schizophrenia spoke of 'no longer [being] able to distinguish how much of myself is in me and how much is already in others. I am a conglomeration, a monstrosity, modeled anew each day' (Freeman et al., 1958, p. 54). A recent study suggests that in some schizophrenic self-narratives, although the narrator correctly uses the first-person pronoun to identify himself as narrator, the narrator will sometimes use a third-person pronoun to designate himself as a character in the narrative (Bernal, 2001). The difference represented by different pronouns may signify precisely a failure of the subject to treat himself as agent of his own narrated actions. Again, this would not be a violation of the immunity principle since it involves, at most, a failure of *objective* identification.

Schizophrenic patients also make mistakes about the agency of various bodily movements. Patients suffering from delusions of control may report that their movements are made or caused by someone or something else. A patient reports: 'The force moved my lips. I began to speak. The words were made for me' (Frith, 1992, p. 66). In this case the patient identifies his own lips as the lips that are moved (he has a sense of ownership for the body parts and for their experienced movement), but he makes an error of identification concerning who produced this movement. Here the sense of agency, rather than the sense of ownership, is disrupted. In the case of thought insertion the schizophrenic subject complains that someone else is inserting thoughts into his stream of consciousness. The thought appears in his mind, manifested within *his own* stream of consciousness, but its presence there is caused by someone else.

The schizophrenic subject is thus able to use the first-person pronoun in a way that does not violate the immunity principle, but that none the less derails the self-narrative. Even in the present tense the subject reports that certain actions that would normally be self-ascribed are in fact not his. How can one explain this disruption in the sense of agency?

In the immediate phenomenology of action, agency is not represented as separate from the action. It is rather felt as an intrinsic property of the action itself and is experienced as a perspectival and embodied source (Marcel, in press; Gallagher & Marcel, 1999). Experimental studies of nonpathological subjects suggest that the sense of agency is based on premotor processes that precede the action and that translate intention into movement, rather than on sensory feedback from movement itself or from peripheral effort associated with such movement (Marcel, in press; Fourneret & Jeannerod, 1998). Other research correlates initial awareness of action with recordings of the lateralized readiness potential and with transcranial magnetic stimulation of the supplementary motor area (Haggard & Eimer, 1999; Haggard & Magno, 1999). These studies strongly suggest that one's initial agentive awareness of a spontaneous voluntary action is based on anticipatory or premovement motor commands.

One model for explaining how such premotor processes relate to the sense of agency involves the idea of a *forward* comparator. This neurological mechanism compares one's intention to move with efference copy of actual motor commands, and does so prior to the actual movement and sensory feedback (Frith et al., 2000). A secondary mechanism involved in motor control compares efference copy of motor commands with the sensory feedback that issues from the movement. This is a slower system that supplements the quicker forward control mechanism. These two mechanisms are dissociated in the case of normal involuntary movement. If, for example, someone pushes me from behind, the movement generates sensory feedback informing me that I am moving. Because the motor system records no intention for that movement, however, the forward mechanism does not register the movement as one caused by me. This suggests that the sense of ownership depends on the sensory-feedback mechanism while the sense of agency depends on the forward mechanism (Gallagher 2000a, 2000b). (The distinction between sense of ownership and sense of agency is a conceptual one. It is often difficult to distinguish between these two senses in intentional action because sensory feedback contributes to and reinforces the sense of agency, just as the forward mechanism contributes to and reinforces the sense of ownership. For example, the sense of ownership often depends on the sense of motor control that is tied to agentive specification (see de Vignemont, 2000, for this point).)

Schizophrenic patients who suffer from delusions of control and from thought insertion have problems with the forward mechanism for motor control, but not with motor control based on sensory feedback (Frith, 1992). Normally, subjects required to use a joystick to follow a target on a computer screen may use either sensory (especially visual) feedback or the forward, premotor system for correction of movement. In the former case, they recognize movement errors based on visual perception of the movement, and correct it well after the movement is underway. When normal subjects are deprived of visual feedback, however, they make quicker and smoother corrections of errors based on the forward mechanism. Experiments show that schizophrenic patients have a problem monitoring their own motor intentions at this forward level (Malenka et al., 1982; Mlakar et al., 1994). Schizophrenic patients, like normal subjects, correct their errors when visual feedback is provided, but, unlike normal subjects, are often unable to correct their mistakes when deprived of visual feedback (Frith & Done, 1988).

These findings are consistent with controlled studies that show abnormal premovement brain potentials in schizophrenia, which Singh and his colleagues associate with elements of a neural network involving supplementary motor, premotor and prefrontal cortexes (Singh et al., 1992). Georgieff & Jeannerod (1998) have proposed that such a network functions as a 'who' system, enabling a subject to attribute an action to its proper origin. When a subject generates action, specific brain areas in that network are activated. Functional brain imagery studies suggest that this system is impaired in schizophrenic subjects who manifest delusions of control and thought insertion (Spence et al., 1997). This evidence is also consistent with the idea that thought insertion, and the disruption of the sense of agency, involve problems with temporal integration, as explicated in the previous section (Chen et al., 1999; Gallagher, 2000b).

Whether or not the problems that pertain to minimal self-awareness and the sense of agency are best explained by faulty comparators or deficiencies in temporal integration, such problems are well-established in schizophrenic patients. They are reflected in schizophrenic self-narrative in the form of the misattribution of action and responsibility for action.

Episodic–autobiographical memory

Both the capacity for temporal integration and the capacity for minimal self-reference seem necessary for the proper working of episodic–autobiographical memory. These capacities are related to two aspects normally understood to define episodic–autobiographical memory: the recollection of the specific time in the past when an event took place, and self-attribution, the specification that the past event involved the person who is remembering it. It is possible, however, that someone who is able to self-attribute actions (for example, when they are occurring) and is also able to specify the proper timeframes for events (for example, in following a set of instructions) still may not be able to acquire memories, or to recollect autobiographical events.

There is a long philosophical tradition, starting with Locke (1690: reprinted 1959), which holds that just such memories form the basis of personal identity. It seems clear that narrative identity is primarily constituted in narratives that recount past autobiographical events. If there is any degree of unity to my life, as Ricoeur (1992) suggests, it is the product of an interpretation of my past actions and of events in the past that happened to me (all of which constitute my life history). If I am unable to form memories of my life history, or am unable to access such memories, then I have nothing to interpret, nothing to narrate that would be sufficient for the formation of self-identity.

The importance of episodic memory for the construction of narrative is also recognized in neuropsychology. Maguire et al. (1999) point out that the successful use of stories to convey and acquire information depends on two factors: that the story makes sense, and that the person who hears the story has access to prior knowledge. The coherence of the story depends on these factors. In the construction of self-narrative, episodic–autobiographical memory provides the prior knowledge out of which the coherent narrative is formed. Markowitsch (see chapter 9, this volume) suggests that the encoding and retrieval of narrative are just the encoding and retrieval of episodic or autobiographical memory, and that such memory provides the contextual environment of former experiences.

It is quite common, in philosophy and neuropsychology, to discuss episodic memory in terms like 'encoding' and 'retrieval', and thus to conceive of memory on the metaphor of information storage. Some psychologists and philosophers, however, propose that memory is not simply a matter of reproduction or retrieval of stored information, but a reconstructive process (Barclay & DeCooke, 1988; Schechtman, 1996; Gallagher, 1998). In this sense the narrative (and self-narrative) process is not simply something that depends on the proper functioning of episodic (and autobiographical) memory, but in fact contributes to the functioning of that memory. Just to the extent that the current contextual and semantic requirements of narrative construction motivate the recollection of a certain event, that recollection will be shaped, interpreted and reconstructed in the light of those requirements. For this reason a variety of issues involved in a discussion of memory are also relevant to our discussion of metacognition in the next section.

A review by Fletcher et al. (1997) summarizes the neurological picture and shows just how complex it is for episodic memory. On the basis of neuroimaging studies, especially PET, neuroscience has been able to define more precisely the network of brain structures involved. From the study of brain-damaged individuals it is well known that the hippocampus, the medial temporal cortex and the prefrontal cortex play essential roles in episodic memory. For example, hippocampal activation has been associated with the creation of associations during encoding of memory and with the experience of conscious recollection (Schacter et al., 1996; Henke et al., 1997). Damage to the medial temporal cortex and hippocampus impairs the acquisition of new memories. Imaging studies confirm that activation of the hippocampus correlates to the encoding of visuospatial and object memory. Encoding for unfamiliar faces and spatial locations activates the left prefrontal cortex, and lesions of the prefrontal cortex affect the retrieval of contextual features of already formed memories. The right prefrontal cortex is activated when there is an intention to retrieve episodic information and again when that retrieval is successful (Fletcher et al., 1997). There is also activation of the right prefrontal cortex in recall involving specific personal qualities in contrast to contents with impersonal qualities (Fink et al., 1996). The network for episodic memory may involve a prefrontothalamocerebellar network (Andreasen et al., 1996; Fink et al., 1996) and retrieval may further involve the parietal cortex and the precuneus (Fletcher et al., 1997). More generally, there is a growing consensus that almost all regions of the brain are involved in memory, and that episodic memories are distributed throughout the neocortex (Fuster, 1997).

Impairment of episodic–autobiographical memory is a cognitive deficit commonly found in schizophrenia. Schizophrenics do not have problems with all types of memory, but they do have a focused deficit in the type of remembering that involves mental reliving of their own actions and experiences (Danion et al., 1999). PET studies show that schizophrenic patients, relative to controls, have reduced hippocampal activation during verbal episodic memory retrieval (Heckers et al., 1998). Activation of the prefrontal cortex during retrieval of poorly encoded content was also different for controls and schizophrenic patients: in contrast to controls who activated one prefrontal area (area 8), schizophrenic patients activated several prefrontal areas anterior to area 8. This study suggests that the more widespread activation of prefrontal areas might be related to the greater effort for retrieval required by the patients. Heckers et al. (1998) also found evidence for hippocampal hyperactivity in the schizophrenic patients they tested, something associated with abnormal thought processes, hallucinations and delusions. They hypothesize that the hyperactivity may interfere with the normal recruitment of the hippocampus during memory retrieval, and suggest that their findings are consistent with the model of abnormal corticohippocampal interaction in schizophrenia (Goldman-Rakic, 1994; Frith et al., 1995; Dolan & Fletcher, 1997).

It seems clear that if schizophrenic patients have problems in either the encoding or the retrieval of memories, they will also have trouble in constructing a viable self-narrative. This is not just a question of whether they can remember their own story. Rather, the episodic–autobiographical memory system delivers content for the construction of self-narrative. If autobiographical content is confused, if it is dramatically incomplete, inaccessible or entirely fleeting, this will be reflected in the self-narrative. The explicit and self-conscious formation of a life story depends on the material provided by memory. Lacking such material, there are at least two possible responses. The first can be seen in some cases of transient global amnesia. A patient may feel completely disoriented and ask such things as 'Where am I?', 'What day is today?' or 'Where are we going?' Here we have questions, but no narrative. A second possible response results in a narrative, but one that is confabulated or extremely enhanced by metacognition that has become hyperreflexive.

Reflective metacognition

The process of interpretation that ordinarily shapes episodic–autobiographical memories into a narrative structure depends on the capacity for reflective metacognition. A life event is not always meaningful in itself, but depends on a narrative structure that lends it context and sees in it significance that goes beyond the event itself. To form a self-narrative, one needs to do more than simply remember life events. One needs to consider them reflectively, deliberate on their meaning and decide how they fit together semantically. Metacognition allows for that reflective process of interpretation. It also enhances the product delivered by episodic–autobiographical memory. As Ricoeur points out, narrative identity 'must be seen as an unstable mixture of fabulation and actual experience' (1992, p. 162). It is possible, for the sake of a unified or coherent meaning, to construe certain events in a way that they did not in fact happen. To some degree, and for the sake of creating a coherency to life, it is normal to confabulate and to enhance one's story. Self-deception is not unusual; false memories are frequent. Whether in any particular case metacognition contributes to this process, or limits it, it is clearly essential for the interpretive process that produces the self-narrative.

Frith (1992) suggests that metacognition is problematic in schizophrenia. Specifically he contends that there is a disruption of self-monitoring in both motor and cognitive domains. Self-monitoring can include introspective metarepresentation, a second-order reflective consciousness, a form of introspection that is disturbed in the schizophrenic. We note, however, that it is possible for metarepresentation to go wrong in at least two ways. Firstly, as Frith emphasizes, it can fail in a way that leaves the schizophrenic without the ability to monitor his or her own experience.

Secondly, however, as Sass (1998, 2000) suggests, metarepresentation and a certain degree of *overmonitoring* of experience can be generated in hyperreflexive experience, when processes that are ordinarily tacit (processes that I normally do not have to monitor explicitly or consciously) come to the subject's attention. (Something like this hyperreflection may generate what Phillips (see chapter 15, this volume) calls 'sick narratives'. Concerning the self-narrative of Mrs M, Phillips suggests that her 'medication, instead of being an automatic ritual that is barely focused on, remains an active object of attention and an active reminder of the painful reality of her mental illness'.) Neurological dysfunctions that might lead a subject to attend to what is ordinarily tacit in experience include the problems outlined in previous sections involving prefrontal cortex, premotor cortex, supplementary motor area, hippocampus, and so forth. Either kind of metacognitive disturbance holds consequences for the schizophrenic self-narrative.

It is possible that the disruption of metacognition can be selectively Frithian and Sassian in succession. Either a failure of self-monitoring, or a hyperreflexive shift, where the subject begins to focus on normally implicit aspects of experience, could motivate the schizophrenic to introspect explicitly about what is absent from or odd about his or her experience. In turn, this introspection can lead to a further, compensatory hyperreflection that may entail a failure to monitor other normally monitored aspects. A schizophrenic may have great difficulties with attention, not because of a complete lack of attention, but because she is attending in a high degree to certain aspects of her experience that are not usually the focus of attention. The failure of self-monitoring may be that there is too much of it going on. This possibility is not unrelated to what Sass calls a central paradox of schizophrenic experience: 'a strange oscillation, or even coexistence, between two opposite experiences of the self: between the loss or fragmentation of self and its apotheosis in moments of solipsistic grandeur' (Sass, 1998, p. 317). The failure of self-monitoring to which Frith attributes thought insertion and symptoms of influence may lead to first-person narrative claims like 'I didn't want to do this, that machine made me'. Such claims none the less require a metacognition to recognize the failure of self-monitoring. Failures of self-attribution that involve a disruption in the sense of agency and a lack of self-monitoring are not sufficient, however, to explain why the subject attributes agency for the action to someone or something else. If in some respect there is a shrinking of the self ('these are not my actions') there is at the same time an expansion of the narrative that accounts for the self – an expansion that includes other people or things. (An example can be found in Mr S's delusional narratives (see chapter 15, this volume).)

It is possible that schizophrenic hyperreflexive experience is motivated by precisely the kind of failures that we have reviewed above. If there is a failure in my sense of agency, and I experience thought insertion, for example, or if there is some experienced lack of temporal integration, it seems likely that certain aspects of my experience, which are usually tacit or implicit, would begin to manifest themselves in an explicit way. That would motivate an introspective search for explanations to account for such experience. Indeed, as Bruner & Kalmar (1998) suggest, the driving force for the formation of narrative in the mode of metacognition is 'trouble', or a sense of jeopardy. Pöppel (1978), in reference to Korsakoff psychosis, suggests that when there is a dissociation between experienced events and the timeframe in which they happened (a problem with episodic memory), the result is likely to be confabulation.

Based on experiments with split-brain patients, Gazzaniga (1995, 1998) suggests that a specific left-hemisphere mechanism, which he calls the 'interpreter', is responsible for the neurological process involved in generating narratives that compensate for missing or distorted information. The interpreter mechanism weaves together autobiographical fact and newly devised fiction to produce a self-narrative that maintains the sense of a continuous self. In agreement with Dennett's characterization of the narrative self, Gazzaniga contends that we have a propensity to enhance our personal narratives with elements that smooth over discontinuities and discrepancies in self-constitution (Gazzaniga & Gallagher, 1998). The greater the discontinuities and discrepancies, as in schizophrenia, the more one's personal narratives involve deliberations, abstractions, withdrawals and confabulations that may include attribution of agency for one's actions to some other agent. (In some cases there are ongoing auditory hallucinations or quasihallucinations known as *running commentary* and/or arguing voices – a heard voice commenting on the patient's ongoing actions or thoughts; or hallucinatory voices discussing the patient in the third person.)

Conclusions

My intent in this chapter has not been to provide a theory of schizophrenia, or a theory of the complete concept of self, but to contribute to an understanding of how self-narratives are generated, and how they can go wrong in schizophrenia. Whatever the specific neurological mechanisms (or dynamical processes) involved in the generation of narrative, it seems clear that a number of things can and in some cases do go wrong in schizophrenia. (Table 16.1). Although schizophrenics are able to use the first-person pronoun in a way that anchors their self-narrative to themselves, they sometimes have problems with self-attribution and the sense of agency for their actions. They attribute such actions to other agents as causes, and this is reflected in the content of schizophrenic self-narratives.

Table 16.1 Correlations amongst phenomenological aspects, cognitive problems, neurological dysfunctions, and narrative effects in schizophrenia

Self-narrative in schizophrenia	Phenomenology	Cognitive problems	Neurological dysfunction	Narrative effects
Temporal structure	Curtailed future perspective; derailed temporal order; impairment of self-temporalization	Dysfunction of working memory; slowed cognitive processing; breakdown of semantic binding	Prefrontal dysfunction	Lack of internal concordance; lack of temporal perspective as narrator; fragmented self-narrative
Minimal self-reference	Lack of sense of self-agency; thought insertion, delusions of control and auditory hallucinations	Dysfunction of *forward* comparator and preaction processes; 'who' system	Abnormal pre-movement brain potentials in SMA, premotor and prefrontal cortexes	Misattribution of agency; objective misidentification
Autobiographical memory	Difficulties remembering past personal events; incomplete and fleeting memories	Encoding and retrieval problems	Reduced hippocampal activation during retrieval; hyperactivation of prefrontal areas	Impoverished content; incoherent contexts
Metacognition	Focus on normally tacit dimensions; attention problems; introverted reflection	Hyperreflection; problems with self-monitoring	Overactivation of left-hemisphere 'interpreter'	Confabulated narratives; 'sick' narratives

SMA, supplementary motor area.

Structural problems are apparent when schizophrenics cannot maintain the serial order or temporal perspective for life events. Essential structures of the narrative process having to do with sequential plot and perspectival timeframes are disrupted in important ways. Even if such temporal frameworks remain intact, however, problems with episodic–autobiographical memory may deprive the subject of the proper or adequate content with which to fill such frames. The lack of structure and/or content may motivate the overactivation of a reflective metacognition that is ordinarily at work in the explicit construction of narrative. It is not the case that in schizophrenia metacognition simply ceases. Indeed, it may become hyperreflexive and lead to the confabulation of unusual self-narratives. Failures in some or in all of these areas help to explain the problems that schizophrenic subjects have in constructing a self-narrative.

REFERENCES

Andreasen, N.C., O'Leary, D.S., Cizadlo, T. et al. (1996). Schizophrenia and cognitive dysmetria: a positron-emission tomography study of dysfunctional prefrontal-thalamic-cerebellar circuitry. *Proceedings of the National Academy of Sciences of the United States of America*, **93**, 9985–90.

Andreasen, N.C., Paradiso, S. & O'Leary, D.S. (1998). 'Cognitive dysmetria' as an integrative theory of schizophrenia: a dysfunction in cortical–subcortical–cerebellar circuitry. *Schizophrenia Bulletin*, **24**, 203–18.

Barclay, C.R. & DeCooke, P.A. (1988). Ordinary memories: some of the things of which selves are made. In *Remembering Reconsidered: Ecological and Traditional Approaches to the Study of Memory*, ed. U. Neisser & E. Winograd, pp. 91–125. Cambridge: Cambridge University Press.

Bermúdez, J. (1996). The moral significance of birth. *Ethics*, **106**, 378–403.

Bermúdez, J. (1998). *The Paradox of Self-Consciousness*. Cambridge: MIT Press.

Bernal, A.L. (2001). *Concordancias Discordantes: Caracterización del Relato Autobiográfico de Pacientes con Diagnóstico de Esquizofrenia*. Dissertation. Universidad del Valle, Escuela de Psicología, Santiago de Cali, Colombia.

Bovet, P. & Parnas, J. (1993). Schizophrenic delusions: a phenomenological approach. *Schizophrenia Bulletin*, **19**, 579–97.

Bruner, J. & Kalmar, D.A. (1998). Narrative and metanarrative in the construction of self. In *Self-Awareness: Its Nature and Development*, ed. M. Ferrari & R.J. Sternberg, pp. 308–31. New York: Guilford Press.

Campbell, J. (1999). Schizophrenia, the space of reasons and thinking as a motor process. *The Monist*, **82**, 609–25.

Carter, C.S., Perlstein, P., Ganguli, R. et al. (1998). Functional hypofrontality and working memory dysfunction in schizophrenia. *American Journal of Psychiatry*, **155**, 1285–7.

Chen, Y., Palafox, G.P., Nakayama, K. et al. (1999). Motion perception in schizophrenia. *Archives of General Psychiatry*, **56**, 149–54.

Cohen, J.D., Barch, D.M., Carter, C.S. & Servan-Schreiber, D. (1999). Schizophrenic deficits in the processing of context: converging evidence from three theoretically motivated cognitive tasks. *Journal of Abnormal Psychology*, **108**, 120–133.

Cutting, J. (1998). *Psychopathology and Modern Philosophy*. London: Forest.

Danion, J.-M., Rizzo, L. & Bruant, A. (1999). Functional mechanisms underlying impaired recognition memory and conscious awareness in patients with schizophrenia. *Archives of General Psychiatry*, **56**, 639–44.

Daprati, E., Franck, N., Georgieff, N. et al. (1997). Looking for the agent: an investigation into consciousness of action and self-consciousness in schizophrenic patients. *Cognition*, **65**, 71–96.

de Gelder, B., Parnas, J., Bovet, P. et al. (1997). Impaired integration of audition and vision in schizophrenics. *Experimental Brain Research*, **117**, 23.

de Gelder, B., Vroomen, J., Annen, J., Matsdhof, E. & Hodiamont, P. (in press). Audiovisual integration in schizophrenia. *Schizophrenia Research*, **1628**.

Dennett, D. (1988). Why everyone is a novelist. *Times Literary Supplement*, **4459**, 1016, 1028–9.

Dennett, D. (1991). *Consciousness Explained*. Boston: Little, Brown.

DePue, R.A., Dubicki, M.D. & McCarthy, T. (1975). Differential recovery of intellectual, associational, and psychophysiological functioning in withdrawal and active schizophrenics. *Journal of Abnormal Psychology*, **84**, 325–30.

de Vignemont, F. (2000). When the 'I think' does not accompany my thoughts. *Consciousness and Cognition*, **9**, 543.

Dilling, C. & Rabin, A. (1967). Temporal experience in depressive states and schizophrenia. *Journal of Consulting Psychology*, **31**, 604–8.

Dolan, R.J. & Fletcher, P.C. (1997). Dissociating prefrontal and hippocampal function in episodic memory encoding. *Nature*, **388**, 582–5.

Dreher, J.-C., Banquet, J.-P., Allilaire, J.-F. et al. (2001). Temporal order and spatial memory in schizophrenia: a parametric study. *Schizophrenia Research*, **51**, 137–47.

Fink, G.R., Markowitsch, H.J., Reinkemeier, M. et al. (1996). Cerebral representation of one's own past: neural networks involved in autobiographical memory. *Journal of Neuroscience*, **16**, 4275–82.

Fleming, K., Goldberg, T.E., Binks, S. et al. (1997). Visuospatial working memory in patients with schizophrenia. *Biological Psychiatry*, **41**, 43–9.

Fletcher, P.C., Frith, C.D. & Rugg, M.D. (1997). The functional neuroanatomy of episodic memory. *Trends in Neuroscience*, **20**, 213–18.

Fourneret, P. & Jeannerod, M. (1998). Limited conscious monitoring of motor performance in normal subjects. *Neuropsychologia*, **36**, 1133–40.

Franck, N., Farrer, C., Georgieff, N. et al. (2001). Defective recognition of one's own actions in patients with schizophrenia. *American Journal of Psychiatry*, **158**, 454–9.

Frith, C.D. (1992). *The Cognitive Neuropsychology of Schizophrenia*. Hillsdale, NJ: Lawrence Erlbaum.

Frith, C.D. & Done, D.J. (1988). Towards a neuropsychology of schizophrenia. *British Journal of Psychiatry*, **153**, 437–43.

Frith, C.D., Friston, K.J., Herold, S. et al. (1995). Regional brain activity in chronic schizophrenic patients during the performance of a verbal fluency task. *British Journal of Psychiatry*, **167**, 343–9.

Frith, C.D., Blakemore, S.-J. & Walpert, D.M. (2000). Explaining the symptoms of schizophrenia: abnormalities in the awareness of action. *Brain Research Reviews*, **31**, 357–63.

Fuster, J.M. (1997). Network memory. *Trends in Neuroscience*, **20**, 451–58.

Fuster, J.M. (1999). Commentary on 'The human self construct and prefrontal cortex in schizophrenia (Vogeley et al.). Association for the Scientific Study of Consciousness: electronic seminar. Available online at: http://www.phil.vt.edu/assc/esem.html

Fuster, J.M., Bodner, M. & Kroger, J.K. (2000). Cross-modal and cross-temporal association in neurons of frontal cortex. *Nature*, **405**, 347–51.

Gallagher, S. (1996). The moral significance of primitive self-consciousness. *Ethics*, **107**, 129–40.

Gallagher, S. (1998). *The Inordinance of Time*. Evanston: Northwestern University Press.

Gallagher, S. (2000a). Philosophical conceptions of the self: Implications for cognitive science. *Trends in Cognitive Science*, **4**, 14–21.

Gallagher, S. (2000b). Self-reference and schizophrenia: a cognitive model of immunity to error through misidentification. In *Exploring the Self: Philosophical and Psychopathological Perspectives on Self-experience*, ed. D. Zahavi, pp. 203–39. Amsterdam: John Benjamins.

Gallagher, S. & Marcel, A.J. (1999). The self in contextualized action. *Journal of Consciousness Studies*, **6**, 4–30.

Gallagher, S. & Meltzoff, A. (1996). The earliest sense of self and others: Merleau-Ponty and recent developmental studies. *Philosophical Psychology*, **9**, 213–36.

Gazzaniga, M. (1995). Consciousness and the cerebral hemispheres. In *The Cognitive Neurosciences*, ed. M. Gazzaniga, pp. 1391–400. Cambridge, MA: MIT Press.

Gazzaniga, M. (1998). *The Mind's Past*. New York: Basic Books.

Gazzaniga, M. & Gallagher, S. (1998). The neuronal Platonist. *Journal of Consciousness Studies*, **5**, 706–17.

Georgieff, N. & Jeannerod, M. (1998). Beyond consciousness of external events: a 'who' system for consciousness of action and self-consciousness. *Consciousness and Cognition*, **7**, 465–77.

Georgieff, N. & Jeannerod, M. (1999). *Deconstruction of Self-consciousness in Schizophrenia*. Discussion of the human self construct and prefrontal cortex in schizophrenia. ASSC Electronic Seminar. Available online at: http://www.phil.vt.edu/assc/esem.html.

Gold, J.M., Carpenter, C., Randolph, C., Goldberg, T.E. & Weinberger, D.R. (1997). Auditory working memory and Wisconsin Card Sorting Test performance in schizophrenia. *Archives of General Psychiatry*, **54**, 159–65.

Goldberg, T.E. & Weinberger, D.R. (1996). Effects of neuroleptic medication on the cognition of patients with schizophrenia: a review of recent studies. *Journal of Clinical Psychiatry*, **57** (suppl. 9), 62–5.

Goldman-Rakic, P.S. (1994). Working memory dysfunction in schizophrenia. *Journal of Neuropsychiatry and Clinical Neuroscience*, **6**, 348–57.

Goldman-Rakic, P.S. (1995). Anatomical and functional circuits in prefrontal cortex of nonhuman primates: relevance to epilepsy. *Advances in Neurology*, **66**, 51–63.

Goldman-Rakic, P.S. & Selemon, L.D. (1997). Functional and anatomical aspects of prefrontal pathology in schizophrenia. *Schizophrenia Bulletin*, **23**, 437–58.

Graybiel, A.M. (1997). The basal ganglia and cognitive pattern generators. *Schizophrenia Bulletin*, **23**, 459–69.

Haggard, P. & Eimer, M. (1999). On the relation between brain potentials and the awareness of voluntary movements. *Experimental Brain Research*, **126**, 128.

Haggard, P. & Magno, E. (1999). Localising awareness of action with transcranial magnetic stimulation. *Experimental Brain Research*, **127**, 102.

Hartmann, E., Milofsky, E., Vaillant, G. et al. (1984). Vulnerability to schizophrenia. Prediction of adult schizophrenia using childhood information. *Archives of General Psychiatry*, **41**, 1050–6.

Heckers, S., Rauch, S., Goff, D. et al. (1998). Impaired recruitment of the hippocampus during conscious recollection in schizophrenia. *Nature Neuroscience*, **1**, 318–23.

Henke, K., Buck, A., Weber, B. & Wieser, H.G. (1997). Human hippocampus establishes associations in memory. *Hippocampus*, **7**, 249–56.

Hume, D. (1975). *A Treatise of Human Nature*. Oxford: Clarendon Press.

Keefe, R.S., Lees-Roitman, S.E. & Dupre, R.L. (1997). Performance of patients with schizophrenia on a pen and paper visuospatial working memory task with short delay. *Schizophrenia Research*, **26**, 9–14.

Levin, S. (1984). Frontal lobe dysfunction in schizophrenia – eye movement impairments. *Journal of Psychiatric Research*, **18**, 27–55.

Locke, J. (1959). *An Essay Concerning Human Understanding.* New York: Dover.

Maguire, E.A., Frith, C.D. & Morris, R.G. (1999). The functional neuroanatomy of comprehension and memory: the importance of prior knowledge. *Brain*, **122**, 1839–50.

Malenka, R.C., Angel, R.W., Hampton, B. & Berger, P.A. (1982). Impaired central error-correcting behaviour in schizophrenia. *Archives of Geneneral Psychiatry*, **39**, 101–7.

Marcel, A.J. (in press). The sense of agency: awareness and ownership of actions and intentions. In *Agency and Self-Awareness*, ed. J. Roessler & N. Eilan. Oxford: Oxford University Press.

Melges, F.T. (1982). *Time and the Inner Future: A Temporal Approach to Psychiatric Disorders.* New York: Wiley.

Melges, F.T. & Freeman, A.M. (1977). Temporal disorganization and inner–outer confusion in acute mental illness. *American Journal of Psychiatry*, **134**, 874–7.

Meltzoff, A. & Moore, M.K. (1977). Imitation of facial and manual gestures by human neonates. *Science*, **198**, 75–8.

Milner, B. (1974). Hemispheric specialization: scope and limits. In *The Neurosciences: Third Study Program*, ed. F.O. Schmitt & F.G. Worden, pp. 75–89. Cambridge: MIT Press.

Minkowski, E. (1970). *Lived Time: Phenomenological and Psychological Studies.* Translated by N. Metzel. Evanston: Northwestern University Press.

Mlakar, J., Jensterle, J. & Frith, C.D. (1994). Central monitoring deficiency and schizophrenic symptoms. *Psychological Medicine*, **24**, 557–64.

Park, S. & Holzman, P.S. (1992). Schizophrenics show spatial working memory deficits. *Archives of General Psychiatry*, **49**, 975–82.

Parnas, J., Bovet, P. & Innocenti, G.M. (1996). Schizophrenic trait features, binding, and cortico-cortical connectivity: a neurodevelopmental pathogenetic hypothesis. *Neurology, Psychiatry and Brain Research*, **4**, 185–96.

Pöppel, E. (1978). Time perception. *Handbook of Sensory Physiology*, **8**, 713–29.

Pöppel, E. (1997). A hierarchical model of temporal perception. *Trends in Cognitive Sciences*, **1**, 56–61.

Pöppel, E. (1994). Temporal mechanisms in perception. *International Review of Neurobiology*, **37**, 185–202.

Pöppel, E. & Schwender, D. (1993). Temporal mechanisms of consciousness. *International Anesthesiology Clinics*, **31**, 27–38.

Ricoeur, P. (1992). *Oneself as Another.* Translated by K. Blamey. Chicago: University of Chicago Press.

Rubin, P., Holm, S.M., Madsen, P.L. et al. (1994). Regional cerebral blood flow distribution in newly diagnosed schizophrenia and schizophreniform disorder. *Psychiatry Research*, **53**, 57–75.

Sartre, J.-P. (1936). *La Transcendance de l'Ego.* Paris: Vrin.

Sass, L. (1992). *Madness and Modernism: Insanity in the Light of Modern Art, Literature, and Thought.* New York: Basic Books.

Sass, L. (1998). Schizophrenia, self-consciousness and the modern mind. *Journal of Consciousness Studies*, **5**, 543–65.

Sass, L. (2000). Furtive abductions: schizophrenia, the lived-body, and dispossession of the self. *Arobase: Journal des Lettres et Sciences Humaines*, **4**, 63–73.

Schacter, D.L., Alpert, N.M., Savage, C.R., Rauch, S.L. & Albert, M.S. (1996). Conscious recollection and the human hippocampal formation: evidence from positron emission tomography. *Proceedings of the National Academy of Science of the USA*, **93**, 321–25.

Schectman, M. (1996). *The Constitution of Selves*. Ithaca: Cornell University Press.

Schwartz, B.D., Maron, B.A., Evans, W.J. & Winstead, D.K. (1999). High velocity transient visual processing deficits diminish ability of patients with schizophrenia to recognize objects. *Neuropsychiatry, Neuropsychology, and Behavioral Neurology*, **12**, 170–7.

Shoemaker, S. (1968). Self-reference and self-awareness. *Journal of Philosophy*, **65**, 555–67.

Singh, J.R., Knight, T., Rosenlicht, N. et al. (1992). Abnormal premovement brain potentials in schizophrenia. *Schizophrenia Research*, **8**, 31–41.

Spence, S.A., Brooks, D. J., Hirsch, S.R. et al. (1997). A PET study of voluntary movement in schizophrenic patients experiencing passivity phenomena (delusions of alien control). *Brain*, **120**, 1997–2011.

Stephens, G.L. & Graham, G. (1994). Self-consciousness, mental agency, and the clinical psychopathology of thought insertion. *Philosophy, Psychiatry, and Psychology*, **1**, 1–12.

Strawson, P.F. (1994). The first person and others. In *Self-Knowledge*, ed. Q. Cassam, pp. 210–15. Oxford: Oxford University Press.

Strous, R.D., Cowan, N., Ritter, W. & Javitt, D. (1995). Auditory sensory ('echoic') memory dysfunction in schizophrenia. *American Journal of Psychiatry*, **152**, 1517–19.

Tauscher-Wisniewski, S. (1999). Cognitive processing speed slows before schizophrenia. Poster session, Society of Biological Psychiatry. Reported by Moon, M.A. *Clinical Psychiatry News*, **27**, 1.

von Steinbüchel, N., Wittman, M. & Pöppel, E. (1996). Timing in perceptual and motor tasks after disturbances to the brain. In *Time, Internal Clocks, and Movement*, ed. M.A. Pastor & J. Artieda, pp. 281–303. London: Elsevier.

Wexler, B.E., Stevens, A.A., Bowers, A.A., Sernyak, M.J. & Goldman-Rakic, P.S. (1998). Word and tone working memory deficts in schizophrenia. *Archives of General Psychiatry*, **55**, 1093–6.

Wittgenstein, L. (1958). *The Blue and Brown Books*. Oxford: Basil Blackwell.

iii Clinical neuroscience

17

Schizophrenia as disturbance of the self-construct

Kai Vogeley

Department of Psychiatry, University of Bonn, Germany and Institute of Medicine, Research Centre Juelich

Abstract
Human self-consciousness can be defined as the capacity to metarepresent one's own mental states, such as perceptions, judgements, beliefs or desires. It is thus closely related to the so-called theory of mind capacity, which requires the ability to model the mental states of others. Other constitutive features of human self-consciousness comprise the experiences of ownership or agency, of egocentric perspectivity and of long-term unity of beliefs and attitudes. These features are assumed to be neurobiologically implemented as episodically active complex neural activation patterns that can be mapped to the brain given adequate operationalizations of these constitutive features. This bundle of constitutive features is called self-construct to distinguish clearly this empirically motivated operationalized approach from classical philosophical concepts. In the pathophysiology of schizophrenia, it is suggested that clinical subsyndromes like cognitive disorganization and derealization syndromes reflect disorders of partial features of self-consciousness. In this chapter the issue of first-person perspective as opposed to third-person perspective is addressed in more detail. With special regard to the psychopathological symptom of hallucinations, the relevance of the self-construct for the pathophysiology of schizophrenia is discussed.

Self-consciousness and potential empirical indicators

Self-consciousness is a central theme in classical philosophy and contemporary philosophy of mind and has also recently become one of the focuses of cognitive neurosciences. If empirical indicators for self-consciousness or at least for some of its constitutive features can be identified, then operationalization and subsequent mapping to neural structures become possible. These paradigms could then potentially provide information on pathophysiological processes in diseases such as schizophrenia, assuming that schizophrenia is based on disturbances of partial features of self-consciousness.

Consciousness in general may be defined as the integrated internal representation of the outer world and the organism in this world. This representation is based on actual experiences, perceptions and memories providing reflected responses to the needs of our environment. Consciousness thus relies upon the integrative, supramodal, sensory-independent, holistic representation of the world. The world model refers to different coordinate systems, both object- and viewer-centred perspectives in space representation, both physical and subjective time scales in time representation, acquired during ontogenetic development. Having invoked these internal representations, consciousness serves as a reliable and robust presentation platform providing 'availability to thought' (Putnam, 1994) for the integration of actual perception and memory in order to generate valid and useful reactions to the environment. Consciousness is a fundamental tool for our world orientation. Self-consciousness refers to the awareness of one's own mental states, such as perceptions, attitudes, opinions, intentions to act, and so forth, that are available for the self-conscious organism. Representing such mental states into one combined framework that allows us to maintain the integrity of our own mind is understood as a metarepresentational cognitive capacity. Essential for such a teleological and functionalistic view on self-consciousness are constitutive features or specific experiences that reflect the involvement of a specific 'sense of self'.

To indicate that this collection of properties is potentially accessible by adequate operationalizations for the purpose of experimental neuropsychological studies without strong philosophical a priori implications, the term 'self-construct' is used. At least, the following essential features of human self-consciousness can be identified (Vogeley et al., 1999):

1. ownership;
2. perspectivity;
3. unity.

Firstly, the experience of ownership (with respect to perceptions, judgements, etc.) or agency (with respect to actions, movements, etc.) relates to the experiential quality, that I am perceiving or judging, having my own perceptions, memories and thoughts, performing my movements for myself. This is reflected by the use of personal pronouns of the first-person singular in language. Secondly, perspectivity refers to the experience that my conscious states appear to be centred around myself and to the experience of embodiment of my mental states, such as memories, perceptions and thoughts incorporated in my own body. This quality is probably closely linked to the body schema or body image (Berlucchi & Aglioti, 1997; Vogeley & Fink, 2003). Thirdly, the experience of unity is associated with long-term coherent wholes of beliefs and attitudes, that are consistent with preexisting autobiographical contexts (Fink et al., 1996).

Following such a neuroscientific research programme, that aims to elucidate neural correlates of higher brain functions, it needs conceptual clarification on the relationship between mind and brain traditionally discussed in the literature on the mind–body problem in philosophy of mind. Philosophically, this analysis is based on the so-called identity theory, according to which mental phenomena can be identified under certain circumstances with neural phenomena (Vogeley, 1995). The dualistic account, traditionally differentiating between physical and mental phenomena, needs to be maintained, as mental phenomena, including psychopathological symptoms (e.g. hearing a voice commenting on the subject's behaviour), are irreducible with respect to corresponding brain states regarding their semantic content. However, this dualistic account is a nonsubstantial account, which means that the mental phenomena ontologically refer to brain phenomena, although they are not reducible to brain phenomena. On the basis of Leibniz' *principium identitatis indiscernibilium* (identity principles of indistinguishability: Leibniz, 1971; originally published 1765), it is not possible to identify corresponding phenomena from different classes directly (mental and brain phenomena), but only statements about phenomena belonging to the different classes of mental phenomena and brain phenomena. In other words, the intention of a mental phenomenon is irreducible, but it refers at the same time to the same extensional basis, which is the nervous system. Only statements or sentences about mental phenomena and statements or sentences about brain phenomena are 'identifiable' in a strict sense in terms of their congruent ontological extensions (brain phenomena).

Following such a naturalistic research programme, a neuronal network as implementation of the self has been postulated, that assigns perspectivity and intentionality to our perception, thus establishing a neuronal 'self-model' as an episodically active complex neural activation pattern in the human brain, possibly based on an innate and hardwired model (Metzinger 1993, 1995; Damasio, 1994; Melzack et al., 1997). The fact that we are never able to detect the model character as such is due to its fast activation which remains unconscious in its model character. Much attention has been paid to cortical oscillation phenomena as temporal coding processes (Engel et al., 1991, 1999; Bressler, 1995), which appear to play a central role in feature binding and heteromodal representations of holistic or synaesthetic perceptions or experiences. This naturalistic account in principle allows the operationalization of different self-associated capacities and the identification of neural correlates, summarized in the self-construct.

Self-perspective

Representing mental states into one combined framework that allows us to maintain the integrity of our own mind is a metarepresentational cognitive capacity, for which the ability to develop and apply a self-perspective appears to be essential (Vogeley et al., 1999, 2001; Vogeley & Fink, 2003). Self-perspective in this context refers to the subjective experiential multidimensional space centred around one's own person. In this basic sense, self-perspective is a constituent of a 'minimal self' defined as 'consciousness of oneself as an immediate subject of experience, unextended in time' (Gallagher, 2000). The correct assignment and involvement of the self-perspective is reflected by the use of personal pronouns ('I', 'my', e.g. perception, opinion, and so forth).

Closely related to the ability to assign and maintain a self-perspective is the capacity to attribute opinions, perceptions or attitudes to others, often referred to as 'mind-reading' (Baron-Cohen, 1995). The latter ability is an essential social skill that plays a crucial role in interindividual communication. The ability to read another person's mind can be reliably assessed in so-called 'theory of mind' (TOM) paradigms (Fletcher et al., 1995), in which mental states or propositional attitudes of an agent with regard to a particular set of informations or propositions are to be modelled. Typically, these propositions can be described as representations of epistemic mental states comprising an agent ('Peter'), an attitude ('knows that') and a proposition (a physical event, p), e.g. 'Peter knows that p' (Wimmer & Perner, 1983; Baron-Cohen et al., 1986). This allows the representation of mental states of an agent, even if the proposition is not true. The propositional attitude 'Peter believes that it is raining' may be true, although the proposition 'it is raining' may be false (Leslie & Thaiss, 1992; Leslie & Roth, 1993). This allows the ascription even of an inadequate perception or judgement in so-called 'false belief' tasks. Self-perspective in this context refers to the special situation, in which oneself ('I') is the agent (e.g. 'I know, believe, that p'. However, when Premack & Woodruff (1978) introduced the concept of TOM, it referred to the attribution of mental states to both oneself and others. It is still a matter of debate whether the attribution of mental states to oneself and to others are different processes or not. This is discussed in the fields of developmental psychology and philosophy in the debate between *simulation theory* and *theory theory*.

According to the *simulation theory*, taking someone else's perspective is based on taking one's own perspective and subsequently projecting one's own attitudes on someone else (Harris, 1992), thus reducing the capacity to take the self-perspective to a subcomponent of a more general TOM capacity. In contrast to this, TOM capacity is based on a distinct body of theoretical knowledge acquired during the individual ontogenic development according to *theory theory* (Gopnik & Wellmann, 1992; Perner & Howes, 1992). An adequate method to address this question is the use of functional imaging studies. On a purely behavioural level, an independent cerebral implementation of the two capacities could only be inferred on the basis of a double dissociation. Such studies have not been reported yet and would require patients who suffer from a deficit in ascribing mental states to others with intact capacity to ascribe mental states to oneself and vice versa. Arguments that try to infer the (in)dependence of two cognitive capacities from the sequential development of these capacities in development are usually inconclusive (Gopnik & Wellman, 1992; Gopnik, 1993; Carruthers, 1996).

Neurophysiological evidence relevant to this debate was provided by Gallese et al. (1996) who demonstrated a 'mirror neuron (MN) system' in macaques which matches observation and execution of goal-related motor actions in the premotor cortex (corresponding to F5). Interestingly, the neurons in this area respond to both observation of a goal-directed action performed by other animals and execution of the same movement. More recent studies have provided strong evidence for the existence of an equivalent MN system in humans (Iacoboni et al., 1999; Buccino et al., 2001). Gallese & Goldman (1998) argued that the existence of the MN system provides empirical evidence in favour of the simulation theory, according to which the understanding and prediction of other person's behaviour, operationalized in TOM paradigms, crucially depend on one's own simulation of this particular be-haviour. However, one central question remains unanswered by the MN concept: what is the basis for the behaviourally and phenomenologically obvious specific difference between the execution and observation of actions? It makes a differ-ence both at a behavioural as well as a phenomenal level of subjective experience whether I perform a specific motor act or whether I observe this particular motor act of another individual, in other words, whether I am involved as generator of a par-ticular movement or not. The specific class of motor representations generated by MNs does not detect whether the subject is involved as generator of motor acts or not. Hence, the MN concept intrinsically implies the involvement of other neuronal networks that provide this essential additional information (Vogeley & Newen, 2002).

The purpose of a functional magnetic resonance imaging (fMRI) study based on an extended TOM paradigm was to study the neural correlates of self-perspective in this context (Vogeley et al., 2001). In a TOM paradigm, a subject has to model the knowledge, attitudes or beliefs of another person. The design of our fMRI experiment addressed the issue of whether taking the self-perspective as opposed to taking the perspective of someone else in a typical TOM design employs the same or different neural mechanisms. Presented by a cartoon or by telling a history, the behaviour of another person had to be modelled prospectively by the test person. For this purpose, we used a well-characterized collection of short stories (Fletcher et al., 1995; Happé et al., 1996, 1999; Gallagher et al., 2000) which comprised different types or short narrative texts that allowed subjects to engage the self-perspective with and without engaging TOM at the same time. In the 'physical story' condition (T−S−), short consistent texts with no perspective taking were shown presenting a short story on a certain physical event. In the 'TOM story' condition (T+S−), stories were presented in which agents play a particular role, to which a mental state (e.g. perception, judgement) had to be ascribed. Two newly developed conditions which engaged the capacity of self-perspective in the presence or absence of TOM were added. These latter conditions incorporated the study participant as one of the agents in the story. In the 'self and other ascription stories', participants had to

		Theory of mind	
		TOM+	TOM−
Self-perspective	Self−	TOM stories (T+S−)	Physical stories (T−S−)
	Self+	TOM and self-perspective stories (T+S+)	Self-perspective stories (T−S+)

Figure 17.1 Grid showing fully factorial design with the two factors of theory of mind (TOM) and self-perspective (S) either present (+) or not present (−).

ascribe adequate behaviour, attitudes or perceptions to themselves in a given plot, similar to 'TOM stories'. In the 'self-ascription stories', persons were asked to report their behaviour, attitudes or perceptions in inherently ambiguous situations. The correct assignment of another person's mental state in the TOM conditions was tested by asking the participants to infer a specific behaviour or attitude of another person in the given context of the story, judged as adequate or inadequate according to Fletcher et al. (1995) and Happé et al. (1996). Correct assignment of the self-perspective was monitored by the use of personal pronouns in the documented answer of the particular story. This enabled us to employ a fully factorial design with the two factors of TOM (either present or not present) and self-perspective (either present or not present) (Figure 17.1).

Stories were presented during the fMRI blood oxygen level-dependent (BOLD) contrast echo planar imaging (EPI) measurements for 25 s on a display, with the question being presented subsequently for 15 s. Subjects were instructed to read the story carefully and to read and answer the subsequent question silently (covertly), during which period volumes were acquired continuously. After each presentation subjects were asked to give the answers overtly. In each of the four experimental conditions and the baseline, eight stories were presented. Image analysis comprised realignment, normalization and statistical analysis. Specific effects were analysed with respect to both a subtractive as well as factorial analysis.

Example of 'physical stories' (T−S−)

A burglar is about to break into a jeweller's shop. He skilfully picks the lock on the shop door. Carefully he crawls under the electronic detector beam. If he breaks this beam it will set off the alarm. Quietly he opens the door of the store-room and sees the gems glittering. As he reaches out, however, he steps on something soft. He hears a screech and something small and furry runs out past him, towards the shop door. Immediately the alarm sounds.

Question: Why did the alarm go off?

Example of 'TOM stories' (T+S−)

A burglar who has just robbed a shop is making his get-away. As he is running home, a policeman on his beat sees him drop his glove. He doesn't know the man is a burglar; he just wants to tell him he dropped his glove. But when the policeman shouts out to the burglar, 'Hey, you! Stop!', the burglar turns round, sees the policeman and gives himself up. He puts his hands up and admits that he did the break-in at the local shop.

Question: Why did the burglar do that?

Example of 'self and other ascription stories' (T+S+)

A burglar who has just robbed a shop is making his get-away. He has robbed your store. But you cannot stop him. He is running away. A policeman who comes along sees the robber as he is running away. The policeman thinks that he is running fast to catch the bus nearby. He does not know that the man is a robber who has just robbed your store. You can talk quickly to the policeman before the robber can enter the bus.

Question: What do you say to the policeman?

Example of 'self-ascription stories' (T−S+)

You go to London for a weekend trip and you would like to visit some museums and different parks around London. In the morning, when you leave the hotel, the sky is blue and the sun is shining. So you do not expect it to start raining. However, walking around in a big park later, the sky becomes grey and it starts to rain heavily. You forgot your umbrella.

Question: What do you think?

The brain activation pattern under the main effect of TOM ([T+S+ plus T+S−] relative to [T−S+ plus T−S−]) demonstrated increases in neural activity predominantly in the right anterior cingulate cortex and left temporopolar cortex

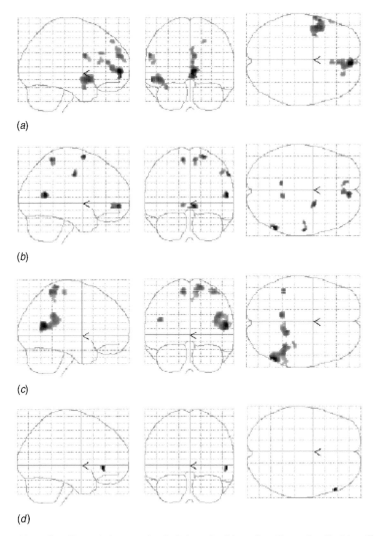

(a)

(b)

(c)

(d)

Figure 17.2   (a) Main effect of theory of mind (TOM); (b) main effect of self; (c) self relative to TOM; (d) interaction of TOM and self.

(Figure 17.2a). The main effect of self-perspective ([T−S+ plus T+S+] relative to [T+S− plus T−S−]) resulted in increased neural activity predominantly in the right temporoparietal junction and in the anterior cingulate cortex. Further significant increases in neural activity associated with self-perspective were observed in the right premotor and motor cortex and in the precuneus bilaterally (Figure 17.2b). When contrasting self-perspective with TOM directly (T−S+ relative to T+S−), activation of the right temporoparietal junction and bilateral precuneus was found, thus corroborating the specific difference between self-perspective and TOM

(Figure 17.2c). The interaction of TOM and self-perspective ([T+S+ relative to T+S−] relative to [T−S+ relative to T−S−]) was calculated to identify those areas activated specifically as a result of the presence of both TOM and self-perspective. This calculation revealed an increase in brain activity in the area of the right lateral prefrontal cortex (Figure 17.2d) (Vogeley et al., 2001).

Our results demonstrate that the ability to attribute opinions, perceptions or attitude to others, often referred to as 'mind-reading' (Baron-Cohen, 1995), and the ability to apply the self-perspective rely on both common and differential neural mechanisms. The cerebral implementation of the TOM capacity is located predominantly in the anterior cingulate cortex whereas the capacity for taking the self-perspective leads to additional neural activations basically in the right temporoparietal junction and the medial aspects of the superior parietal lobe, i.e. the precuneus. The fact that differential brain loci in different brain lobes are activated associated with the attribution of self-perspective or with 'mind-reading' of others suggests that these components are implemented at least in part in different brain modules and thus constitute distinct psychological processes. This is supported by the observation of a significant interaction between TOM and self-perspective in the right prefrontal cortex, a region which has previously been implicated in 'supervisory attentional' mechanisms (Shallice & Burgess, 1996) or monitoring situations that involve conflict of senses (Fink et al., 1999).

While the anterior cingulate cortex seems to be the key structure for assigning a mental state to someone else (irrespective of whether self-perspective is involved in the situation), our results also imply that activation of this brain region is not sufficient when the ability to apply self-perspective is required. In addition to anterior cingulate activation, taking self-perspective draws upon right inferior temporoparietal cortex, irrespective of whether subjects need to assign TOM at the same time or not. This finding is of considerable interest as lesions to the right temporoparietal junction typically result in visuospatial neglect, a neuropsychological deficit which often involves a disturbed (egocentric) frame of reference (Vallar et al., 1999). The activation of the temporoparietal junction during self-perspective is also compatible with evidence for the implementation of our body image in this region (Berlucchi & Aglioti, 1997; Vogeley & Fink, 2003), suggesting that taking the self-perspective may draw on a body representation as the centre of an egocentric experiential space. This conjecture in turn is in good accordance with reports on increased neural activity of right inferior parietal cortex involving visuospatial attention, e.g. navigation through virtual-reality scenes (Maguire et al., 1998) or assessment of the subjective midsagittal plane (Vallar et al., 1999).

Our data also contribute to the above-mentioned debate on simulation theory and theory theory. In the case of exclusive validity of simulation theory, all mental states requiring TOM, attributed to someone else or to oneself, should activate the same brain region. This prediction is in contrast to the results of our study, that show an additional specific activation site under self-perspective not present under TOM besides a marked overlap with shared activity increases in both self-perspective and TOM. That TOM and self-perspective involve at least in part distinct neural mechanisms is further corroborated by the finding of a significant interaction between both factors. Thus, our data clearly reject both simulation and theory theory in their pure form. Rather, our results are in favour of a mixture of both concepts. Whereas the theory theory component appears to be associated with increased activity in the anterior cingulate cortex, the simulation theory component appears to be primarily associated with increased brain activity in the area of the right temporoparietal junction, in which an egocentric reference frame is computed. It thus appears that 'knowledge of another's subjectivity is going to have to involve one's own' (Bolton & Hill, 1996, p. 135).

A central issue of the self-model is the experience of perspectivity in a spatial sense centred around my own body, as worked up by Piaget & Inhelder (1975; originally published 1948) concerning its genetic aspects. This feature depends on an internal representation of the organism's body, named body schema, body image or corporeal awareness, and is realized in the brain by a source of continuously generated input about internal milieu data, at least partly genetically determined (Melzack et al., 1997). Whenever experiences of perspectivity occur, this continual source of interoceptive and proprioceptive input is activated in parallel, presenting a spatial model of one's own body independent of external input and which becomes the centre of the experiential space. As Damasio worked out in his 'somatic marker hypothesis', this body image involves activation of the right parietal region and of the prefrontal cortex (Damasio, 1996). This is anatomically reflected in the strong relationship to diverse constituents of the limbic system, especially paralimbic cortical regions like cingulate, parahippocampal gyri and orbitofrontal cortex. Data about the internal milieu of the organism become available to the prefrontal cortex on the basis of prefrontal–temporolimbic cortical connectivity (Mesulam, 1985; Cummings, 1993; Van Hoesen et al., 1996; Fuster, 1997). This linkage then serves judging situations on the basis of former emotional reactions to similar situations in order to 'constrain the decision-making space by making that space manageable for logic-based, cost–benefit analyses' (Damasio, 1996, p. 1415). This 'body in the brain' was reviewed by Berlucchi & Aglioti (1997) as 'a mental construct that comprises the sensory impressions, perceptions and ideas about the dynamic organisation of one's own body and its relations to that of other bodies'. Teleologically, this serves survival of the whole organism by continuously representing the functional states of the body image, which is represented in the somatosensory region of the right parietal cortex (Damasio, 1994). The rapid and repetitive generation of the body image is based on a prefrontoparietal network, which is unconscious as such as it is continuously reconstituted in its process (Damasio, 1994, 1996; Metzinger, 1995).

Schizophrenia as clinical disorder of self-consciousness

In the pathophysiology of schizophrenia, it is suggested that clinical subsyndromes like cognitive disorganization and derealization syndromes reflect disorders of partial features of the self-construct, as defined in chapter 2 of this volume and in Vogeley et al. (1999). Psychiatric diseases are of special interest in this respect, as they present with different psychopathological symptoms that might be reconstructed as pathological conditions of the self-construct. A disturbance of ownership or agency correlates with the symptoms of thought insertion or thought-broadcasting experiences, the loss of the experience of being the agent of one's own actions, and the experience of hallucinations which are no longer experienced as self-induced internal perceptions. A disturbance of perspectivity, as disturbance in the single, co-herent and temporally stable model of reality centred around a single phenomenal subject, would result in depersonalization and derealization syndromes. A disturbance of unity could result in the experience of no longer being one single person identical over time, as in depersonalization or in ego-dystonic symptoms. According to this general framework, psychopathological symptoms can be reconstructed as disorders of partial features of the self-construct. This is shown in more detail for the symptom of hallucination (Vogeley, 1999).

The characteristic feature of a hallucination is the experiential quality of being world-induced, although this subjectively convincing impression of the hallucinating person cannot be corroborated from an observer's viewpoint. Hallucinations must be considered as internally generated perceptions without an objective correlate in the outer world. The subjective location of the hallucinated content is usually external, but may also be reported to be located internally in the head (David, 1994). Schizophrenic patients suffering from hallucinations exhibit a general bias towards misattributing internal events to an external source (Bentall et al., 1991a, Baker & Morrison, 1998). Hallucinations can be described along several dimensions, including their clarity or distinctness, their intensity, the degree of certainty or confidence. They are mostly context-adequate and embedded in real perceptual contexts. Concerning the high subjective certainty, that the perceived content is 'real', they resemble normal perceptions. In normal perception there is an objective correlate in the outer world that causes the sensory-rich perceptual content. The object perceived is again experienced as real, and this judgement is corroborated from an observer's viewpoint. Imagination is an interesting cognitive capacity in this context as they are lacking an appropriate stimulus in the environment and are at the same time adequately experienced as self-induced. They can thus be regarded as 'intermediate' or 'virtual' perceptions. Based on memory contents they play a considerable role in our world orientation (Richardson, 1995). In comparison to normal perception, Sartre explored a valuable distinction between imagination and perception in *L'Imaginaire* (1940), referring to visual perception. He emphasized that we can be deceived in normal perception regarding the perception of details, so that we can never be sure whether the perceived object is really what we think it is. We can never exclude that our perception is a very good 'copy' of the 'original', whereas during imagination we are always certain that we have evoked an imagination of the original object. In contrast, however, imaginations are usually sensory-poor (Sartre, 1940). Teleologically, imagination can be assumed to be an important step in information processing by providing schemes on which background new informations are analysed (Brown, 1985, p. 351). It appears that normal perception, imagination and hallucination have some overlap in their key properties of source monitoring and reality judgement. Source monitoring refers to the ability to judge correctly where the source of this perceptual content 'comes from'. Reality judgement refers to the ability to judge correctly whether this percept represents an object that is 'really out there'. This initiated the concept of a perceptual continuum integrating perception, imagination and hallucination (Brown, 1985; Behrendt, 1998).

Neurobiologically, primary projection and association cortices considerably participate in the generation not only of perception and imagination, but also of hallucinatory phenomena (Silbersweig et al., 1995; McGuire et al., 1996). It could be shown that hallucinatory experience is correlated with an increased activity in the regions of primary and associative cortices, which are responsible for auditory and speech information processing (Suzuki et al., 1993), suggesting a common neuroanatomic basis constituting a 'conservation principle' (Cohen et al., 1996). According to this, brain areas overlap, on which different perceptual capacities supervene. This hallucination-associated activation correlates with reduced activity in these areas in hallucinating patients on imaginary tasks (McGuire et al., 1996), suggesting that cortical areas are competitively recruited.Empirical studies on the visual system were the basis for developing the neurobiological hypothesis of a functional equivalence of perception and imagery (Shepard & Metzler, 1971; Kosslyn, 1994; Cohen et al., 1996). According to this hypothesis, considerable similarities exist between imagery and perception in functional as well as in anatomical respects of their neural correlates (Farah, 1985; Kosslyn, 1994; Ishai & Sagi, 1995; Cohen et al., 1996). These data provide additional neurobiological plausibility for the concept of a perceptual continuum.

Formally, this perceptual continuum can be understood as a representational system, in which the perceiving person as the representational system is embedded in his/her environment to be represented. This is an asymmetric relation between the person as representing system and the represented environment or aspects of it: a portrait may represent a person, but this person does not represent his portrait (Schumacher, 1997). The various modality-specific perceptual and cognitive capacities are realized by various functional systems in the brain and constitute the representing system. Notably, such a representational system includes the possibility of error or misrepresentation. On this basis, hallucinations can be interpreted as misrepresentations, in which the subjective reality judgement ('Is the perceived object real?') and the objective reality status ('The object does not exist' from an observer's standpoint) are discordant. It has been argued that the development of hallucinations is due to a self-monitoring disturbance that can be defined as a disturbance of the ability to 'distinguish sensations, thoughts, movements caused by their own actions from those that arise from external influences' (Frith, 1995).

However, this concept does not fully explain the high degree of confidence with which schizophrenic patients make judgements on the reality status of their hallucinations and the frequency with which they occur. It is not a necessary consequence of a self-monitoring deficit that internally generated perceptions are misattributed to someone else. This concept thus only provides a necessary, but not sufficient theoretical account of how hallucinations are generated. Focusing on how subjects are modelling reality, Joelle Proust (1999) suggested understanding the capacity of reality judgement or reality modelling as a capacity to represent and modify perceptions in such a way that the organism or the system is enabled reliably to reidentify the world around him/her for the purpose of world orientation. Whereas in simpler organisms such world representations may be 'proximal' (confined to their outer borders or membranes), organisms with increasing complexity might become able to develop the capacity additionally to represent 'distal' events or objects that are 'out there' in the world. This mechanism of integrating world information provides an internal representation of the world as a coherent and consistent model. Information no longer needs to be limited to the perceiving organism, but the organism can develop a reliable body of knowledge on the outer world as a world model or reality model. The integrity of such a world model depends on the capacity of adequately modifying sensory informations to be integrated into the preexisting world model.

A defective world-modelling instance might additionally promote misrepresentational processes such as hallucinations. It was suggested that an abnormality in the representational system generating moment-by-moment predictions of subsequent sensory inputs might result in a weakening of contextually elicited inhibitory processes (Hemsley, 1994). This deficit would involve a disturbance in prediction, in turn resulting in a failure to relate current sensory inputs to stored data of the world model. Hallucinations might thus be the result of a failure to inhibit long-term memory contents due to unstructured sensory inputs. In accordance with this general framework, it can be shown that schizophrenic patients ascribe more global, stable and external origins to events when making causal inferences (Bentall et al., 1991b) and that they favour externality over internality (Bolton & Hill, 1996, p. 341). The fact that schizophrenic patients tend to interpret an internal event as an external one could be explained as a pathologically increased 'permeability' between the individual and the environment. In addition to the highly plausible self-monitoring deficit, one could argue that a deficit in the reality model that provides a reliable and consistent world model could be a additional factor that further facilitates misrepresentational phenomena such as hallucinations.

Future strategies in schizophrenia research

As suggested above, a full understanding of hallucinations is possible as misrepresentation in the context of a representational system that includes the possibility of misrepresentation. Hallucinations might result from a deficit either in the capacity of self-monitoring, providing correctly assigned experiences of ownership, or in the capacity of reality modelling, constituting a reliable consistent model of the outer world, or both. This hypothetical explanation of hallucinations affecting both self and reality modelling or, at least, being induced by an imbalance in the communication of these two systems (Vogeley, 1999) is concordant with different other hypotheses and theoretical accounts of the pathogenesis of hallucinations (Bentall, 1990; Behrendt, 1998). This reconstruction of one of the most prominent symptoms in schizophrenia might illustrate the heuristic importance of the self-construct and its putative disturbances for the understanding of psychopathological phenomena.

This hypothesis of a self–reality imbalance hypothesis underlying the generation of hallucinations may be the basis for further experimental paradigms to be developed in both neuropsychological and functional imaging branches of schizophrenia research. Combined paradigms that operationalize partial features of the above-mentioned self-construct and of the capacity for reality modelling are to be developed. Operationalizations of the first-person perspective as opposed to the third-person perspective might serve as potentially useful paradigms (Vogeley et al., 2001). On the basis of the proposed concept, it can be predicted that hallucinatory experience as a key symptom in schizophrenia is probably facilitated if either self-monitoring or reality modelling is made more difficult for the test person in an experimental design. This type of experiment could be based on perceptual tasks which progressively increase in degree of difficulty with respect to self-monitoring and/or reality discrimination. With increasing degree of difficulty, hallucinatory experience is assumed to emerge or at least to be facilitated. The study of the relative impact of both domains could also serve to differentiate between the two theoretical concepts postulating either a disturbance of both domains or a disturbance of the communication between both domains. A consistent relative pattern of both domains would be in favour of the first variant, whereas changing patterns of the relative participation of both domains would be in favour of the imbalance variant of the proposed hypothesis.

With respect to the neurobiological correlates, Frith speculated that the self-monitoring disturbance is due to a disconnection or communicative disturbance of the prefrontal cortex and posterior brain regions (Frith, 1995). In fact, there is now converging evidence for schizophrenia as a disconnectivity syndrome (Vogeley & Falkai, 1998) and for the involvement of the prefrontal cortex (Vogeley et al., 1999). This could be especially relevant for the parietal lobe, which is the implementation site of the body image and body-centred spatial concepts (Berlucchi & Aglioti, 1997; Melzack et al., 1997). Our own data support this speculation of a frontoparietal interplay, that is related, in more general terms, to the capacity of distinguishing between myself and others. In terms of a pathomechanism it was speculated that hallucinations could arise from a nervous system with increased cortical 'associativity' (Behrendt, 1998). With respect to the two alternative concepts of a 'disconnectivity' or a 'hyperassociativity' mechanism explaining the pathogenesis of hallucinations, empirical data do not provide conclusive evidence for one or other concept. However, both variants do in fact propose a disturbance in the communication between different brain regions, probably between prefrontal and parietal brain regions. This underlines the heuristic value of the proposed account of a self-construct disturbance in general and an imbalance of some sort between self-monitoring and reality modelling domains in hallucinatory experience in particular.

Future research has to focus on the neuropsychological reconstruction of psychopathology in relation to brain sites and functions. Establishing experimental paradigms that operationalize the first-person as opposed to the third-person account is a first step. It would be useful to have a whole set of different experimental approaches available focusing on the different partial features of the self-construct.

REFERENCES

Baker, C.A. & Morrison, A.P. (1998). Cognitive processes in auditory hallucinations: attributional biases and metacognition. *Psychological Medicine*, **28**, 1199–208.

Baron-Cohen, S. (1995). *Mindblindness*. Cambridge, MA: MIT Press.

Baron-Cohen, S., Leslie, A. & Frith, U. (1986). Mechanical, behavioral and intentional understanding of picture stories in autistic children. *British Journal of Developmental Psychology*, **4**, 113–25.

Behrendt, R.P. (1998). Underconstrained perception: a theoretical approach to the nature and function of verbal hallucinations. *Comprehensive Psychiatry*, **39**, 236–48.

Bentall, R.P. (1990). The illusion of reality: a review and integration of psychological research on hallucination. *Psychological Bulletin*, **107**, 82–95.

Bentall, R.P., Baker, G.Y. & Havers, S. (1991a). Reality monitoring and psychotic hallucinations. *British Journal of Clinical Psychology*, **30**, 213–22.

Bentall, R.P., Kaney, S. & Dewey, M.E. (1991b). Paranoia and social reasoning: an attribution theory analysis. *British Journal of Clinical Psychology*, **30**, 13–23.

Berlucchi, G. & Aglioti, S. (1997). The body in the brain: neural bases of corporeal awareness. *Trends in Neuroscience*, **20**, 560–4.

Bolton, D. & Hill, J. (1996). *Mind, Meaning and Mental Disorder. The Nature of Causal Explanation in Psychology and Psychiatry*. Oxford: Oxford University Press.

Bressler, S.L. (1995). Large-scale cortical networks and cognition. *Brain Research Reviews*, **20**, 288–304.

Brown, J.W. (1985). Hallucinations. Imagery and the microstructure of perception. In *Handbook of Clinical Neurology*, vol. 1(45). *Clinical Neuropsychology*, ed. P. J. Vinken, pp. 351–72. Amsterdam: North Holland.

Buccino, G., Binkofski, F., Fink, G.R. et al. (2001). Action observation activates premotor and parietal areas in a somatotopic manner: an fMRI study. *European Journal of Neuroscience*, **13**, 400–5.

Carruthers, P. (1996). Simulation and self-knowledge: a defence of theory–theory. In *Theories of Theories of Mind*, ed. P. Carruthers & P.K. Smith, pp. 22–38. Cambridge: Cambridge University Press.

Cohen, M.S., Kosslyn, S.M., Breiter, H.C. et al. (1996). Changes in cortical activity during mental rotation. A mapping study using functional MRI. *Brain*, **119**, 89–100.

Cummings, J.L. (1993). Frontal-subcortical circuits and human behavior. *Archives of Neurology*, **50**, 873–80.

Damasio, A.R. (1994). *Descartes' Error. Emotion, Reason and the Human Brain*. New York: G.P. Putnam's Son.

Damasio, A.R. (1996). The somatic marker hypothesis and the possible functions of the prefrontal cortex. *Philosophical Transactions of the Royal Society: Biologic Sciences*, **351**, 1413–20.

David, A.S. (1994). The neuropsychological origin of auditory hallucinations. In *Neuropsychology of Schizophrenia*, ed. A.S. David & J. Cutting, pp. 269–313. London: Lawrence Erlbaum.

Engel, A.K., König, P., Kreiter, A.K. & Singer, W. (1991). Interhemispheric synchronization of oscillatory neuronal responses in cat visual cortex. *Science*, **252**, 1177–79.

Engel, A.K., Fries, P., König, P., Brecht, M. & Singer, W. (1999). Temporal binding, binocular rivalry, and consciousness. *Consciousness and Cognition*, **8**, 128–51.

Farah, M.J. (1985). Psychophysical evidence for a shared representational medium for mental images and percepts. *Journal for Experimental Psychology (General Psychology)*, **114**, 91–103.

Fink, G.R., Markowitsch, H.J., Reinkemeier, M. et al. (1996). Cerebral representation of one's own past: neural networks involved in autobiographical memory. *Journal of Neuroscience*, **16**, 4275–82.

Fink, G.R., Marshall, J.C., Halligan, P.W. et al. (1999). The neural consequences of conflict between intention and the senses. *Brain*, **122**, 497–512.

Fletcher, P., Happé, F., Frith, U. et al. (1995). Other minds in the brain: a functional imaging study of 'theory of mind' in story comprehension. *Cognition*, **57**, 109–28.

Frith, C.D. (1995). The cognitive abnormalities underlying the symptomatology and the disability of patients with schizophrenia. *International Journal of Psychopharmacology*, **10**, 87–98.

Fuster, J. (1997). *The Prefrontal Cortex. Anatomy, Physiology, and Neuropsychology of the Frontal Lobe*. New York: Lippincott-Raven.

Gallagher, I. (2000). Philosophical conceptions of the self: implications for cognitive science. *Trends in Cognitive Science*, **4**, 14–21.

Gallagher, H.L., Happé, F., Brunswick, N. et al. (2000). Reading the mind in cartoons and stories: an fMRI study of 'theory of mind' in verbal and non-verbal tasks. *Neuropsychologia*, **38**, 11–21.

Gallese, V. & Goldman, A. (1998). Mirror neurons and the simulation theory of mind-reading. *Trends in Cognitive Science*, **2**, 493–501.

Gallese, V., Fadiga, L., Fogassi, L. & Rizzolatti, G. (1996). Action recognition in the premotor cortex. *Brain*, **119**, 593–609.

Gopnik, A. (1993). How we know our minds: the illusion of first-person-knowledge of intentionality. *Behavioral and Brain Sciences*, **16**, 1–14.

Gopnik, A. & Wellmann, H. (1992). Why the child's theory of mind really is a theory. *Mind and Language*, **7**, 145–51.

Happé, F., Ehlers, S., Fletcher, P. et al. (1996). 'Theory of mind' in the brain. Evidence from a PET scan study of Asperger syndrome. *Neuroreport*, **8**, 197–201.

Happé, F.G.E., Brownell, H. & Winner, E. (1999). Acquired 'theory of mind' impairments following stroke. *Cognition*, **70**, 211–40.

Harris, P.L. (1992). From simulation to folk psychology: the case for development. *Mind and Language*, **7**, 120–44.

Hemsley, D.R. (1994). Cognitive disturbance as the link between schizophrenic symptoms and their biological bases. *Neurology, Psychiatry and Brain Research*, **2**, 163–70.

Iacoboni, M., Woods, R.P., Brass, M. et al. (1999). Cortical mechanisms of human imitation. *Science*, **286**, 2526–8.

Ishai, A. & Sagi, D. (1995). Common mechanisms of visual imagery and perception. *Science*, **268**, 1772–4.

Kosslyn, S.M. (1994). *Image and Brain: The Resolution of the Imagery Debate*. Cambridge, MA: MIT Press.

Leibniz, G.W. (1971) (originally published 1765). *Neue Abhandlungen über den menschlichen Verstand*. Hamburg: Philosophische Bibliothek, Felix Meiner Verlag.

Leslie, A. & Roth, D. (1993). What can autism teach us about metarepresentation? In *Understanding Other Minds: Persepctives from Autism*, ed. S. Baron-Cohen, H. Tager-Flusberg and D. Cohen. Oxford: Oxford University Press, 83–111.

Leslie, A. & Thaiss, L. (1992). Domain specificity in conceptual development: evidence from autism. *Cognition*, **43**, 225–31.

Maguire, E.A., Burgess, N., Donnett, J.G. et al. (1998). Knowing where and getting there: a human navigation network. *Science*, **280**, 921–4.

McGuire, P., Silbersweig, D.A., Wright, I. et al. (1996). The neural correlates of inner speech and auditory verbal imagery in schizophrenia: relationship to auditory verbal hallucinations. *British Journal of Psychiatry*, **169**, 148–59.

Melzack, R., Israel, R., Lacroix, R. & Schultz, G. (1997). Phantom limbs in people with congenital limb deficiency or amputation in early childhood. *Brain*, **120**, 1603–20.

Mesulam, M.M. (1985). *Principles of Behavioral Neurology*. Philadelphia: FA Davis.

Metzinger, T. (1993). *Subjekt und Selbstmodell*. Paderborn: Schöningh.

Metzinger, T. (1995). Ganzheit, Homogenität und Zeitkodierung. In *Bewußtsein. Beiträge aus der Gegenwartsphilosophie*, ed. T. Metzinger, pp. 595–633. Paderborn: Schöningh.

Perner, J. & Howes, D. (1992). 'He thinks he knows': and more developmental evidence against simulation (role taking) theory. *Mind Language*, **7**, 72–86.

Piaget, J. & Inhelder, B. (1975). Die Entwicklung des räumlichen Denkens beim Kinde (1948). In *Gesammelte Werke*. Stuttgart: Klett Verlag.

Premack, D. & Woodruff, G. (1978). Does the chimpanzee have a theory of mind? *Behavioral and Brain Sciences*, **4**, 515–26.

Proust, J. (1999). Mind, space and objectivity in non-human animals. *Erkenntnis*, **5**, 141–58.

Putnam, H. (1994). Sense, nonsense, and the senses: an inquiry into the powers of the human mind. *Journal of Philosophy*, **XCI**, 445–517.

Richardson, J.T.E. (1995). The efficacy of imagery mnemonics in memory remediation. *Neuropsychologia*, **33**, 1345–57.

Sartre, J.P. (1980). *L'Imaginaire*, 2nd edn. Rowohlt: Reinbek.

Schumacher, R. (1997). Philosophische Theorien mentaler Repräsentationen. *Deutsche Zeitschrift für Philosophie*, **45**, 785–815.

Shallice, T. & Burgess, P. (1996). The domain of supervisory processes and temporal organization of behaviour. *Philosophical Transactions of the Royal Society: Biologic Sciences*, **351**, 1405–11.

Shepard, R.N. & Metzler, J. (1971). Mental rotation of three-dimensional objects. *Science*, **171**, 701–3.

Silbersweig, D.A., Stern, E., Frith, C. et al. (1995). A functional neuroanatomy of hallucinations in schizophrenia. *Nature*, **378**, 176–9.

Suzuki, M., Yuasa, S., Minabe, Y., Murata, M. & Kurachi, M. (1993). Left superior temporal blood flow increases in schizophrenic and schizophreniform patients with auditory hallucination: a longitudinal case study using 123I-IMP SPECT. *European Archives for Psychiatry and Clinical Neurosciences*, **242**, 257–61.

Vallar, G., Lobel, E., Galati, G. et al. (1999). A fronto-parietal system for computing the egocentric spatial frame of reference in humans. *Experimental Brain Research*, **124**, 281–6.

Van Hoesen, G.W., Morecraft, R.J. & Semendeferi, K. (1996). Functional neuroanatomy of the limbic system and prefrontal cortex. In *Neuropsychiatry*, ed. B.S. Fogel, R.B. Schiffer & S.M. Rao. Baltimore: Williams & Wilkins.

Vogeley, K. (1995). *Repräsentation und Identität. Zur Konvergenz von Hirnforschung und Gehirn-Geist-Philosophie*. Berlin: Duncker und Humblot.

Vogeley, K. (1999). Hallucinations emerge from an imbalance of self monitoring and reality modelling. *The Monist*, **82**, 626–44.

Vogeley, K. & Falkai, P. (1998). The cortical dysconnectivity hypothesis of schizophrenia. *Neurology, Psychiatry and Brain Research*, **6**, 113–22.

Vogeley, K. & Fink, G.R. (2003). Neural correlates of first-person-perspective. *Trends in Cognitive Science*, **7**, 38–42.

Vogeley, K. & Newen, A. (2002). Mirror neurons and the self construct. In M. Stamenov & V. Gallese: *Mirror Neurons and the Evolution of Brain and Language*. John Benjamins Publishers.

Vogeley, K., Kurthen, M., Falkai, P. & Maier, W. (1999). Essential features of the human self model are implemented in the prefrontal cortex. *Consciousness and Cognition*, **8**, 343–63.

Vogeley, K., Bussfeld, P., Newen, A. et al. (2001). Mind reading: neural mechanisms of theory of mind and self-perspective. *NeuroImage*, **14**, 170–81.

Wimmer, H. & Perner, J. (1983). Beliefs about beliefs: representation and constraining function of wrong beliefs in young children's understanding of deception. *Cognition*, **13**, 103–28.

18

Action recognition in normal and schizophrenic subjects

Marc Jeannerod, Chloe Farrer, Nicolas Franck, Pierre Fourneret, Andres Posada, Elena Daprati and Nicolas Georgieff

Institut des Sciences Cognitives, Bron, France

Abstract

The ability to attribute an action to its proper agent and to understand its meaning when it is produced by someone else are basic aspects of human social communication. Several psychiatric symptoms, such as those of schizophrenia, relate to a dysfunction of the awareness of one's own action as well as of recognition of actions performed by others. Such syndromes thus offer a framework for studying the determinants of the sense of agency, which ultimately allows one to attribute correctly actions to their veridical source. This chapter will report a series of experiments in normal subjects and schizophrenic patients dealing with the recognition of actions. The basic paradigm used in these experiments was to present the subject with simple actions which may or may not correspond to those they currently execute. Systematic distortions have been introduced, such that the threshold for accepting an action as one's own could be determined. In normal subjects, this threshold is relatively high, indicating the existence of a specific mode of processing for action signals, independent from visual processing used in other perceptual activities. In schizophrenic patients, this threshold is further increased, with a strong tendency to self-attribute actions which do not correspond to those they have performed. The results reveal a clear distinction between patient groups with and without hallucinations and/or delusions of influence. Influenced patients show a higher rate of self-attributions. These results point to schizophrenia and related disorders as a paradigmatic alteration of a 'who?' system for action monitoring and self-consciousness.

Introduction: the sense of agency

The mechanism by which one becomes aware of one's own actions, and can distinguish them from those of other people, is a critical one, for a number of reasons. Firstly, the ability to recognize oneself as the agent of an action is one way by which the self builds as an entity independent from the external world. Secondly, the ability to attribute an action to its proper agent is a prerequisite for establishing social communication. Ultimately, functions such as understanding the meaning of an action and inferring the intention of its agent may be determined by these more elementary abilities.

Agency versus ownership

Being aware of one's own actions is not a straightforward process. Following Gallagher (2000), awareness of action may involve at least two components: indeed, an agent may be aware of the fact that he or she is moving (the sense of ownership) without being necessarily aware that he or she has a causal role in controlling the movement (the sense of agency). Although in many circumstances the two components coincide, there are situations where they dissociate. This is the case for movements caused by external forces, like reflex responses, for example, where the subject feels being the owner of the movement without feeling that he or she is the author of the response. In experimental conditions, movements caused by brain stimulation may also enter this category. Stimulation of cortical motor centres in the awake subject (using transcranial magnetic stimulation or TMS) produces brisk small movements which the subject may see and feel without having the least impression of having intended them (Jeannerod, 1997). Finally, pathological conditions offer many examples of abnormal movements due to impairments of the motor system, and the cause of which clearly lies outside a conscious sense of agency.

To illustrate this difference between sense of ownership and sense of agency it may be interesting to refer briefly to classical discussions among physiologists in the nineteenth century. Some of them, like Alexander Bain, thought that the conscious sensation arising from a movement had its sole origin in the centrally generated efferent discharges to the muscles, in the 'outgoing stream of nervous energy' (Bain, 1855). Others, however, expressed a more balanced view. Duchenne de Boulogne (1855), for example, distinguished between what he called 'muscular consciousness', originating from the effect of will on muscular contractions, and 'muscular sense', the set of peripheral sensations generated by the displacement of the limb. He conjectured that muscular consciousness should exist independently of muscular sensations, in patients with complete anaesthesia of one limb, for example. In a similar vein, Lewes introspectively considered that the complex experience arising from a voluntary movement was the sum of both the 'sense of effort' (of central origin) and the 'sense of effect' (of peripheral origin) (Lewes, 1878; Jeannerod, 1993). According to the above definition, the sense of effort and the sense of effect would approximately superimpose with Gallagher's sense of agency and sense of ownership, respectively.

The general idea of this chapter is that the sense of agency and the ability to attribute an action to its proper agent are tightly connected processes. The discussion in the previous paragraph has stressed the role of internal cues (under the terms of muscular consciousness or sense of effort) in signalling the willed or intentional nature of an action. Thus, the presence of these internal cues during generation of an action should induce from the agent both a feeling of agency and a judgement of self-attribution for that action. By contrast, in their absence, no sense of agency should be experienced by the agent, and the action should be attributed to someone else. More generally, according to a widely accepted hypothesis (Jeannerod, 1990; Wolpert et al., 1995), the above internal cues are thought to contribute to an internal model of the action to be performed in order to reach a desired goal. This internal model serves as a reference against which the sensory signals arising from execution of the action are compared, such that the match between the two indicates completion of the intended action. Note that this general hypothesis has further implications on the issue of attribution. If an internal model is present and the action-related sensory signals match it, this will be interpreted as an action that has been intended and executed by the agent. Conversely, if sensory signals arise, but no internal model is present, this will be interpreted as an externally generated event.

The distinction between self-generated movements and movements produced by other agents, and the corresponding attribution judgements, however, cannot be drawn from this simplistic model. What renders this distinction more difficult is the existence of a third possibility for the state of the internal model: this is the situation where an internal model has been generated but no action-related sensory signals arise. This possibility corresponds to the case where the action is imagined or intended, but not executed. Here, the available information for self-attributing the action is entirely internal to the self, based on the internal model which has been built in correspondence to the agent's intention. But, even if the goal of the movement remains a virtual one, and no possibility exists for matching the end result with the internal model, the above internal cues which are responsible for the sense of agency should nevertheless be present and the action should be attributed to the self. In addition, a further difficulty arises from the situation where a subject observes the action performed by another agent. This situation cannot be reduced to the existence of sensory signals without an internal model. As will be stressed below, it is likely that the observer also builds a representation of the action he or she sees, which he or she will use for understanding its meaning, inferring the agent's intentions and, ultimately, establishing social communication. Yet, no sense of agency should arise in the observer and the action should be attributed to the external agent.

The simulation hypothesis

There is a further potential confound between situations where actions are represented but not executed, for both conceptual and empirical reasons. Firstly, conceptually, recent theories on represented actions (e.g. intended, imagined or observed) have insisted on the idea that these actions undergo the same processing as effect-ively executed actions, except that they are not executed. Accordingly, many of the properties of motor images have been tentatively explained by the possibility that they would be 'quasiactions' blocked from execution by an additional, inhibitory mechanism (Jeannerod, 1994). Concerning observed actions, the theory goes on to say that they would activate within the observer's brain the same mechanisms that would be activated, were that action intended or imagined by that observer. In turn, this representation in the brain of the observed movements influences the interpretation made by the observer. In other words, the observer would use an implicit strategy of putting him- or herself 'in the shoes of the agent'. This theory (see Gallese and Goldman, 1998, for review), which posits that actions performed by others can be understood by an observer to the extent that they can be 'simulated' by that observer, would represent the basis for a broad spectrum of cognitive func-tions, ranging from understanding others' actions to learning by observation and imitation.

Secondly, this concept of simulation is now used, in neural terms, as an ex-planatory framework for the finding that both forms of motor representations (imagined and observed actions) involve a subliminal activation of the motor sys-tem (Jeannerod, 1999, 2001; Jeannerod & Frak, 1999). Brain-mapping experiments (using positron emission tomography (PET) or functional magnetic resonance imaging (fMRI) show activation of a partially overlapping cortical and subcorti-cal network during motor imagery and action observation. This network involves structures directly concerned with motor execution, such as motor cortex, dorsal and ventral premotor cortex, lateral cerebellum, and basal ganglia; it also involves areas concerned with action planning, such as dorsolateral prefrontal cortex and posterior parietal cortex. A recent metaanalysis of these data (Grèzes & Decety, 2001) reveals that the degree of overlap between different modalities of represen-tations varies from one cortical area to another. Concerning primary motor cortex itself, fMRI studies unambiguously demonstrate that pixels activated during con-traction of a muscle are also activated during imagery of a movement involving the same muscle (Roth et al., 1996). There are also indications for a similar effect during action observation (Hari et al., 1998), which is further demonstrated by direct mea-surement of corticospinal excitability by TMS of motor cortex (Fadiga et al., 1995). In premotor cortex and supplementary motor area (SMA), the overlap between imagined and observed actions is almost complete, as it is also in the posterior parietal cortex. By contrast, action observation largely involves the inferotemporal cortex, which is not the case for action imagination. Although the cortical networks pertaining to each form of covert (or represented) actions do not entirely overlap with each other, there are large cortical zones which are common to both. This relative similarity of neurophysiological mechanisms accounts for both the fact that actions can normally be attributed to their veridical author, and that action attribution remains a fragile process. Indeed, there are in everyday life ambiguous situations where the cues for the sense of agency become degraded and which obviously require a subtle mechanism for signalling the origin of an action. As the experiments below will show, situations can be created where normal subjects fail to recognize their own actions and misattribute to themselves actions performed by another agent. This may also be the case in situations created by interactions between two or more individuals (e.g. joint attention, matched actions or mutual imitation) or situations pertaining to the domain of human–machine interactions (e.g. telemanipulation, virtual-reality systems). A neural mechanism for explaining these difficulties will be presented at the end of the chapter.

Failure of the attribution mechanisms

Pathological conditions offer many examples of misattributions: a typical case is that of schizophrenia. Among the wide range of manifestations characterizing this disease, the so-called 'first-rank symptoms' have been considered critical for its diagnosis. According to Schneider (1955), these symptoms refer to a state where patients interpret their own thoughts or actions as due to alien forces or to other people and feel they are controlled or influenced by others. First-rank symptoms might reflect the disruption of a mechanism which normally generates consciousness of one's own actions and thoughts and allows their correct attribution to their author. Thus a study of attribution behaviour in schizophrenic patients would not only help to understand the factors responsible for misattribution in the patients, but also shed light on this critical function in normal life.

The pattern of misattributions due to agency disturbances in schizophrenic patients is twofold. Firstly, patients may attribute to others rather than to themselves their own actions or thoughts (underattributions); secondly, patients may attribute to themselves the actions or thoughts of others (overattributions). According to the French psychiatrist Pierre Janet (1937), these false attributions reflected the existence in each individual of a representation of others' actions and thoughts, in addition to the representation of one's own actions and thoughts: false attributions were thus due to an imbalance between these two representations. A typical example of underattributions is hallucinations. Hallucinating schizophrenic patients may show a tendency to project their own experience on to external events. Accordingly, they may misattribute their own intentions or actions to external agents. During auditory hallucinations, the patient will hear voices that are typically experienced as coming from an external powerful entity, but which in fact correspond to sub-vocal speech produced by the patient (Gould, 1949). The voices are often comments where the patient is addressed in the third person, and which include commands and directions for action (Chadwick & Birchwood, 1994). The patient may declare that he or she is being acted upon by an alien force, as if his or her thoughts or acts were controlled by an external agent. The so-called mimetic behaviour observed at the acute stage of psychosis also relates to this category.

The reverse pattern of misattribution can also be observed. Overattributions were early described by Janet (1937): what this author called 'excess of appropriation' corresponded for the patient to the illusion that actions of others are in fact initiated or performed by him/her and that he/she is influencing other people. In this case, patients are convinced that their intentions or actions can affect external events, for example, that they can influence the thought and actions of other people. Accordingly, they tend to misattribute the occurrence of external events to themselves. The consequence of this misinterpretation would be that external events are seen as the expected result of their own actions. This type of error by overattribution is an exaggeration of what can be observed in normal subjects who, according to Nielsen (1963), also attribute to themselves actions performed by others when they are presented in ambiguous conditions.

In the next sections, several possible explanations for these attribution impairments will be explored. The problem will be to determine whether they relate to a general deficit of executive mechanisms, impairing cognitive functions such as anticipation or working memory or, alternatively, whether they relate to a more specific problem dealing with action recognition *per se*. In light of the mechanisms described in the previous section, the hypothesis has been developed that schizophrenics would fail to monitor their willed intentions, including those related to the expression of thought. The consequence of this failure in self-monitoring would make them unable to disentangle actions arising from the external world from those generated as a consequence of their own cognitive functioning (Frith et al., 2000). This hypothesis will be further developed and integrated within a different framework, which includes a prominent, and perhaps neglected, aspect of schizophrenia, namely its intersubjective dimension.

A disturbance of executive mechanisms in schizophrenia

Investigators using neuropsychological methods for testing cognitive abilities in schizophrenic patients have established the deficiency in explicit and conscious modalities of processing information as a dominant characteristic of the disease (see Kuperberg & Heckers, 2000, for review). Accordingly, such patients have consistently been shown to perform poorly in cognitive tasks where working memory is likely to be involved, like learning abstract sequences (Dominey and Georgieff, 1997), management of rules (Laws, 1999), attention tasks (Bernard et al., 1997), processing of context (Servan-Schreiber et al., 1996) or semantic processing (Kuperberg et al., 1998). This behavioural evidence, however, is only partially consistent with neuroimaging data. Because in normal subjects working memory has often been associated with activation of the frontal lobes (Koechlin et al., 1999; Prabhakaran et al., 2000), one should expect that schizophrenic subjects should not show this pattern of cortical activity. As a matter of fact, fMRI studies in patients do not systematically show frontal lobe deactivation during working memory tasks (Stevens et al., 1998; Manoach et al., 1999). It has been claimed that the difference in frontal activation with respect to normal subjects is too modest to support the idea of a frontal lobe dysfunction (Zakzanis & Heinrichs, 1999). Future work in this field will have to focus on broader task-related neural networks linking cortical (Fletcher, 1999) and subcortical areas (Andreasen, 1999). Dysfunction of these networks, including defective inhibition or disinhibition, may be responsible for the working memory impairment.

It remains that such an impairment would probably affect the ability to interpret correctly the origin of an action. Recognition of a self-produced action implies that its goal and potential consequences are anticipated by the agent. Anticipation, in turn, requires short-term storage of the parameters encoded during the early stages of action execution, or even prior to execution. Self-attribution of the action will rely on the degree of match between these parameters and the final appearance of the action. This type of predictive behaviour is at work in nearly all human everyday activities.

Examining the ability of schizophrenic patients to anticipate forthcoming events therefore seems to be a legitimate start for understanding how they can monitor their own actions and, by extension, those of other people. One possible experimental approach to this problem consists in studying responses of subjects in tasks where they can manipulate advanced information either provided to them or acquired through learning. The ability to produce anticipatory responses should reflect the elementary process which ultimately allows predictive behaviour in natural situations.

An experimental study of anticipation in schizophrenia

Anticipation was studied using a simple situation where subjects had to learn a sequence of colours appearing on a computer screen: a subject who knows that the colours appear in a fixed order learns the sequence voluntarily, simply by watching the computer screen and repeating the colour names verbally. If, during this process of learning, the subject is instructed to press a specific key each time a given colour appears on the screen, the time to press the key sharply decreases after the complete sequence has been consciously disclosed and verbalized. As a matter of fact, keys are now pressed *before* the next colour is shown.

A group of 20 schizophrenic patients, and a group of matched control subjects ran experiments where stimuli were presented as temporal sequences

(Posada et al., 2001). Schizophrenic symptoms were assessed by the Scale for Assessment of Positive Symptoms (SAPS) (Andreasen, 1984) and the Scale for Assessment of Negative Symptoms (SANS) (Andreasen, 1983). The total SAPS score was 28.8 ± 15.2, and the total SANS score was 36.5 ± 22.4.

All subjects were first tested in a condition where they knew the existence of the sequence and had to learn it; subsequently, after they had acquired the sequence, they were tested for their ability to anticipate their responses with respect to the appearance of the stimuli. Although patients were found to be able to acquire the sequence almost normally, they proved to be impaired in using their explicit knowledge to produce anticipatory responses.

During the experiment, subjects were seated in front of a computer screen where sequences of coloured (yellow, green or blue) rectangles were displayed. Whenever a rectangle appeared, subjects were instructed to push the corresponding colour button on a button box. Response time (RT) was recorded. For each trial, a feedback was given after the subject's response. In the first condition (sequence learning), the subject was instructed to try to disclose the sequence and to report it verbally to the experimenter. Whenever a subject could not find the sequence after seven blocks, he/she was helped by the experimenter until he/she discovered the sequence. In the anticipation conditions, the repetitive sequences were explicitly given to the subject before the experiment. The subject received the instruction to try to push the correct buttons before the next element of the sequence appeared on the screen.

In the first condition of the experiment (learning), the number of blocks necessary to disclose and explicitly to report the sequence was determined. Subjects who failed to disclose the sequence after seven blocks were reported as 'failures'. Schizophrenic subjects needed 3.4 ± 1.6 blocks ($n = 14$; six failures) to find the temporal sequence. Controls needed 2.6 ± 1.61 blocks ($n = 18$; two failures) to find the temporal sequence. No significant difference was found in the number of blocks between groups for the temporal sequences (t-test, $P = 0,2$).

No significant difference in RTs between groups was found. In block 1, when subjects completely ignored the sequence, the two groups had nearly identical RTs, showing that schizophrenic subjects did not differ from normal subjects for what concerns pure reaction times to visual stimuli. In the following three blocks (4–6) where subjects knew the sequence and received the instruction to anticipate, control subjects showed a highly significant decrease in RTs with respect to schizophrenic subjects. The RTs in control subjects dropped to 280 ms, but only to 680 ms for the schizophrenic group. In a final random sequence block (R), where no anticipation was possible, RTs grew for both groups, but significantly less so in schizophrenics than in controls.

In the other condition (anticipation), where subjects explicitly received the sequence information at the beginning of the test, the response pattern was very

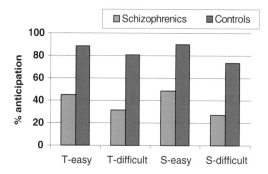

Figure 18.1   Percentage of anticipatory responses given by control subjects and schizophrenic patients. Subjects were tested in several versions of the colour sequence experiment. T, the colour sequence is presented as a temporal sequence; S, the colours appear sequentially in different spatial locations. Easy and difficult refer to short or long sequences, respectively. Reproduced from Posada et al. (2001).

similar between groups, but RTs were higher for schizophrenic subjects. Control subjects had mean RTs between 100 and 200 ms and schizophrenic subjects between 600 and 700 ms, except in the easiest condition, where the RTs were around 350 ms. In both groups, response times remained stationary during the blocks with instruction to anticipate (blocks 1–7). The analysis of variance (ANOVA) analysis showed a highly significant difference between groups but no interaction between groups and blocks. Finally, RTs increased for the random sequence block. Although this increase was much more marked in the control group, the fact that the schizophrenic patients also increased their RTs for the random sequence clearly indicates that they were still presenting some degree of anticipation.

The group mean of the percentages of anticipation (e.g. the mean difference between RTs for the anticipation blocks and RTs in the random sequence block) is shown in Figure 18.1. There was a significant reduction in the capacity of anticipation in schizophrenic subjects. Control subjects showed percentages of anticipation between 70 and 90% and schizophrenic subjects, between 30 and 50% only.

A working memory impairment?

The above results reveal a deficit in anticipatory behaviour in the group of schizophrenic patients. This deficit cannot be the consequence of impairments in elementary perceptual or motor functions. The patients had no difficulty performing the basic sensorimotor task of associating a colour displayed on the computer screen with the corresponding colour button; they also showed normal values of reaction times when they responded to presentation of colours before knowing the sequence. The number of errors remained low, not significantly different from that of control subjects. In addition, all patients were able, more or less rapidly, to learn and to remember the target sequences in each of the experimental conditions. Although control subjects typically required two blocks to acquire the sequence, patients needed three blocks. Failures (inability to acquire the sequence after seven blocks) were about three times more frequent in patients than in controls: however, those who had not been able to disclose the sequence by themselves, when properly trained by the experimenter, were able to memorize it. These results indicate that, although patients learned more slowly than controls, they had retention abilities compatible with task execution.

The major impairment in the schizophrenic patients in dealing with the learned colour sequences appeared when the instruction to respond in anticipation to the colours was introduced. In this condition, patients could only partly reduce their response times in comparison with their performance prior to learning. Whereas control subjects produced response times in the range of 100–200 ms (i.e. well below typical reaction times), patients were barely able to perform better than 600–700 ms. Note, however, that some degree of anticipation persisted in patients, as demonstrated by the fact that, in all conditions, their RTs were shorter than their purely reactive RTs in the random sequence blocks. Thus, the patients in this experiment, although they were strongly impaired in using the explicit knowledge they had available about the sequences to anticipate the occurrence of the next event, had retained the ability to understand and to perform the task.

To anticipate an incoming event is a cognitive process which requires the knowledge of regularities in the temporal unfolding of external events. In the particular process of anticipating the next incoming colour, subjects must use simultaneously the notion of a repetitive sequence, the sequence information stored in memory, the instruction to anticipate and the perception of the colour of the stimulus. All these components are integrated to produce a motor representation which activates the motor command to push the correct button. This integrative process, which has received considerable interest in neuropsychology, fits the definition of the 'working memory' which operates at the interface between memory, attention and perception (Baddeley, 1998).

The behavioural and clinical consequences of lack of anticipation

A deficit in using available information to anticipate correctly an incoming event probably represents an explanatory framework for some of the pathological aspects of schizophrenic behaviour. Such a deficit may be particularly deleterious in the domain of action, where a lack of anticipation may create situations where the consequences of actions are not properly evaluated. When planning (or intending) to move his/her hand to the right, for example, a normal individual anticipates seeing and feeling it moving in that direction. If the anticipation process is impaired, the direction in which the hand is seen to move may appear to be unrelated to the desired direction. This might be the sort of situations schizophrenic patients are faced with: in the above example, the patient may feel that his/her hand was displaced by an external agent, or even that it was an alien hand. When asked to whom this hand belongs, or who was the author of this movement, the patient may adopt different strategies: he or she may attribute the hand and/or the movement to an external agent, or he or she may use a default strategy by attributing the movement to him- or herself. Both strategies correspond to frequently observed clinical symptoms in certain categories of schizophrenic patients. In other studies, to be described below, we have repeatedly shown that such patients tend to overattribute to themselves movements performed by other agents (Daprati et al., 1997) and have increased thresholds for detecting movements differing from those they have actually performed (Franck et al., 2001). Lack of anticipation would thus preclude the normal match of actions with their internal representations, with the consequence that self-performed actions would not be recognized and would be misattributed. This hypothesis appears to be complementary with the more general theory of Gray et al. (1991), who suggested that such patients may fail to use, in processing new information, stored regularities about the external world: hence their inability to anticipate forthcoming events (Frith et al., 2000).

It may appear tempting to generalize this reasoning to other schizophrenic symptoms. An abnormal time integration has been proposed to participate in the production of schizophrenic symptoms (Minkowski, 1927). Impairment of patients in matching executed and represented actions could lead to the production of positive symptoms, such as incongruous actions or hallucinations, as well as to negative symptoms like impossibility in acting, apathy or lack of social interactions. It remains, however, that defective working memory and defective anticipation cannot represent a sufficient explanation for schizophrenic symptoms: it has also been found in other nonpsychotic categories of patients (e.g. patients with frontal lobe lesions), who show no attribution problems.

Dysfunction of a specific mechanism for recognizing action

Whether a lack of anticipation can represent the final explanation for misattribution of actions in schizophrenic patients thus seems highly doubtful. Misattributions are far from being evenly distributed among patients. Instead, this type of symptom is observed preferentially (if not exclusively) in one particular class of patients. For this reason, we will now investigate an alternative possibility, that of the disruption of a specific system for perceiving, recognizing and attributing actions.

Our argument is based on the existence of the already mentioned Schneiderian symptoms in schizophrenic patients. These symptoms include insertion of thought, auditory–verbal hallucinations, delusion of reference and delusions of alien control. They represent false beliefs which lead to a feeling of depersonaliza-tion by impairing the distinction between the self and the external world. The fact that these symptoms pertain to the realm of action is strongly supported by a set of clinical and experimental arguments based on the study of hallucinations. It has been known for some time that auditory–verbal hallucinations in schizophrenic patients are related to the production of speech by the patient. Some hallucinated patients even show muscular activity in their laryngeal muscles (David, 1994). Thus, auditory–verbal hallucinations represent a typical example of misattribution, where patients perceive their inner speech as voices arising from an external source. Ex-periments using neuroimaging techniques have greatly contributed to this problem by studying brain activation during hallucinations, or during inner speech in pa-tients predisposed to hallucinations and subjects experiencing no hallucinations. The results show that, during hallucinations (as signalled by the patients), brain metabolism is increased in the primary auditory cortex (Heschl gyrus) on the left side (Dierks et al., 1999), as well as in the basal ganglia (Silbersweig et al., 1995). By contrast, subjects predisposed to hallucinations show decreased activity in speech temporal areas during inner speech and auditory–verbal imagery, as compared to other subjects (McGuire et al., 1996). The clearest result from these conflicting data is that, during verbal hallucinations, the auditory temporal areas remain active, which suggests that the nervous system in these patients behaves as if it were actually processing the speech of an external speaker. Patients perceive their own thinking as originating from the outside world. This explanation would be consistent with the idea (Frith et al., 2000) that the normal mechanism for attributing thought to its internal origin is a comparison between the executive commands leading to speech and the anticipated sensory consequences of these commands. Inner speech would normally be accompanied by a mechanism that decreases activity at the level of primary auditory cortex, perhaps via an inhibitory projection from the frontal lobe. Because in verbal hallucinations the inner speech is usually not uttered, this hypothesis would be consistent with the notion that the sense of agency must be functioning even in the absence of comparison with external reafferences, and that actions can be monitored at the level of their representation, not only at the level of their execution. As a matter of fact, in clinical practice the Schneiderian symptoms almost exclusively concern nonexecuted actions. Hallucinations, once considered as a perception without an object, should therefore be reevaluated as an action without a subject.

Other types of hallucinations, such as mental automatism and delusions of alien control might also correspond to an impairment of recognition of action. Spence et al. (1997) examined cortical activity in schizophrenic patients with experience of delusional control. During the scan, the patients were required voluntarily to move a joystick and freely to select the direction of the movement. Most of them reported vivid experiences of alien control when performing the motor task. Brain activation was found to be increased in a cortical network including the left pre-motor cortex and the right inferior parietal lobule and angular gyrus, at the level of areas 40 and 39. This right parietal hyperactivity in deluded subjects is particularly interesting: it is noteworthy that lesions at this level frequently result in altered awareness (neglect) of the contralateral limbs and space, and denial of the disease (anosognosia); conversely, transient hyperactivity (during epileptic fits, for example) may produce impressions of an alien phantom limb (Spence et al., 1997).

In an effort to quantify the degree of misattribution in schizophrenic subjects, we designed experimental situations where subjects had to produce agency judgements about hand movements that were shown to them and that corresponded, or not, to their own movements. These experiments are described below.

A pilot study of agency in normal and schizophrenic subjects

In this section, we will present data from an experiment where the performance of groups of schizophrenic patients was compared to those of matched controls (Daprati et al., 1997). A situation was created where the subjects were shown movements of a hand of an uncertain origin, that is, a hand that could equally likely belong to them or to someone else, using a paradigm directly borrowed from the study of voluntary movement by Nielsen (1963). Subjects were instructed to determine explicitly whether they were the author of the hand movements they saw. In order to give such a response, they had to use all available cues to compare the current movement of their unseen hand with the movement that was displayed to them.

Sixty subjects participated in the study, including 30 normal control subjects and 30 schizophrenic patients. Hallucinations were present in 13 patients; delusion of control was reported by seven patients; finally, delusion of control and hallucinations were both present in six cases. During the experiment, the subject's hand and the experimenter's hand were filmed with two different cameras. By changing the position of a switch, one or the other hand could be briefly (5 s) displayed on the video screen seen by the subject. A mirror with an inclination of 30° in the vertical plane was placed at 40 cm from a table, and at 35 cm from the subject's frontal plane. Subjects positioned their right hand on the table, below the mirror. A camera filmed the subject's hand, the image of which appeared on a TV-screen located on a shelf, 15 cm over the subject's head and was reflected by the mirror (Figure 18.2). Thus, looking at the mirror, subjects had the impression that they watched their own hand as through a window. A second camera, placed in another part of the room, filmed the experimenter's hand. The display allowed the experimenter to match the image of her hand exactly with that of the subject's hand before the beginning of

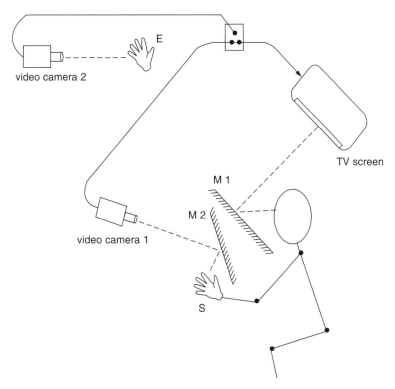

Figure 18.2 Schematic diagram of experimental set-up used in Daprati et al. (1997) experiment. M1 and M2, mirrors used to reflect the image of the subject's hand; S, subject; E, experimenter.

each trial. The experimenter's and the subject's hands were covered with identical gloves, in order to minimize the effects of gross morphological differences.

The task for the subjects was to perform a requested movement with their right hand, and to monitor its execution by looking at the image in the mirror. At the beginning of each experimental trial, a blank screen was presented. An instruction to perform a movement was given and the subject and the experimenter had to execute the requested movement at an acoustic signal. Once the movement was performed and the screen had returned blank, a question was asked of the subject: 'You have just seen the image of a moving hand. Was it your own hand? Answer *yes* if you saw your own hand performing the movement you have been executing. Answer *no* in any other case, that is, if you doubt that it was your own hand or your own movement'. One of four possible movements of the fingers was required in each trial: (1) extend thumb; (2) extend index; (3) extend index and middle finger; and (4) open hand wide. One of three possible images of the hand could be presented to the subjects in each trial: (1) the subject's own hand (condition: Subject); (2) the experimenter's hand performing the same movement (condition: Experimenter Same); and (3) the experimenter's hand performing a different movement (condition: Experimenter Different).

A descriptive analysis of the results showed that hallucinating patients made more recognition errors (median value 24) than nonhallucinating patients (11) and controls (5). Similarly, patients experiencing delusion of control made more recognition errors (median value 24) than the rest of the patients (18) and controls (5). The present analysis focuses only on patients experiencing delusion of control. The total number of recognition errors was significantly different between groups. Errors occurred especially in the condition Experimenter Same, i.e. in the trials where the hand on the screen performed the same movement that was required from the subject but was not his/her own, the median for error rate was 5 in the control group, 17 in the nondelusional group and 23 in the delusional group, whereas virtually no errors occurred when subjects saw their own hand, or a hand performing a different movement. Differences between the three groups for the condition Experimenter Same showed a strong trend to significance (comparison controls versus nondelusional $P = 0.006$; controls versus delusional $P = 0.001$; nondelusional versus delusional $P = 0.07$, Mann–Whitney U-test). All these differences were clearly significant by using the criterion of hallucinations instead of delusions.

In this experiment, normal control subjects were able unambiguously to determine whether the moving hand seen on the screen was theirs or not, in two conditions. Firstly, when they saw their own hand (trials from the condition Subject), they correctly attributed the movement to themselves. Secondly, when they saw the experimenter's hand performing a movement which departed from the instruction they had received (condition Experimenter Different), they denied seeing their own hand. By contrast, their performance degraded in the condition Experimenter Same, that is, in trials where they saw the experimenter's hand performing the same movement as required by the instruction: in this condition, they misjudged the hand as theirs in about 30% of cases.

It is also in that particular condition that the rate of incorrect responses increased in schizophrenic patients. The error rate amounted to 77% in the group of patients with hallucinations or 80% in the group with delusional experiences, whereas in the nonhallucinating group, it was around 50%. The fact that all patients gave nearly correct responses in the other two conditions (the error rate remained 1–7%) shows that the effect observed in trials Experimenter Same was not due to factors unrelated to the task, such as lack of attention. The explanation for this effect therefore should be found in a deficit of the mechanism which is normally used for controlling and recognizing one's own movements.

The pattern of responses that we recorded in our condition Experimenter Same (in both normal controls and schizophrenics) could be explained by the paucity of movement-related cues available to the comparator mechanism. Because the subject's (invisible) hand and the experimenter's (visible) hand both executed the same movement, some mismatch occurred between the anticipated and the perceived final hand postures. The only available cues were the dynamic signals generated during the movements themselves. Slight differences in timing and kinematic pattern between the intended movement and that perceived by visual and kinaesthetic channels had to be used in order to give the correct response. A decrease in sensitivity of this mechanism would explain the greater difficulties met by the schizophrenic patients. Even normal subjects misjudged the ownership of the experimenter's hand in about 30% of trials. This finding suggests that the mechanism for recognizing actions and attributing them to their true origin operates with a relatively narrow safety margin: in conditions where the visual cues are degraded or ambiguous, it is barely sufficient for making correct judgements about the origin of action, although it remains compatible with correct determination of agency in everyday life.

A parametric study of agency in normal and schizophrenic subjects

The above experiment by Daprati et al. (1997) demonstrates that the clinical difficulty in identifying the origin of an action observed in patients with delusion of influence can be experimentally provoked. The procedure used in this experiment, however, did not allow the determination of those cues, used by normal subjects to give correct attribution responses, that were missing in the influenced schizophrenic patients. Another experiment was therefore designed to answer this question (Franck et al., 2001). Using a situation similar to that of Daprati et al., a realistic virtual hand was used, instead of the hand of an experimenter, and this was superimposed on to the subject's hand. Not only did this device allow more standard experimental conditions; it also allowed the systematic distortion of the movements of the virtual hand with respect to those of the subject's hand. The results fully support the existence of impaired attributions of action in schizophrenia, especially in influenced patients.

Twenty-nine schizophrenic subjects and 29 normal controls participated in the study. During the experiment itself, five schizophrenic subjects revealed they were unable to perform the task correctly and, for this reason, were not further included in the study. None of them were influenced or hallucinated. Accordingly, all data reported below only bear on the 24 patients who completed the task. At the time of testing, six patients were classified as 'influenced'. The remaining 18 'noninfluenced' patients scored 2 or less at this subscale. Finally, the patients underwent neuropsychological testing to assess their spatial perception abilities. To this aim, the Birmingham Object Recognition Battery (BORB) (Riddoch & Humphreys, 1993) was used. The patients' performances were within normal range.

During the experiment an image of an electronically reconstructed hand was presented to the subjects. A specially designed program run on a PC computer synthesized pictures of a hand holding a joystick according to the real position of a joystick actually held by the subject and connected to the computer. This design allowed the dynamic representation of the movements of the joystick held by the subject with an intrinsic delay inferior to 30 ms. Temporal or angular biases could be introduced in this representation (see below), modifying the apparent direction or the degree of synchrony of the movement actually performed by the subject with respect to the movement displayed on the computer screen. The computer monitor on which the virtual image appeared was placed face-down on a metallic support. A horizontal mirror, located 18 cm below the monitor screen, reflected the image. The joystick was placed below the mirror on a table supporting the apparatus, so that the subject's hand holding the joystick was located approximately 18 cm below the mirror. Thus, when subjects looked at the mirror, they saw the image of a virtual hand moving a joystick just above their own unseen hand actually doing that.

Subjects held the joystick with their right hand, with their elbow resting on the table. The position of their forearm was adjusted so as to coincide with the direction of the virtual forearm seen in the mirror. Subjects were instructed to maintain fixed the position of their fingers on the joystick and to restrict their movements to the wrist joint. The task consisted in executing a series of simple movements with the joystick from the resting position, in the straight-ahead direction, to the right or to the left. Each trial started with a dark screen. A green spot was displayed for 1 s on the left, on the right or on the top of the screen. The image of the virtual hand then appeared for 2 s, during which subjects had to execute a movement of the joystick in the direction indicated by the position of the green spot. Immediately after the trial, subjects had to answer the question: 'Did the movement you saw on the screen exactly correspond to that you have made with your hand?' They had to answer *yes* or *no*.

Three categories of trials were used:

1. Neutral trials: movements of the virtual hand seen on the screen exactly replicated those made by the joystick.
2. Trials with angular bias: movements of the virtual hand were deviated by a given angular value with respect to those made by the joystick. Seven values of angular bias from 5° to 40°, either to the right or to the left, were used.
3. Trials with a temporal bias: movements of the virtual hand were delayed by a given time with respect to those made by the joystick. Seven values of temporal bias from 50 to 500 ms were used.

Verbal responses of the subjects were recorded. According to whether trials were with or without bias, subjects could potentially make two types of errors: *yes* responses in trials with a bias, and *no* responses in neutral trials. The maximum number of errors was 12 for the neutral trials and 84 for the trials with an angular or a temporal bias. Presentation of the results below will focus on the *yes* responses, because this type of response reflects the subjects, ability to recognize a movement as their own.

Control subjects and patients gave *yes* (correct) responses in nearly all neutral trials. The median value of erroneous *no* responses was equally small ($n = 1$) for the control subjects and for the influenced and noninfluenced patient subgroups. The distribution of *yes* responses for the biased trials, although it clearly differed between groups, as will be shown below, kept a relatively similar pattern across groups. In both control subjects and patients, the number of *yes* responses was higher for the smaller temporal and angular biases, and became lower as the biases increased. In other words, only the shape of the distribution differed between groups.

Influenced schizophrenic patients gave globally more *yes* responses than noninfluenced schizophrenic patients and normal controls in both the trials with angular and temporal bias. Figure 18.3 reveals the main characteristic of these results, namely that the differences between the control group and the two patients groups varied as a function of the amplitude of the biases. It shows the number of *yes* responses for trials with an angular bias. Whereas noninfluenced patients showed a sharp decrease in erroneous *yes* responses (down to 50% of maximum number of errors) already for a bias between 15° and 20°, a value not very different from that of controls, influenced patients did not reach the same score until the bias increased to 30 – 40°. The results were different for the temporal bias. Whereas control subjects showed a clear decrease in *yes* responses for a relatively small bias (100–150 ms), both influenced and noninfluenced patients followed a similar trend and did not show a decrease in the rate of *yes* responses until the bias reached 300 ms. Statistical comparison showed that both groups of patients produced significantly more errors than the control group in the trials with a temporal bias for delays longer than 100 ms. In the trials with an angular bias, the difference with the control group was significant for angles larger than 10° for the influenced patients and for the 30° and 40° angles only for noninfluenced patients.

The results from this experiment provide an insight to the cues used to recognize one's own actions. Control subjects still recognized as their own a movement delayed by up to 150 ms with respect to the movement they actually executed. Similarly, if normal subjects saw their movement rotated from its actual trajectory by about 15°, they still accepted it as their own. This result shows that the accuracy for detecting the features of one's own movement is limited, and that this limitation is far beyond perceptual thresholds of the visual system for detecting temporal gaps or angular deviations (Fourneret & Jeannerod, 1998). These results clarify the findings of Daprati et al. (1997) where normal subjects failed in about 30% of cases to recognize an alien hand as distinct from their own hand, when the two hands

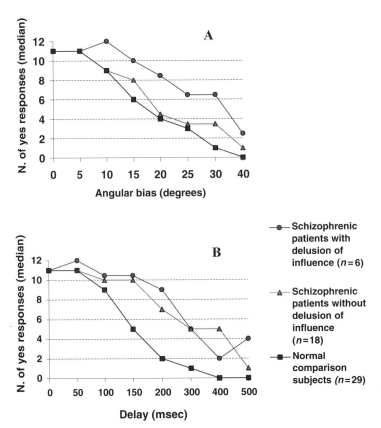

Figure 18.3   A parametric study of attribution responses in control subjects and schizophrenic patients (Franck et al., 2001). Single movements performed by subjects were shown to them through a mirror. The appearance of the movement might be deviated from its actual course. Subjects were instructed to answer *yes* if they considered that the movement they saw corresponded to the one they executed. At 0° (no deviation), all subjects correctly responded *yes*. Control subjects tolerated deviations of up to 15° before they consistently rejected the movement they saw as corresponding to their actual movement. One group of schizophrenic patients (with delusions of influence) continued to give *yes* responses up to 30° deviations.

performed nearly synchronous movements. As delays between the two hands and movement trajectories were not measured in Daprati et al.'s experiment, one can only speculate on those cues that were missing for the subjects to identify a hand as alien. However, the present results indicate that these misattributions were likely to occur when the delays between the two movements were below 150 ms, or their trajectories deviated from each other by less than 15°.

In the present experiment, the patients were clearly worse than controls at recognizing as distinct from their own movements that were delayed or deviated. All 24 schizophrenic patients responded at chance when a time delay up to 300 ms was introduced. For angular deviations, only the influenced patients responded at chance up to 30°, whereas noninfluenced patients presented an error rate comparable to normal controls, i.e. became aware of the angle around 15°. Defective perceptual or attentional factors seem to be ruled out by the fact that all patients (including the influenced ones) performed well in the BORB test, indicating that they had retained a normal ability to discriminate small angular differences. In the case of temporal biases, one could argue that schizophrenic patients are known to be slow in many tasks and that their reaction times are globally increased, a feature which can be categorized among the negative symptoms (Cadenhead et al., 1997). In fact, our temporal delay condition is quite different from a reaction time task (see below). Finally, the fact that the same patients performed differently in the two tasks is a good indication that they were not influenced by unspecific factors when giving their responses.

Neural constraints on action recognition in the social context

Experimental manipulations of the appearance of one's own movements impair the correct self-attribution of these movements, an effect which is dramatically increased in schizophrenic patients. It seems likely to attribute these difficulties in detecting differences between self-produced and externally produced movements, in the absence of other obvious visual deficit, to an impairment of a specific neural system devoted to perception of actions produced by living organisms and singularly by human beings, and operating during interactions between several people.

Perception of biological movements

One of the prerequisites for the functioning of such a system is that it can distinguish biological movements from those produced by mechanical devices. Biological movements involve specific kinematic properties and regularities which make them recognizable to other people (Johansson, 1977). This property is illustrated by recent psychophysical experiments. These experiments tested the perception of apparent motion from static pictures of an object presented at different locations. If the object is a human figure (for example, alternating static pictures of a model with his arm positioned behind his head and in front of his head) the time between the two static pictures will have to increase up to 400 ms in order for the observer to report a biologically plausible trajectory (the arm moving around the head). Below this threshold, the observer will report the most direct trajectory (the arm across the head) (Shiffrar & Freyd, 1990; Ramachandran et al., 1998; Stevens et al., 2000). This is consistent with the present results showing that the attribution system operates with a temporal and spatial resolution which is relatively low with respect to the capabilities of the visual system.

The effect of introducing a temporal delay between the observed movement and the actual movement can be discussed first. As stated above, this impairment is different from slowness to respond; it expresses a difficulty in the perception of slight temporal differences. Recent findings in schizophrenic patients might represent a rationale for the difficulty met by the patients from the present study: such patients are unable to discriminate between two different velocities of a moving vertical grating (Chen et al., 1999) and they cannot discriminate fast motions of a moving dot (Schwartz et al., 1999). Such inabilities might not be unique to schizophrenic patients: indeed, similar results have been obtained in autism (Gepner et al., 1995). Thus, there is a possibility that psychotic patients in general are unable to integrate time cues in their perception of movement, efficiently and this would account for our finding that all patients in the present study, irrespective of their clinical symptomatology, were impaired in detecting delays in their own movements. Although this impairment probably contributes to the high rate of misattributions observed here, it may not represent the core of the problem, mainly because it does not differentiate between influenced and noninfluenced patients.

The deficit in detecting movement direction might be a better determinant of difficulties in attribution met by these patients. One of the main findings of the experiments of Franck et al. (2001) is that only influenced patients were impaired in attributing movements with angular biases. Coding the direction of a movement is indeed a critical condition for an agent to reach an object precisely in peripersonal space. Perceiving the direction of a movement is also useful information for an observer to understand the action of the agent of this movement: during a movement, the arm points to the goal of the action and its direction may reveal the intention of the agent. It is thus not surprising that a patient deprived of this information will misinterpret the intention displayed by others in their movements, and that this will have consequences on understanding interactions between people. In the present study, the fact that influenced patients tended to self-attribute movements, the direction of which was distorted, illustrates this problem. In Daprati et al.'s experiment (Daprati et al., 1997), influenced patients were also worse than noninfluenced ones at differentiating the movements they executed with their own hand from movements executed more or less synchronously by another hand. The discrepancies between movements performed by the two agents, although they were perceptible to normal subjects and, to a large extent, to noninfluenced patients, were far too small, as we know from the above parametric study, to be detected by influenced patients.

The situations used in our experiments privileged self-attribution responses. Only one hand was present at a time to the patient: thus, the situation always referred to the patient as the agent of the action. If another agent were clearly involved in the situation, this might leave the possibility for the patient to produce the opposite type of response, i.e. a response of underattribution. This possibility has been tested in our laboratory. An experiment where the patient's hand was shown along with another hand revealed that influenced patients tended to make more attribution errors and that their errors were more frequently misattributions to the other than to the self. Normal controls and noninfluenced patients made an equal number of errors in both directions (Farrer et al., 2002).

A neural hypothesis for action recognition: the 'who' system

We have therefore created the experimental conditions for the study of social cognition and its disorders in psychotic patients. In this concluding section, we briefly present a framework for integrating social cognition to the neural substrate. Our present conception of action recognition (Georgieff & Jeannerod, 1998; Jeannerod, 1999) is based on the existence of neural networks subserving the various forms of representation of an action. Accordingly, each representation entails a corticosubcortical network including, to varying extent, activation of interconnected neural structures. Some of these networks have been described in an earlier section of this chapter. Although these ensembles are clearly distinct from one form of representation to another (e.g. the representation of a self-generated action versus the representation of an action observed or predicted from another agent), they partly overlap: posterior parietal and premotor areas, for example, are activated during both. When two agents socially interact with one another, this overlap creates 'shared representations', i.e. neural structures that are simultaneously activated in the brains of the two agents. In normal conditions, however, the existence of nonoverlapping parts, as well the existence of possible differences in intensity of activation between the activated zones, allows each agent to discriminate between representations activated from within from those activated from outside, and to disentangle which belongs to him or her from that which belongs to the other. This process would thus be the basis for correctly attributing a representation (or the corresponding action) to the proper agent or, in other words, for answering the question of 'who' is the author of an action. The flow chart shown in Figure 18.4 is a tentative illustration of the many interactions between two agents. Each agent builds in his or her brain a representation of both his or her own intended actions, using internal cues like his/her own beliefs and desires, and the potential actions of the other agent with whom he/she interacts. These partly overlapping representations are used by each agent to built a set of predictions and estimates about the social consequences of the represented actions, if and when they would be executed. Indeed, when an action comes to execution, it is perceived by the other agent as a set of social signals which confirm (or not) his or her predictions and possibly modifies his or her beliefs and desires.

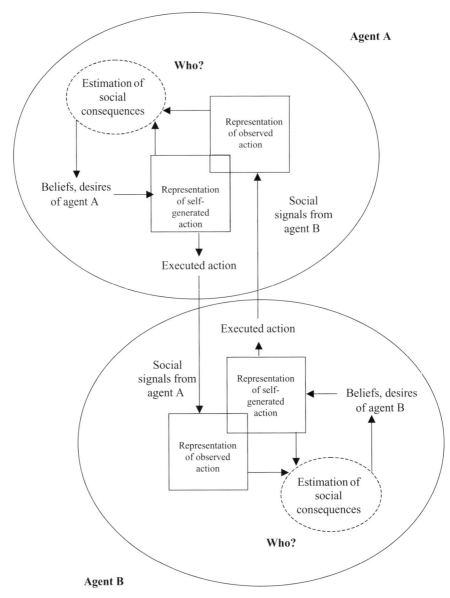

Figure 18.4 A flow chart of the interplay between two agents. For explanation, see text.

This concept allows us to make hypotheses about the nature of the dysfunction responsible for misattribution of actions by schizophrenic patients. Changes in the pattern of cortical connectivity could alter the shape of the networks corresponding to different representations, or the relative intensity of activation in the areas composing these networks. Several examples in relation to verbal hallucinations or alien control of movements have been described in the present chapter. Unfortunately, little is known on the functional aspects of cortical connectivity underlying the formation of these networks and, a fortiori, on their dysfunction in schizophrenia. Among the relevant studies, several have pointed to the prefrontal cortex as one of the possible sites for perturbed activation: not only is it hypoactive in many patients (Weinberger & Berman, 1996), its morphological aspect has also been shown to be modified on postmortem examination (Goldman-Rakic & Selemon, 1997). Because prefrontal areas are known normally to exert an inhibitory control on other areas involved in various aspects of motor and sensorimotor processing, an alteration of this control in schizophrenic patients might result in aberrant representations for actions. Referring to Figure 18.4, one of the two agents would become 'schizophrenic' if, due to an alteration in the pattern of connectivity of the corresponding networks, the degree of overlap between the representations in his brain increased in such a way that the representations would become undistinguishable from each other. The pattern of misattribution in this patient would be a direct consequence of this alteration: for example, decreased self-attribution if frontal inhibition were too strong, or increased self-attribution if it were too weak.

Other deficits in executive mechanisms, like reduced memory span and inability to anticipate forthcoming events, are also likely to contribute to the impairment in action recognition. Lack of anticipation impairs the comparison of an executed action with its internal representation and may therefore render self-attribution of that action more difficult. However, misattribution in schizophrenic patients also holds for inner speech, thoughts, intentions and other forms of nonexecuted actions, which cannot be explained by a mechanism based on the processing of overt action signals. The problem should rather be looked for at the level of an internal mechanism which would include both simulation of the action (intended, imagined or observed) and of its expected consequences. A mismatch between the two would have dramatic consequences on the attribution of the intention to its real agent.

REFERENCES

Andreasen, N.C. (1983). *The Scale for the Assessment of Negative Symptoms (SANS)*. Iowa City, IA: University of Iowa.

Andreasen, N.C. (1984). *The Scale for the Assessment of Positive Symptoms (SAPS)*. Iowa City, IA: University of Iowa.

Andreasen, N.C. (1999). A unitary model of schizophrenia. *Archives of General Psychiatry*, **56**, 781–7.

Baddeley, A. (1998). Recent developments in working memory. *Current Opinion in Neurobiology*, **8**, 234–8.

Bain, A. (1855). *The Senses and the Intellect.* London: Parker.

Bernard, D., Lancon, C. & Bougerol, T. (1997). Attention models in evaluating schizophrenia. *Encephale*, **23**, 113–18.

Cadenhead, K.S., Geyer, M.A., Butler, R.W. et al. (1997). Information visual processing deficits of schizophrenia patients: relationship to clinical ratings, gender and medication status. *Schizophrenia Research*, **28**, 51–62.

Chadwick, P. & Birchwood, M. (1994). The omnipotence of voices. A cognitive approach to auditory hallucinations. *British Journal of Psychiatry*, **164**, 190–201.

Chen, Y., Palafox, G.P., Nakayama, K. et al. (1999). Motion perception in schizophrenia. *Archives of General Psychiatry*, **56**, 149–54.

Daprati, E., Franck, N., Georgieff, N. et al. (1997). Looking for the agent: an investigation into consciousness of action and self-consciousness in schizophrenic patients. *Cognition*, **65**, 71–86.

David, A.S. (1994). The neuropsychological origin of auditory hallucinations. In *The Neuropsychology of Schizophrenia*, ed. A.S. David & J.C. Cutting, pp. 269–313. Hove: Lawrence Erlbaum.

Dierks, T., Linden, D.E.J., Jandl, M. et al. (1999). Activation of the Heschl's gyrus during auditory hallucniations. *Neuron*, **22**, 615–21.

Dominey, P. & Georgieff, N. (1997). Schizophrenic learn surface but not abstract structure in a serial reaction time task. *Neuroreport*, **8**, 2877–82.

Duchenne de Boulogne (1855). *De l'Éléctrisation Localisée et de son application à la Physiologie et à la Médecine.* Paris: Baillère.

Fadiga, L., Fogassi, L., Pavesi, G. & Rizzolatti, G. (1995). Motor facilitation during action observation. A magnetic stimulation study. *Journal of Neurophysiology*, **73**, 2608–11.

Farrer, C., Franck, N., Georgieff, N. et al. (2002). Confusing the self and the other. Impaired attribution of actions in patients with schizophrenia. *Schizophrenia Bulletin* (in press).

Fletcher, P. (1999). Abnormal cingulate modulation of fronto-temporal connectivity in schizophrenia. *Neuroimage*, **9**, 337–42.

Fourneret, P. & Jeannerod, M. (1998). Limited conscious monitoring of motor performance in normal subjects. *Neuropsychologia*, **36**, 1133–40.

Franck, N., Farrer, C., Georgieff, N. et al. (2001). Defective recognition of one's own actions in schizophrenia. *American Journal of Psychiatry*, **158**, 454–9.

Frith, C.D., Blakemore, S. & Wolpert, D.M. (2000). Explaining the symptoms of schizophrenia: abnormalities in the awareness of action. *Brain Research Reviews*, **31**, 357–63.

Gallagher, S. (2000). Philosophical conceptions of the self: implications for cognitive science. *Trends in Cognitive Science*, **4**, 14–21.

Gallese, V. & Goldman, A. (1998). Mirror neurons and the simulation theory of mind reading. *Trends in Cognitive Science*, **2**, 493–501.

Georgieff, N. & Jeannerod, M. (1998). Beyond consciousness of external reality: a "who" system for consciousness of action and self-consciousness. *Consciousness and Cognition*, **7**, 465–77.

Gepner, B., Mestre, D., Masson, G. & de Schonen, S. (1995). Postural effects of motion vision in young autistic children. *Neuroreport*, **6**, 1211–14.

Goldman-Rakic, P.S. (1994). Working memory dysfunction in schizophrenia. *Journal of Neuropsychiatry and Clinical Neurosciences*, **6**, 348–57.

Goldman-Rakic, P.S. & Selemon, L.D. (1997). Functional and anatomical aspects of prefrontal pathology in schizophrenia. *Schizophrenia Bulletin*, **23**, 437–58.

Gould, L.N. (1949). Auditory hallucinations in subvocal speech: objective study in a case of schizophrenia. *Journal of Nervous and Mental Diseases*, **109**, 418–27.

Gray, J.A., Feldon, J., Rawlins, J.N.P., Hemsley, D.R. & Smith, A.D. (1991). The neuropsychology of schizophrenia. *Behavioral and Brain Sciences*, **14**, 1–84.

Grèzes, J. & Decety, J. (2001). Functional anatomy of execution, mental simulation, and verb generation of actions: a meta-analysis. *Human Brain Mapping*, **12**, 1–19.

Janet, P. (1937). Les troubles de la personnalité sociale. *Annales Médico-Psychologiques*, II, 149–200.

Jeannerod, M. (1990). The representation of the goal of an action and its role in the control of goal-directed movements. In *Computational Neuroscience*, ed. E. Schwartz, pp. 352–65. Cambridge: MIT Press.

Jeannerod, M. (1993). A theory of representation driven actions. In *The perceived Self: Ecological and Interpersonal Sources of Self-knowledge*, ed. U. Neisser, pp. 89–101. Cambridge: Cambridge University Press.

Jeannerod, M. (1994). The representing brain. Neural correlates of motor intention and imagery. *Behavioral and Brain Sciences*, **17**, 187–245.

Jeannerod, M. (1997). *The Cognitive Neuroscience of Action*. Oxford: Blackwell.

Jeannerod, M. (1999). To act or not to act: perspectives on the representation of actions. *Quarterly Journal of Experimental Psychology*, **A52**, 1–29.

Jeannerod, M. (2001). Neural simulation of action: a unifying mechanism for motor cognition. *Neuroimage*, **14**, S103–9.

Jeannerod, M. & Frak, V. (1999). Mental imaging of motor activity in humans. *Currrent Opinions in Neurobiology*, **9**, 735–9.

Johansson, G. (1977). Studies on visual perception of locomotion. *Perception*, **6**, 365–76.

Koechlin, E., Basso, G., Pietrini, P., Panzer, S. & Grafman, J. (1999). The role of the anterior prefrontal cortex in human cognition. *Nature*, **399**, 148–51.

Kuperberg, G. & Heckers, S. (2000). Schizophrenia and cognitive function. *Current Opinion in Neurobiology*, **10**, 205–10.

Kuperberg, G.R., McGuire, P.K. & David, A.S. (1998). Reduced sensitivity to linguistic context in schizophrenic thought disorder: evidence from on-line monitoring for words in linguistically anomalous sentences. *Journal of Abnormal Psychology*, **107**, 423–34.

Laws, K.R. (1999). A meta analytic review of Wisconsin card sort studies in schizophrenia: general intellectual deficit in disguise? *Cognitive Neuropsychiatry*, **4**, 1–35.

Lewes, G.H. (1878). Motor feelings and the muscular sense. *Brain*, **1**, 14–28.

Manoach, D.S., Press, D.Z., Thangaraj, V. et al. (1999). Schizophrenic participants activate dorsolateral prefrontal cortex during a working memory task, as measured by fMRI. *Biological Psychiatry*, **45**, 1128–37.

McGuire, P.K., Silbersweig, D.A. & Frith, C.D. (1996). Functional neuroanatomy of verbal self-monitoring. *Brain*, **119**, 907–17.

Minkowski, E. (1927). *La Schizophrénie. Psychopathologie des Schizoïdes et des Schizophrènes*. Lausanne: Editions Payot & Rivages.

Nielsen, T. (1963). Volition: a new experimental approach. *Scandinavian Journal of Psychology*, **4**, 225–30.

Posada, A., Franck, N., Georgieff, N. & Jeannerod, M. (2001). Anticipating incoming events: an impaired cognitive process in schizophrenia. *Cognition*, **81**, 209–25.

Prabhakaran, V., Narayanan, K., Zhao, Z. & Gabrieli, D.E. (2000). Integration of diverse information in working memory within the frontal lobe. *Nature Neuroscience*, **3**, 85–9.

Ramachandran, V.S., Armel, C., Foster, C. & Stoddard, R. (1998). Object recognition can drive motion perception. *Nature*, **395**, 852–3.

Riddoch, M.J. & Humphreys, G.W. (1993). *BORB: Birmingham Object Recognition Battery*. Hove: Lawrence Erlbaum.

Roth, M., Decety, J., Raybaudi, M. et al. (1996). Possible involvement of primary motor cortex in mentally simulated movement. A functional magnetic resonance imaging study. *Neuroreport*, **7**, 1280–4.

Schneider, K. (1955). *Klinische Psychopathologie*. Stuttgart: Thieme Verlag.

Schwartz, B.D., Maron, B.A., Evans, W.J. & Winstead, D.K. (1999). High velocity transient visual processing deficits diminish ability of patients with schizophrenia to recognize objects. *Neuropsychiatry, Neuropsychology and Behavioural Neurology*, **12**, 170–7.

Servan-Schreiber, D., Cohen, J.D. & Steingard, S. (1996). Schizophrenic deficits in the processing of context. *Archives of General Psychiatry*, **53**, 1105–12.

Shiffrar, M. & Freyd, J. (1990). Apparent motion in the human body. *Psychological Science*, **1**, 257–64.

Silbersweig, D.A., Stern, E., Frith, C. et al. (1995). A functional neuroanatomy of hallucinations in schizophrenia. *Nature*, **378**, 176–9.

Spence, S.A., Brooks, D.J., Hirsch, S.R. et al. (1997). A PET study of voluntary movements in schizophrenic patients experiencing passivity phenomena (delusions of alien control). *Brain*, **120**, 1997–2011.

Stevens, A.A., Goldman-Rakic, P.S., Gore, J.C., Fulbright, R.K. & Wexler, B.E. (1998). Cortical dysfunction in schizophrenia during auditory word and tone working memory demonstrated by functional magnetic resonance imaging. *Archives of General Psychiatry*, **55**, 1097–103.

Stevens, J.A., Fonlupt, P., Shiffrar, M. & Decety, J. (2000). New aspects of motion perception: selective neural encoding of apparent human movements. *NeuroReport*, **11**, 109–15.

Weinberger, D.R. & Berman, K.F. (1996). Prefrontal function in schizophrenia: confounds and controversies. *Philosophical Transactions of the Royal Society B*, **351**, 1495–503.

Wolpert, D.M., Ghahramani, Z. & Jordan, M.I. (1995). An internal model for sensorimotor integration. *Science*, **269**, 1880–2.

Zakzanis, K.K. & Heinrichs, R.W. (1999). Schizophrenia and the frontal brain: a quantitative review. *Journal of International Neuropsychological Society*, **5**, 556–66.

19

Disorders of self-monitoring and the symptoms of schizophrenia

Sarah-Jayne Blakemore and Chris Frith

Wellcome Department of Cognitive Neurology, Institute of Neurology, University College London, London, UK

Abstract

In this chapter we attempt to explain one class of symptoms associated with schizophrenia. We concentrate on symptoms that are characterized by a confusion between the self and other, such as auditory hallucinations and delusions of control. We propose that such symptoms arise because of a failure in the mechanism by which the predicted consequences of self-produced actions are derived from an internal forward model. Normally the forward model predicts and cancels the sensory consequences of self-produced actions. We argue that an impairment in this prediction and cancellation mechanism can cause self-produced sensations to be classified as externally produced. This problem leads to a number of behavioural consequences, such as a lack of central error correction, many of which have been observed in patients with delusions of control and related symptoms. At the physiological level, delusions of control are associated with overactivity in the parietal cortex. We suggest that this overactivity results from a failure to attenuate responses to sensations of limb movements even though these sensations can be anticipated on the basis of the movements intended. The lack of attenuation may arise from corticocortical disconnections which prevent inhibitory signals arising in the frontal areas which generate motor commands from reaching the appropriate sensory areas.

Introduction

Auditory hallucinations and passivity symptoms in schizophrenia

Rather than attempting to elucidate a biological basis for schizophrenia, our aim in this chapter is to try and explain one class of symptoms. We shall concentrate on symptoms that are characterized by a confusion between the self and other, such as auditory hallucinations and delusions of control (Table 19.1). Auditory hallucinations are common in schizophrenia, and normally consist of hearing spoken speech or voices (Hoffman, 1986; Johnstone, 1991). Certain types of auditory hallucinations are included as 'first-rank' features in schizophrenia, features that have been regarded as pathognomonic of the disorder in most circumstances (Schneider, 1959). These features have much in common with the 'nuclear syndrome of

Table 19.1 Examples of auditory hallucinations and passivity symptoms

Symptom	Example
Auditory hallucinations	• One female patient said she could hear God talking to her, saying things like 'Shut up and get out of here' • 'I hear a voice saying "He's an astronomy fanatic…He's getting up now. He's going to wash. It's about time"'
Thought insertion	• 'Thoughts are put into my mind like "Kill God". It's just like my mind working, but it isn't. They come from this chap, Chris. They're his thoughts'
Thought withdrawal	• 'It doesn't allow me to think about what I want to think about. It blocks my mind'
Passivity experiences	• 'My fingers pick up the pen, but I don't control them. What they do is nothing to do with me…The force moved my lips. I began to speak. The words were made for me' • 'My grandfather hypnotized me and now he moves my foot up and down' • 'They inserted a computer in my brain. It makes me turn to the left or right' • 'It's just as if I were being steered around, by whom or what I don't know'
Made emotions	• 'It puts feelings into me: joy, happiness, embarrassment, depression. It just puts it in and I feel the glow spread over me'
Somatic passivity experiences	• 'I have tingling feelings in my legs caused by electric currents from an alternator'

Quotations from Mellors (1970).

schizophrenia' described by the present state examination (PSE/Catego system (Wing et al., 1974)).

Passivity experiences or delusions of alien control are further first-rank features in schizophrenia (Schneider, 1959). The essence of this symptom is that the subject experiences his or her own actions as being created by some outside force (Wing et al., 1974). The actions in question can be very trivial, such as picking up a cup or combing one's hair. Patients describe their thoughts, speech and/or actions as having been influenced or even replaced by those of external agents rather than being produced by themselves (Table 19.1). Other examples of passivity include thoughts or emotions being made for the patient by outside forces.

Evidence for misattribution of self-generated action in schizophrenia

There is evidence that the auditory hallucinations experienced by schizophrenic patients are caused by their own inner speech. Originally Gould (1949) amplified the subvocal activity observed in a hallucinating schizophrenic patient with a microphone. He found that this activity represented whispered speech that was qualitatively different from the patient's own voluntary whispers. Moreover, what the whispered voice said corresponded to the report given by the patient of her hallucinations. Green & Preston (1981) have more recently replicated this result. Further evidence suggesting that hallucinations are the consequence of subvocal speech came from studies showing that it is possible to suppress them (and hence reduce the number of auditory hallucinations significantly) by occupying the speech musculature by holding the mouth wide open (Bick & Kinsbourne, 1987). There is also evidence that hallucinating schizophrenics show defects in tasks that require self-monitoring. For example, they are more likely than normal controls to attribute to the experimenter items that they themselves generated a week earlier (Bentall et al., 1991). Another example of misattribution of self-generated action in schizophrenia comes from a study that examined the effect of distorted auditory feedback on patients' perception of their own voice. In the acute phase of illness, the patients reported hearing another person speaking when they spoke. This tendency to attribute their own voice to another person was significantly correlated with the severity of their current delusions (Cahill et al., 1996).

Frith (1992; Frith et al., 2000a, 2000b) suggested that these abnormal experiences arise through a lack of awareness of intended actions. Such an impairment might cause thoughts or actions to become isolated from the sense of will normally associated with them. This would result in the interpretation of internally generated voices or thoughts as external voices (auditory hallucinations and thought insertion) and of one's own movements and speech as externally caused (passivity or delusions of control). In this chapter we explore the components of an 'internal model' of motor control that normally allows us to recognize the sensory consequences of our own actions, and describe how an impairment in this type of internal model might be associated with auditory hallucinations and passivity experiences.

Thinking as a type of action

The model we describe in this chapter was originally put forward to explain how we control and learn motor actions. Here, we propose that this type of model might also apply to thoughts, if thinking is accepted as a type of action. There is much precedence for this assumption. Locke refers to thinking and willing as 'the two great and principal Actions of the Mind' (Locke, 1690). Hughlings Jackson suggested that thinking may be considered the highest and most complex form of motor activity (Hughlings Jackson, 1932). Watson (1914) regarded the thought process as consisting of slight muscular movements, especially (but not exclusively) speech movements. Feinberg later proposed that the corollary discharge mechanisms of control and integration of movements are also present in thinking (Feinberg, 1978). Our model assumes that thoughts, in so far as they are intended and self-generated, are kinds of actions and have to match the subject's intention to feel self-generated, as in the case of a motor action. However, whether a single mechanism under-lies our ability to recognize as our own all self-generated events, including our own thoughts, is the subject of philosophical debate (Zahavi, 2000). There is no direct evidence that thoughts are monitored by the same process as limb move-ments. However, there would be an evolutionary advantage of a single mechanism controlling all events in which a distinction between self and other is useful or necessary.

Detecting the sensory consequences of our own actions

Our sensory systems are constantly bombarded by a multitude of sensory stimuli, from which it is important to extract the few stimuli that correspond to important changes within the environment. One class of stimuli that are in most circumstances of lesser biological importance are those that arise as a necessary consequence of our own motor actions. Humans can readily detect whether sensory signals are the result of self-generated actions or other environmental events. It has been proposed that information about intentions is used to distinguish the sensory consequences of our own actions from externally produced sensory stimulation (Jeannerod, 1988, 1997; Frith, 1992; Wolpert et al., 1995; Decety, 1996; Wolpert, 1997). In order to achieve this, some kind of internal predictor has been postulated (Wolpert et al., 1995, 2001). It is proposed that an *efference copy* of the motor command (Von Holst, 1954) is used to make a prediction of the sensory consequences (*corollary discharge*; Sperry, 1950) of the motor act. This prediction is then used to cancel the sensory effect of the motor act. These mechanisms have been the subject of much investigation, mainly in the oculomotor domain.

Von Helmholtz (1867) noted that, when making eye movements, the percept of the world remains stable, despite the movement of the retinal image. He suggested that the *effort of will* involved in making eye movements contains information about the sensory consequences of the eye movement, which is sent to the visual areas in order for perceptual compensation to occur. Von Holst (1954) investigated this hypothesis and suggested that, when sending motor commands to move the eyes, the motor areas of the brain send a parallel efference copy to the visual areas. This predicts the sensory consequences (corollary discharge) of the movement and this prediction is the signal used to compensate for retinal displacement during eye movements (Sperry, 1950).

Although these mechanisms have mainly been studied with reference to eye movements, it appears that sensory predictions produced in conjunction with motor commands are not restricted to eye movements, but also provide perceptual stability in the context of all self-produced actions. Our ability to monitor, and recognize as our own, self-generated limb movements, touch, speech and thoughts suggests the existence of a more general 'self-monitoring' mechanism (Feinberg, 1978; Frith, 1992).

Internal forward models of the motor system

It has recently been suggested that this self-monitoring mechanism involves an internal representation of the motor system (Frith et al., 2000a, 2000b). This ability to recognize actions as our own depends upon internal representations of the motor system that mimic aspects of the external transformations. Such internal representations are known as *internal models* because they model the motor system and the external world. One type of internal model, known as a *forward model*, captures the forward or causal relationship between actions and their sensory outcomes. It is proposed that self-produced events can be recognized and discounted by using the sensory prediction errors made by an internal forward model (Wolpert et al., 1995).

When a sensation occurs, its source can be determined by predicting the sensory consequences of self-generated movements based on the efference copy of the motor command. The predicted sensory consequences are then compared with the actual sensory feedback from the movement. Self-produced sensations can be correctly predicted on the basis of motor commands, and there will therefore be little or no sensory discrepancy resulting from the comparison between the predicted and actual sensory feedback. In contrast, externally generated sensations are not associated with any efference copy and therefore cannot be predicted by the model and will produce a higher level of sensory discrepancy. By using such a system it is possible to cancel out sensations induced by self-generated movement and thereby distinguish sensory events due to self-produced motion from sensory feedback caused by the environment, such as contact with objects.

Perception of the sensory consequences of actions in normal subjects

If the action were actually executed, the content of the motor representation would not reach consciousness because it would be cancelled as soon as the corresponding movements were executed (perhaps by the incoming signals generated by the execution itself) (Jeannerod, 1994).

Evidence suggests that the sensory consequences of some self-generated movements are perceived differently from identical sensory input when it is externally generated. An example of such differential perception is the phenomenon that people cannot tickle themselves (e.g. Weiskrantz et al., 1971; Claxton, 1975). It has been argued that efference copy produced in parallel with the motor command underlies this phenomenon. In Weiskrantz et al.'s (1971) psychophysical study, a tactile stimulus that transversed the sole of the subject's foot was administered by the experimenter, the subject or both. Subjects rated the self-administered tactile stimulus as less tickly than the externally administered tactile stimulus. When the stimulation was associated with passive arm movements, tickle strength was reduced, but not to the level of the self-administered tactile stimulus. The authors attributed the differences in response to the mode of delivery: self-administered tactile stimulation produces both efference copy in accordance with the motor command and reafference pro-duced by the arm movement; passive arm movement produces only reafference and externally administered tactile stimulation produces neither efference copy nor reafference. The authors therefore concluded that, although reafference plays a role, the attenuation signal is based mainly on the efference copy signal produced in concordance with a self-generated movement.

One explanation of these results is that there is a general 'gating' of all in-coming sensory stimulation during self-generated movement. Indeed, this kind of movement-induced sensory gating has been documented in humans (Angel & Malenka, 1982; Chapman et al., 1987; Milne et al., 1988; Collins et al., 1998). Such findings suggest that the perception of sensory stimulation might be attenuated simply if self-generated movement occurs simultaneously with the stimulus – the movement might not necessarily have to produce the sensory stimulus in order for it to be attenuated. This, however, is inconsistent with the theoretical approach of forward models we have outlined, which posits that in order for sensory attenuation to occur, the specific sensory consequences of the movement must be accurately predicted.

To investigate this, we asked subjects to rate the sensation of a tactile stimulus on the palm of their hand, and examined the perceptual effects of altering the correspondence between self-generated movement and its sensory (tactile) conse-quences. This was achieved by introducing parametrically varied degrees of delay or trajectory rotation between the subject's movement and the resultant tactile stimu-lation. The result of increasing the delay or trajectory rotation is that the sensory stimulus no longer corresponds to that which would be normally expected based on the efference copy produced in parallel with the motor command. Therefore as the delay or trajectory rotation increases, the sensory prediction becomes less accurate. This has three possible effects on the sensation. Firstly, if sensory attenuation is due to a general movement-induced sensory gating, then since movement occurs under all delays and trajectory rotations, the sensation would remain at the same level of attenuation under all conditions. Secondly, if sensory attenuation relies on a completely accurate prediction of the sensation, then no attenuation would occur under any delay or trajectory rotation. Thirdly, sensory attenuation could be proportional to the accuracy of the prediction, in which case as the delay or trajectory rotation is increased, the intensity of the sensation should increase.

A robotic interface was employed to produce the delays and trajectory rotations. Subjects moved a robotic arm with their left hand and this movement caused a second foam-tipped robotic arm to move across their right palm. Thus, motion of the left hand determined the tactile stimulus on the right palm. By using this robotic interface so that the tactile stimulus could be delivered under remote control by the subject, *delays* of 100, 200 and 300 ms were introduced between the movement of the left hand and the tactile stimulus on the right palm. In a further condition *trajectory rotations* of 30°, 60° and 90° were introduced between the direction of the left-hand movement and the direction of the tactile stimulus on the right palm. Under all delays and trajectory rotations the left hand made the same sinusoidal movements and the right hand experienced the tactile stimulus. Only the temporal or spatial correspondence between the movement of the left hand and the sensory effect on the right palm was altered.

The results showed that subjects rated the self-produced tactile sensation as being significantly ($P < 0.001$) less tickly, intense and pleasant than an identical stimulus produced by the robot (Blakemore et al., 1999a). Furthermore, subjects reported a progressive increase in the tickly rating as the delay was increased between 0 ms and 200 ms ($P < 0.0005$) and as the trajectory rotation was increased between 0 and 90°($P < 0.01$). These results support the hypothesis that the perceptual attenuation of self-produced tactile stimulation is due to precise sensory predictions, rather than a movement-induced nonspecific attenuation of all sensory signals. When there is no delay or trajectory rotation, the model correctly predicts the sensory consequences of the movement, so no sensory discrepancy ensues between the predicted and actual sensory information and the motor command to the left hand can be used to attenuate the sensation on the right palm. As the sensory feedback deviates from the prediction of the model (by increasing the delay or trajectory rotation), the sensory discrepancy between the predicted and actual sensory feedback increases, which leads to a decrease in the amount of sensory attenuation.

Behavioural evidence for problems of self-monitoring in schizophrenia

It has been suggested that the experience of passivity arises from a lack of awareness of the predicted limb position based on the forward model (Frith et al., 2000a). In the absence of such awareness the patient cannot correct errors prior to peripheral feedback and is not aware of the exact specification of the movement. Thus the patient is aware of the intention to move and of the movement having occurred, but is not aware of having initiated the movement. It is as if the movement, although intended, has been initiated by some external force. In a variation on this theme,

Spence (1996) has suggested that the problem is to do with the timing of awareness. The awareness of the actual outcome of the movement precedes the awareness of the predicted outcome, which is contrary to the normal experience of our own agency.

In a reformulation of an earlier model (Frith, 1987), we suggest that the experience of alien control arises from a lack of awareness of the predicted limb position. Such patients are aware that the action matches their intention, but they have no awareness of initiating the action or of its predicted consequences (Frith et al., 2000a). In parallel, the patient's belief system is faulty so that he or she interprets this abnormal sensation in an irrational way. Patients with delusions of control therefore feel as if their intentions are being monitored and their actions made for them by some external force (Figure 19.1). This could arise if there were

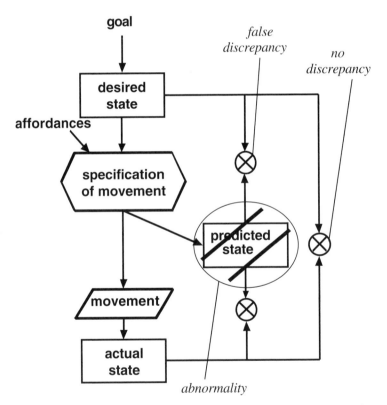

Figure 19.1 The proposed underlying disorder leading to auditory hallucinations and passivity phenomena. The patient formulates the action or thought appropriate to his/her intention and the action or thought is successfully performed. The patient is aware that the action or thought matches the intention, but has no awareness of initiating the action or thought or of its predicted consequences. The patient therefore feels as if his/her intentions are being monitored and his/her actions made for him/her by some external force.

an impairment of either the prediction or the comparison process of the forward model. For example, if the comparison process were impaired and always produced a high level of sensory discrepancy despite the accuracy of the sensory prediction, then self-produced sensations would be associated with high levels of sensory discrepancy despite being accurately predicted. In this way, self-produced stimulation could be interpreted as being externally produced. Self-produced events could also be confused with externally generated events if the former were not predicted accurately.

There is nothing obviously abnormal in the motor control of schizophrenic patients. However, there are subtle problems consistent with a lack of awareness of predicted actions. Two experiments, in which subjects had to correct their errors very rapidly in the absence of visual feedback, found evidence that central monitoring is faulty in schizophrenia (Malenka et al., 1982; Frith & Done, 1989). Normal control subjects were adept at this task, suggesting that they monitor the response intended (via corollary discharge) and do not need to wait for external feedback about the response that actually occurred. Failure to correct their errors in the absence of feedback was characteristic of schizophrenic patients with passivity symptoms in the study by Frith & Done (1989).

Such patients have difficulty remembering the precise details of actions made in the absence of visual feedback (Mlakar et al., 1994; Stirling et al., 1998). They also have difficulty distinguishing between correct visual feedback about the position of their hand and false feedback when the image of the hand they see is in fact that of another person attempting to make the same movements as the patient (Daprati et al., 1997). Recent evidence demonstrates that patients with schizophrenia are more likely than normal control subjects to believe that they read aloud words they actually read silently (Franck et al., 2000). Patients who were hallucinating at the time of the experiment performed significantly worse – they confused reading silently and aloud more – than nonhallucinating patients. This was taken to support the suggestion that such patients are unable to discriminate correctly between inner and outer speech, and that this might play a role in the onset of their hallucinations. Hallucinating schizophrenic patients are more likely than normal controls to attribute to the experimenter items that they themselves generated a week earlier (Bentall et al., 1991). Patients with auditory hallucinations are more likely to confuse the source of their speech when their speech is distorted in pitch (Cahill et al., 1996; Johns & McGuire, 1999; Johns et al., 2001; see chapter 20, this edition).

Jeannerod (1999) has suggested that conscious judgement about a movement requires a different form of representation from that needed for unconscious comparisons of predictions and outcomes within the motor system. Following Barresi & Moore (1996; see also Frith, 1995) he suggests that conscious judgements about movements require 'third-person' information while control of movement depends upon private 'first-person' information. Jeannerod suggests that schizophrenic patients fail to monitor the third-person signals that enable them to make judgements about their own actions. Frith et al. (2000a) suggest that, in schizophrenia, something goes awry with the mechanism that translates the first-person representations that are involved in motor control into the third-person representations that are needed for conscious monitoring of the motor control system. This is part of a more general problem that these patients have in escaping from a first-person, egocentric view of the world. They have great difficulty in seeing the world from any viewpoint other than their own.

The perception of self-produced sensory stimuli in patients with auditory hallucinations and passivity

To test the hypothesis that certain symptomatology associated with schizophrenia is due to a defect in self-monitoring, we investigated whether patients with auditory hallucinations and/or passivity experiences are abnormally aware of the sensory consequences of their own movements. Age-matched patients with a diagnosis of schizophrenia, bipolar affective disorder and depression were divided into two groups on the basis of the presence ($n = 15$) or absence ($n = 23$) of auditory hallucinations and/or passivity experiences according to the positive and negative symptom scale (PANSS) interview (Kay et al., 1987). These patient groups and 15 age-matched normal control subjects were asked to rate the perception of a tactile sensation on the palm of their left hand. The tactile stimulation was either self-produced by movement of the subject's right hand or externally produced by the experimenter. In order to obtain an objective assessment of the ability of subjects to rate a tactile sensation, in a control task subjects were asked to rate the 'roughness' of four objective grades of sandpaper on a scale. Data from subjects who failed to rate the sandpaper in the correct order of roughness were excluded from the analysis.

The results demonstrated that normal control subjects and patients with neither auditory hallucinations nor passivity symptoms experienced self-produced stimuli as less intense, tickly and pleasant than identical, externally produced tactile stimuli. In contrast, patients with these symptoms did not show a decrease in their perceptual ratings for tactile stimuli produced by themselves as compared to those produced by the experimenter (Blakemore et al., 2000). Figure 19.2 shows the difference between the ratings for self-produced and externally produced tactile stimulation for the three subject groups. These results support the proposal that auditory hallucinations and passivity experiences are associated with an abnormality in the forward model mechanism that normally allows us to distinguish self-produced from externally produced sensations. It is possible that the neural

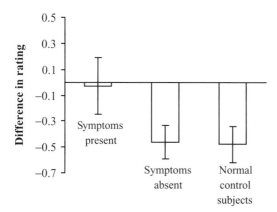

Figure 19.2   Graph showing mean combined perceptual rating differences between self-produced and externally produced tactile stimulation conditions for the three subject groups: patients with auditory hallucinations and/or passivity experiences, patients without these symptoms and normal control subjects. There was no significant difference between the perceptual ratings in these two conditions in patients with auditory hallucinations and/or passivity experiences, hence the mean rating difference was close to zero. In contrast, there was a significant difference between the perceptual ratings in the two conditions in patients without these symptoms and in normal control subjects: both groups rated self-produced stimulation as significantly less tickly, intense and pleasant than externally produced stimulation.

system associated with this mechanism, or part of it, operates abnormally in people with such symptoms.

The physiological basis of the perceptual modulation of self-produced sensory stimuli

Neurophysiological data demonstrate that neuronal responses in somatosensory cortex are attenuated by self-generated movement. Active touch is 'gated' in the primary somatosensory cortex of rats (Chapin & Woodward, 1982) and monkeys (Chapman & Ageranioti-Belanger, 1991; Jiang et al., 1991; Chapman, 1994) compared with passive and external touch of an identical tactile stimulus. For example, neuronal activity in somatosensory areas 3b, 1 and 2 in monkeys was attenuated when monkeys scanned their hand over a surface texture compared to when their hand was passively moved over the same surface, or when the surface moved underneath their hand (Chapman, 1994). It is possible that this movement-induced somatosensory gating is the physiological correlate of the decreased sensation associated with self-produced tactile stimuli in humans. In order for somatosensory cortex activity to be attenuated to self-produced sensory stimuli, these stimuli need to be predicted accurately. The cerebellum is a possible site for a forward model of the motor apparatus that provides predictions of the sensory consequences of motor commands. This proposal has been supported by computational (Ito, 1970;

Paulin, 1989; Miall et al., 1993; Wolpert et al., 1998), neurophysiological (Oscarsson, 1980; Gellman et al., 1985; Andersson & Armstrong, 1985, 1987; Simpson et al., 1995) and functional neuroimaging data (Imamizu et al., 2000).

To investigate the hypothesis that the somatosensory cortex and the cerebellum are involved in modulating the sensation of a self-produced tactile stimulation, we used functional magnetic resonance imaging (fMRI) to examine the neural basis of self- versus externally produced tactile stimuli in humans (Blakemore et al., 1998). Normal subjects were scanned while a tactile stimulation device allowed a tactile stimulus (a piece of soft foam) to be applied to the subjects' left palm either by their right hand or by the experimenter. To examine the neural correlates of self-produced tactile stimuli we employed a factorial design with the factors of firstly, self-generated movement of the right hand versus rest, and secondly, tactile stimulation on the left palm versus no stimulation. Using this design we were able to assess the difference in brain activity during self-generated relative to externally generated tactile stimulation while factoring out activity associated with self-generated movement and tactile stimulation.

The results showed an increase in activity of the secondary somatosensory cortex (SII) and the anterior cingulate cortex (ACC; Brodmann areas 24/32) when subjects experienced an externally produced tactile stimulus relative to a self-produced tactile stimulus. The reduction in activity in these areas to self-produced tactile stimulation might be the physiological correlate of the reduced perception associated with this type of stimulation. The activity in the ACC in particular may have been related to the increased tickliness and pleasantness of externally produced compared to self-produced tactile stimuli. Previous studies have implicated this area in affective behaviour and positive reinforcement (Vogt et al., 1992; Porrino, 1993; Vogt & Gabriel, 1993). Alternatively the activity in ACC might be related to the requirement to monitor the sensations the subjects were experiencing (Lane et al., 1997; Frith & Frith, 1999).

While the decrease in activity in SII and ACC might underlie the reduced perception of self-produced tactile stimuli, the pattern of brain activity in the cerebellum suggests that this area is the source of the SII and ACC modulation. In SII and ACC, activity was attenuated by all movement: these areas were equally activated by movement that did and that did not result in tactile stimulation. In contrast, the right anterior cerebellar cortex was selectively deactivated by self-produced movement that resulted in a tactile stimulus, but not by movement alone, and significantly activated by externally produced tactile stimulation. This pattern suggests that the cerebellum distinguishes between movements depending on their specific sensory consequences. Further psychophysiological interaction analysis showed that the cerebellum may be involved in providing the signal that is used to attenuate the somatosensory response to self-produced tactile stimulation

(Blakemore et al., 1999b). A recent positron emission tomography (PET) study found that regional cerebral blood flow (rCBF) in the cerebellum is correlated with the accuracy of sensory prediction (Blakemore et al., 2001). Using a robotic interface, computer-controlled delays (between 0 and 300 ms) were introduced between the movement of one hand and its sensory (tactile) consequences on the other hand. As the sensory stimulation diverged from the motor command producing it, rCBF in the right cerebellar cortex increased. In this study, the delays were not detected by the subjects. Thus the cerebellum appears to be involved in detecting discrepancies between one's intentions and their consequences at an unconscious level.

Physiological abnormalities associated with delusions of control

If patients with delusions of control fail to predict the sensory consequences of their actions, then, at the physiological level, we would expect to see overactivity in regions concerned with analysis of the relevant sensations. Spence et al. (1997) scanned patients with delusions of control while they performed a simple motor task in which they were required to move a joystick in one of four directions, chosen at random, in time with a pacing tone. In comparison to a control task involving routine joystick movements this task activates prefrontal and superior parietal cortex. The patients experienced their delusions in association with the performance of this task. They also showed overactivity in superior parietal cortex relative to normal controls and to patients who did not have delusions of control. Activity in the parietal cortex is more typical of passive movements than active ones (Weiller et al., 1996). Thus, at the experiential level, when the patient makes an active movement it can feel like a passive movement. It is this feeling that leads to the belief about alien control. Overactivity has also been observed in left superior temporal gyrus in schizophrenic patients performing auditory–verbal tasks (Dolan et al., 1995; Frith et al., 1995). These observations could be relevant to the experience of auditory hallucinations, but we do not know if this overactivity is related to specific symptoms.

We presume that the overactivity observed in these studies does not result from some abnormality intrinsic to the area in which the overactivity is observed. The overactivity arises through the lack of an inhibitory signal that normally attenuates activity associated with stimuli that can be predicted. The fundamental abnormality associated with the symptom is likely to be found in the system that generates this inhibitory signal. Before we can locate this abnormality it will probably be necessary to locate more precisely the brain regions concerned with developing the forward model and representing the predicted consequences of action. A possible clue comes from the observation in many studies of underactivity in the prefrontal cortex and/or anterior cingulate cortex of patients with schizophrenia (see Ebmeier et al., 1995, for a review). In the study of Spence et al. (1998) underactivity of frontal cortex was observed in both groups of patients with schizophrenia, whether or not they had delusions of control. The patients were retested after an interval of several weeks when the delusions were no longer in evidence. At this time both the overactivity in parietal cortex and the underactivity of frontal cortex were no longer present and the overall pattern of brain activity was normal.

We might speculate that there is a causal link between the overactivity in parietal cortex and the underactivity in prefrontal cortex. A number of studies have found evidence for abnormal connectivity between frontal cortex and more posterior regions in patients with schizophrenia (see McGuire & Frith, 1996, for a review). In normal control subjects the interactions between these areas is reciprocal in the sense that high activity in the frontal region goes with reduced activity in the posterior regions. In patients with schizophrenia this relationship is not observed and activity in anterior and posterior regions is independent, suggesting a lack of connectivity. These observations are consistent with the notion that, normally, signals arising in prefrontal cortex where actions are initiated inhibit activity in posterior regions where the sensory consequences of actions are received. This might be the mechanism by which responses to new states are suppressed when that state has been correctly predicted on the basis of the forward model. This suppression seems not to be happening in patients with schizophrenia. We could also speculate that different symptoms arise as a result of slightly different disconnections. Failure to suppress activity in parietal cortex would lead to delusions of control, while failure to suppress activity in temporal cortex would lead to hallucinations or thought insertion. At present we do not know the precise route of these connections between frontal regions and sensory association cortex. It is likely that the basal ganglia and the cerebellum might form important stages.

Acknowledgements

The research was supported by the Wellcome Trust. S-J Blakemore was supported by a Wellcome Trust 4-year PhD programme in neuroscience at University College London.

REFERENCES

Andersson, G. & Armstrong, D.M. (1985). Climbing fibre input to b zone Purkinje cells during locomotor perturbation in the cat. *Neuroscience Letters Supplement*, **22**, S27.

Andersson, G. & Armstrong, D.M. (1987). Complex spikes in Purkinje cells in the lateral vermis of the cat cerebellum during locomotion. *Journal of Physiology (London)*, **385**, 107–34.

Angel, R.W. & Malenka, R.C. (1982). Velocity-dependent suppression of cutaneous sensitivity during movement. *Experimental Neurology*, **77**, 266–74.

Barresi, J. & Moore, C. (1996). Intentional relations and social understanding. *Behaviour and Brain Science*, **19**, 107–54.

Bentall, R.P., Baker, G.A. & Havers, S. (1991). Reality monitoring and psychotic hallucinations. *British Journal of Clinical Psychology*, **30**, 213–22.

Bick, P.A. & Kinsbourne, M. (1987). Auditory hallucinations and subvocal speech in schizophrenic patients. *American Journal of Psychiatry*, **144**, 222–5.

Blakemore, S.-J., Wolpert, D.M. & Frith, C.D. (1998). Central cancellation of self-produced tickle sensation. *Nature Neuroscience*, **1**, 635–40.

Blakemore, S.-J., Frith, C.D. & Wolpert, D.W. (1999a). Spatiotemporal prediction modulates the perception of self-produced stimuli. *Journal of Cognitive Neuroscience*, **11**, 551–9.

Blakemore, S.-J., Wolpert, D.M. & Frith, C.D. (1999b). The cerebellum contributes to somatosensory cortical activity during self-produced tactile stimulation. *NeuroImage*, **10**, 448–59.

Blakemore, S.-J., Smith, J., Steel, R., Johnstone, E. & Frith, C.D. (2000). The perception of self-produced sensory stimuli in patients with auditory hallucinations and passivity experiences: evidence for a breakdown in self-monitoring. *Psychological Medicine*, **30**, 1131–9.

Blakemore, S.-J., Frith, C.D. & Wolpert, D.W. (2001). The cerebellum is involved in predicting the sensory consequences of action. *NeuroReport*, **12**, 1879–85.

Cahill, C., Silbersweig, D. & Frith, C.D. (1996). Psychotic experiences induced in deluded patients using distorted auditory feedback. *Cognitive Neuropsychiatry*, **1**, 201–11.

Chapin, J.K. & Woodward, D.J. (1982). Somatic sensory transmission to the cortex during movement: gating of single cell responses to touch. *Experimental Neurology*, **78**, 654–69.

Chapman, C.E. (1994). Active versus passive touch: factors influencing the transmission of somatosensory signals to primary somatosensory cortex. *Canadian Journal of Physiology and Pharmacology*, **72**, 558–70.

Chapman, C.E. & Ageranioti-Belanger, S.A. (1991). Comparison of the discharge of primary somatosensory cortical (SI) neurones during active and passive tactile discrimination. *Proceedings of the Third IBRO World Congress of Neuroscience*, p. 317. Oxford: Pergamon.

Chapman, C. E., Bushnell, M.C., Miron, D., Duncan, G.H. & Lund, J.P. (1987). Sensory perception during movement in man. *Experimental Brain Research*, **68**, 516–24.

Claxton, G. (1975). Why can't we tickle ourselves? *Perceptual and Motor Skills*, **41**, 335–8.

Collins, D.F., Cameron, T., Gillard, D.M. & Prochazka, A. (1998). Muscular sense is attenuated when humans move. *Journal of Physiology*, **508**, 635–43.

Daprati, E., Franck, N., Georgieff, N. et al. (1997). Looking for the agent: an investigation into consciousness of action and self-consciousness in schizophrenic patients. *Cognition*, **65**, 71–86.

Decety, J. (1996). Neural representation for action. *Reviews in the Neurosciences*, **7**, 285–97.

Dolan, R.J., Fletcher, P., Frith, C.D. et al. (1995). Dopaminergic modulation of an impaired cognitive activation in the anterior cingulate cortex in schizophrenia. *Nature*, **378**, 180–3.

Ebmeier, K.P., Steele, J.D., MacKenzie, D.M. et al. (1995). Cognitive brain potentials and regional cerebral blood flow equivalents during two- and three-sound auditory 'oddball tasks'. *Electroencephalography and Clinical Neurophysiology*, **95**, 434–43.

Feinberg, I. (1978). Efference copy and corollary discharge: implications for thinking and its disorders. *Schizophrenia Bulletin*, **4**, 636–40.

Franck, N., Rouby, P., Daprati, E. et al. (2000). Confusion between silent and overt reading in schizophrenia. *Schizophrenia Research*, **41**, 357–64.

Frith, C.D. (1987). The positive and negative symptoms of schizophrenia reflect impairments in the perception and initiation of action. *Psychological medicine*, **17**, 631–48.

Frith, C.D. (1992). *The Cognitive Neuropsychology of Schizophrenia.* Hove, Sussex: Lawrence Erlbaum Associates.

Frith, C.D. (1995). Consciousness is for other people. *Behavioural and Brain Sciences*, **18**, 682–3.

Frith, C.D. & Done, D.J. (1989). Experiences of alien control in schizophrenia reflect a disorder in the central monitoring of action. *Psychological Medicine*, **19**, 359–63.

Frith, C.D. & Frith, U. (1999). Interacting minds – a biological basis. *Science*, **286**, 1692–5.

Frith, C.D., Friston, K.J., Herold, S. et al. (1995). Regional brain activity in chronic schizophrenic patients during the performance of a verbal fluency task. *British Journal of Psychiatry*, **167**, 343–9.

Frith, C.D., Blakemore, S.-J. & Wolpert, D.M. (2000a). Explaining the symptoms of schizophrenia: abnormalities in the awareness of action. *Brain Research Reviews*, **31**, 357–63.

Frith, C.D., Blakemore, S.-J. & Wolpert, D.M. (2000b). Abnormalities in the awareness and control of action. *Philosophical Transactions of the Royal Society of London: Biological Sciences*, **355**, 1771–88.

Gellman, R., Gibson, A.R. & Houk, J.C. (1985). Inferior olivary neurons in the awake cat: detection of contact and passive body displacement. *Journal of Neurophysiology*, **54**, 40–60.

Gould, L.N. (1949). Auditory hallucinations and subvocal speech. *Journal of Nervous and Mental Disease*, **109**, 418–27.

Green, P. & Preston, M. (1981). Reinforcement of vocal correlates of auditory hallucinations by auditory feedback: a case study. *British Journal of Psychiatry*, **139**, 204–8.

Hoffman, R.E. (1986). Verbal hallucinations and language production processes in schizophrenia. *Behavioral and Brain Sciences*, **9**, 503–17.

Hughlings Jackson, J. (1932). *Selected Writings of John Hughlings Jackson.* London: Hodder & Stoughton.

Imamizu, H., Miyauchi, S., Tamada, T. et al. (2000). Human cerebellar activity reflecting an acquired internal model of a new tool. *Nature*, **403**, 192–5.

Ito, M. (1970). Neurophysiological aspects of the cerebellar motor control system. *International Journal of Neurology*, **7**, 162–76.

Jeannerod, M. (1988). *The Neural and Behaviourial Organisation of Goal-directed Movements.* Oxford: OUP.

Jeannerod, M. (1994). The representing brain – neural correlates of motor intention and imagery. *Behavioral and Brain Sciences*, **17**, 187–202.

Jeannerod, M. (1997). *The Cognitive Neuropsychology of Action.* Cambridge: Blackwell.

Jeannerod, M. (1999). To act or not to act: perspectives on the representation of actions. *Quarterly Journal of Experimental Psychology A*, **52**, 981–1020.

Jiang, W., Chapman, C.E. & Lamarre, Y. (1991). Modulation of the cutaneous responsiveness of neurones in the primary somatosensory cortex during conditioned arm movements in the monkey. *Experimental Brain Research*, **84**, 342–54.

Johns, L.C. & McGuire, P.K. (1999). Verbal self-monitoring and auditory hallucinations in schizophrenia. *Lancet*, **353**, 469–70.

Johns, L.C., Rossell, S., Frith, C. et al. (2001). Verbal self-monitoring and auditory verbal hallucinations in patients with schizophrenia. *Psychological Medicine*, **31**, 705–15.

Johnstone, E.C. (1991). Defining characteristics of schizophrenia. *British Journal of Psychiatry*, **13**, (suppl.) 5–6.

Kay, S., Fiszbein, A. & Opler, L. (1987). The positive and negative symptom scale for schizophrenia. *Schizophrenia Bulletin*, **13**, 261–76.

Lane, R.D., Fink, G.R., Chua, P.M. & Dolan, R.J. (1997). Neural activation during selective attention to subjective emotional responses. *Neuroreport*, **8**, 3969–72.

Locke, J. (1690). *Essay Concerning Human Understanding*, II.VI.2. Oxford: Clarendon Press (reprinted 1989).

Malenka, R.C., Angel, R.W., Hampton, B. & Berger, P.A. (1982). Impaired central error-correcting behavior in schizophrenia. *Archives of General Psychiatry*, **39**, 101–7.

McGuire, P.K. & Frith, C.D. (1996). Disordered functional connectivity in schizophrenia. *Psychological Medicine*, **26**, 663–7.

Mellors, C.S. (1970). First-rank symptoms of schizophrenia. *British Journal of Psychiatry*, **117**, 15–23.

Miall, R.C., Weir, D.J., Wolpert, D.M. & Stein, J.F. (1993). Is the cerebellum a Smith predictor? *Journal of Motor Behaviour*, **25**, 203–16.

Milne, R.J., Aniss, A.M., Kay, N.E. & Gandevia, S.C. (1988). Reduction in perceived intensity of cutaneous stimuli during movement: a quantitative study. *Experimental Brain Research*, **70**, 569–76.

Mlakar, J., Jensterle, J. & Frith, C.D. (1994). Central monitoring deficiency and schizophrenic symptoms. *Psychological Medicine*, **24**, 557–64.

Oscarsson, O. (1980). Functional organization of olivary projection to the cerebellar anterior lobe. In *The Inferior Olivary Nucleus: Anatomy and Physiology*, ed. J. Courville, C. DeMontigny & Y. Lamarre. New York: Raven Press.

Paulin, M.G. (1989). A Kalman filter theory of the cerebellum. In *Dynamic Interactions in Neural Networks: Models and Data*, ed. E.M.A. Arbib & E.S. Amari, pp. 241–59. Berlin: Springer-Verlag.

Porrino, L.J. (1993). Functional consequences of acute cocaine treatment depend on route of administration. *Psychopharmacology Berlin*, **112**, 343–51.

Schneider, K. (1959). *Clinical Psychopathology*. New York: Grune & Stratton.

Simpson, J.L., Wylie, D.R. & De Zeeuw, C.I. (1995). On climbing fiber signals and their consequence(s). *Behavioural and Brain Sciences*, **19**, 384.

Spence, S.A. (1996). Free will in the light of neuropsychiatry. *Philosophy, Psychiatry and Psychology*, **3**, 75–90.

Spence, S.A., Brooks, D.J., Hirsch, S.R. et al. (1997). A PET study of voluntary movement in schizophrenic patients experiencing passivity phenomena (delusions of alien control). *Brain*, **120**, 1997–2011.

Spence, S.A., Hirsch, S.R., Brooks, D.J. & Grasby, P.M. (1998). Prefrontal cortex activity in people with schizophrenia and control subjects. Evidence from positron emission tomography for remission of 'hypofrontality' with recovery from acute schizophrenia. *British Journal of Psychiatry*, **172**, 316–23.

Sperry, R.W. (1950). Neural basis of spontaneous optokinetic responses produced by visual inversion. *Journal of Comparative Physiological Psychology*, **43**, 483–9.

Stirling, J.D., Hellewell, J.S.E. & Quraishi, N. (1998). Self-monitoring dysfunction and the schizophrenic symptoms of alien control. *Psychological Medicine*, **28**, 675–83.

Vogt, B.A., Finch, D.M. & Olson, C.R. (1992). Functional heterogeneity in cingulate cortex: the anterior executive and posterior evaluative regions. *Cerebral Cortex*, **2**, 435–43.

Vogt, B.A., & Gabriel, M. (eds) (1993). *Neurobiology of Cingulate Cortex and Limbic Thalamus*. Boston: Birkauser.

Von Helmholtz, H. (1867). *Handbuch der Physiologischen Optik*, 1st edn. Hamburg, Germany: Voss.

Von Holst, E. (1954). Relations between the central nervous system and the peripheral organs. *British Journal of Animal Behaviour*, **2**, 89–94.

Watson, J.B. (1914). *Behavior: An Introduction to Comparative Psychology*. New York: Holt.

Weiller, C., Juptner, M., Fellows, S. et al. (1996). Brain representation of active and passive movement. *NeuroImage*, **4**, 105–10.

Weiskrantz, L., Elliot, J. & Darlington, C. (1971). Preliminary observations of tickling oneself. *Nature*, **230**, 598–9.

Wing, J.K., Cooper, J.E. & Sartorius, N. (1974). *Description and Classification of Psychiatric Symptoms*. London: Cambridge University Press.

Wolpert, D.M. (1997). Computational approaches to motor control. *Trends in Cognitive Sciences*, **1**, 209–16.

Wolpert, D.M., Miall, R.C. & Kawato, M. (1998). Internal models in the cerebellum. *Trends in Cognitive Sciences*, **2**, 338–47.

Wolpert, D.M., Ghahramani, Z. & Jordan, M.I. (1995). An internal model for sensorimotor integration. *Science*, **269**, 1880–2.

Wolpert, D.M., Ghahramani, Z. & Flanagan, R. (2001). Perspectives and problems in motor learning. *Trends in Cognitive Sciences*, **5**, 487–94.

Zahavi, D. (ed.) (2000). *Advances in Consciousness Research*. Amsterdam: John Benjamins.

20

Hearing voices or hearing the self in disguise? Revealing the neural correlates of auditory hallucinations in schizophrenia

Cynthia H.Y. Fu and Philip K. McGuire

Institute of Psychiatry, London, UK

Abstract

In this chapter we have explored the model of impaired self-monitoring which has been proposed to underlie the pathophysiology of auditory hallucinations and delusions in schizophrenia. We begin with an overview of the model from its beginnings in sensorimotor literature to its elaboration by Chris Frith. We then review the neuropsychological support and functional neuroimaging data of verbal self-monitoring in healthy individuals, inner speech and auditory hallucinations. A summary of our most recent data of overt verbal self-monitoring as measured by functional magnetic resonance imaging in healthy individuals as well as in patients with schizophrenia, both acutely psychotic and in remission, follows. We complete the chapter with a proposal for the neural circuitry involved in self-monitoring based on our behavioural and neuroimaging data and proposals for future research.

Introduction

That we recognize our thoughts, even the most bizarre and unpleasant ones, as arising from our own minds is a phenomenon which we take for granted. Associated with this is our ability to distinguish ourselves from others at a basic physical level and in terms of more nebulous concepts like ideas, beliefs and values. Yet most of us can also recall moments, such as upon wakening, when we've wondered if an experience was real or a dream. The experience of psychosis may represent an extreme example of this uncertainty. A hallucination, one of the cardinal features of psychosis, is a perception which occurs in the absence of a corresponding sensory stimulus. When this perception involves hearing, the hallucination is described as auditory. Although an auditory hallucination can involve almost any type of sound, including simple noises and music (Cutting, 1997), in schizophrenia, hallucinations of speech (auditory–verbal hallucinations) are particularly common (Wing et al., 1974). The *sine qua non* symptom of schizophrenia has classically been hallucinations in the form of voices, discussing the patient in the third person

(Schneider, 1959). However, voices directly addressing the patient in the second person occur more frequently (Goodwin et al., 1971; Nayani & David, 1996; Cutting, 1997), with a variable, but most often derogatory, content (Goodwin et al., 1971; Nayani & David, 1996). Over a century ago, Maudsley (1886) proposed that auditory–verbal hallucinations originate from an individual's own thoughts. More recently, converging evidence from functional imaging data has clarified how such experiences are mediated in the brain (Cleghorn et al., 1992; McGuire et al., 1993; Suzuki et al., 1993; Silbersweig et al., 1995; Dierks et al., 1999; Shergill et al., 2000a). These studies indicate that auditory–verbal hallucinations are not, as once supposed, generated by random firing in the temporal cortex, but involve an extensive cortical and subcortical network implicated in the generation and perception of language.

How could one's personal thoughts (or 'inner speech') be perceived as overt verbal commands, running commentaries and criticisms, delivered in another person's voice? A variety of cognitive theories have been proposed to explain the phenomena of auditory–verbal hallucinations or 'hearing voices', as patients typically describe these experiences. Our research has focused on the model of impaired 'self-monitoring' which has been elegantly elucidated by Chris Frith (1992).

This model of auditory–verbal hallucinations evolved from work on sensorimotor function. It is widely held that the control of somatic movement involves internal models which predict and correct the motor command prior to its effective output as a physical action (Wolpert et al., 1995). Although the precise neural components of the systems responsible for motor monitoring remain a subject of debate, the general consensus is that it involves some form of a 'corollary discharge' (Helmholtz, 1866; Sperry, 1950; McCloskey et al., 1974; McCloskey & Torda, 1975), 'efference copy' (von Holst, 1954), or 'forward model' (Wolpert et al., 1995) which accompanies motor intent, as well as sensory feedback loops (Evarts, 1971; Wolpert et al., 1995). If the generation of language and thought can be considered as analogous to production of movements, perhaps comparable internal 'monitors' and 'feedback' loops exist for the activity of thinking: a notion proposed by such seemingly diverse theorists as Freud and Hughlings Jackson in the early 1900s (Fuster, 1997, p. 226). Following from this, the monitoring of thought generation may contribute to the conscious awareness of thought and play a role in distinguishing self from nonself (Feinberg, 1978).

Irwin Feinberg (1978) suggested that an impairment of the corollary discharge accompanying conscious thought (an internal feedback circuit) is responsible for the 'psychosis of thinking' and in particular the positive symptoms of schizophrenia: auditory hallucinations, delusions and formal thought disorder. Chris Frith (Frith & Done 1987; Frith 1992, p. 82) further developed and refined these theories in his model of 'cognitive self-monitoring'. He proposed a circuit in which goals and plans become willed intentions, then intended actions, and terminate as a motor response (Frith, 1992). According to this model, self-awareness arises from an internal 'self-monitor' that receives information about an intended action, but following from the sensorimotor literature, there is an additional direct line of information about goals and plans through some form of a corollary discharge. Furthermore, goals and plans are also made known to external perception (an external monitor) via a comparator signal that indicates expected actions, and this occurs at an 'unconscious' level (Frith, 1992, p. 87). Thus, if hallucinations arise from inner speech, then the problem is not that inner speech is being generated but that there is impaired self-monitoring: the ability to recognize its origin as being from oneself, and a subsequent misattribution to external sources (Frith, 1992, p. 73). Defective self-monitoring might thus underlie the symptoms of auditory hallucinations and delusions of thought insertion, withdrawal and control. Frith (1992, p. 84) also suggested that this self-monitoring system is specific to 'speech acts' while an analogous system exists for limb movements.

While this model can explain how auditory–verbal hallucinations may be derived from a patient's thoughts, it doesn't explain why some thoughts (such as derogatory ones) appear to be more likely to be perceived as hallucinations than others (Goodwin et al., 1971; Nayani & David, 1996). Furthermore, if inner speech is usually in the first person (Hulburt et al., 1994), why are auditory–verbal hallucinations typically experienced in the second or third person, while first-person phenomena such as thought echo and *Gedankenlautwerden* (hearing one's thoughts aloud) are relatively rare (Goodwin et al., 1971; Nayani & David, 1996; Cutting, 1997)? The predominance of both speech with a negative content and a nonself grammatical form may reflect a bias towards attributing inner speech which is incongruous to the patient's beliefs or wishes (inner speech he/she doesn't want to 'hear') to an external source (Hoffman, 1986; Morrison et al., 1995). In support of this is evidence that patients who are prone to auditory–verbal hallucinations are more likely to attribute self-generated words to an external source when the content is emotional (Morrison & Haddock, 1997; Johns & McGuire, 1999).

Following from these cognitive theories, investigations of the neural correlates of auditory–verbal hallucinations have aimed to reveal the underlying pathophysiology, asking, where is the self in auditory–verbal hallucinations at a neurobiological level? Functional neuroimaging provides an in vivo examination of neural activity in individuals. Using these techniques, investigators have 'captured' the neural correlates of auditory hallucinations while they were being experienced by patients (McGuire et al., 1993; Silbersweig et al., 1995; Dierks et al., 1999; Shergill et al., 2000b).Findings from these studies have revealed an intriguing overlap with cortical regions involved in language and speech processes. Moreover, in order to examine directly the question of whether auditory–verbal hallucinations do arise from an individual's own thoughts, McGuire et al. (1995, 1996a, 1996b) investigated the process of inner speech in a series of studies in healthy persons and, more specifically,

'Distorted Self' Feedback

'Other' Feedback

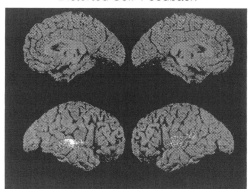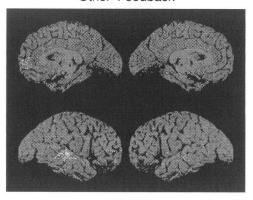

Figure 20.1   Positron emission tomography data showing areas of increased brain blood flow when healthy subjects spoke aloud and heard either a distorted version of their own speech, or another person saying what they were articulating. In both cases, relative to speaking aloud normally, there was bilateral engagement of the lateral temporal cortex. Reproduced from McGuire et al. (1996b), with permission.

in persons with schizophrenia. While undergoing positron emission tomography (PET) scans with $H_2{}^{15}O$, which provides a measurement of regional cerebral blood flow (rCBF), subjects generated sentences with single adjectives that were presented on a screen, a paradigm that approximates inner speech. The adjectives were personally descriptive and most were derogatory (e.g. 'stupid', 'ugly'). Subjects were required to incorporate these adjectives into sentences of the form 'You are...', reproducing the form and content of typical auditory verbal hallucinations (Goodwin et al., 1971; Nayani & David, 1996; Cutting, 1997). Subjects were further required to imagine these sentences being spoken in an unknown, expressionless alien voice, mimicked from a prepared tape recording prior to scanning (auditory–verbal imagery). Compared to the baseline task of silently reading the adjectives aloud, both experimental conditions were associated with increased activity in the left inferior frontal region (Broca's area) which probably corresponds to the silent articulation component that is common to both tasks. Interestingly, in the auditory–verbal imagery task, additional areas of activation were recruited in the left middle temporal gyrus, supplementary motor area (SMA) and medial prefrontal cortex in healthy subjects. However, subjects with schizophrenia and persistent hallucinations ('hallucinators') showed reduced activation in these areas, while those subjects with schizophrenia but no history of hallucinations ('nonhallucinators') had the same pattern of activation as healthy subjects. Furthermore, 'hallucinators' had decreased activation in the cerebellum as compared to 'nonhallucinators' (Figure 20.1).

Using functional magnetic resonance imaging (fMRI), which has greater temporal and spatial resolution than PET, Shergill et al. (2000b) have replicated and

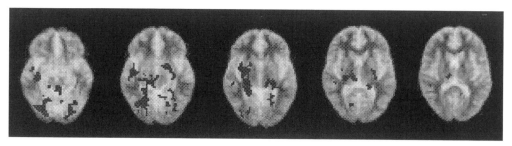

Figure 20.2 Functional magnetic resonance imaging data showing areas differentially activated when patients with schizophrenia who suffered from hallucinations imagined another person speaking. Compared to healthy volunteers, these patients showed significantly reduced activation in the lateral and medial temporal cortex and in the cerebellar cortex. Reproduced from Shergill et al. (2000b), with permission.

expanded these findings, and have also examined auditory–verbal imagery in the first, second and third person (Figure 20.2). Complementing the results of the PET studies, these fMRI data have revealed additional activation during the generation of inner speech in the SMA, left superior temporal/inferior parietal cortex and right cerebellum. These regions were also engaged during the auditory–verbal imagery paradigms, which were associated with further activation in the left premotor, middle temporal and inferior parietal cortices. These additional activations are consistent with the notion that imagining another's speech places more demands on covert articulation and verbal self-monitoring than covertly generating the same material in one's own 'inner voice' (Shergill et al., 2000b). As in the PET studies, 'hallucinators' showed less activation than controls in the temporal cortex and cerebellum during auditory–verbal imagery (Shergill et al., 2000b).

In the above studies, although there were some important between-group differences in activation, all subjects, those with schizophrenia with or without hallucinations and healthy controls, engaged a similar set of frontal and temporal areas across a series of tasks that involved the processing of inner speech. This suggests that the neural dysfunction in hallucinations is unlikely to reflect an abnormality in the processing of inner speech per se. Imagining a sentence being spoken in another person's voice entails the generation of inner speech but also implicitly engages the monitoring of this output. When imagining alien speech, hallucinators displayed a normal left inferior frontal response, but failed to recruit areas engaged by nonhallucinators and healthy controls, such as the temporal cortex and the cerebellum. As these regions have been implicated in normal verbal self-monitoring (McGuire et al., 1996b; Blakemore et al., 1998), this functional difference may reflect an impairment in this process in hallucinators and a propensity to misconstrue inner speech as arising from an external source.

Cahill et al. (1996) devised a more direct means of examining the process of verbal self-monitoring, based on the premise that auditory verbal hallucinations are the result of a failure in monitoring the intention to generate speech (Frith, 1992; Cahill et al., 1996). When we speak, we normally recognize that what we hear is our own voice. This ability arises from two sources: the external sensory feedback (the sounds of our own voice plus feedback via bone conduction) and self-monitoring of the intention to speak (Frith, 1992; Cahill et al., 1996). If there is an impairment in self-monitoring, then recognition and identification depend primarily on external sensory feedback. Thus, if the external feedback is corrupted, for example through acoustic distortion, within a system which is already compromised by impaired self-monitoring, erroneous attributions should occur (Cahill et al., 1996). In their task, individuals with schizophrenia spoke with the experimenter and into a microphone while wearing headphones through which they heard their own voice (auditory–verbal feedback). This feedback was then modified by distortion of the pitch of their voice. In the presence of distorted feedback, patients tended to misattribute externally the source of the feedback, believing that it was produced by someone else. In particular, schizophrenic patients with delusions made the greatest errors in external misattributions (Cahill et al., 1996). Johns & McGuire (1999) subsequently used a similar paradigm to compare schizophrenic patients with and without active hallucinations and controls. Patients with current hallucinations and delusions made errors about the source of their speech when it was distorted, and misattribution was particularly likely when they articulated derogatory adjectives (Johns & McGuire, 1999; Johns et al., 2001). Furthermore, both studies found a direct correlation between the likelihood of misattribution and the magnitude of pitch distortion (Cahill et al., 1996; Johns & McGuire, 1999; Johns et al., 2001) (Figure 20.3).

These studies have tested the chain of events that underlie speech production and self-recognition, beginning from the intention to speak to overt vocalization, and then hearing this vocalization, which is a form of auditory feedback. At each stage, information may be available about whether the source of the output arises from the self or not, and Frith (1992) has suggested that an internal 'self-monitor' uses this information to makes this distinction. Levelt (1983) proposed that this process occurs at three levels: (1) with the intention to speak; (2) when the intended output has been formulated, but not yet articulated; and (3) following vocalization, when the speech is perceived. If self-monitoring is impaired in individuals with hallucinations and/or delusions, distorting the auditory–verbal feedback may interfere with monitoring at the level of sensory feedback and reveal the underlying deficit. The existing data are consistent with such a mechanism.

What are the neural correlates of this self-monitoring system? Blakemore et al. (1998) addressed this question in an fMRI study which examined why we laugh

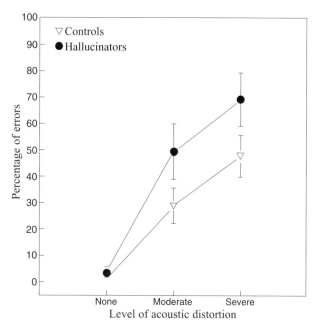

Figure 20.3 Effect of acoustic distortion on the ability of subjects to recognize their own speech online. Patients who suffer from hallucinations are more likely than controls to misidentify their own speech as alien. Both groups make more errors as the level of distortion is increased. Reproduced from Johns et al. (2001), with permission.

when tickled by someone else, but not when we make the same movements ourselves (Weiskrantz et al., 1971; see chapter 19, this volume). In healthy volunteers, they compared the effect of self-generated versus externally generated tactile stimulation, a tickle with soft foam on their palm, at various delays with the longer delays producing the highest tickly ratings (Blakemore et al., 1998). When the stimuli were self-generated, less activity was found in the somatosensory, cerebellar and anterior cingulate cortices. Blakemore et al. (1998) suggested that the specific site in which sensory consequences of motor commands are predicted is the right anterior lobe of the cerebellum as it was selectively deactivated by self-produced movements associated with a tactile sensation, in contrast to the somatosensory and anterior cingulate cortices. Effectively, they propose that the cerebellum acts as the self-monitor, distinguishing between self- and externally generated motor actions. In the condition of a self-produced tickle, the predicted sensory feedback, mediated by the cerebellum, matches that experienced by the somatosensory cortex which is revealed as a decreased activation (relative to externally produced stimuli) and experienced as being less tickly.

Self-monitoring has also been examined in the verbal modality. Frith speculated that the anterior cingulate cortex has a key role in controlling vocalization through Broca's area while also producing a corollary discharge to Wernicke's area, thereby modifying speech perception, and it itself is modified by the striatal loop which includes the thalamus (Frith, 1992, p. 92). The neural circuit that Frith and Done (1987; Frith, 1992, p. 92) proposed to underlie the self-monitoring of speech processes comprised the anterior cingulate, Broca's and Wernicke's areas, the supplementary motor area and basal ganglia. Gray et al. (1990) also included the parahippocampal region with the hippocampus at its hub. McGuire et al. (1996a) investigated overt verbal self-monitoring in healthy volunteers with PET using $H_2{}^{15}O$ and found that activation in the lateral temporal cortex was associated with 'alien' feedback as compared to distorted feedback of the subject's own speech. An additional component of the neural response was maximal when subjects first encountered distorted feedback, but diminished over subsequent trials. This activation was localized to the hippocampal region.

We have recently extended this approach to verbal self-monitoring using fMRI, which permits the acquisition of a greater amount of data than with PET, and provides a better temporal resolution, facilitating the detection of time-dependent changes in activation (Fu et al., 2000). However, a key disadvantage of fMRI is the production of high-amplitude acoustic noise (about 110 dB) during image acquisition. This makes it difficult for subjects to hear auditory stimuli and their own voice – not an ideal environment for the investigation of auditory–verbal feedback. In order to avoid the confounding effects of scanner noise, we have developed an event-related fMRI acquisition sequence in which images are collected in a discontinuous manner, such that there are periods within the acquisition sequence when the scanner is silent. It is during these 'windows' that trials of the self-monitoring task are performed, allowing subjects to speak and hear their overt verbal feedback in the absence of scanner noise.

During each fMRI session, subjects performed an overt verbal self-monitoring task which involved the experimental manipulation of auditory–verbal feedback. The baseline condition consisted of reading single nouns aloud and hearing one's own voice (as normal). Single adjectives were presented on a computer screen with their frequency and imageability of each word matched across tasks (Gilhooly & Logie, 1980). Subjects' speech was recorded by a nonmagnetic microphone and fed back to them, in real time, via headphones incorporated into ear defenders. There were three experimental conditions, presented in a randomized order (with the baseline condition): (1) reading aloud with pitch distortion: the subject reads aloud while hearing his/her own speech whose pitch has been lowered by four semitones; (2) reading aloud with 'alien' feedback: the subject reads aloud while hearing the words spoken by another person, synchronous with his/her own speech; and (3) reading aloud with distorted 'alien' feedback: the 'alien' speech was also lowered by four semitones. During each experimental condition, the subject decided whether the feedback he/she heard was: (1) his/her own voice; (2) someone else's; or (3) that he/she was uncertain of the source, by pressing the corresponding button on a three-button box with the possible choices displayed on the lower portion of the display screen. Preliminary data have revealed activations in the hippocampus, bilateral temporal cortices, prefrontal regions and cerebellum associated with this process (Fu et al., 2001). These regions encompass and extend those found in the previous PET study (McGuire et al., 1996b).

It is unclear whether there is a singular entity for all cognitive self-monitoring (independent of modality) or there are separate monitors for different processes, such as speech and limb movements, as suggested by Frith (1992, p. 84). However, independent studies of motor and verbal self-monitoring suggest that both processes normally involve the cerbellar cortex, and that the engagement of this region is attenuated in patients with psychotic phenomena (McGuire et al., 1996b; Blakemore et al., 1998; Shergill et al., 2000b). At the same time, these studies implicate the lateral temporal cortex in verbal self-monitoring, and the somatosensory cortex in motor monitoring. It may be that there are some brain regions which participate in cognitive self-monitoring, independent of the modality of the monitored process, and others which are modality-specific, localized to areas implicated in sensory processing in that modality.

REFERENCES

Blakemore, S.J., Wolpert, D.M. & Frith, C.D. (1998). Central cancellation of self-produced tickle sensation. *Nature and Neuroscience*, **1**, 635–40.

Cahill, C., Silbersweig, D., & Frith, C. (1996). Psychotic experiences induced in deluded patients using distorted auditory feedback. *Cognitive Neuropsychiatry*, **1**, 201–11.

Cleghorn, J.M., Franco, S., Szechtman, B. et al. (1992). Towards a brain map of auditory hallucinations. *American Journal of Psychiatry*, **149**, 1062–9.

Cutting, J. (1997). *Principles of Psychopathology*. Oxford: Oxford University Press.

Dierks, T., Linden, D.E., Jandl, M. et al. (1999). Activation of Heschl's gyrus during auditory hallucinations. *Neuron*, **22**, 615–21.

Evarts, E.V. (1971). Central control of movement. V. Feedback and corollary discharge: a merging of the concepts. *Neuroscience Research Program Bulletin*, **9**, 86–112.

Feinberg, I. (1978). Efference copy and corollary discharge: implications for thinking and its disorders. *Schizophrenia Bulletin*, **4**, 636–40.

Frith, C.D. (1992). *The Cognitive Neuropsychology of Schizophrenia*. Hove, East Sussex, UK: Erlbaum.

Frith, C.D. & Done, D.J. (1987). Towards a neuropsychology of schizophrenia. *British Journal of Psychiatry*, **153**, 437–43.

Fu, C.H.Y., Ahmad, F., Amaro, E., Jr et al. (2000). An event-related fMRI study of overt verbal self-monitoring. *Neuroimage*, **11**, S76.

Fu, C.H.Y., Brammer, M.J., Williams, S.C.R. et al. (2001). Hearing voices or the self in disguise? Neural correlates of impaired self-monitoring in schizophrenia. *Schizophrenia Research*, **49**, 176.

Fuster, J.M. (1997). *The Prefrontal Cortex: Anatomy, Physiology, and Neuropsychology of the Frontal Lobe*, 3rd edn. Philadelphia, PA: Lippincott-Raven.

Gilhooly, K.J. & Logie, R.H. (1980). Age of acquisition, imagery, concreteness, familiarity, and ambiguity measures for 1944 words. *Behavioral Research Methods and Instruments*, **12**, 395–427.

Goodwin, D., Alderson, P. & Rosenthal, R. (1971). Clinical significance of hallucinations in psychiatric disorders. *Archives of General Psychiatry*, **24**, 76–80.

Gray, J.A., Feldon, J., Rawlins, J., Hemsley, D. & Smith, A. (1990). The neuropsychology of schizophrenia. *Behaviour Brain Science*, **14**, 1–84.

Helmholtz, H. (1866). *Handbuch der Physiologischen Optik*. Leipzig: Voss.

Hoffman, R.E. (1986). Verbal hallucinations and language production processes in schizophrenia. *Behaviour and Brain Science*, **9**, 503–48.

Hulburt, R.T., Happe, F. & Frith, U. (1994). Sampling the form of inner experience in three adults with Asperger's syndrome. *Psychological Medicine*, **24**, 385–95.

Johns, L.C. & McGuire, P.K. (1999). Verbal self-monitoring and auditory hallucinations in schizophrenia. *Lancet*, **353**, 469–70.

Johns, L.C., Rossell, S., Frith, C. et al. (2001). Verbal self-monitoring and auditory verbal hallucinations in patients with schizophrenia. *Psychological Medicine*, **31**, 705–15.

Levelt, W.J.M. (1983). Monitoring and self-repair in speech. *Cognition*, **14**, 41–104.

Maudsley, H. (1886). *Natural Causes and Supernatural Seemings*. London: Kegan Paul, Trench.

McCloskey, D.I. & Torda, T.A. (1975). Corollary motor discharges and kinaesthesia. *Brain Research*, **100**, 467–70.

McCloskey, D.I., Ebeling, P. & Goodwin, G.M. (1974). Estimation of weights and tensions and apparent involvement of a 'sense of effort'. *Experimental Neurology*, **42**, 220–32.

McGuire, P.K., Shah, G.M.S. & Murray, R.M. (1993). Increased blood flow in Broca's area during auditory hallucinations in schizophrenia. *Lancet*, **342**, 703–6.

McGuire, P.K., Silbersweig, D.A., Wright, I. et al. (1995). Abnormal perception of inner speech: a physiological basis for auditory hallucinations. *Lancet*, **346**, 596–600.

McGuire, P.K., Silbersweig, D.A., Murray, R.M. et al. (1996a). Functional anatomy of inner speech and auditory verbal imagery. *Psychological Medicine*, **26**, 29–38.

McGuire, P.K., Silbersweig, D.A. & Frith, C.D. (1996b). Functional neuroanatomy of verbal self-monitoring. *Brain*, **119**, 907–17.

Morrison, A.P. & Haddock, G. (1997). Cognitive factors in source monitoring and auditory hallucinations. *Psychological Medicine*, **27**, 669–79.

Morrison, A.P., Haddock, G. & Jarrier, N. (1995). Intrusive thoughts and auditory hallucinations: a cognitive approach. *Behavioural Cognitive Psychotherapy*, **22**, 259–64.

Nayani, A. & David, A.S. (1996). The auditory hallucination: a phenomenological survey. *Psychological Medicine*, **26**, 177–95.

Schneider, K. (1959). *Clinical Psychopathology*. New York: Grune & Stratton.

Shergill, S.S., Brammer, M.J., Williams, S.C., Murray, R.M. & McGuire, P.K. (2000a). Mapping auditory hallucinations in schizophrenia using functional magnetic resonance imaging. *Archives of General Psychiatry*, **57**, 1033–88.

Shergill, S.S., Bullmore, E., Simmons, A., Murray, R. & McGuire, P. (2000b). Functional anatomy of auditory verbal imagery in schizophrenic patients with auditory hallucinations. *American Journal of Psychiatry*, **157**, 1691–3.

Silbersweig, D.A., Stern, E., Frith, C. et al. (1995). A functional anatomy of hallucinations in schizophrenia. *Nature*, **378**, 176–9.

Sperry, R.W. (1950). Neural basis of the spontaneous optokinetic response produced by visual inversion. *Journal of Comparative Physiology and Psychology*, **43**, 482–9.

Suzuki, M., Yuasa, S., Minabe, Y., Murata, M. & Kurachi, M. (1993). Left superior temporal blood flow increases in schizophrenic and schizophreniform patients with auditory hallucination: a longitudinal case study using ^{123}I-IMP SPECT. *European Archives of Psychiatry and Clinical Neuroscience*, **242**, 257–61.

von Holst, E. (1954). Relations between the central nervous system and the peripheral organs. *British Journal of Animal Behaviour*, **2**, 89–94.

Weiskrantz, L., Elliott, J. & Darlington, C. (1971). Preliminary observations on tickling oneself. *Nature*, **230**, 598–9.

Wing, J.K., Cooper, J.E. & Sartorius, N. (1974). *The Measurement and Classification of Psychiatric Symptoms*. Cambridge: Cambridge University Press.

Wolpert, D.M., Ghahramani, Z. & Jordan, M.I. (1995). An internal model for sensorimotor integration. *Science*, **269**, 1880–2.

21

The cognitive neuroscience of agency in schizophrenia

Henrik Walter and Manfred Spitzer

Universitätsklinik für Psychiatrie, ULM, Germany

Abstract

Agency is the *sense* of ownership, i.e. the personal *experience* of being the originator of one's thoughts and actions (Walter, 2001). Disorders of agency are prominent in schizophrenia and may also be part of several other neuropsychiatric disorders and syndromes, e.g. alien-hand syndrome, drug-induced psychoses or anosognosia. In recent years, cognitive neuroscience has made considerable progress in understanding the neural basis of agency. In this chapter, current neurocognitive theories of agency are reviewed which are based on the assumption that an internal monitoring deficit lies at the core of disorders of agency in schizophrenia. It is demonstrated how they fail to explain several features of disturbed agency. A complementary theory is proposed which takes into account the experiences of reference and insertion of personal relatedness as well as the acknowledged role of dopamine for schizophrenia and its role as a neuromodulator regulating signal-to-noise ratio.

The psychopathology of agency in schizophrenia

Schizophrenic patients often report the immediate experience of someone else controlling their thoughts and actions. In addition, sometimes they feel they are in control of external events or are convinced they know what other people think. They think that things or events are related to themselves in a special way, have a personal significance or are made especially for them. The German psychiatrist Kurt Schneider emphasized these types of ideation as criteria for the diagnosis of schizophrenia, and because of their relative homogeneity and recognizability, they are frequently referred to as Schneiderian first-rank symptoms. In German psychopathology, these symptoms are called *Ichstörungen*, i.e. (literally) 'disorders of the I'. In British psychopathology, these experiences are sometimes called 'passivity phenomena', whereas in Anglo-American psychiatry they are subsumed under the category of delusions, e.g. as 'delusions of alien control'. However, German as well as British psychopathologists emphasize that these (primary) 'disorders of experience' should be distinguished from the concept of delusions as false beliefs (Spitzer, 1990; Frith, 1992).

The functional neuroanatomy of agency

Recently, neurocognitive theories about agency in schizophrenia have been proposed. Frith (1992) suggested that an *internal monitoring deficit* causes delusions of alien control. In the normal state of mind, actions are monitored by comparing internal predictions and actual outcome of actions using feedback loops. If the monitoring process is disturbed, the experience of loss of control results. Behavioural studies have shown that delusions of alien control in schizophrenic patients correlate with the patients' failure to correct their own motor errors in the absence of visual feedback (Frith & Done, 1989). Patients with delusions of alien control also show impaired memory for their own motor acts (Mlakar et al., 1994). An internal monitoring deficit of self-generated internal speech was postulated to be the cause of verbal hallucinations in schizophrenic patients (Frith, 1996). According to Frith, this self-monitoring process also operates on thoughts.

Spence et al. (1997) used a motor task to study schizophrenic patients with passivity phenomena with positron emission tomography (PET). Patients were compared to: (1) healthy controls; (2) schizophrenic patients without passivity phenomena; and (3) themselves studied again upon remission. Passivity phenomena were associated with hyperactivity in the right inferior parietal cortex and the anterior cingulate cortex. Because the parietal cortex is a region in which information about the body and the external space is integrated, possibly giving rise to the egocentric coordinate space, the dysfunction of this region may explain the abnormal experience of not being in control of one's actions. Lesions of the anterior cingulate sometimes result in the alien-hand syndrome, i.e. the experience that the movement of one's hand is not under one's volitional control (Gasquoine, 1993).

Based on animal experiments, Frith & Done (1988) have proposed that the monitoring deficit is localized in the parahippocampal gyrus or in the anterior cingulate which normally transmits prefrontally generated intentions to the hippocampus. Using a delayed-feedback paradigm in a self-tickling functional magnetic resonance imaging (fMRI) experiment, Blakemore et al. (1999) argue that the cerebellum may be a crucial structure in comparing predicted and performed movement (see chapter 19, this volume).

Jeannerod et al. have proposed a slightly different version of this self-monitoring theory (Georgieff & Jeannerod, 1998). As shown by several PET experiments (e.g. Decety et al. 1997), specific prefrontal areas are only active during simulation and observation of actions, but not during the execution of actions. In the monkey, neurons have been described which are active during the observation of movements of others (mirror neurons: Gallese et al., 1996). Georgieff & Jeannerod propose that in schizophrenic patients the representation of actions is less selective than in normal subjects. Patients no longer distinguish properly between their own actions and actions of others. In experiments with a data glove, simulating an alien hand, the authors have shown that schizophrenic patients are not very good at judging whether a hand movement on a computer screen was made by themselves or by someone else (Daprati et al., 1997).

Although these theories explain *passivity phenomena*, they cannot explain the flip-side of the coin of *Ichstörungen*, i.e. 'experiences of reference' (EoR). This is the phenomenon that external events are experienced as personally meaningful and specifically related to the patient. To account for EoR, Frith invokes an additional explanation which was originally developed to explain autism. He proposes that there is a 'theory of mind (TOM) module' in the human brain which is dysfunctioning in schizophrenic patients (Frith, 1996). According to TOM, humans develop between the age of 3 and 4 the concept of other people having minds, enabling them to understand behaviour on the basis of beliefs (mind-reading) and thereby to understand the concept of cheating and lying. Based on neuroimaging studies in humans with PET which show an activation of the left medial prefrontal cortex during TOM tasks (Goel et al., 1995), Frith believes that this area (BA9) is a possible neuroanatomical candidate for the TOM module. However, recent studies with schizophrenic patients show that it is rather formal thought disorder than paranoid symptoms which correlate with poor performance in TOM tasks (Greig et al., 1999). Additionally, studies in brain-lesioned patients show an association of poor performance in TOM tasks only with bilateral orbitofrontal lesions and not with dorsolateral or dorsomedial lesions (Stone et al., 1998).

Apart from these inconsistencies, it is very unsatisfying to explain a core symptom like *Ichstörungen* within two different theoretical frameworks. Moreover, neither Frith nor Jeannerod relates their ideas to the acknowledged role of dopamine in positive schizophrenic symptoms. Finally, both theories do not take into account the profound affective changes associated with these experiences, which are clinically referred to as delusional mood and anxiety. In sum, according to our point of view, the question of a neurobiologically plausible and parsimonious account of *Ichstörungen* has not found a satisfying answer yet.

Neuromodulation and *Ichstörungen*

Spitzer (1995) proposed a theory that accounts for the occurrence of disorders of experience in schizophrenic patients in terms of the neuromodulatory effects of dopamine (and noradrenaline (norepinephrine)). Neuromodulators influence the action of neurotransmitters like glutamate and gamma-aminobutyric acid (GABA). Neuromodulatory neurons are small in number, have diffuse projections and act rather slowly, as the effects of neuromodulatory agents are G-protein-coupled rather than ion-channel-coupled. We may understand the difference between neurotransmitters and neuromodulators by likening their actions to the functions of a TV set. Fast glutamatergic information processing corresponds to the signal determining the details of the picture. Neuromodulatory effects correspond to general variables like brightness, contrast and colour saturation.

Dopamine (and noradrenaline) have been demonstrated to amplify strong signals and to dampen weak ones. Hence, the net effect of their action is to enhance the signal-to-noise ratio. To go back to the TV analogy: noradrenaline and dopamine appear to control the contrast of the picture, i.e. the difference between signal determining the brightness of individual pixels and the noise, i.e. random background activity of the system.

Within this framework of a neuromodulatory function of dopamine, the question of how to relate dopaminergic function and schizophrenic symptoms arises – in particular, how the activity of dopamine and noradrenaline may affect thought processes, and how disordered thought in schizophrenia may be conceived.

If the dopaminergic tone is low, the signal-to-noise ratio is below the normal level. Access to stored information is unreliable, because activations of cortical representations are less focused and overlap. In normal people, such a neuromodulatory state of low signal-to-noise ratio may increase the likelihood of creativity and change. In the pathological range, formal thought disorder with loosening of associations may result.

In contrast, if there is too much dopamine, the signal-to-noise ratio is high. Access to stored information is focused and reliable, but change becomes unlikely. *Ichstörungen* may occur as a result of pathological hyperfocusing. Small signals (i.e. perceptions to which we would normally pay little or no attention at all) may be amplified to a degree that is much higher than usual. This may result in experiences of significant events when in fact merely ordinary events happen. Once such spurious meanings have been activated and thereby become relevant to further thought processes, they are less likely to be discarded, as the likelihood of change of cortical representations decreases with increasing signal-to-noise. Competing concepts, ideas and hypotheses about reality are less likely to be activated. Furthermore, it is known that increased anxiety and a high neuromodulatory tone of dopamine and noradrenaline are associated.

On the basis of these ideas it becomes possible to explain both types of experiences in *Ichstörungen*: when *external* events are experienced as unusually significant, 'delusions' of *reference* may result. If *internal* events, e.g. mismatch signals, are experienced as unusually significant, 'delusions' of *alien control* may develop. But why does the issue of personal relatedness play such a prominent role in these symptoms? To answer this question we will take a look at two neuropsychiatric syndromes in which symptoms which are highly similar to *Ichstörungen* occur.

Personal relatedness, right hemisphere and dopamine

Delusional misidentification syndromes (DMS) are conditions in which a patient incorrectly identifies or reduplicates persons, places, objects and events (see reviews in Feinberg & Roane, 1997; Moselhy & Oyebode, 1997). These syndromes are reported to have an incidence of between 0.001 and 4%, and are predominantly found in patients with schizophrenia and affective psychosis. In 25–40% of cases, however, they occur in organic brain disease. While some evidence suggests that a right-hemispheric lesion can be both necessary and sufficient to produce DMS, the bulk of cases supports the argument that a right-hemispheric lesion is much more likely to be associated with DMS in the context of bifrontal or diffuse cortical pathology. Numerous explanations for DMS, ranging from psychoanalytical theories to visuospatial problems and difficulties in face processing, have been proposed.

Capgras syndrome and the Fregoli syndrome are the two most common DMS. In Capgras syndrome, patients believe that a familiar person has been replaced by a double or an imposter. In Fregoli syndrome, unfamiliar people are believed to be familiar ones, even if there is no physical resemblance. The symmetric picture of these two syndromes has led several authors to propose a dichotomization of DMS. Some authors see the difference between Capgras and Fregoli syndrome in hypo- versus hyperidentification, while others have interpreted them within the framework of familiarity versus unfamiliarity. Most recently, Feinberg & Roane (1997) proposed that the distinguishing feature between both syndromes is *personal relatedness*, which may be either withdrawn or inserted. In conclusion, these two delusional syndromes share a right hemisphere pathology, and may be regarded as resembling experiences of alien control (withdrawal of personal relatedness) and experiences of reference (insertion of personal relatedness).

Additional data from cognitive neuroscience studies may be taken as evidence that the right hemisphere plays a special role in personal relatedness. Such right-hemispheric involvement in personal relatedness has been shown in investigations of decision making in brain-lesioned patients (Damasio, 1994; Bechara, 1999), in PET studies of autobiographical memory (Fink et al., 1996) and in studies with transcranial magnetic stimulation on self-recognition in normal subjects (Keenan et al., 2000) as well as in patients with depersonalization (Keenan et al., 2000). Moreover, several authors have regarded the right hemisphere, and the parietal lobe in particular, as a possible origin of 'alienation' (Angyal, 1936; Nasrallah, 1985; Cutting, 1989).

Another neuropsychiatric syndrome of interest for our discussion is anosognosia, i.e. denial of illness. The most common form is denial of hemiplegia resulting from a lesion of the right hemisphere compromising the right parietal lobe. When anosognosic patients are asked if they are paralysed they rigorously deny it. If forced to move or to attend to their inabilities they will ignore the obvious evidence of their paralysis and rationalize away problems in using their arms. Several explanations have been proposed for this condition.

Recently, Ramachandran & Blakeslee (1998) formulated a hypothesis postulating an anomaly detector in the right hemisphere. They argue that anosognosic behaviour is a result of an imbalance of the different information-processing strategies of both hemispheres. Healthy people tend to ignore small incongruities in their experience of the world that do not fit into their world model. Incongruities are normally forced into a world model because we have been evolutionarily designed to have a consistent world-view in order to be able to decide and act. According to Ramachandran & Blakeslee, this strategy is mainly adopted by the left hemisphere. However, if significant incongruities emerge, there must be a mechanism which forces a change in our model of the world. The authors suggest that the right hemisphere serves this very function. Because the right hemisphere works in a more holistic manner, it is more susceptible to overall changes and may serve as an anomaly detector: if anomalies cross a certain threshold the right hemisphere intervenes and forces a paradigm shift. Instead of discarding or distorting evidence, an attempt is made to question the status quo and to construct a new model. As the right hemisphere is damaged in patients with anosognosia, denial and rationalization prevail in the clinical picture.

The neuromodulatory theory of *Ichstörungen* and the role of the right hemisphere for anomaly detection and personal relatedness may be put together within the framework of different hemispheric modes of information processing, as proposed by Stephen Kosslyn (Kosslyn et al., 1992; Brown & Kosslyn, 1993, see also Oepen et al., 1988): Whereas the left hemisphere is characterized by smaller receptive fields resulting in focused, conjunctive coding, the right hemisphere is characterized by larger, overlapping receptive fields resulting in a coarse coding. This may explain the dominance of the right hemisphere for information processing of spatially and temporally distributed features of reality. Although this hypothesis has not yet been proven decisively, it can explain why dopamine affects the right hemisphere more than the left: if the main effect of dopamine is to focus signals it will affect a system which relies on coarse coding, i.e. the right hemisphere, more prominently than a system which relies on conjunctive coding, i.e. the left hemisphere.

In the case of *Ichstörungen* the anomaly detector in the right hemisphere might be hyperactive because of the increased dopaminergic tone. Ordinary events are experienced as highly significant because internal or external signals are hyperfocused. Depending on which signals are processed a loss or an insertion of personal relatedness occurs. Because the right hemisphere signals 'something is wrong' – which is accompanied by high levels of anxiety – the left hemisphere begins to construct explanations resulting in what we call delusions. However, it is highly probable that the dysfunction is not localized in one region, e.g. the right parietal cortex, but rather that the interaction of different right-hemispheric regions and the left hemisphere is disturbed.

There is already some experimental evidence for this hypothesis: in a series of papers Spitzer et al. have shown that schizophrenic patients with formal thought disorder show increased indirect semantic priming (Spitzer, 1997). This can be explained by a reduced level of dopamine resulting in a reduced ability to focus information processing with consecutive loosening of associations. If positive symptoms, including *Ichstörungen*, are associated with an increased dopaminergic tone we should find normal or even reduced priming effects in such patients. Actually, this result has been found in paranoid patients (Henik et al., 1992). Additionally, the application of L-dopa in healthy subjects shows the same effect (Kischka et al., 1996). That the right hemisphere is specialized for less focused information processing has recently been demonstrated by electrophysiological methods: indirect semantic priming elicits event-related potentials (ERP) priming effects only over the right hemisphere (Kiefer et al., 1998). Finally, there is evidence from animal research that dopamine receptors and dopamine levels show hemispheric asymmetry (Nowak, 1989).

Summary

Contemporary neurocognitive theories explain disorders of agency in terms of internal monitoring deficits. However, they neither account for the experiences of reference and of significance nor for the insertion of personal relatedness. Furthermore, they do not consider the acknowledged role of dopamine in positive symptoms. In contrast to these views, we have proposed a special role of the neuromodulator dopamine for *Ichstörungen* and the right hemisphere. There are experimental ways to test this hypothesis and first results are in accordance with it. The cognitive neuroscience approach to psychiatry (Spitzer & Casas, 1997; Walter, 1998) should not be regarded as opposed to psychopathology but rather as a promising road to explain what our patients experience phenomenologically.

REFERENCES

Angyal, A. (1936). The experience of the body-self in schizophrenia. *Archives of Neurology and Psychiatry*, **35**, 1029–53.

Bechara, A. (1999). Emotionen und Entscheidungsfindung nach Frontalhirnläsionen: Ansätze zum Verständnis bestimmter psychiatrischer Erkrankungen. *Nervenheilkunde*, **18**, 54–9.

Blakemore, S.J., Frith, C.D. & Wolpert, D.M. (1999). The cerebellum is involved in predicting the sensory consequences of action. *Neuroimage*, **9**, S445.

Brown, H.D. & Kosslyn, S.M. (1993). Cerebral lateralization. *Current Opinion in Neurobiology*, **3**, 183–6.

Cutting, J. (1989). Body image disorders: comparision between unilateral hemisphere damage and schizophrenia. *Behavioral Neurology*, **2**, 201–10.

Damasio, A.R. (1994). *Descartes's Error*. New York: Putnam's.

Daprati, E., Franck, N., Georgieff, N. et al. (1997). Looking for the agent: an investigation into consciousness of action and self-consciousness in schizophrenic patients. *Cognition*, **65**, 71–86.

Decety, J., Grezes, J. & Costes, N. (1997). Brain activity during observation of action. Influence of action content and subject's strategy. *Brain*, **120**, 1763–77.

Feinberg, T.E. & Roane, D.M. (1997). Misidentification syndromes. In *Behavioral Neurology and Neuropsychology*, ed. T.E. Feinberg & M.J. Farah, pp. 391–7. New York: McGraw Hill.

Fink, G.R., Markowitsch, H.J., Reinkemeier, M. et al. (1996). Cerebral representation of one's own past: neural networks involved in autobiographical memory. *Journal of Neuroscience*, **16**, 4275–82.

Frith, C.D. & Done, D.J. (1988). Towards a neuropsychology of schizophrenia. *British Journal of Psychiatry*, **153**, 437–43.

Frith, C.D. & Done, D.J. (1989). Experiences of alien control in schizophrenia reflect a disorder in the central monitoring of action. *Psychological Medicine*, **19**, 359–63.

Frith, C.D. (1992). *The Cognitive Neuropsychology of Schizophrenia*. Hillsdale, NJ: Erlbaum.

Frith, C.D. (1996). The role of the prefrontal cortex in self-consciousness: the case of auditory hallucinations. *Philosophical Transactions of the Royal Society of London B*, **351**, 1505–12.

Gallese, V., Fadiga, L., Fogassi, L. et al. (1996). Action recognition in the premotor cortex. *Brain*, **119**, 593–609.

Gasquoine, P.G. Alien hand sign. *Journal of Clinical and Experimental Neuropsychology*, **15**, 663–7.

Georgieff, N. & Jeannerod, M. (1998). Beyond consciousness of external reality: a 'who' system for consciousness of action and self-consciousness. *Conscious Cognition*, **7**, 465–77.

Goel, V., Grafman, J., Sadato, N. et al. (1995). Modeling other minds. *NeuroReport*, **6**, 1741–6.

Greig, T.C., Bell, M.D. & Bryson, G.J. (1999). 'Theory of mind' impairment in schizophrenia. Cognitive and symptom correlates. *Schizophrenia Research*, **36**, 168.

Henik, A., Priel, B. & Umansky, R. (1992). Attention and automaticity in semantic processing of schizophrenic patients. *Neuropsychiatry, Neuropsychology and Behavioral Neurology*, **5**, 161–9.

Keenan, J.P., Wheeler, M.A., Gallup, G.G. Jr. et al. (2000). Self-recognition and the right prefrontal cortex. *Trends in Cognitive Science*, **4**, 338–44.

Kiefer, M., Weisbrod, M., Kern, I. et al. (1998). Right hemisphere activation during indirect semantic priming: evidence from event-related potentials. *Brain and Language*, **64**, 377–408.

Kischka, U., Kammer, T., Maier, S. et al. (1996). Dopaminergic modulation of semantic network activation. *Neuropsychologia*, **34**, 1107–13.

Kosslyn, S.M., Chabris, C.F., Marsolek, C.J. et al. (1992). Categorical versus coordinate spatial relations: computation analyses and computer simulations. *Journal of Experimental Psychology: Human Perception and Performance*, **18**, 562–77.

Mlakar, J., Jensterle, J. & Frith, C.D. (1994). Central monitoring deficiency and schizophrenic symptoms. *Psychological Medicine*, **24**, 557–64.

Moselhy, H., & Oyebode, F. (1997). Delusional misidentification syndromes: a review of the anglophone literature. *Neurology and Psychiatry and Brain Research*, **5**, 21–6.

Nasrallah, H.A. (1985). The unintegrated right cerebral hemispheric consciousness as alien intruder: a possible mechanism for Schneiderian delusions in schizophrenia. *Comprehensive Psychiatry*, **26**, 273–82.

Nowak, G. (1989). Lateralization of neocortical dopamine receptors and dopamine level in normal Wistar rats. *Polish Journal of Pharmacology and Pharmacy*, **41**, 133–7.

Oepen, G., Harrington, A., Spitzer, M. et al. (1988). 'Feelings' of conviction. On the relation of affect and thought disorder. In *Psychopathology and Philosophy*, ed. M. Spitzer., F.A. Uehlein & G. Oepen, pp. 43–55. Berlin: Spinger.

Ramachandran, V.S. & Blakeslee, S. (1998). *Phantoms in the Brain*. New York: Morrow.

Spence, S.A., Brooks, D.J., Hirsch, S.R. et al. (1997). A PET study of voluntary movement in schizophrenic patients experiencing passivity phenomena (delusions of alien control). *Brain*, **120**, 1997–2011.

Spitzer, M. (1990). On defining delusions. *Comprehensive Psychiatry*, **31**, 377–97.

Spitzer, M. (1995). A neurocomputational approach to delusions. *Comprehensive Psychiatry*, **36**, 83–105.

Spitzer, M. (1997). A cognitive neuroscience of thought disorder. *Schizophrenia Bulletin*, **23**, 29–50.

Spitzer, M. & Casas, B. (1997). Project for a scientific psychopathology. *Current Opinion in Psychiatry*, **10**, 395–401.

Stone, V.E., Baron-Cohen, S. & Knight, R.T. (1998). Frontal lobe contributions to theory of mind. *Journal of Cognitive Neuroscience*, **10**, 640–56.

Walter, H. (1998). Emergence and the cognitive neuroscience of psychiatry. *Zeitschrift für Naturforschung*, **53c**, 723–37.

Walter, H. (2001). *Neurophilosophy of Free Will*. Cambridge, MA: MIT Press.

22

Self-consciousness: an integrative approach from philosophy, psychopathology and the neurosciences

Tilo Kircher[1] and Anthony S. David[2]

[1] Department of Psychiatry, University of Tübingen, Germany
[2] Institute of Psychiatry and Maudsley Hospital, London, UK

Abstract

In this chapter, we want to try and integrate the divergent lines introduced in the other parts of this book. We propose a model of self-consciousness derived from phenomenology, philosophy, the cognitive and neurosciences. We will then give an overview of research data on self-processing from various fields and link it to our model. Some aspects of the disturbances of the self in pathological states such as brain lesions and schizophrenia will be discussed. Finally, the clinically important concept of insight into a disease and its neurocognitive origin will be introduced. We argue that self-consciousness is a valid construct and, as shown in this chapter, it is possible that it can be studied with the instruments of cognitive neuroscience.

Introduction

The *self* as an entity distinct from the *other* has entered western thought through Greek philosophy (see chapter 1, this volume, for details). Throughout history, a myriad of different notions, starting from theology, philosophy, psychoanalysis, to early psychological concepts, psychopathology, the social sciences, and, more recently, cognitive psychology, neurology and the neurosciences have been developed. With the advent of scientific interest in consciousness towards the end of the twentieth century, self-consciousness has also become a topic taken up by the neuroscientific community. As a first phenomenological approximation based on commonly shared experience, we know that we are the same person across time, that we are the author of our thoughts/actions, and that we are distinct from the environment. These 'feelings' are so fundamental to our human experience that we hardly ever think about them. However, there are neuropsychiatric conditions where this basic tone of selfhood loses its natural givenness, with subsequent changes in the perception of oneself and the environment.

In the following, we wish to introduce a model of self-consciousness which will serve as a framework for the understanding of most of the chapters in this book. We then present examples of neuroscientific studies of the *self*. We will further discuss selectively clinical cases with an alteration of 'selfhood' and will focus particularly on schizophrenia, applying our model to some of its symptoms such as hallucinations and delusions of alien control. Another important aspect to altered states of self-consciousness is a loss of insight into one's own state. The study of pathological states is particularly helpful, because tacit assumptions during the construction of explanatory models for the faculty in question may be exposed.

A model of consciousness and self-consciousness

Due to the elusiveness of the *self*, we need a conceptual framework before we can begin to map out its neural basis and its disorders. Then it will be possible to generate testable hypotheses. Since the scientific study of consciousness and particularly self-consciousness is still very young, and there is not as yet a vast amount of empirical data, we need to investigate findings and concepts from different sources such as philosophy, cognitive psychology, neuroscience and psychopathology. Phenomenology may serve as a starting point. With the help of detailed phenomenological analysis, the foundations of scientific psychology (W. Wundt, W. James) and later psychiatry (K. Jaspers) were outlined. In the study of self-consciousness phenomenology will now again serve as the appropriate defining base on which the sciences may develop their starting point. The model we present below is derived from phenomenological (for further details see Henry, 1963, 1965; Merleau-Ponty, 1965) and analytical philosophy (for further details see Bermudez et al., 1995; Metzinger, 1995; Block et al., 1997), cognitive psychology, psychopathology and the neurosciences. It will serve as an initial framework and is meant to be largely descriptive. Later we will focus on some of the details of its subcomponents.

What do we mean by 'consciousness'? We have a certain, privileged access to our own mental states that nobody else has and that cannot be accessed from the outside in its primary subjective givenness. When I look at the colour of the sky, the experience of the blueness is something of which I myself am immediately aware. It is the subjective, prereflexive givenness of any experience that nobody else can have in my particular form. In the philosophical literature, these conscious experiences are variously called 'phenomenal consciousness', 'raw feelings', 'qualia' or 'first-person perspective' (see chapters 2 and 17). We will use the word 'qualia' here in the sense of 'purely subjective, prereflexive, first-person experience' (Figure 22.1).

Every experience – the humming of the computer, the smell of perfume, the numbness of my foot, the memory of yesterday's dinner or a vague feeling – is the content of phenomenal consciousness. It is the characteristic feature of qualia that they exist only through their content. We may at some point be able to characterize

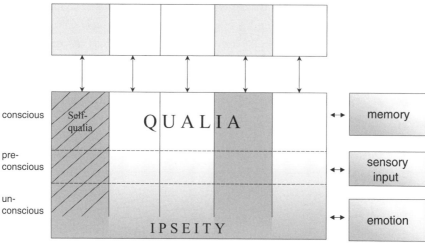

Figure 22.1   A model of consciousness and self-consciousness. The contents of phenomenal consciousness (intentionality) are prereflexive, raw feelings, qualia. They may be sensory experiences,
memories and emotions. Their content is on a continuum of high (grey) or low (white) self-
valence (e.g. perception of one's own face versus stranger's face). They may be conscious,
when they are attended to; preconscious, when they are not attended to; or unconscious
(e.g. information from the autonomous nervous system, such as heart rate or blood oxygen
level). Ipseity is the unifying 'basic tone' of the first-person givenness of all experiences.
There is a special type of self-qualia, responsible for the feeling of unity, coherence, self-
affectability and agency. If we reflect on qualia (i.e. think about primary experiences), the
content enters introspective consciousness.

fully the brain state (or third-person perspective) that corresponds to a 'raw feeling';
however, even the most thorough description will entirely lack the subjective experience that only I have. The blueness of the sky is nothing but light waves of a
certain length; the experience of the colour only becomes real in my mind. An even
better example might be pain: the feel of a pinprick is only in my mind; without the
subjective feeling of pain, it is not pain. It is not the firing of neurons in my spinal
cord or in my brain that constitutes pain, but the awareness of a sensation in only
my consciousness.

These phenomenal states are something special, different from physical (chemi-
cal, neurobiological) states, because they are characterized by 'transparency',
'presence', and 'perspectiveness' (Metzinger, 1995). *Transparency* means that the
brain constructs our reality, but the mechanism of this construction is not represented in it. The representational character of phenomenal consciousness is not
accessible to consciousness. We cannot be aware of how our brain constructs qualia
in terms of its neurocomputational mechanisms. If we did, neuroscience would

be trivial or may not even exist at all. Transparency leads to a 'naive realism', the tacit assumption that the content of phenomenal consciousness has a direct contact to the environment, and is not a mere construct whose effects may have stronger implications for the behaviour than the 'true' content. If parts of the representational system, e.g. the right parietal lobe or Wernicke's area (left superior temporal lobe), are lesioned, the patient may be unaware of the resulting deficit (hemineglect, aphasia), which leads to a lack of insight into the illness (see below). Transparency is also a prerequisite for the development of hallucinations.

Conscious states are further characterized by their *presence*, i.e. they are in the focus of our attention. Once we accept that phenomenological states are present, it follows logically that there are others that are not present at the moment. There are preconscious experiences which can enter phenomenological consciousness once we direct our attention to them. When I focus on the blueness of the sky (quale A), I am usually not aware of the ground pressing against my feet (quale B). We would argue that there are mental phenomena that may never enter phenomenal consciousness, but still may influence our behaviour. For example, there is now evidence from functional brain-imaging studies for the unconscious processing of sensory stimuli in healthy subjects (Srinivasan et al., 1999; Dehaene & Naccache, 2001; Rees, 2001). These results show that stimuli are processed in specific brain areas but do not enter phenomenal consciousness. Unconscious states encompass all mental activity that is not accessible to consciousness (e.g. sensorimotor self-monitoring; see chapters 18 and 19).

A third factor is important, if we wish to understand what phenomenal consciousness is. This is the fact that experiences are always and only experiences of an 'I'. It is me who realizes the blueness of the sky, the smell of perfume, the taste of wine. This notion is called the *perspectiveness* of phenomenal consciousness. Further, we suggest that we have to distinguish two types of perspectiveness: *ipseity* and *self-qualia*. Let us first consider what philosophers mean by ipseity. The *I* in every experience (qualia, raw feelings) is implicitly and prereflectively present in the field of awareness and is crucial to the whole structure. The *I* is not yet a 'pole' but more a field, through which all experiences pass. This basic self does not arise from any inferential reflection or introspection, because it is not a relation, but an intrinsic property of qualia. When I have a perception of pain, this perception is simultaneously a tacit self-awareness, because my act of perception is given to me in the first-person perspective, from my point of view and only in my field of awareness. This basic dimension of subjecthood, ipseity, is a medium in which all experience, including more explicit and thematic reflection, is rendered possible and takes place (see chapters 3, 11 and 12; also Henry, 1963, 1965; Parnas, 2000). What is this particular functional property of ipseity that makes it the centre of phenomenal consciousness? Ipseity might be granted in the brain by a continuous source of internally generated input. Each and every time when there is conscious experience (i.e. when we are awake), there is the tacit existence of internal proprioceptive input. The perpetual flow of background cerebral activity is the centre of phenomenal consciousness. The content of this background activity is the continuous flow of unconscious 'thoughts' (Dennett, 1991) and maybe even more so, a representation of a (spatial) model of our body independently of somatosensory input, the 'background buzz of somatosensory input' (Kinsbourne, 1995). It is this feeling of ipseity that makes our experiences feel a united, single being (see chapter 5).

Besides this tacit ipseity, there are also very particular types of qualia that might be called 'self-qualia' or '(phenomenal) self-consciousness'. Their content is the pervasive feeling of *self* and its different aspects. Depending on the author, the content of phenomenal self-consciousness may differ somewhat, but basically it is: (1) self-agency, the sense of the authorship of one's actions; (2) self-coherence, the sense of being a physical whole with boundaries; (3) self-affectivity, experiencing affect correlated with other experiences of self; and (4) self-history (autobiographical memory), a sense of enduring over time. Self-qualia are not different from any other type of qualia in the way they are transparent, present and perspective. Usually their content is preconscious and also encompasses unconscious activity (e.g. auditory or sensorimotor self-monitoring; see chapters 6, 18 and 19). How does the pervasive feeling of selfhood (see chapter 10 for the role of emotion), the sum of the experience of all self-qualia (the self-construct) arise? Because self-qualia, like other qualia, are transparent. The representational structure is not represented in the generation of these self-experiences. In the same way that we think we are in direct contact with the world, although it is a mere construct in our brain, we feel in direct contact with ourselves. We do not at all realize that it is just a construct that can be overthrown, for example in depersonalization or delusions of alien control.

So far we have described the first level of consciousness, i.e. phenomenal self-consciousness. At a second level, we can reflect about the content of phenomenal consciousness: it is a reflective awareness of qualia. Versions of this 'introspective consciousness' can be found in the works of John Locke (1959), William James (1950), David Armstrong (1980), Paul Churchland (1995), William Lycan (1997) and others. It is also called 'higher-order thought', 'perception of the mental', 'second-person perspective' (see chapter 2), 'second-order thoughts' and may be conceptualized as a perception-like, higher-order representation of our own mental states. For example, I can reflect about the pain of a pinprick, or the blueness of the sky. It may still be a preverbal thought; once I verbalize the reflected content (Kircher et al., 2000), I can communicate it to somebody else (see chapter 4 for linguistic implications).

For a coherent self-structure across time, an unimpaired memory system is necessary (see chapter 9). We would claim that all phenomenal experiences, be they memories, feelings or sensory perceptions, can be processed on a self versus nonself continuum, depending on the self-valence of its content. For example, the autobiographical content of being in love has a high self-valence, whereas the insignificant event of a bee landing on a flower (observed by you) has a low self-valence. This means that the content of phenomenal consciousness and introspective consciousness is processed on a self versus nonself dimension. We will later report some experiments investigating this point.

Data from neuroscience

Once we have accepted that there are experiences of selfhood (phenomenal self-consciousness), we can start to look at their neural correlates. What has been done in neuroscience thus far is mostly investigating the cognitive and neural structures of phenomenal consciousness, triggered by external sensory stimuli with little or no self-valence (vision, hearing, memory, attention). More recently, not commonly shared subjective experiences such as emotion processing have drawn attention. There is reason to believe that the most subjective experiences, *self-qualia*, are also amenable to scientific research. Having introduced a model of consciousness, we can frame experimental results and concepts from neuroscience within it. We will focus on phenomenal self-consciousness, introspective self-consciousness and the question of self-valence. Most studies in this context have entailed processing of stimuli with high versus low self-valence, including autobiographical memory, as well as sensorimotor and auditory self-monitoring, theory of mind and perspective taking (ego- and allocentric space processing).

In our model we have proposed that all information can be processed on a self versus nonself continuum (self-valence). We propose that self processing is domain-specific, i.e. a deficit in a particular function does not imply a deficit in another function (McGlynn & Schacter, 1989). In terms of our model, for example, a loss of autobiographical memory does not change somatosensory or verbal self-monitoring. What brain areas might correspond to particular functions of our model? Regarding neurological instantiation, it is known that lesions in the posterior parietal and prefrontal regions produce a lack of awareness of deficits (Keefe, 1998), that is, the ability to reflect upon one's own abilities is impaired. We therefore suggest that these areas constitute an important part of a network subserving self-processing. The basic level of self-processing (pre- or unconscious self-qualia) involves sensory integrative functions of the sort carried out by the parietal lobes. Lesions in these areas lead to neglect phenomena. Visuospatial neglect is associated with right, language-related neglect with left temporoparietal lesions

(Leicester et al., 1969). Also at this level is 'internal information', such as mental images or inner speech, recognized as self-produced via efference-copy mechanisms (see chapters 18 and 19; Sperry, 1950; von Holst & Mittelstaedt, 1950). Operations on this level are highly overlearned and not necessarily conscious. A second level of self-processing (introspective self-consciousness) is associated with the executive control functions of the lateral prefrontal cortex. Here, complex behaviour is governed and this requires active decisions and involves conscious processes. The two primary symptoms in almost every patient with a lesion in the prefrontal regions (Luria, 1969), including leucotomy (Walsh & Darby, 1999), are: (1) a disturbed critical attitude toward and inadequate evaluation of one's own state or deficits and (2) a loss of spontaneity. We therefore suggest that it is a crucial region in introspective self-consciousness.

Facial self-recognition

The face is our most distinct external feature. The ability to recognize oneself in the mirror is regarded as a test for 'self-awareness' in animals (see chapter 7). Mirror self-recognition does not occur in humans before 18 months or in other primates, except adult great apes (Gallup, 1970; Parker et al., 1994). In order to recognize oneself in the mirror, a concept of the *self* is necessary. The existence of 'phenomenal self-consciousness' (conscious self-qualia) is a prerequisite for self-recognition, giving rise to the pervasive feeling of *self*. Whether introspective self-consciousness is necessary is still a matter of debate. The ability to solve theory of mind tasks is also dependent on functioning phenomenal self-consciousness, because only when a being has a stable self-concept, can s/he infer mental states of others. Theory of mind refers to the ability to infer mental states of other persons (see e.g. Hong et al., 1995; Povinelli & Preuss, 1995). This faculty is impaired in schizophrenia (Sarfati & Hardy Bayle, 1999) and autism (Pilowsky et al., 2000).

In a series of experiments, we tested whether one's own face is processed differently from other faces (see chapter 8). One major problem when studying self-face processing is to control for emotional salience and overlearnedness, since both are known to influence processing (Klatzky & Forrest, 1984; Young et al., 1985; Valentine & Bruce, 1986). We tried to overcome this by using the face of each subject's partner for comparison. The idea behind these experiments was to investigate cognitive processes involved in qualia experiences with very high self-valence that would trigger phenomenal and introspective self-consciousness. The other idea was that qualia with high self-valence (own face) is processed differently from qualia with lower self-reference (partner's face). We presented adult, healthy subjects with either their own face, their partner's face or an unknown face, one at a time, on a computer screen and measured reaction time and accuracy of recognition by button press. In different experiments, with different groups of subjects, we presented the faces: (1) centrally on a screen; (2) to one or other hemifield; (3) subliminally (for an average of 32 ms using backward masking); and (4) morphed with another identity (Kircher et al., 2001b; Yoon 2001). As expected, we found faster reaction times for the recognition of familiar (self and partner) versus unfamiliar faces. There was however no robust difference in response time or error rate between the 'self' and 'partner' conditions.

To explore the neural correlates of phenomenal and introspective self-consciousness, we used functional magnetic resonance imaging (fMRI) to measure brain activation while subjects viewed morphed versions of either their own or their partner's face, alternating in blocks with presentation of an unknown face. When subjects viewed themselves (minus activation for viewing an unknown face), activation was detected in right limbic (hippocampal formation, insula, anterior cingulate), left prefrontal and superior temporal cortex. In the partner (versus unknown) experiment, only the right insula was activated (Kircher et al., 2001b). The activation consequent upon recognizing one's own face was more extensive and the pattern striking. The right limbic regions, which were extensively activated when self was contrasted with novel, are known to be engaged in pleasant and unpleasant emotional responses (Lane et al., 1997; Phillips et al., 1997). We interpret the activation of the right limbic system in our study as a unique, strong emotional response to seeing our own face. The left prefrontal cortex, which was only activated by self-faces, is thought to have an important role in executive processes such as the conscious integration of information to form a coherent 'whole' from multimodal inputs (Miller, 1992; Vandenberghe et al., 1996). The combination of right limbic and left cortical activation could underlie human self-recognition. Experiments with split-brain patients (Preilowski, 1979; Sperry et al., 1979; Gallois et al., 1988) have shown that, although rudimentary self-recognition occurs in the disconnected right hemisphere, only transcallosal transfer of information enables the sensory experience to reach awareness.

The onset of self-recognition in human infancy correlates with the myelination of fibres in the frontal lobe (Kinney et al., 1988). Isolated failures of self-recognition have yet to emerge in the neurological/psychiatric literature. Such failure does not seem to occur following isolated frontal lesions or in cases of amnesia with profound loss of autobiographical memory (Tulving, 1993b) where there is a preservation in phenomenal self-consciousness. The relatively widespread and bilateral activation we have demonstrated in response to self-stimuli suggests that many processes contribute to self-perception with some built-in redundancy, hence the resistance to disruption by common neurological lesions. We suggest that a neural network involving the right limbic system in conjunction with left-sided associative and executive regions enables the integration of self-valent affect and cognition to produce the unique experience of phenomenal and introspective self-consciousness.

Autobiographical semantic memory

The facts about oneself, William James' 'me', must be stored in the memory system and can be reflected upon in introspective consciousness (see chapter 9). The memory system components of relevance here are episodic and semantic memory (Tulving, 1991). Semantic memory is concerned with acquisition, retention and use of organized information in the broadest sense; its principal function is cognitive modelling of the world. For example, our knowledge that Rome is the capital of Italy is processed via semantic memory. Episodic memory depends on semantic memory for many of its operations; its purpose is to retain the memory for events (e.g. facts about my recent holiday in Italy).

Evidence suggests that memories about ourselves are stored and divided according to these categories. Episodic or autobiographical memory enables the individual to remember personally experienced events in subjective time as embedded in a matrix of other personal happenings, for example the circumstances of our last holiday, yesterday's departmental meeting and today's lunch. An aspect of semantic memory is personal semantic memory: this comprises information about ourselves, our personality and who we are. The validity of this distinction between episodic and semantic self-knowledge stems from behavioural, brain lesion and functional imaging studies. In an experiment by Klein & Loftus (1993), subjects were presented with a personality trait word and asked to perform one of three tasks: to indicate whether the word is self-descriptive (describe), to retrieve an autobiographical memory related to the word (remember) or to define the semantic meaning of the word (define). In a second step, they were asked to perform either the same or different task from the first one. The paradigm is based on the following premise: if, in the process of performing the first task, information relevant to performing the second task is made available, then the time required to perform the second task should be less than if that information were not available. The authors found that the autobiographical memory task did not influence performance (response time) on the self-descriptive task, nor did the self-descriptive task influence performance on the autobiographical memory task. These results indicate that subjects do not search autobiographical episodic memory to come up with a judgement about themselves, nor do they access abstract (semantic) self-knowledge whilst retrieving autobiographical memories.

These experiments can be questioned on the grounds that these memory systems may interact with each other to perform the task and it is therefore difficult to demonstrate compellingly that the two systems are independent. However, there are amnesic patients with intact semantic but impaired access to episodic memory. Of interest is the case described by Hodges & McCarthy (1993) of a then 67-year-old male garage owner who sustained bilateral paramedian thalamic infarctions. General intellectual functioning, language and immediate memory were relatively normal. However, he had a profound deficit in autobiographical memory, believing himself to be currently serving in the Navy – in fact he served from 1941 to 1946. He could recall virtually no events, personal or public, after 1945; he confused his grown-up children and could not say which were married, had children and so on. On the other hand, he was able to provide answers rich in detail to questions about famous people from all eras but not equally famous events. How can this pattern be explained? The authors argue that a simple account in terms of loss of stored information is not adequate but instead suggest that retrieving information organized by personal themes (high self-valence) may be specifically disrupted by thalamic lesions.

There are case studies which are illuminating in regard to the distinction between semantic and episodic self-knowledge (Kapur et al. 1995). One patient, KC, was involved in a motorcycle accident at the age of 30 (Tulving, 1993a). As a result, he suffered from anterograde and retrograde amnesia. Besides the amnesia, the brain damage produced a profound change in his personality from outgoing, adventurous and gregarious to a now passive, cautious and reticent man. He does not remember a single event or happening from his life and does not know how he behaved in any particular instance. Does this patient know what kind of person he is? To test this, he and his mother were given the same list of trait adjectives and both were asked to rate their own and the other's personality (after the accident). The mother's ratings of the patient's personality were consistent with his own and vice versa. Since the accident that caused profound amnesia and a change in personality, KC has relearned his personality traits despite the fact that he cannot access any recollection of his own behaviour and so is unable to infer traits from behaviour.

Another case is WJ, an 18-year-old female college student who suffered temporary loss of episodic memory following a head injury – a dense retrograde amnesia of 6–7 months (Kapur et al., 1995). During this time and despite being unable to remember anything about college or anything else happening at around that time, she was able to describe herself accurately, according to friends' ratings and her own rating on recovery when her memory returned to the preinjury level. Despite all the limitations of single case approaches, it is shown here that semantic self-knowledge is represented in a memory system other than episodic memory.

The question remains whether semantic self-knowledge is different from semantic knowledge about other persons. In a typical experiment designed to answer this question, participants are given lists of personality trait words which they have to judge for self or other descriptiveness. When recall is tested subsequently (usually 0–10 min after encoding), self-descriptive traits are better remembered (for review, see Symons & Johnson, 1997). Thus, a person remembers the word 'friendly' better after answering the question 'Does the word "friendly" describe you?' than after answering the question 'Does the word "friendly" describe your father?' (Lord, 1980; Ferguson et al., 1983; Keenan & Baillet, 1983). This has been termed the self-reference effect (Rogers et al., 1977). Related work has shown a reaction time advantage in decision tasks for self-descriptive versus nonself-descriptive personality traits (Markus, 1977). The most commonly given explanation for the self-descriptive effect is that it promotes *elaborative* processing (Rogers et al., 1977; Keenan, 1993). Elaboration is the 'breadth, extensiveness and amount of processing that occurs at any particular level of depth of analysis' (Eysenck & Eysenck, 1979). During elaborative processing, multiple associations between the stimulus word and other material are evoked (Anderson & Reder, 1979; Klein & Loftus, 1988). Furthermore, it has been argued that this elaboration occurs incidentally, i.e. without the wilful act of self-reference processing (Markus, 1977; Symons & Johnson, 1997). From this research it has been concluded that semantic self-structure in memory is highly elaborated and organized, invokes multiple associations and is continually and incidentally updated, well learned and often used (Kihlstrom, 1993; Maki & Carlson, 1993; Symons & Johnson, 1997).

Surprisingly, very little is known about the cerebral structures involved in semantic autobiographical processing. In our own study, we used fMRI to delineate significant changes in blood oxygenation level-dependent contrast as an index of changes in local neuronal activity in human volunteers (Kircher et al., 2002). Our aim was to probe the model described above and test whether there was differential cerebral activation for incidental (preconscious) and intentional (introspective) semantic self-processing. In two individually tailored experiments, we measured localized MRI signal changes while subjects judged personality and physical trait words, differing in the amount of self-valence.

In the first experiment (intentional semantic self-processing), subjects were presented with personality trait adjectives and made judgements as to their self-descriptiveness (versus nonself-descriptiveness). In the second experiment (incidental semantic self-processing), subjects categorized words according to whether they described physical versus psychological attributes, while unaware that the words had been arranged in blocks according to self-descriptiveness. Regarding our consciousness model (Figure 22.1), we probed the neural correlates of preconscious qualia with high versus low self-valence retrieved from semantic autonoetic memory. In both the intentional and incidental experiment, preconscious self-qualia are evoked automatically. The subjects had previously rated the words for self-descriptiveness 6 weeks prior to the scanning session. A reaction time advantage was present in both experiments for self-descriptive trait words, suggesting a facilitation effect (Markus, 1977). Common areas of activation for the two experiments included the left superior parietal lobe, with adjacent regions of the lateral prefrontal cortex also active in both experiments. Differential signal changes were present in the left precuneus for the intentional and the right middle temporal gyrus for the incidental experiment. The results suggest that self-processing involves distinct processes and can occur on more than one cognitive level with corresponding functional neuroanatomic correlates in areas previously implicated in awareness of one's own state.

Overall, the results of both our experiments show that self-descriptive compared to nonself-descriptive traits evoke a unique pattern of neural activation. When subjects process self-descriptive words (versus nonself-descriptive words), whether intentional or incidental, they activate the superior parietal cortex and left inferior frontal gyrus. This result confirms our predictions based on the model presented. We suggest that information is processed on a self versus nonself dimension in multimodal integration areas (superior parietal and inferior frontal gyri). We speculate that the rich associations evoked by self-relevant processing are integrated in the inferior frontal and superior parietal lobe (Markus, 1977). The reason that such a specific self-activation network might have developed is perhaps the biological need to distinguish between self and other or the outstanding subjective importance of the self.

The area solely activated in our intentional self (minus nonself) condition included the precuneus. This structure has previously been identified in memory encoding and retrieval paradigms in functional imaging studies (Shallice et al., 1994; Fletcher et al., 1995; Krause et al., 1999; Wiggs et al., 1999). The paradigm employed in the incidental experiment was essentially a semantic categorization task, yet we argue that self-relevant words evoke memories automatically, hence the overlap with content-neutral studies of memory retrieval. We suggest that the precuneus plays a crucial role in memory processes that involve processing with high self-valence, as in episodic memory, and that the self component is an important factor in its involvement.

In a related positron emission tomography (PET) study by Craik et al. (1999), trait adjectives were presented in different sets of scans and participants had to judge on a four-point scale whether the adjective described themselves, Brian Mulroney (former Canadian prime minister), the general social desirability of the trait or instead they were requested to indicate the number of syllables in the word. They found a small increase in activation only in the self versus general conditions, but not in any of the other direct comparisons in the right anterior cingulate. Comparing self versus syllable, the left inferior frontal gyrus was activated, similar to our signal changes in the intentional experiment. However, they did not tailor their stimuli to the individual participants, which could explain the lack of differential activation. Computations for high and low self-valence would both be present in their self-condition, thus diluting the effect.

Social self

Using introspective consciousness, we can reflect on our own mental states. We can retrieve memory traces from our memory stores about past events, other people and ourselves, and think about them. We have a stable mental representation of a particular person – ourselves – and as such this is part of the individual's wider knowledge concerning objects and events in his or her world. The knowledge of ourselves and its organization is usually called *self-concept* in social science and personality psychology. An early debate revolved around the question of whether the self-concept is unitary (Snygg & Combs, 1949; Allport, 1955) or multidimensional (for review see Kihlstrom & Cantor, 1984; Marsh & Hattie, 1996). Early multidimensional models were proposed by social psychologists Cooley (1902) and Mead (1934), who suggested that the individual perceives him- or herself largely through the reaction of others. Each person possesses as many selves as there are significant other persons in the environment. Nowadays, multidimensional models in various forms are favoured (Neisser, 1988). Here, different aspects of the self-concept, like physical, academic, social, family and emotional self-concept, are grouped as hierarchical, correlated or independent factors. Just as the theories and definitions of self-concept have varied widely across times and researchers, so has the assessment methodology taken many forms. For example, semantic differentials, adjective checklists, drawing tasks, projective tests, actual–ideal measures and third-party reports have been used (for review, see Keith & Bracken, 1996). Several validated self-report questionnaires, usually based on one of the multidimensional models, have been developed (for review, see Wylie, 1989; Hattie, 1992).

Recent work in the field of social cognition and abnormal psychology has thrown up at least two relevant and heuristic constructs: self-complexity (Linville, 1987) and self-discrepancy (Higgins, 1987). Self-complexity could be regarded as the number of (integrated) selves one defines oneself by or at least the number of social roles one has. High self-complexity seems to protect the individual against stress. Crudely, if a person defines herself as doctor, mother, wife, singer, runner, cook, councillor, etc., then a disruption or loss of one of these roles will be buffered by the presence of those remaining. Someone with low self-complexity would be more vulnerable.

The self-discrepancy model (Higgins, 1987) has been taken up by Bentall and colleagues (Bentall et al., 1994) as a basis for persecutory delusions (see chapter 14). Higgins subdivides the self-concept into different domains: (1) the actual self, which is my representation of attributes I believe I possess; (2) the ideal self, which is my representation of the attributes that I would like to possess; and (3) the ought self, which is my representation of the attributes that I believe I should or ought to possess. Bentall et al. (1994) explain persecutory delusions through a discrepancy between the content of these domains. If there is a mismatch between the actual self and the ideal self, triggered by an external event, (deluded) patients try (unconsciously) to diminish this painful discrepancy at the expense of perceiving others as having a negative view of themselves (Kinderman & Bentall, 1996). They do not see themselves in an unfavourable light, but externalize this feeling on to others.

Schizophrenia

Generally, neuroscientific investigations have so far mostly dealt with the processing of sensory stimuli. They can be well controlled and the experiences are commonly shared by healthy subjects (blue is usually blue for you and me). The investigations become more difficult with higher-order, intrinsically generated phenomena. Even more difficult is the investigation of genuinely subjective experiences, such as emotions, self-valence or the feeling of selfhood. An intrinsic problem of phenomenal self-consciousness in general is that it can only be mediated through introspective consciousness, which requires a great amount of reflectivity and verbal–intellectual capacity. Thorough, easy-to-understand descriptions of the feeling of self or self-qualia in particular are further hampered by its 'immediate givenness, wholeness and embodiment'. This means it is a fundamental, affective tone of mental, emotional and bodily unity which is so basic to our experience that it is very difficult to grasp. Descriptions of phenomenal self-consciousness are the realm of phenomenology. Edmund Husserl (1922) and Maurice Merleau-Ponty (1965), in particular, have described subtle intrapsychic phenomena on the basis of a 'pure I', where through self-consciousness the connection of experiences is given. The problem with their descriptions is that they are not intuitively understandable but require some effort from the reader. This, their subjective givenness and the complexity of the phenomena are the reason why they have not been the focus of much scientific research.

Consciousness and self-consciousness are probably the most complex phenomena we know of. An intrinsic problem in the investigation of phenomenal consciousness is its transparency, i.e. the structure of its representation is not represented (see above). That means, if we want to know something about the cognitive structure and brain states correlated with the perceptual experience of 'greenness' it does not help to reflect on 'greenness' via introspective consciousness, but only to do neuroscientific experiments (e.g. on the visual cortex). Another possibility is to interview and test patients with impairments in the experience in question. We can then compare their experiences and test results with those of healthy controls and thus generate tentative models of the underlying neurocognitive structure, correlating with the experience.

Phenomenology of ego-disorders in psychosis

One way of understanding self-qualia is to look at pathological states of phenomenal self-consciousness and to develop systematic descriptions and models. Here we want to focus especially on schizophrenia, arguably the best-known, most prevalent and most severe disorder of the self. Schizophrenic disorders were described at the turn of the twentieth century (see chapter 1). Eugen Bleuler (Bleuler, 1916, p. 434) considered in schizophrenia 'the whole personality loosened, split and forfeit its natural harmony'. All the other basic and accessory symptoms would be a result of this core pathology. Kraepelin (1913) claimed that a disunity of consciousness ('orchestra without a conductor') was the core feature of the illness. The disunity was closely linked to 'a peculiar destruction of the psychic personality's inner integrity, whereby emotion and volition in particular are impaired' (1913, p. 668, my translation). A contemporary of Bleuler and Kraepelin, Joseph Berze (1914) was the first to propose explicitly that *a basic alteration of self-consciousness*, a peculiar change, a diminished luminosity and 'affectability' of self-awareness, was a primary disorder of schizophrenia. He presented a number of case histories with patients complaining: 'I have no self-consciousness', 'I think I have a diminished, unclear I-feeling', '...a diminishing of the feeling of being a centre of connection of a present organisation...' (p. 62).

The most influential classification of self-disturbance (*Ichstörung*) was proposed by Jaspers (1913, 1963), which was further elaborated by Scharfetter (see chapter 13; Scharfetter, 1980, 1981). These classifications are primarily based on examining the various self-disturbances in schizophrenic patients, drawing inferences from these observations onto the 'normal' self-experience. This seems reasonable, since unimpaired people are inclined to take the basic dimensions for granted and entertain no doubts about them. Among different translators, the original German '*Ich*' ('I') was variably translated as 'self' or 'ego': these terms are therefore here used synonymously. The German '*Ich*' ('I') has a more philosophical connotation than in English when it is used as a noun ('*das Ich*'; 'the I'), therefore '*Ich-Störungen*' ('ego-disturbances', which in English is more connected to the psychoanalytical tradition, in contrast to German.) The 'I' 'refers to the certainty of experience. It is I myself: living, functioning on my own, unified and coherent, delineated by a boundary open for communication in an afferent direction, self-identical through the course of life and in various situations' (Scharfetter, 1980).

There are five basic unimpaired dimensions of ego-consciousness: these would be the different self-qualia in our model presented above. The pathology of *ego-vitality* (Jaspers' *Daseinsbewußtsein*: awareness of existence) can result in the patients' experience (or fear) of their own death, the ruin of the world, humanity, the universe. Being in this state, 'the individual, although existing, cannot feel his/her existence any more. Descartes' "cogito ergo sum" can only be superficially thought, but it is no longer a factual experience' (Jaspers, 1963). Ego-vitality is heightened in mania. The concept of *ego-activity* is probably best known and had its forerunners (besides Jasper's *Vollzugsbewuβtsein*: awareness of one's own performance) in Kronfeld (1922), Gruhle (1932) and Schneider (1967). Its disturbance results in a lack of one's own ability for self-determined acting, thinking, feeling and perceiving. Secondary to this, delusions are formed of alien control, made or stopped feelings, thoughts, perceptions. Clinically, psychomotor slowing to the point of stupor might occur. The disturbance of *ego-consistency* (Jasper's *Einheit des Ich*: unity of the self) resulted in the invention of the term schizophrenia by Bleuler. It is conceptualized as the destruction of the coherence of one's self, the body and soul, as a unitary being; the connection of thinking and feeling is disrupted. Diverging and ununifiable feelings and thoughts are experienced simultaneously. Multiple personality or heautoscopy is sometimes given as an example of this disturbance (Sims, 1988). But disturbance of ego-consistency is not 'to be confused with the so called "double personality", which appears objectively in alternating states of consciousness' (Jaspers, 1963, p. 125). In cases of 'double personalities or alternating consciousness [the] dissociated psychic life appears so richly developed that it feels as if one is dealing with another personality' (ibid., p. 404). In the condition of multiple personality, each of the distinct personalities has a feeling of a cohesive whole (David et al., 1996). Heautoscopy is an optical phenomenon of seeing oneself outside oneself, yet at the same time retaining one's ego-experience intact. If *ego-demarcation* (Jaspers' *Ichbewuβtsein im Gegensatz zum Auβen*: self distinct from the outside world) is impaired, the patient can no longer distinguish between inner and outer; he/she feels defencelessly abandoned to all manner of external influences. Patients may believe that they themselves experience what they see or hear from others, e.g. 'I have to suffer everything that other patients on this ward have to undergo'. Disturbed *ego-identity* (Jaspers' *Identität des Ich*: identity of the self) manifests itself in a loss or change concerning the own identity in respect of gestalt, physiognomy, gender, genealogical origin and biography. This is often accompanied by disturbances of bodily experience, of ego-consistency and ego-vitality. As a secondary formation of delusions, a new identity, often of higher status, can take over the patient's lost one.

Kurt Schneider (1967) addressed self-disorders in his description of passivity phenomena, allegedly reflective of a loss of 'ego-boundaries'. Detailed descriptions of self-disturbances, usually associated with the explorations of the sense and the nature of self, are to be found in phenomenologically oriented work (see chapters 11 and 12). The main implication is that self-disorders represent the *core feature* of schizophrenia, conferring on it a unique gestalt and reflecting its pathogenic nucleus. Because these psychopathological phenomena are difficult to grasp in clinical work, there has been little empirical research done on them so far.

When patients experience profound alterations of themselves and their environment, coupled with strong affects, it is only natural that their self-construct (in the terminology of social psychology) changes. Due to hospitalization, symptoms and changes in personality due to the disease process, their course of life and their self-narrative can be strongly affected (see chapters 15 and 16).

Self-recognition in schizophrenia

From phenomenological observation we have learnt that at least some patients with schizophrenia have a profound alteration of phenomenal and introspective self-consciousness. Earlier in this chapter we showed that an intact phenomenal self-consciousness is related to the ability to recognize oneself in the mirror and that facial self-recognition results in a unique pattern of cerebral activation. In another study we wanted to test whether there is an impairment in facial self-recognition in patients with schizophrenia as a result of disturbed self-functions.

Twenty right-handed patients with schizophrenia and 20 matched healthy controls were required to indicate by button press whether a face presented on a computer screen depicted themselves, their same-sex first-degree relative (as a control face for familiarity and emotional salience) or a stranger's face (Kircher et al., 2002). The faces were presented individually for 100 ms to one hemifield, so that only one cerebral hemisphere would process the stimulus initially. Hemifield presentation was introduced, because, as discussed earlier, we have suggested that an interplay between the two hemispheres is crucial in facial self-processing (Kircher et al., 2001b). Reaction times did not differ within the two groups across the identities for lateralized presentation. Similarly, there was no difference in the error rate across the identities for left-hemispheric presentation within both groups. However, there was a significant interaction for group × hemifield ($P = 0.04$) and group × identity ($P = 0.02$) in the error rate. This was due largely to the patients showing an increase in error rate for the recognition of their own face presented to the right hemifield/left hemisphere compared to the other identities ($P = 0.004$). Recognition of their own face presented to the left hemisphere was selectively impaired in patients with schizophrenia. We interpret this finding as evidence for a disturbance in self-processing, resulting from an alteration of self-awareness (phenomenal self-consciousness and introspective self-consciousness).

Self-monitoring

One fundamental cognitive ability is to attribute events observed in the environment to one's own or somebody else's actions. Most results with regard to self-monitoring have been obtained in neuropsychological studies investigating patient groups that were suspected of having some deficits in self-monitoring. Frith (1982) and Feinberg (1978) proposed that certain symptoms of schizophrenia, such as delusions of control and hallucinations, are due to deficits in self-monitoring. Delusions of control refer to movements, thoughts or emotions being inserted or controlled from outside. In this theory such passivity phenomena (or ego-disorders, which are subsumed under 'bizarre delusions' in the Anglo-American literature) are explained by a failure in the anticipatory control of one's own movements. A problem with this theory is that movements are treated like thoughts. The core assumptions of the theory are similar to the ones made by the corollary discharge (Sperry, 1950) or efferent copy model (von Holst & Mittelstaedt, 1950). These models were devised to explain how the central nervous system compensates for eye movements in order to enable a stable perception of the visual world. They assume that an efference copy is derived from each motor command to be executed which predicts the sensory consequences of the command. In the case of eye movements this prediction can be used to keep the perceived visual world stable. It has been shown that predictions of sensory consequences are also derived from other motor systems (Wolpert et al., 1995). Comparisons of the predictions with changes in the sensory input allow the self-monitoring system to determine which of these changes are due to one's own actions. Several studies have been conducted to provide evidence for this assumption (Frith & Done, 1989; Daprati et al., 1997; Franck et al., 2001). Failures in the prediction itself or the comparison of the prediction with the sensory input can lead to some of the symptoms of schizophrenia, like delusions of control, because they lead to incorrect attributions to self or other (see chapters 18 and 19).

There are at least two further patient groups that seem to have problems with monitoring the relation between their own movements and their perceived consequences. A study with the alien-hand task showed that apraxic patients with lesions in the left parietal cortex more often confuse the experimenter's hand with their own hand than healthy controls (Sirigu et al., 1999). Sirigu and coworkers interpret this result as evidence that apraxic patients have problems with generating and maintaining a kinaesthetic model of their movements.

Patients with lesions of the prefrontal cortex also have problems with self-monitoring. Slachevsky and coworkers (2001) compared this patient group with healthy subjects on their performance on a task originally devised by Fourneret & Jeannerod (1998). The task was to trace a straight line by moving a stylus on a writing pad. Their hand was hidden behind a mirror that reflected a computer monitor displaying the line to be traced and the line produced by the participants. In some trials, angular perturbations between the actual movement and the visual consequences observed on the screen were introduced. Frontal patients and healthy participants were able to compensate well for smaller perturbations. However, frontal patients had more problems compensating for larger perturbations. Slachevsky and her coworkers concluded from the first result that an automatic compensation mechanism is still intact in frontal patients. The second result was explained by the assumption that frontal patients remain unaware of larger perturbations that require the conscious monitoring system to become involved and therefore have more problems in compensating them.

In a series of experiments we have further explored self-monitoring in healthy participants – in particular, the sensitivity for detecting changes in mapping between their movement and their visual consequences (Knoblich & Kircher, 2002). There are essentially three possible mechanisms for monitoring the relationship between these two sources of information. The first and simplest assumption is that proprioceptive and visual information can be directly compared if the task at hand makes such a comparison necessary. As soon as these two information sources diverge to a certain extent, an external influence is inferred. A second possible assumption is that the execution of a motor command automatically leads to a prediction of the sensory consequences, including changes in the visual input. This prediction is compared to the sensory input. As soon as there is a certain amount of divergence between the predicted consequences and the actual input, an external influence is inferred (Blakemore et al., 1998a). The third possibility is that there are actually two separate processes (Jeannerod, 1999; Slachevsky et al., 2001). The first process operates on representations that are not cognitively penetrable and automatically uses deviations between a prediction of the sensory consequences of an action and the actual sensory input to adjust future motor commands (this process would be very similar to the one described in the second assumption above). The second process operates on representations that are cognitively penetrable, namely expected and actually observed events, and leads to explicit attribution of events to oneself within a certain range of deviation.

We investigated the sensitivity for mapping changes between movements and their consequences. In several experiments, participants drew circles on a writing pad and observed a moving dot on a computer screen that exactly reproduced their movements. At some point, the mapping between the movement and its visual consequences (the movement of the dot) was changed to different extents. Participants were instructed to lift the pen immediately when they detected a change. The main results were that the sensitivity was surprisingly low, even for large mapping changes, and that the participants compensated for these changes without noticing that they did so. This pattern was found under a number of different conditions, e.g. different drawing velocities. The results support the assumption that self-monitoring is based on a comparison between intended and observed events and not on a comparison between visual and proprioceptive information.

Regarding our model on self-consciousness presented above, self-monitoring is part of the unconscious self-states (Figure 22.1). It is likely that self-monitoring is domain-, i.e. modality-specific (sensory, motor, verbal, etc.), and that there is no single brain region responsible for self-monitoring in general. Functional brain-imaging studies in healthy people have shown the cerebellum to be involved in predicting the sensory consequences of movements (Blakemore et al., 1998b) and prefrontal, premotor, motor and parietal cortical regions to be responsible for the generation of self-paced movements (Spence et al., 1997). Together, these areas might be responsible for intact sensory motor self-monitoring. In patients with schizophrenia and passivity phenomena, cingulate and parietal regions were hyperactivated in the study by Spence et al. (1997), suggesting an anatomical substrate for the misattribution of internally generated acts to external sources. Verbal self-monitoring (Indefrey & Levelt, 2000), which is considered to be impaired in patients with schizophrenia suffering particularly from hallucinations and formal thought disorder, has been attributed to the superior temporal regions (Kircher et al., 2001a; McGuire et al., 1995).

Insight in psychopathology

General considerations

Insight in psychosis has been conceptualized as a multidimensional construct which encompasses at least three elements (David, 1990):
1. awareness that one is suffering from a mental illness;
2. the capacity to relabel psychotic experiences as such;
3. understanding the need for, and compliance with, treatment.

Many factors must contribute to the acquisition of insight, including the social milieu of the individual and his/her notions of illness and illness attribution – clearly a matter influenced by culture, education, factual knowledge, upbringing and wider social norms beside the individual's perspective (Amador & David, 1997). Nevertheless, at its heart lies the notion of self-awareness: the individual, ego (or part thereof) observing his or her own thoughts, perceptions and beliefs and coming to a view about them in a second-person perspective. To achieve this, that is, to 'expect a patient to arrive at a conclusion that his illness is nervous we are in many cases expecting a very remarkable exercise from him' (Lewis, 1934). Aubrey Lewis goes on:

The hysteric brings to bear on his symptoms . . . a hysterical mind, not a healthy mind with a limited separable disturbance . . . The obsessional brings his repetitive self-torturing mind to bear on his condition . . . The schizophrenic, the manic or the depressive patient . . . all contemplate their apprehensive change with that disturbed mind. His judgements and attitude can therefore never be the same as ours because his data are different, and his machine for judging is different in some respects.

Such a feat requires that certain psychological functions of judgement or appraisal or 'insight' must be separable, to an extent, or, to use modern terminology, 'modular'

(Fodor, 1983). The plausibility of such a state of affairs is given credence by the kind of dissociations between functions reported in the neuropsychological literature, including those relating to deficits in awareness (see below).

One might even ask, is insight possible for a person with schizophrenia? Jaspers did not think so. He believed that 'in psychosis there is no lasting or complete insight' (Jaspers, 1913). After all, how can one be deluded, that is, hold incorrigibly to a belief in the face of evidence to the contrary and yet also hold a belief that the other belief is false? Of course, not all deluded people do have insight, yet this paradoxical situation is seen in many patients with delusions when questioned at length. Garety & Hemsley (1987) have studied delusions along various dimensions and have shown that such variables as 'conviction' and 'plausibility' correlate weakly at best. Strauss (1969) not only interviewed deluded patients at length but, significantly, over time. He reported a state of 'double awareness', particularly during recovering from psychosis in which belief and nonbelief seemed to coincide (see also Stanton & David, 2000). It is perhaps easier to accept that a person may doubt his or her delusions and oscillate between total and partial conviction. If so, one only has to accept that such oscillations could be so frequent as to amount to dual awareness.

Such paradoxical situations are hard to grasp but we can begin to approach this from the point of view of a common experience such as being engrossed in a book or movie. Imagine watching a well-made film about aliens from outer space, such as 'ET: the extra-terrestrial'. The plight of ET as he is being chased or as he lies dying inside an oxygen tent is genuinely moving. This does not necessarily imply that we 'believe' in ET or confuse fantasy (or film) with reality. Further, our response to the story is both intellectual and emotional, not merely conditioned by the dramatic tension, music and images manipulated by a skilful director like Steven Spielberg – although that certainly helps. It appears as if we believe in the characters of the film, yet a moment's reflection would leave no doubt that we know that it is 'just a film'. Indeed, such an act of reflection would be provoked by the mere posing of the question: is this real? It appears, though, that in the absence of such an interruption, we are in a state of double awareness.

Is lack of insight a cognitive deficit?

If self-awareness is to some extent a natural cognitive function or skill, is lack of self-awareness, or specifically, lack of awareness of the self as mentally ill, a cognitive deficit? The pathophysiological basis of poor insight, or the analogy with anosognosia or 'frontal lobe deficits' of neurological patients has, as noted above, some attractions as a framework (David, 1990). The first formal test of this was by Young et al. (1993), who found a correlation between insight as assessed from a semistructured interview (Amador et al., 1993) and measures obtained from the

Wisconsin Card Sorting Test, a traditional executive or 'frontal lobe' test. However, several attempts to replicate this have been unsuccessful. In fact, the bulk of the results go against this idea (Cuesta & Peralta, 1994; Cuesta et al., 1995; David et al., 1995; Collins et al., 1997; Dickerson et al., 1997; but see Lysaker et al., 1998; Mohamed et al., 1999; Smith et al., 2000). Another way of showing that lack of insight cannot be equated with a global cognitive deficit or even a deficit in 'mental illness detection' is the work employing case vignettes. The procedure is to ask psychotic patients to read a description of a person with delusions or hallucinations and behavioural disorder and to ask whether they would regard such a person as suffering from a mental illness. Such responses can then be correlated with an insight score from some rating scale or, more specifically, the patient's own psychopathology can be rated in the same way. The aim of the task is to test the individual's awareness of the 'self as a mentally ill person'. This approach has shown that psychotic patients have a very similar model of mental illness (Chung et al., 1997), including the need for medical treatment, as do mental health professionals, but this is entirely separate from their own illness awareness (Swanson et al., 1995; Startup, 1997). The problem is that such patients (like the rest of us) tend to think that mental illness is something that happens to other people. That self-perception is protected from objective scrutiny – presumably in order to preserve self-esteem (see chapter 14). In other words: 'They are mad; he is mentally ill; I am under stress/misunderstood/a loveable eccentric'.

Conclusions

In this chapter we have introduced a new model of the self based on concepts of philosophy, the cognitive and neurosciences as well as the normal and the abnormal. The scientific study of this topic is just emerging, but we have tried to give an overview of the current positions. Sources of data and theory come from experimental studies of normal volunteers, functional neuroimaging and clinical studies of patients with focal brain damage and psychiatric disorders, particularly schizophrenia. Just as in any other young field of research, established definitions and concepts do not yet exist and an all-encompassing view must remain somewhat speculative. More data must be accumulated and, along this course, new and refined models will emerge. We believe self-consciousness, and, in particular, the 'feeling of selfhood' (self-qualia) is a valid construct and its neurocognitive–emotional basis will be understood in the near future.

Acknowledgements

The authors would like to thank Henner Giedke, Dirk Leube and Thomas Hünefeld for their helpful comments.

REFERENCES

Allport, G.W. (1955). *Becoming.* New Haven, CT: Yale University Press.

Amador, X.F. & David, A.S. (1997). *Insight and Psychosis.* New York: Oxford University Press.

Amador, X.F., Strauss, D.H., Yale, S.A. et al. (1993). Assessment of insight in psychosis. *American Journal of Psychiatry*, **150**, 873–9.

Anderson, J.R. & Reder, L.M. (1979). An elaborative processing explanation of depth of processing. In *Levels of Processing in Human Memory*, ed. L.S. Cermak & F.I.M. Craik, pp. 385–403. Hillsdale, NJ: Erlbaum.

Armstrong, D. (1980). *The Nature of Mind and Other Essays.* Ithaca, NY: Cornell University Press.

Bentall, R.P., Kinderman, P. & Kaney, S. (1994). The self, attributional processes and abnormal beliefs: towards a model of persecutory delusions. *Behavioral Research and Therapy*, **32**, 331–41.

Bermudez, J.L., Marcel, A. & Eilan, N. (1995). *The Body and the Self.* Cambridge, MA: MIT Press.

Berze, J. (1914). *Die primäre Insuffizienz der psychischen Aktivität.* Leipzig: Franz Deuticke.

Blakemore, S.J., Goodbody, S.J. & Wolpert, D.M. (1998a). Predicting the consequences of our own actions: the role of sensorimotor context estimation. *Journal of Neuroscience*, **18**, 7511–18.

Blakemore, S.J., Wolpert, D.M. & Frith, C.D. (1998b). Central cancellation of self-produced tickle sensation. *Nature and Neuroscience*, **1**, 635–40.

Bleuler, E. (1916). *Lehrbuch der Psychiatrie.* (Reprinted 1983.) Berlin: Springer.

Block, N., Flanagan, O. & Güzeldere, G. (1997). *The Nature of Consciousness.* Cambridge, MA: MIT Press.

Chung, K.F., Chen, E.Y.H., Lam, L.C.W., Chen, R.Y.L. & Chan, C.K.Y. (1997). How are psychotic symptoms perceived? A comparison between patients, relatives and the general public. *Australian and New Zealand Journal of Psychiatry*, **31**, 756–61.

Churchland, P. (1995). *The Engine of Reason, the Seat of the Soul: A Philosophical Journey into the Brain.* Cambridge, MA: MIT Press.

Collins, A.A., Remington, G.J., Coulter, K. & Birkett, K. (1997). Insight, neurocognitive function and symptom clusters in chronic schizophrenia. *Schizophrenia Research*, **27**, 37–44.

Cooley, C.H. (1902). *Human Nature and the Social Order.* New York: Scribner.

Craik, F.I.M., Moroz, T.M., Moscovitch, M. et al. (1999). In search of the self: a positron emission tomography study. *Psychological Science*, **10**, 26–34.

Cuesta, M.J. & Peralta, V. (1994). Lack of insight in schizophrenia. *Schizophrenia Bulletin*, **20**, 359–66.

Cuesta, M.J., Peralta, V., Caro, F. & De Leon, J. (1995). Is poor insight in psychotic disorders associated with poor performance on the Wisconsin Card Sorting Test? *American Journal of Psychiatry*, **152**, 1380–2.

Daprati, E., Franck, N., Georgieff, N. et al. (1997). Looking for the agent: an investigation into consciousness of action and self-consciousness in schizophrenic patients. *Cognition*, **65**, 71–86.

David, A.S. (1990). Insight and psychosis. *British Journal of Psychiatry*, **156**, 798–808.

David, A., van Os, J., Jones, P. et al. (1995). Insight and psychotic illness. Cross-sectional and longitudinal associations. *British Journal of Psychiatry*, **167**, 621–8.

David, A., Kemp, R., Smith, L. & Fahy, T. (1996). Multiple personality and schizophrenia. In *Methods in Madness: Case Studies in Cognitive Neuropsychiatry*, ed. P. Halligan & J. Marshall, pp. 123–46. East Sussex: Lawrence Erlbaum.

Dehaene, S. & Naccache, L. (2001). Towards a cognitive neuroscience of consciousness: basic evidence and a workspace framework. *Cognition*, **79**, 1–37.

Dennett, D. (1991). *Consciousness Explained*. Boston: Little, Brown.

Dickerson, F.B., Boronow, J.J., Ringel, N. & Parente, F. (1997). Lack of insight among outpatients with schizophrenia. *Psychiatric Services*, **48**, 195–9.

Eysenck, M.W. & Eysenck, M.C. (1979). Processing depth, elaboration of encoding, memory stores, and expended processing capacity. *Journal of Experimental Psychology: Human Learning and Memory*, **5**, 472–84.

Feinberg, I. (1978). Efference copy and corollary discharge: implications for thinking and its disorders. *Schizophrenia Bulletin*, **4**, 636–40.

Ferguson, T.J., Rule, G.R. & Carlson, D. (1983). Memory for personally relevant information. *Journal of Personal and Social Psychology*, **44**, 251–61.

Fletcher, P.C., Frith, C.D., Grasby, P.M. et al. (1995). Brain systems for encoding and retrieval of auditory-verbal memory. An in vivo study in humans. *Brain*, **118**, 401–16.

Fodor, J. (1983). *The Modularity of Mind*. Cambridge, MA: MIT Press Bradford Books.

Fourneret, P. & Jeannerod, M. (1998). Limited conscious monitoring of motor performance in normal subjects. *Neuropsychologia*, **36**, 1133–40.

Franck, N., Farrer, C., Georgieff, N. et al. (2001). Defective recognition of one's own actions in patients with schizophrenia. *American Journal of Psychiatry*, **158**, 454–9.

Frith, C.D. (1992). *The Cognitive Neuropsychology of Schizophrenia*. Hove, UK: Lawrence Erlbaum.

Frith, C.D. & Done, D.J. (1989). Experiences of alien control in schizophrenia reflect a disorder in the central monitoring of action. *Psychological Medicine*, **19**, 359–63.

Gallois, P., Ovelacq, E., Hautecoeur, P. & Dereux, J.F. (1988). Disconnexion et reconnaissance des visages. [Disconnection and recognition of faces. A case with lesions of the left visual cortex and the splenium.] *Revue Neurologique de Paris*, **144**, 113–19.

Gallup, G.G. (1970). Chimpanzees: self-recognition. *Science*, **167**, 86–7.

Garety, P.A. & Hemsley, D.R. (1987). Characteristics of delusional experience. *European Archives of Psychiatry and Neurological Science*, **236**, 294–8.

Gruhle, H.W. (1932). Die Schizophrenie: Allgemeine Symptomatologie. Die Psychopathologie. In: *Handbuch der Geisteskrankheiten*, ed. O. Bumke, pp. 135–210. Berlin: Springer Verlag.

Hattie, J. (1992). *Self-concept*. Hillsdale, NJ: Erlbaum.

Henry, M. (1963). *L'essence de la manifestation*. Paris: PUF.

Henry, M. (1965). *Philosophie et phénoménologie du corps*. Paris: PFU.

Higgins, E.T. (1987). Self-discrepancy: a theory relating self and affect. *Psychological Review*, **94**, 319–40.

Hodges, J.R. & McCarthy, R.A. (1993). Autobiographical amnesia resulting from bilateral paramedian thalamic infarction. A case study in cognitive neurobiology. *Brain*, **116**, 40.

Hong, C.C., Gillin, J.C., Dow, B.M., Wu, J. & Buchsbaum, M.S. (1995). Localized and lateralized cerebral glucose metabolism associated with eye movements during REM sleep and wakefulness: a positron emission tomography (PET) study. *Sleep*, **18**, 570–80.

Husserl, E. (1922). *Ideen zu einer reinen Phänomenologie. Augemeine Einführung in die reine Phänomenologie*, vol. 1, 2nd edn, p. x–323. Halle an der Saale: Max Niemeyer.

Indefrey, P. & Levelt, W.J.M. (2000). The neural correlates of language production. In *The New Cognitive Sciences*, ed. M.S. Gazzaniga, Boston, MA: pp. 845–64. MIT Press.

James, W. (1950). *Principles of Psychology*. New York: Dover Publications.

Jaspers, K. (1913). *Allgemeine Psychopathologie*. Berlin: Springer.

Jaspers, K. (1963). *General Psychopathology*. Manchester: Manchester University Press.

Jeannerod, M. (1999). The 25th Bartlett lecture: to act or not to act: perspectives on the representation of actions. *Quarterly Journal of Experimental Psychology*, **52**, A, 1–29.

Kapur, S., Craik, F.I., Jones, C. et al. (1995). Functional role of the prefrontal cortex in retrieval of memories: a PET study. *Neuroreport*, **6**, 1880–4.

Keefe, R.S.E. (1998). The neurobiology of disturbances of self. In *Insight and Psychosis*, ed. X.F. Amador & A.S. David, pp. 142–73. New York: Oxford University Press.

Keenan, J.M. (1993). An exemplar model can explain Klein and Loftus' results. In *Advances in Social Cognition*, ed. T.K. Srull & R.S. Wyer, pp. 69–78. New York: Erlbaum.

Keenan, J.M. & Baillet, S.D. (1983). Memory for personally and socially significant events. In *Attention and Performance*, ed. R.S. Nickerson, pp. 651–69. Hillsdale, NJ: Erlbaum.

Keith, L.K. & Bracken, B.A. (1996). Self-concept instrumentation: a historical and evaluative review. In *Handbook of Self-Concept*, ed. B.A. Bracken, pp. 91–171. New York: John Wiley.

Kihlstrom, J.F. (1993). What does the self look like? In *Advances in Social Cognition*, ed. T.K. Srull & R.S. Wyer, pp. 79–90. New York: Erlbaum.

Kihlstrom, J.F. & Cantor, N. (1984). Mental representations of the self. *Advances in Experimantal and Social Psychology*, **17**, 1–47.

Kinderman, P. & Bentall, R.P. (1996). Self-discrepancies and persecutory delusions: evidence for a model of paranoid ideation. *Journal of Abnormal Psychology*, **105**, 106–13.

Kinney, H.C., Brody, B.A., Kloman, A.S. & Gilles, F.H. (1988). Sequence of central nervous system myelination in human infancy. II. Patterns of myelination in autopsied infants. *Journal of Neuropathology and Experimental Neurology*, **47**, 217–34.

Kinsbourne, M. (1995). Awareness of one's own body: an attentional theory of its nature, development and brain basis. In *The Body and the Self*, ed. J.L. Bermudez, A. Marcel & N. Eilan, pp. 205–23. Cambridge, MA: MIT Press.

Kircher, T.T.J., Brammer, M.J., Simmons, A. & McGuire, P.K. (2000). Pausing for thought: Activation of left superior temporal sulcus when subjects pause during speech. submitted

Kircher, T.T.J., Liddle, P.F., Brammer, M.J. et al. (2001a). Neural correlates of formal thought disorder in schizophrenia. *Archives of General Psychiatry*, **58**, 769–74.

Kircher, T., Baar, S., Plewnia, C. & Bartels, M. (2002a). Impaiment of facial self recognition in schizophrenia. in preparation.

Kircher, T.T.J., Brammer, M.J., Bullmore, E. et al. (2002b). The neural correlates of intentional and incidental self processing. *Neuropsychologia*, **40**, 683–92.

Kircher, T.T.J., Senior, C., Phillips, M.L. et al. (2001b). Recognising one's own face. *Cognition*, **78**, B1–15.

Klatzky, R.L. & Forrest, F.H. (1984). Recognizing familiar and unfamiliar faces. *Memory and Cognition*, **12**, 60–70.

Klein, S.B. & Loftus, J. (1988). The nature of self-referent encoding: the contributions of elaborative and organizational processes. *Journal of Personal and Social Psychology*, **55**, 5–11.

Klein, S.B. & Loftus, J. (1993). The mental representation of trait and autobiographical knowledge about the self. In *The Mental Representation of Trait and Autobiographical Knowledge about the Self. Advances in Social Cognition*, ed, T.K. Srull & R.S. Wyer, pp. 1–49. Hillsdale, USA: Lawrence Erlbaum.

Knoblich, G. & Kircher, T. (2002). Deceiving oneself about control: sensitivity for mapping changes between movements and their consequences. submitted

Kraepelin, E. (1913). *Ein Lehrbuch für Studierende und Ärzte*. Leipzig: Barth.

Krause, B.J., Schmidt, D., Mottaghy, F.M. et al. (1999). Episodic retrieval activates the precuneus irrespective of the imagery content of word pair associates. A PET study. *Brain*, **122**, 255–63.

Kronfeld, A. (1922). Ueber schizophrene Veränderungen des Bewutseins der Aktivität. *Zeitschrift für die gesamte Neurologie und Psychiatrie*, **74**, 15–68.

Lane, R.D., Reiman, E.M., Bradley, M.M. et al. (1997). Neuroanatomical correlates of pleasant and unpleasant emotion. *Neuropsychologia*, **35**, 1437–44.

Leicester, J., Sidman, M., Stoddard, L.T. & Mohr, J.P. (1969). Some determinants of visual neglect. *Journal of Neurology, Neurosurgery and Psychiatry*, **32**, 580–7.

Lewis, A. (1934). The psychopathology of insight. *Br. J. Med. Psychol.*, **14**, 332–48.

Linville, P.W. (1987). Self-complexity as a cognitive buffer against stress-related illness and depression. *Journal of Personal and Social Psychology*, **52**, 663–76.

Locke, J. (1959). *An Essay Concerning Human Understanding*. New York: Dover Publications.

Lord, C.G. (1980). Schemas and images as memory aids: two models of processing social information. *Journal of Personal and Social Psychology*, **38**, 257–69.

Luria, A.R. (1969). Frontal lobe syndromes. In *Handbook of Clinical Neurology*, ed. P.J. Vinken & G.W. Bruyn, pp. 725–57. Amsterdam: North Holland.

Lycan, W.G. (1997). *Consciousness and Experience*. Cambridge, MA: MIT Press.

Lysaker, P.H., Bell, M.D., Bryson, G. & Kaplan, E. (1998). Neurocognitive function and insight in schizophrenia: support for an association with impairments in executive function but not with impairments in global function. *Acta Psychiatrica Scandinavica*, **97**, 297–301.

Maki, R.H. & Carlson, A.K. (1993). Knowledge of the self: is it special? In *Advances in Social Cognition*, ed. T.K. Srull & R.S. Wyer, pp. 101–110. New York: Erlbaum.

Markus, H. (1977). Self-schemata and processing information about the self. *Journal of Personal and Social Psychology*, **35**, 63–78.

Marsh, H.W. & Hattie, J. (1996). Theoretical perspectives on the structure of self-concept. In *Handbook of Self-Concept*, ed. B.A. Bracken. New York: John Wiley.

McGlynn, S.M. & Schacter, D.L. (1989). Unawareness of deficits in neuropsychological syndromes. *Journal of Clinical and Experimental Neuropsychology*, **11**, 143–205.

McGuire, P.K., Silbersweig, D.A., Wright, I. et al. (1995). Abnormal monitoring of inner speech: a physiological basis for auditory hallucinations. *Lancet*, **346**, 596–600.

Mead, G.H. (1934). *Mind, Self and Society*. Chicago: University of Chicago Press.

Merleau-Ponty, M. (1965). Phänomenologie der Wahrnehmung. Berlin: Walter de Gruyter.

Metzinger, T. (1995). *Conscious Experience*. Paderborn: Schöningh-Verlag.

Miller, L.A. (1992). Impulsivity, risk-taking, and the ability to synthesize fragmented information after frontal lobectomy. *Neuropsychologia*, **30**, 69–79.

Mohamed, S., Fleming, S., Penn, D.L. & Spaulding, W. (1999). Insight in schizophrenia: its relationship to measures of executive functions. *Journal of Nervous and Mental Disease*, **187**, 525–31.

Neisser, U. (1988). Five kinds of self-knowledge. *Philosophical Psychology*, **1**, 35–59.

Parker, S.T., Mitchell, R.W. & Boccia, M.C. (1994). *Self Awareness in Animals and Humans.* Cambridge: Cambridge University Press.

Parnas, J. (2000). The self and intentionality in the pre-psychotic stages of schizophrenia. In *Exploring the Self*, ed. D. Zahavi, pp. 115–47. Amsterdam: John Benjamin.

Phillips, M.L., Young, A.W., Senior, C. et al. (1997). A specific neural substrate for perceiving facial expressions of disgust. *Nature*, **389**, 495–8.

Pilowsky, T., Yirmiya, N., Arbelle, S. & Mozes, T. (2000). Theory of mind abilities of children with schizophrenia, children with autism, and normally developing children. *Schizophrenia Research*, **42**, 145–55.

Povinelli, D.J. & Preuss, T.M. (1995). Theory of mind: evolutionary history of a cognitive specialization. *Trends in Neuroscience*, **18**, 418–24.

Preilowski, B. (1979). Consciousness after complete surgical section of the forebrain commissures in man. In *Structure and Function of Cerebral Commissures*, ed. I.S. Russell, M.W. van Hoff & G. Berlucchi, pp. 411–20. London: Macmillan Press.

Rees, G. (2001). Neuroimaging of visual awareness in patients and normal subjects. *Current Opinion in Neurobiology*, **11**, 150–6.

Rogers, T.B., Kuiper, N.A. & Kirker, W.S. (1977). Self-reference and the encoding of personal information. *Journal of Personal and Social Psychology*, **35**, 677–88.

Sanz, M., Constable, G., Lopez-Ibor, I., Kemp, R. & David, A. (1997). A comparative study of insight scales and their relationship to psychopathological and clinical variables. *Psychological Medicine*, **28**, 437–46.

Sarfati, Y. & Hardy Bayle, M.C. (1999). How do people with schizophrenia explain the behaviour of others? A study of theory of mind and its relationship to thought and speech disorganization in schizophrenia. *Psychological Medicine*, **29**, 613–20.

Scharfetter, C. (1980). *General Psychopathology.* Cambridge: Cambridge University Press.

Scharfetter, C. (1981). Ego-psychopathology: the concept and its empirical evaluation. *Psychological Medicine*, **11**, 273–80.

Schneider, K. (1967). *Klinische Psychopathologie*, 8th edn. Stuttgart: Thieme Verlag.

Shallice, T., Fletcher, P., Frith, C.D. et al. (1994). Brain regions associated with acquisition and retrieval of verbal episodic memory. *Nature*, **368**, 633–5.

Sims, A. (1988). *Symptoms in the Mind. An Introduction to Descriptive Psychopathology.* London: WB Saunders.

Sirigu, A., Daprati, E., Pradat Diehl, P., Franck, N. & Jeannerod, M. (1999). Perception of self-generated movement following left parietal lesion. *Brain*, **122**, 74.

Slachevsky, A., Pillon, B., Fourneret, P. et al. (2001). Preserved adjustment but impaired awareness in a sensory-motor conflict following prefrontal lesions. *Journal of Cognitive Neuroscience*, **13**, 332–40.

Smith, T.E., Hull, J.W., Israel, L.M. & Willson, D.F. (2000). Insight, symptoms, and neurocognition in schizophrenia and schizoaffective disorder. *Schizophrenia Bulletin*, **26**, 193–200.

Snygg, D. & Combs, A.W. (1949). *Individual Behaviour*. New York: Harper & Row.

Spence, S.A., Brooks, D.J., Hirsch, S.R. et al. (1997). A PET study of voluntary movement in schizophrenic patients experiencing passivity phenomena (delusions of alien control). *Brain*, **120**, 1997–2011.

Sperry, R.W. (1950). Neural basis of the spontaneous optokinetic response produced by visual inversion. *Journal of Comparative and Physiological Psychology*, **43**, 482–9.

Sperry, R.W., Zaidel, E. & Zaidel, D. (1979). Self recognition and social awareness in the deconnected minor hemisphere. *Neuropsychologia*, **17**, 153–66.

Srinivasan, R., Russell, D.P., Edelman, G.M. & Tononi, G. (1999). Increased synchronization of neuromagnetic responses during conscious perception. *Journal of Neuroscience*, **19**, 5435–48.

Stanton, B. & David, A.S. (2000). First person accounts of delusions. *Psychiatric Bulletin*, **24**, 333–6.

Startup, M. (1997). Awareness of own and others' schizophrenic illness. *Schizophrenia Research*, **26**, 203–11.

Strauss, J.S. (1969). Hallucinations and delusions as points on continua function. *Archives of General Psychiatry*, **21**, 581–6.

Swanson, C.L., Freudenreich, N.J., McEvoy, J.P. et al. (1995). Insight in schizophrenia and mania. *Journal of Nervous and Mental Disease*, **183**, 752–5.

Symons, C.S. & Johnson, B.T. (1997). The self-reference effect in memory: a meta-analysis. *Psychological Bulletin*, **121**, 371–94.

Tulving, E. (1991). Concepts of human memory. In *Memory: Organisation and Locus of Change*, ed. G. Squire, G. Lynch, N.M. Weinberger & J.L. McGaugh. Oxford University Press, New York.

Tulving, E. (1993a). Self-knowledge of an amnesic individual is represented abstractly. In *The Mental Representation of Trait and Autobiographical Knowledge about the Self. Advances in social cognition*, ed. T. Srull & R.S. Wyer, p. viii. Hillsdale, NJ: Lawrence Erlbaum.

Tulving, E. (1993b). Self-knowledge of an amnesic is represented abstractly. In *The Mental Representation of Trait and Autobiographical Knowledge about the Self. Advances in Social Cognition*, ed. T.K. Srull & R.S. Wyer, pp. 147–56. Hillsdale, NJ: Erlbaum.

Valentine, T. & Bruce, V. (1986). Recognizing familiar faces: the role of distinctiveness and familiarity. *Canadian Journal of Psychology*, **40**, 300–5.

Vandenberghe, R., Price, C., Wise, R., Josephs, O. & Frackowiak, R.S. (1996). Functional anatomy of a common semantic system for words and pictures. *Nature*, **383**, 254–6.

von Holst, E. & Mittelstaedt, H. (1950). Das Reafferenzprinzip (Wechselwirkungen zwischen Zentralnervensystem und Peripherie). *Naturwissenschaften*, **37**, 464–76.

Walsh, K. & Darby, D. (1999). *Neuropsychology. A Clinical Approach*, 4th edn. Edinburgh: Churchill Livingstone.

Wiggs, C.L., Weisberg, J. & Martin, A. (1999). Neural correlates of semantic and episodic memory retrieval. *Neuropsychologia*, **37**, 103–18.

Wolpert, D.M., Ghahramani, Z. & Jordan, M.I. (1995). An internal model for sensorimotor integration. *Science*, **269**, 1880–2.

Wylie, R.C. (1989). *Measures of Self-concept.* Lincoln, NE: University of Nebraska Press.

Yoon, H.U. (2001). *Ich selbst oder ein anderer? Vertraut oder fremd? Untersuchungen zur Gesichter-erkennung.* Doctoral dissertation. University of Tübingen.

Young, A.W., Hay, D.C., McWeeny, K.H., Flude, B.M. & Ellis, A.W. (1985). Matching familiar and unfamiliar faces on internal and external features. *Perception*, **14**, 737–46.

Young, D.A., Davila, R. & Scher, H. (1993). Unawareness of illness and neuropsychological performance in chronic schizophrenia. *Schizophrenia Research*, **10**, 117–24.

Index